THE BIBLE OF ALTERNATIVE MEDICINE

HUNDREDS OF NATURAL REMEDIES FOR NEARLY EVERY AILMENT

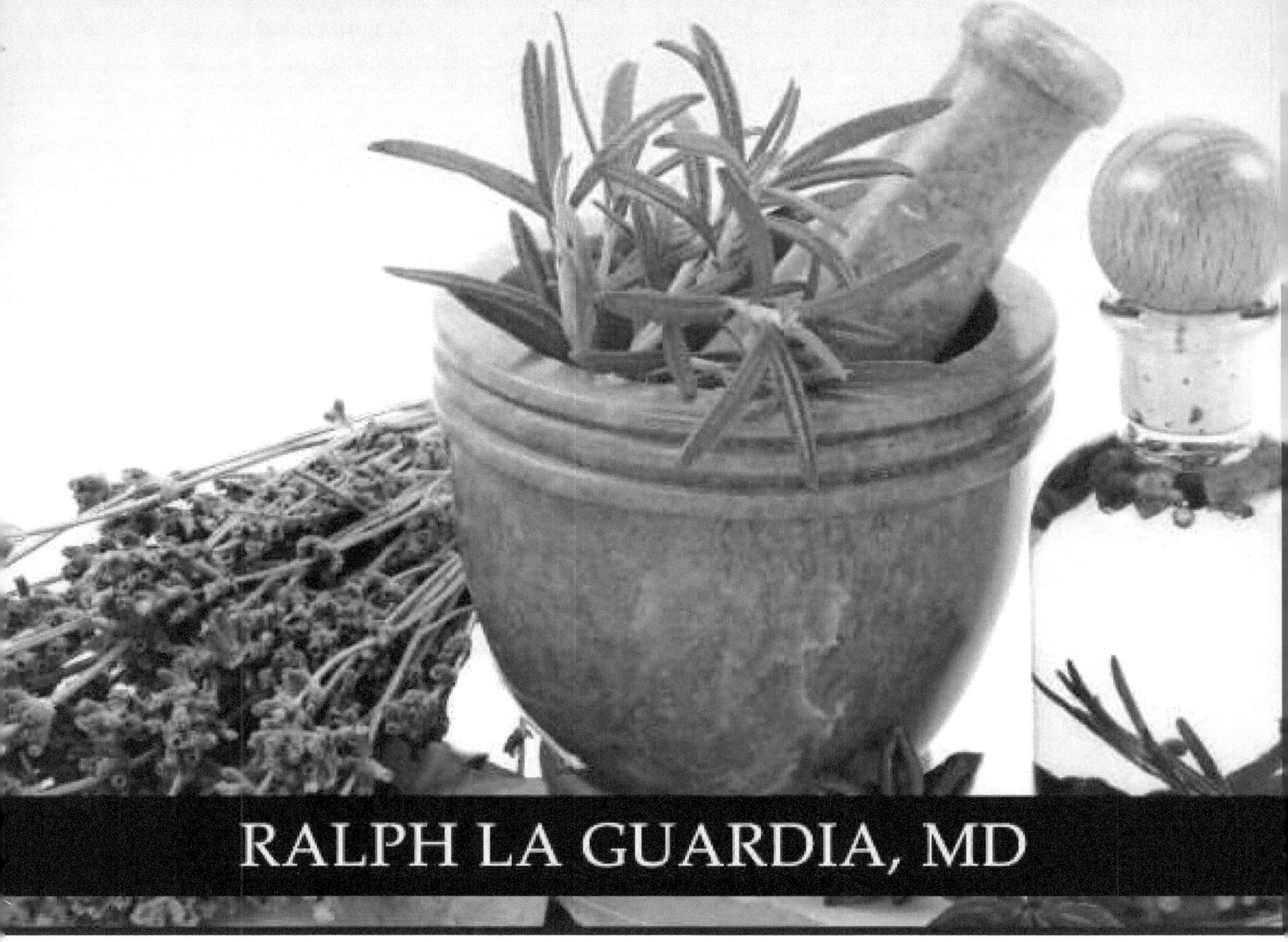

RALPH LA GUARDIA, MD

DISCLAIMER FOR THE BIBLE OF ALTERNATIVE MEDICINE

The information given and the opinions voiced by the author in this volume are for educational and entertainment purposes only, and in no way does it constitute medical advice or the practice of medicine, nor does it establish any doctor–patient relationship either explicit or implied between the publisher, author, and the readers. This book is meant in no way to substitute or replace the advice of your personal physician or other health care provider. The author and the publisher strongly urge their readers to seek up-to-date, standard medical care from certified practitioners whenever possible. Medicine is always changing and many of the recommendations in this book might not be as effective as currently available treatments. The reader should never delay seeking medical advice or disregard or discontinue medical advice or treatment from their health care provider because of information in this book or any of the resources cited in this book.

This book is intended solely to stimulate discussion and learning. Some of the actions it describes may be illegal in your jurisdiction, while others are potentially dangerous. The reader has the total responsibility to use the information provided in this book wisely, safely, and legally. The medical information in this book is of a general nature and is not meant to substitute for the advice of a qualified professional such as a physician, dentist, nurse practitioner or physician's assistant, or any other health care provider. No actions should be taken based on the information provided in this book.

The opinions and information contained in this book are believed to be accurate and sound, based on the best information available to the author, but readers who fail to consult the appropriate health authorities assume the risk of any injuries or illness incurred from the use of this book. Medicine is a constantly growing and changing discipline and as such, the author and the publisher cannot be held responsible for perceived errors or omissions.

Although the author has carefully researched available sources to ensure accuracy and completeness, he assumes no responsibility for errors, omissions, and completeness about the information provided in this book (including doses, methods of mixing and preparing medications and treatments, treatment times, etc.). Neither does the author or publisher assume liability for any harm caused by the use or the misuse of any methods, products, instructions, or information in this book or any of the resources cited in this book, including but not exclusively other books, websites, or references.

THE BIBLE OF ALTERNATIVE MEDICINE

DEDICATION

I dedicate this book to our Lord Jesus Christ. You are the creator of it all, you are the alpha and the omega, everything else is meaningless. I am so grateful for everything you have done for me and continue to do for me every day of my life. I can only hope that you continue to love us all and continue to shed your love and grace upon all of mankind.

I also dedicate this book to my loving parents; my late father, Dominick, who taught me the value of discipline and hard work by his never ending example, and my mother, Mary, who taught me from a young age that you can do anything you put your mind to and who has always had undying faith in "her son the doctor". As we used to sing, "We will stick together through thick and thin, we will love each other through thick and thin".

And to my wife, Lynne, who never fails to love and support me and put up with my endless idiosyncrasies."You are my moon and stars". You are a saint and I will love you forever. Your beautiful smile lights up my world and always will.

And to my son, Marcus, with whom I have had so many adventures and hope to have so many more, and who carries my DNA into the future, nobody will ever love you like I do.

I also dedicate this book to all those courageous physicians who have gone before me, refusing to accept the prevailing dogma, thinking outside the box, doing their own research and incredibly finding answers where others failed miserably. You suffered the wrath and ridicule of your colleagues and yet soldiered on, it is to all of you that the Alternative Medicine community owes so much and for all your perseverance we are so grateful, for without you this book would not be possible.

THANK YOU:

A special thanks to the following people for their invaluable help in the writing and preparation of this book:

To Deb Intagliata:Thanks for your help with all my endless computer snafu's, as well as your invaluable assistance in the final editing. Thanks so much for your endless patience with my computer incompetence and for working tirelessly on manuscripts I send to you in "formatting hell". You are the best.

To Linda Longobardi: Thank you for your continuous stream of interesting articles and your research, I do goof on you a lot, but I do appreciate it.

To my lovely wife Lynne: Thanks for your endless patience with my "writing" for hours in my office on end. Without you I would get nothing done, you are my true love and a source of endless inspiration.

TABLE OF CONTENTS

PART ONE
THE BASICS YOU NEED TO KNOW

CHAPTER ONE

ESSENTIAL HEALTH PRACTICES

INTRODUCTION

TABLE OF CONTENTS

In this first chapter I want to teach you all of the essential health practices that you need to know to keep yourself and your family healthy. Many of these are well known to most of you; however I want to insure that you understand all of these guiding principles for your health. They all are important in their own regard; the more of these you can follow and incorporate into your lifestyle the better your health will be.

One of the guiding principles of this book is to empower you the patient to better understand what is happening to you thus allowing you to immediately intervene in any problem that may arise, thereby shortening the illness and speeding up your recovery.

Infections of all types; viral, bacterial and fungal are by far the most common medical problems that you and your family will encounter, so let's start with health practices that will strengthen your immune system to prevent these and also to supercharge your immunity to wipe out any infection you might contract.

I will teach you all the current methods for non-antibiotic treatment of infections; some are very well known and accepted, others are controversial and/or relatively unknown to both physicians and the general public. I would stockpile as many of these as you can afford. Most are relatively inexpensive. Once your alternative medicine chest is fully loaded with these you will be able to treat almost any infection that may arise.

I have spent decades reading obscure medical books and journals to find many of these incredibly effective treatments. I have been a practicing physician "in the trenches" with sick patients for more than twenty- five years.

During that time I have been guilty, along with the vast majority of my colleagues, for the overtreatment of patients with antibiotics. Despite my awareness of antibiotic resistance as a growing problem, I am guilty of prescribing a Z Pak (Zithromax) for a patient calling up with cold symptoms who does not want to come in to be seen. More than likely this patient has a viral infection (viruses are not affected by antibiotics, only bacteria are) and the Z Pak will do nothing for them, but patients push physicians for antibiotics and all too often we give in. This is a major problem in the United States, but a much larger problem internationally, where too often patients do not even need a prescription but can go into any local pharmacy and buy antibiotics that they ask for or the local pharmacist suggests to them. This is compounded by patients who frequently stop taking their antibiotics when they feel better, not for the prescribed length of time. What this in effect is doing is selecting out the weak bacteria by quickly killing them and leaving bacteria that are resistant. Now these strong resistant bacteria that remain flourish and rapidly take over the infected area. This very quickly leads to bacterial resistance to the antibiotic in question and problems like MRSA (Methicillin Resistant Staphylococcus Aureus). MRSA (pronounced Murse-ah) is a growing problem in hospitals in the United States as well as internationally. It is very difficult to eradicate and has led to many serious infections and deaths of patients. It is made worse by inadequate hygiene on the part of doctors and nurses, who are not washing their hands and are thus spreading the infection. It has also been estimated that up to 4 percent of the health care workers are carriers of MRSA, usually in their noses, thus also contributing to its transmission to others.

Ironically, this has created a situation in which hospitals are one of the most dangerous places for patients in terms of contracting infectious diseases.

All of the above misuses of antibiotics on the part of patients and doctors pale in comparison to the abuse of antibiotics on the part of farmers and ranchers. Big Agribusiness is by far the greatest consumer of antibiotics in the United States; currently they are using over 70 percent of all antibiotics to feed their livestock. This misuse of antibiotics to protect their livestock is insane, and leading to antibiotic resistance on a huge scale, pouring these resistant bugs into contaminated waterways and sending out contaminated meat to consumers nationwide. MRSA-contaminated pork has been routinely found in various studies from samples taken all over the United States. Whether this contamination is originally from the meat or from human handlers is unclear, but either way, we are being exposed to this on a routine basis. MRSA currently kills more than 18,000 Americans annually; this is more than the AIDS virus. One study at the University of Minnesota found that from 25 to 39 percent of the hogs carry MRSA, although as of yet there are no proven cases of humans getting MRSA from contaminated meat. It has been known to enter the ground water adjacent to hog farms and contaminate it with MRSA. There is also a new strain called ST398 that recently emerged that has been found on hog farms.

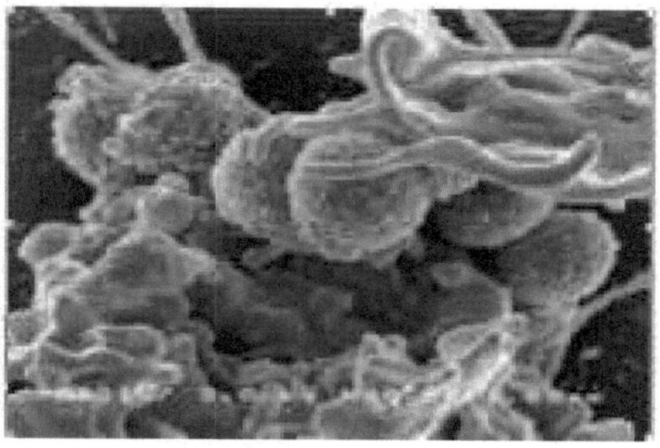

Photo above shows the interaction between a white blood cell and MRSA bacteria.

This all paints a very ominous picture of antibiotic resistant bacteria emerging much faster than new antibiotics can be developed. What does this mean for us? It means that we have to learn other methods for treating infections that do not involve the use of antibiotics. We have to be smarter and use all the means at our disposal, thus this chapter. In this chapter I will teach you all the methods currently available for the treatment of any infection that may rear its ugly head. Historically and continuing right up to present day, the major thrust by medicine for the treatment of infections has been purely offensive. We attack infections with antibiotics and hope to eradicate them. This has worked since World War II when the first antibiotics were released for use by the public after a horrific fire in a night club in Boston called the Coconut Grove.

A candle caught the curtains and the fake palm trees on fire and the crowd stampeded for the exits. Unfortunately, in those days the exit doors opened inward; the crowd pressed against the doors and kept anyone from opening the doors. The victims piled up like firewood against the doors and died in droves. The survivors were severely burned and required antibiotics to prevent overwhelming infections from killing them. Penicillin was released to the local hospitals and was hailed as a miracle drug. That began our war with the bacterial world, a world that includes the oldest living organisms on earth, and by far the most numerous. There is no niche on the planet not inhabited by some form of bacteria, from the coldest ice to the saltiest water, to volcanic vents on the ocean floor. They all reproduce the same way, by dividing themselves in two, thus one could make the argument that these current bacteria are descendants of the original organisms! They have outsmarted our every effort to eradicate them, and will continue to do so. Eradication of bacteria is an unobtainable goal and one that would be suicidal for mankind. We humans have coevolved with bacteria and require them to survive.

They cover our entire skin and every orifice of our bodies. They live in our guts and are responsible for much of our immunity, our digestion, and our assimilation of foods. They produce vitamins for us and in a limited way they help make minerals organic and thus we are able to absorb them. We could not live without bacteria, and our bodies harbor 100x more bacteria than human cells. Even our DNA includes many bacterial genes! We have to fight bacteria more intelligently than we currently are attempting. Our battle with bacteria has been going on about seventy years and we are starting to lose the war quite badly.

THE ARGUMENT FOR PREVENTION

We will always get infections, and we will have to deal with the ones we contract, but in the meantime a strategy that will best serve us is prevention. We have been purely on the offensive for almost seventy years and it is not working! It is time we add a defensive strategy to our game plan. Benjamin Franklin was right, "an ounce of prevention is worth a pound of cure". That is just as true today as it was in Ben's time and believe me it will be just as true tomorrow.

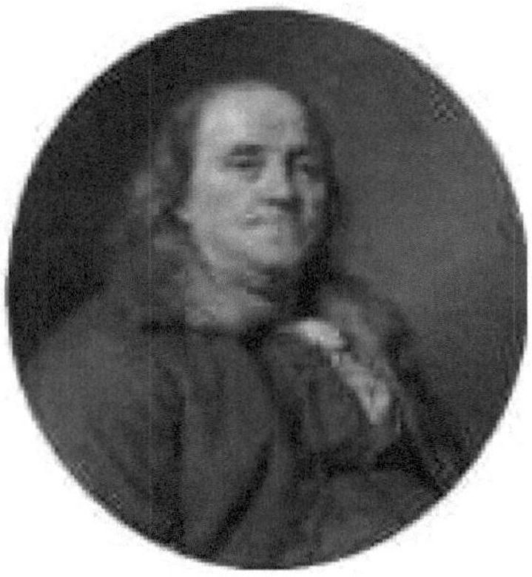

Prevention starts with good personal hygiene; hand washing, and isolation of infected patients to prevent transmission. That also means boosting our immune system with excellent nutrition, minerals, trace elements and vitamins all included with fresh clean water and lots of sunlight. The cornerstone to prevention is the immune system; anything that boosts the immune system is health-enhancing. Here I am going to give you an entire menu of ways to do just that!

Always keep this in mind… infection is only caused by a compromised immune system. A healthy individual with a robust immune system and a positive attitude will be impervious to even the most virulent infection. Diseases are the result of two processes going on simultaneously, depression of your immune system and cellular malfunction. Cells are dysfunctional (do not function like they should) as a consequence of several possible problems or a combination of several problems. For example, cells need adequate oxygen, hydration, and the proper pH. They also need a wide variety of vitamins, minerals, and trace elements.

We have evolved from the ancient oceans where we were literally immersed in a sea of nutrients that provided every mineral and trace element. Consequently our blood contains all of the same minerals and trace elements. This is not a weird coincidence, it is by design. To insure proper health and cellular function you need to provide your body with the same broad spectrum of those same minerals and trace elements. Think of it as arming your defense!

In this section I will teach you all the methods currently known to boost your immunity and augment your immune system's fight against any possible invaders. I will also teach you all of the methods available other than Antibiotics for the treatment of any infections you might contract in this brave new world.

ESSENTIAL PRACTICES FOR GOOD HEALTH

There are several good health practices that if followed will always enhance your immunity and promote good health. These should be universally followed to enhance the health of your family and lower the transmission rate of any infections that they might be exposed to. If you want to be vigorously healthy follow as many of these as you can, all would be outstanding.

In the following section are all the fundamental ways for you to stay healthy. Some, like vitamins, I did not repeat in the section under what to do if you think you are coming down with an infection, assuming you will max out all of these suggestions such as hydration and vitamins, etc.

Personal Hygiene

Bathing a minimum of once a week should be mandatory, and this should involve scrubbing any dirt or grime off of your body with soap and a brush or a face cloth. It also involves cleaning yourself from head to toe and washing your hair with soap or a shampoo. That is a minimum; more often will be helpful. Daily bathing is a luxury and not a necessity. If water is an issue, use grey water from rain spouts and rain barrels, not sterile water, which is a waste of resources and unnecessary. Stream or lake water can also be used. Remember, this is not for drinking; only bathing.

As far as shampoos go, studies show the expensive ones are no different, just packaged nicer. Even dish detergent works just fine for shampoo and will do the intended job for a lot less money.

Bathing of your face and anus and genital areas more often is ideal, and should be done daily if you have the luxury of enough grey water and time, etc. This will keep many infections at bay and make you much more comfortable. Your body entrances such as your mouth and your anus are points of entry of bacterial, fungal, and viral infectious agents. Water and soap are highly underrated for cleansing the human body. Water also works to dissolve many toxins and dilute them as well as wash them away. Antiseptics, on the other hand, may help prevent infections but may delay adequate wound healing. Your first line should be old-fashioned soap and water, lathering up your skin from head to toe and rinsing it off thoroughly.

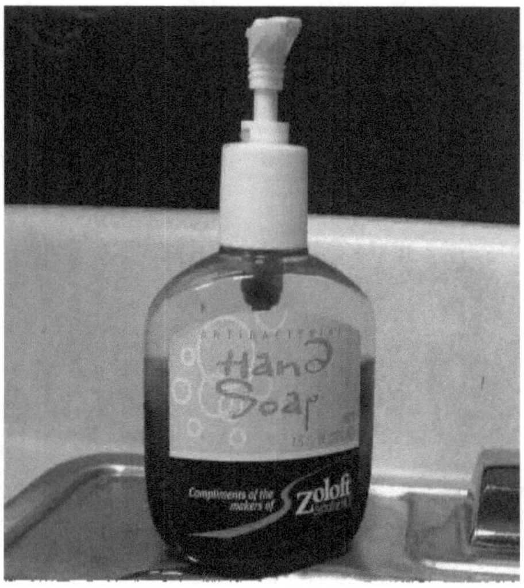

As far as antibiotic soaps go, they are not of much use, are more expensive, and are doing the same thing as injudicious use of antibiotics; they are selecting out for bacterial resistance. Stay away from them, they are not only unnecessary but are harmful and dangerous. Mothers who are busy sterilizing every surface with antiseptic sprays, using antibacterial hand soaps, and keeping their children impeccably clean and off the "dirty" floor are not only wreaking havoc with the local bacteria, selecting out for resistance, but even more importantly they are harming the very children they are trying so hard to protect. What we have learned from studies of children worldwide with allergies is that children brought up with more siblings, pets, and especially farm animals, and in less than hygienic conditions had significantly less problems with allergies and asthma. The reason is that their immune systems were challenged from birth with allergens and antigens and bacteria, viruses, fungi, and parasites ....exactly what your immune system was designed to handle, and guess what happened? They handled it wonderfully without problems and developed a robust immune system that was better able to determine self from foreign invader and had less of an allergic response.

Hand Washing

Frequent hand washing with soap is essential for the prevention of disease transmission as well as personal health.

After every bowel movement a patient should wash their hands. Many diseases are transmitted via the fecal to oral route. Also, before any food preparation, you should wash your hands thoroughly. Studies show that a good hand washing with soap will reduce diseases due to diarrhea by 50 percent, respiratory illness by 25 percent. Hand washing with soap will also significantly reduce the incidence of skin infections, eye infections, and the transmission of parasites. Hand washing for just these two situations will go a long way towards maintaining the health of your family. Also remember to have your family member's keep their nails relatively short and to clean beneath their nails routinely; this is often a hot spot for microbial growth.

Dental Care

There are no people with bad teeth in good health; the two just do not go together. There is a reason for that, if your mouth is full of rotten teeth, that means they are being colonized by pathogenic or disease causing bacteria, viruses, and even fungal infections such as thrush. Now instead of a mouth full of healthy, disease-preventing bacteria that are acting as your body's first line of defense, you have a mouth full of rotten teeth and bad bacteria. Disease-causing bacteria and viruses find a nice acidic home in mouths with poor dentition and will flourish there. Those same disease-causing pathogens, in turn, seed throughout your body and have to be dealt with by your immune system.

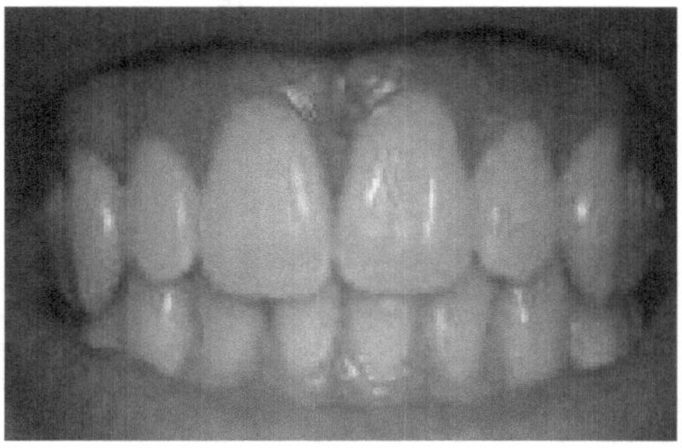

This constant barrage of bacteria and other pathogens on your immune system preoccupies it and squanders its scarce resources to fight off these infections. Your immune system will also be constantly attacking the infected mouth and attempting to regain that lost territory. Eventually the bacteria begin to win and gain other footholds in your body and disease spreads as your body steadily weakens.

This can all easily be prevented by brushing your teeth vigorously at least once a day; more is even better. Rinsing your mouth out with a 50 percent solution of hydrogen peroxide and water and then flossing and brushing your teeth is the best method for cleansing your mouth. The hydrogen peroxide also helps prevent plaque formation on your teeth and will keep them nice and white.

I just recently rewatched the movie Papillon with Steve McQueen. There is one scene where he is put in solitary for two years for his first escape attempt. Upon being put in his cell, he immediately paces it off to figure out his exercise space and then spends time every day brushing his teeth with a strip of rag pulled off his tattered prison uniform. He intuitively knew the best way to keep himself healthy was to exercise and keep a positive attitude and also to keep his teeth healthy. Even if you have to chew the ends of a small branch, do it and make it into a toothbrush; your efforts will be well rewarded. Many of the infections we contract are done so through our mouths and eliminating this source will serve you all very well.

Sleep

Proper sleep for health maintenance is very under appreciated. The average American gets much less sleep than is needed, and this leads to all kinds of problems that you probably never imagined, such as obesity, strokes, sudden death, and many others. It also leads to innumerable deaths from accidents both in the work place and also at home, and especially on the roads. Americans as a group are chronically sleep deprived. You should aim for eight good hours of solid uninterrupted sleep.. A minimum of six hours and a maximum of nine hours of sleep nightly is the proper range. You should also practice good sleep hygiene, meaning you should not watch TV in bed, talk on the phone or stay on your computer, your bed should be for sex and sleep only.

Contrary to popular perceptions, a good night's sleep promotes weight loss not weight gain. This goes back to what your mother told you as a child about getting sleep so you would grow. As with many "old wives' tales", it has a factual basis. When you go into a nice, deep sleep you enter a level during which your body releases growth hormone. This, as the name implies, leads to growth in height (until you are an adult), the buildup of muscle, and the breakdown of fat. The result is a net weight loss, as well as a nice refreshed, rejuvenated feeling the next day.

When I was in medical school, we all studied around the clock. After a while I learned that pushing me to continue trying to absorb all that information when I was nodding out was counterproductive. It was not working at that point and I was just wasting my time. I learned that when I was nodding out, it was time to go to bed for the evening. My most productive time for the absorption of complex medical concepts with large amounts of information was first thing in the morning upon awakening. My well rested mind was like a sponge soaking up everything effortlessly.

Sunshine

The sun is good for you; ignore everything you have been told about avoiding the sun. Our ancestors were out in the sun all year round, without sunblock, and did not develop skin cancer like modern man.

The reason is they were always out there, so they were not getting burned. Sunburns are a modern problem, even for the fairest-skinned among us (excluding albinos, of course). Modern man is for the most part an indoor creature, and the last few generations have seen that accelerating as kids watch TV and play video games rather than playing outside in the sun and fresh air (depending on where you live—I grew up in New Jersey, two miles from New York City, so there was no fresh air for us).

When they do go out and go to the beach their skin has not seen the sun since the previous August and they burn to a crisp. Most of our ancestors were involved in farming, hunting, fishing, and herding, which involved them being outside for most of the year.

When they weren't trying to produce food they were outside for festivals and for repairing of their homes and barns, etc. Their skin was well tanned and never burned. This also provided them with a nice, steady source of vitamin D for most of the year, which boosted their immune system and helped their bone health and prevented cancers, it also helps mood, although I am not claiming they were necessarily in good moods…!

In my practice here in New England it is rare that I see anyone with normal vitamin D levels from October to May, and for most not even during the summer months. For patients with dark skin types it is even worse; blacks and dark-skinned Hispanics are always vitamin D deficient due to large amounts of melanin, or skin pigment, which blocks the sunshine thus preventing vitamin D production from cholesterol. That brings up another little known fact, sunbathing causes a drop in your cholesterol levels by diverting that cholesterol to the production of vitamin D. Cholesterol is the skeleton used by the body for the production of vitamin D and many hormones.

BUILDING BLOCKS OF GOOD NUTRITION

Many times in this book I talk about the importance of good nutrition. You have to provide your body with all of its nutritional needs in order for it to build and repair itself and to maintain a vigorous immune system. The building blocks you will need include the following:

Hydration

Adequate hydration with fresh, clean water is critical. Ideally water with a slightly alkaline pH is best for you, high in minerals and trace elements also helps but is difficult to find. As long as you have clean water you can always supplement it by adding a complete mineral and trace element supplement such as Supreme Fulvic, which also contains fulvic acid (see following section for complete details).

Minerals and Trace Elements

A mineral source should contain all the minerals, and especially important is all of the trace elements. A humic shale source is best; this will contain both humic and fulvic acids, both of which are essential for good health.

Fulvic acid will make your body's cell membranes more permeable and facilitate the entry of those minerals, vitamins, and trace elements to the inside of the cell, where they can be used by the cell to produce the thousands of different chemicals that cells need and are capable of producing. A lack of any of these minerals or trace elements will result in some cellular dysfunction (not working properly) and eventually, disease.

Ideally you should get your minerals and trace elements from plants or animals (that eat plants) that you are eating, but since our food is grown on severely depleted soils that are missing many minerals and trace elements, we have no choice but to supplement our diets with a humic shale-derived mineral source. Of course, the better option is to heal your soil by providing either rock dust or Azomite or some other form of minerals and feed those all-important soil microbes, and they will do their job and convert inorganic minerals to organic minerals to feed your garden plants, from which you will now get your minerals in an ideal form ….from plants.

Essential Amino Acids

Amino acids are building blocks to protein. Your body carries out the vast majority of its activities by way of proteins that it manufactures. Essential amino acids are amino acids that your body cannot synthesize on its own and must be obtained in your diet. There are nine essential amino acids and six conditionally essential amino acids, meaning that they become essential given the right conditions such as a premature birth.

Most of your body is built on protein. Your muscles and your enzymes are mostly proteins, so having the full complement of amino acids to build this immense variety of proteins is absolutely essential. Protein deficiencies affect all of the body's organs and systems, especially the developing brain (iodine is also essential for the developing brain, a lack of which leads to cretinism), immune system, the GI tract, heart, liver, and kidney function.

The Native Americans used the "three sisters" to meet all their amino acids needs. The three sisters were corn, beans, and squash. These three plants provided the full complement of amino acids that they needed in order to not only survive but thrive. Native Americans were vigorously healthy before they adopted an American diet; since then they have been ravaged by diabetes, hypertension, obesity, and many of the other degenerative illnesses.

Essential Fatty Acids

Essential Fatty Acids are fatty acids that cannot be made by your body and just like essential amino acids; they can only come from your diet.

There are only two essential fatty acids that your body needs and they are alpha-linolenic and linoleic acid. Alpha-linolenic acid is an omega-3 fatty acid and linoleic acid is an omega-6 fatty acid. Both of these fatty acids are found in plant food.

A good supply of good fats are fine; do not be afraid of animal fats, you just need a balance. Fish oil, hemp oil, black seed oil, flaxseed oil, walnut oil, olive oil, and coconut oil are all excellent sources of a broad spectrum of the fatty acids that your body needs.

Eczema is a classic example of the results of a diet deficient in essential fatty acids; giving patients with eczema a combination of a good fatty acid source, zinc, and sunshine will cure the vast majority of these patients. Depression, ADHD and other mental illnesses are all helped by a diet high in essential fatty acids and fish oil.

I am of the school of thought that these patients need to have all of these building blocks to good health before they are put on steroids and SSRIs (selective serotonin reuptake inhibitors). If we did such nutritional interventions first or even concurrently with pharmaceuticals that hopefully later could be withdrawn, we would have a much greater success rate. This I have proven innumerable times in my practice.

Your body also needs a healthy balance of omega-3 and omega-6 fatty acids. Since fatty acids are essential to the production of many signaling molecules and messengers that control inflammation, mood, behavior, cell signaling and many other processes, if there is an imbalance of these fatty acids there will be problems with inflammation, cell function, and mental processes.

People are fat phobic and there is no need to be, you cannot survive without fats. I go into this further in the section on seed oils such as hemp oil and black seed oil. I would stockpile several of these oils in order to provide you and your group with a nice broad spectrum of essential fats.

The fat phobia that people have is because of the mistaken assumption that obesity is due to fat intake, they point out that a gram of fat has nine calories whereas protein and carbohydrates are four calories per gram. The difference is that carbohydrate ingestion causes insulin to be released. Insulin is essentially a fat storage hormone; it diverts excessive carbohydrate calories into new fat production as well as the protection of existing fat. Americans have been cutting their fat intake with low-fat and fat-free foods for the last several decades only to find themselves progressively more obese. If you look at a graph of high fructose corn syrup it can be superimposed on a graph of obesity during the same years. Carbohydrates are the problem, not fat.

Intermittent fasting for sixteen-hour stretches and/or fasting for two days a week produce greater results in weight loss than any other dietary strategy I know of. I am not a novice in treating obesity, I am board certified in bariatrics, which is the science of weight loss. I have used many different kinds of diets on my patients over the course of my long career and I can say unequivocally that eating a diet of low glycemic foods, which are foods which do not release their sugar content rapidly and thus avoid spikes in your insulin levels, works better than any other diet yet devised. Two days a week, restrict yourself to 600 calories if you are a male and 500 calories if you are a female, of low glycemic foods; the other days eat pretty much whatever you normally would.

This will result in a profound change for the better in your body chemistry and steady, sustained weight loss due to basically two days a week with low insulin levels. It is simple, does not involve calorie counting, and is a realistic diet that can be sustained indefinitely. There is an excellent book outlining this diet called *The Fast Diet* by Dr. Michael Mosley and Mimi Spencer.

Healthy Carbohydrates

Healthy carbohydrates are ideally from organic fruits, vegetables, whole grains, and beans. Unhealthy carbohydrates are from processed foods and highly refined foods such as cakes, pastries, breads, pastas, and foods high in sugar. Whole grains are healthier due to their fiber content as well as other phytonutrients, vitamins, minerals and trace elements.

Beans are a healthy source of both soluble and insoluble fiber as well as being high in protein. Fruits and vegetables are also packaged with lots of fiber and other healthy plant-derived nutrients.

If you have to choose a bread or a pasta (and I fully understand this, being Italian), then stay away from white breads and pastas. Remember the saying, "the whiter the bread, the sooner you're dead". Choose whole grain pastas which have up to three times as much fiber as the white varieties. Multigrain bread is much healthier for similar reasons in addition to which you get more nutrition from the multiple grain sources.

If you absolutely have to have a snack, then popcorn is one of the better choices since, believe it or not, it too is a whole grain. Some food manufacturers go to incredible lengths to make junk food sound healthy as evidenced by the ad for vitamin donuts below. Yes, the fortification with B1 is a good idea, but it is far outweighed by the refined sugar content, trans- fats, chemicals and preservatives in the rest of the donut.

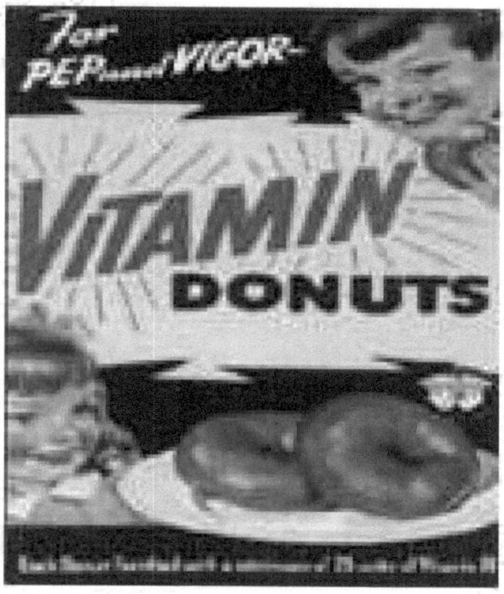

We need to keep ourselves in good health and this will require healthy, organically grown fruits and vegetables as well as grass fed, free- range animals and livestock. Organic alone will not work if the soils are still depleted; you need to also feed the soil.

Growing plants in your garden or orchard and applying pesticides, herbicides, and chemical fertilizers is the most foolish thing you can do. The fungicides, herbicides, and pesticides kill off all that rich, wonderful microbial life in the soil.

That microbial world in your soil is filled with beneficial fungi and bacteria which break down all the leaves, branches, and other vegetable matter in the soil and change it into rich black dirt, filled with humic and fulvic acids, which are essential for health. These same microorganisms also convert inorganic minerals into an organic form so your body can assimilate them.

Our bodies cannot utilize minerals and trace elements in an inorganic form. The beneficial gut flora in your body convert some of these minerals into an organic form, they also produce essential vitamins for you and help your immune system as well as aiding in digestion. The conversion rate of inorganic minerals to organic by your gut is quite small.

Your body was designed in a jungle garden where there were large amounts of fruits, wild edible plant matter of various types, and nuts. Meat and fish were also in abundance. There is even a theory that the development of the brain of Homo sapiens (modern man) was kick-started by a movement to the shores of lakes and the ocean and the incorporation of large quantities of shellfish and other fish and along with them a very high omega-3 fatty acid content. Until the last hundred years or so we only had organically grown fruits and vegetables; then industrial farming, using chemicals of all types, began. With those organic vegetables and fruits came large doses of humic and fulvic acids. These humates also help the binding and elimination of toxins and heavy metals from our bodies. Currently our bodies are undergoing an unprecedented attack of toxins and heavy metals in our air, water, and food. We are also exposed to large quantities of toxins from seemingly "harmless" sources such as fire retardant chemicals on our rugs, bedspreads, and furniture, and toxins in your cosmetics and personal hygiene products. Many toxins come from plastic containers, leaching toxic chemicals and estrogen-like hormones that eventually enter our bodies and must be detoxified and eliminated.

This current toxic onslaught is new. Over millions of years as we evolved there were not any of the toxins we are currently exposed to. Our bodies need help in ridding themselves of these toxins, but the best way to help your body is to lower its toxic load exposure, and nothing does this better than fresh, clean, organic food. Remember, health begins in the soil. If you are eating food that is grown in ground soaked in chemical pesticides, herbicides, and fungicides, it is devoid of microbial life and only provides you with a skeleton of a plant lacking in minerals and trace elements and humic and fulvic acids, all of which are essential for good health. Our bodies evolved with the full complement of amino acids, fatty acids, minerals, vitamins, humic acid (including fulvic acid) and trace elements; restoring these will restore health and prevent many of the acute and chronic degenerative diseases we currently are afflicted with.

We will only survive if we follow the ideal plan God has designed here on this incredible planet. Why try to recreate the wheel, it is a beautiful, balanced system designed to provide us with our every need.

Vitamins

Your body also needs the full spectrum of vitamins: Vitamins A, D, E, and K are fat soluble, and B complex and vitamin C are water soluble. Vitamins are best assimilated from organic sources, i.e. fruits, nuts, and vegetables. Remember, soluble means what they dissolve in. All vitamins are fat soluble except B and C which dissolve in water. All of the fat soluble vitamins need to be taken with a fatty meal in order to be absorbed, otherwise they are going straight through you. Vitamins B and C can be taken on an empty stomach because they are water soluble; since your body is mostly water, your GI tract always contains enough water to properly dissolve them.

I would certainly stockpile at least a year's worth of a good multivitamin and a years' worth of vitamin C for each member of your family. Vitamin C is so very essential to good health and helps boost your immune system as part of the antioxidant cascade, along with alpha lipoid acid, vitamin E, CoQ10 and glutathione. Alpha lipoic acid is an essential substance for your body's health; it is able to enter every cell of your body and cross barriers such as the blood-brain barrier and the cell membrane due to its unique property of being both fat and water soluble. ALA, as it is abbreviated, is the only substance known to have both fat and water solubility and I think this speaks volumes as to its importance in the body.

HALL OF FAME OF IMMUNE SYSTEM BOOSTERS

Here is a list of some of the most powerful nutrients to boost your immune system. These take prevention to an entirely new dimension. I have not included old classics like vitamin C and other antioxidant vitamins, since I reviewed them above. The assumption is that you have already maxed out all of the modalities above, and now we are taking it to another level. Keep in mind that these are mostly for prevention, but some also treat certain illnesses.

Here are the Hall of Famers:

Astaxanthin

Astaxanthin is pronounced asta-zan-thin. Astaxanthin is a carotenoid, similar to carotene which gives carrots their characteristic orange color, and it is this astaxanthin that gives krill and salmon their pink/red color. Like other carotenoids, astaxanthin is fat soluble; therefore you have to take it with fat to absorb it. Astaxanthin is also found in microalgae, yeast, trout, shrimp, crayfish, crustaceans, and the feathers of some birds. Unlike other carotenes, astaxanthin is not a precursor of vitamin A and therefore is not converted to vitamin A in humans.

The primary commercial source of astaxanthin is from a microalgae named Haematococcus pluvial, which has the highest concentration of astaxanthin found in nature. Lobsters and crabs among other animals feed on this microalgae and get their characteristic red color from them.

Astaxanthin is a very powerful antioxidant and is 550 times stronger than vitamin E and 6,000 times stronger than citamin C! It works as an anti- inflammatory as well interfering with five different inflammation-producing pathways. Astaxanthin therefore is very useful in the treatment of any inflammatory condition, and as a potent antioxidant it also boosts your immunity and will help prevent infections and fight off any you might contract. Since it is such a potent anti-inflammatory agent it also works to control pain. Astaxanthin works to block cox2 enzymes and as such works like the cox2 inhibitors such as Celebrex and Mobic that are used in the treatment of arthritis.

Astaxanthin also works for endurance; it is highly concentrated in the muscles of salmon, for example, and is responsible for their incredible feats of strength as they swim upstream to spawn annually. Incidentally, astaxanthin also works for vision, helping macular degeneration, diabetic retinopathy, eye fatigue, and strain. Astaxanthin also helps you recover from fatigue and even helps problems like sunburn.

Colostrum

Colostrum is also called first milk or beestings. It is produced by mammals in late pregnancy and is the first milk they give to their offspring. It is lower in fat (infants have a hard time digesting fat) and higher in protein than normal breast milk and more importantly it is full of antibodies to protect the newborn from disease.

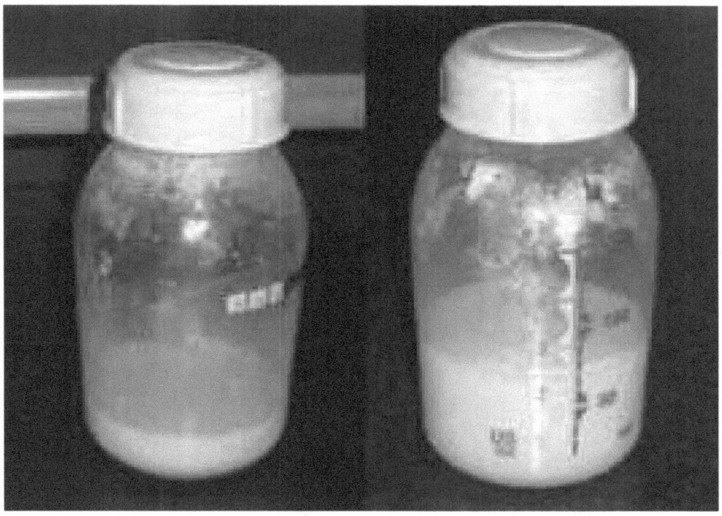

Colostrum (on the left) and Breast Milk

Colostrum from both cows and humans is thick, sticky, and yellowish in color; it is also chock full of carbohydrates, minerals, and vitamins. Bovine colostrum from pasture fed cows is full of antibodies to nineteen human pathogens such as E. Coli, staphylococcus, shigella, salmonella, cryptosporidium and rotavirus (which cause diarrhea in infants), and others.

Prior to the introduction of antibiotics in the 1940s the use of antibody-rich colostrum was one of the only means of fighting infections. Colostrum also contains lactoferrin, complement, lysosomes, lacto peroxidase, and proline-rich polypeptides (PRPs), all of which help fight infections.

PRPs are interesting due to their immune- modulating effect upon the immune system. PRPs have the ability to boost the immune system in one direction to fight an infection and also dampen it down in the other direction once the infection has passed, helping to prevent autoimmune diseases. That effect on the immune system in either direction is what is known as modulating.

Colostrum also contains antioxidants like hemopexin (which binds free heme in the body from damaged red blood cells) and lactoferrin (which binds iron, preventing bacterial infections because bacteria require iron to reproduce). It also has antifungal activity against many fungal infections including Candida albicans. Antibody levels in colostrum are one hundred times higher than breast or cow's milk! Colostrum can also be administered rectally to treat cases of colitis.

Researchers have injected cows with various disease-causing organisms, so they will develop antibodies to these diseases. The colostrum of these cows is known as Hyperimmune Bovine Colostrum. This sounds like a wonderful idea but in practice it has not proven to be as useful as physicians originally had hoped. If you have an allergy to cow's milk or dairy products you probably will be allergic to colostrum as well.Colostrum has proved very effective for the treatment of infectious diarrhea. The usual dose is 10 to 20 grams a day for approximately ten days. Colostrum also contains large amounts of the secretory immunoglobulin A which protects the newborns' throats, lungs, and intestinal tract from infections. Colostrum also has a mild laxative effect; this helps induce the infant's first bowel movement, or meconium. This meconium helps eliminate bilirubin, which is a byproduct of the large quantity of dead red blood cells that are normally produced at birth; this helps prevent jaundice in newborns.

Colostrum also has a beneficial effect on the normal good bacteria in the intestinal tract allowing them to colonize your intestines. These beneficial bacteria are also known as probiotics, and they help the immune system, as well as competing with pathogenic or harmful bacteria and preventing them from colonizing your colon.

Colostrum is helpful for all babies, but is especially useful to help premature infants survive and thrive. Colostrum is only for prevention and will not treat any infections.

Stolle's Milk

Stolle's milk was originally developed by a business man named Ralph Stolle (yet another great Ralph) who was looking to improve his own health. He believed the best way to do so was by improving his immune system. Ralph Stolle owned a large dairy farm in Lebanon, Ohio, where he developed a method of injecting pathogens (germs) directly into the bloodstream of cows in order to stimulate their immune systems and to increase their production of specific antibodies to human diseases. He was wealthy and used his wealth to finance a large experiment where he gave away to over 8,000 patients his Stolle's milk. It was very successful in the treatment of a large variety of conditions. His patients reported a decrease in arthritic complaints, fatigue, and their cholesterol levels, as well as a boosting of their immune systems with resulting decrease in infections of all types. Apparently it is cheap to produce and can be done so even in third-world countries. It is completely safe to use and can be taken orally. It offers protection against a wide variety of different organisms including bacteria, yeasts, fungi, protozoa, viruses, rickettsia, amoeba, and parasites. It is also reported to accelerate healing of injuries and increases energy and stamina. It can easily be delivered as an oral vaccine.

Ralph Stolle eventually went into partnership with a company from New Zealand and around 1999 he was bought out and it is now produced by SMBI, or Stolle's Milk Biologics, Inc.

For newborn mammals of any type, colostrum and Stolle's milk will provide a huge survival advantage by providing an acquired or adaptive immunity. SMBI currently produces milk as a 26-in-1 polyvalent vaccine. They do this by producing in a laboratory the twenty-six most common human pathogens and then heat-killing them and then injecting this product into cows, thus producing antibodies in the cow to all twenty-six pathogens. SMBI also claims that this contains an anti- inflammatory factor that helps reduce inflammation from allergies and infections, thus reducing pain, swelling, itching, and redness.

Stolle's milk also contains macrophage-activating factor which activates macrophages which ingest bacteria and other invaders as well as boosting immunity. They also claim that it helps reduce atherosclerosis (hardening of the arteries) and therefore heart disease.

Keep in mind that both colostrum and Stolle's milk are for prevention only; they are useless in the treatment of a disease you have already been infected with. SMBI also has patents on their Stolle's milk to lower blood pressure, anti-aging effects, prevention of lung infections, prevention of tooth decay, prevention of rheumatoid arthritis, lung protection, gastrointestinal protection, and even the prevention of body odor!!!

Stolle's milk is currently freeze-dried by a patented method and is produced in a powder in packets that you rehydrate by adding either warm or cold water. Do not use hot water -- it will inactivate the antibodies.

Garlic

Garlic (or the Stinking Rose as it is sometimes referred to), or Allium sativum has many benefits for your health and your immune system; man has been using garlic for over five thousand years. Garlic is a member of the lily family that also includes onions, chives, and leeks.

To get the most health benefit from garlic you should eat it either as an aged extract (Kyolic), chopped, whole, or crushed. Garlic contains many health giving compounds, most of which are sulfur-rich compounds such as its most potent compound, allicin. Allicin is destroyed by cooking, especially greater than 350F, so either crush or chop your garlic or eat it whole.

If you do cook it, do so for as short a time as possible, ideally less than ten minutes and never greater than 250F, which will conserve the allicin. Allicin will remain viable if crushed or chopped for between two and a half days. If removed and purified as an extract it will last from two to sixteen hours at room temperature. Allicin is very unstable and will not last long once activated by crushing or chopping. The exception to this is Kyolic, which is an aged garlic extract that preserves garlic activity without any garlic smell.

Garlic is a seleniferous plant, meaning it will uptake selenium actively from the soil, even if the selenium is scarce; thus it is a great source of selenium. Selenium is important for hundreds of selenium-dependent enzyme systems in your body, including changing thyroid hormone from its inactive T4 form to its active T3 form. Selenium-poor diets are also notoriously high in cancer; perhaps this is the reason for some of garlic's reported anticancer benefits.

Garlic has many extraordinary health benefits, but one of its most useful for our needs is its strong antibacterial effects. It has been utilized down through time immemorial for the treatment of wounds and infections. It has been used as recently as both world wars; in fact, the Russians utilized it topically on wounds in the form of crushed garlic juice when their other antibiotics ran out; it was even called Russian Penicillin.

Garlic has been shown by researchers to slow the growth and sometimes kill outright over sixty species of mold and twenty species of bacteria, even MRSA.The chief antibiotic compound in garlic is allicin, it also gives garlic its strong smell. One milligram of allicin is equal to approximately fifteen standard units of penicillin. Using that formula, approximately 100 mg of allicin would be equivalent to a single dose of penicillin. Allicin kills MRSA and many other super-bugs that have developed antibiotic resistance.

Garlic boosts your immune system and helps prevent as well as treat infections, has been used for generations for the common cold as well as more serious infections. Garlic works against both bacterial infections and viral infections as well as yeast and fungal infections, and intestinal parasites like worms.

Garlic also lowers your blood pressure by providing polysulfides (sulfur- rich compounds) that are utilized by the body's red blood cells to make hydrogen sulfide gas. Hydrogen sulfide gas causes the blood vessels to expand and therefore lowers blood pressure and has a cardio-protective effect. Fresh garlic is also an excellent source of vitamin C, B 6 and manganese (as well as the selenium I mentioned earlier). Garlic is also an excellent source of the mineral sulfur, which is frequently deficient in the American diet and has many health benefits. Garlic also lowers bad fats in your blood like triglycerides and total cholesterol from 5 to 15 percent. Garlic is also a potent anti-inflammatory agent as well as being a good antioxidant. Inflammation is the basis for most noninfectious chronic diseases.

All of garlics sister plants such as leeks, onion, and chives also have similar benefits as garlic, but to a lesser degree. All should be included in your survival garden and included in raw crushed or chopped form in your diet or taken as an extract form like Kyolic. I would keep several bottles of Kyolic in my alternative medicine chest to use for any bad colds or infections that may arise.

Kyolic also comes in powder form. Kyolic has no allicin, but has over 200 other beneficial sulfur-rich compounds found in garlic, and thus retains many of garlic's health benefits. Kyolic is also made from organic garlic without any exposure to pesticides, herbicides, fungicides, and chemical fertilizers, etc.

As always, you will get the most benefit from the raw form of garlic or any of its relatives such as chives, leeks, and onions; once cooked, the enzymes and other beneficial compounds in these raw vegetables are destroyed. Most enzymes in food are destroyed by cooking raw foods at 125 degrees F or greater for more than twenty minutes. Most foods are better for you when they are raw due to their enzyme, mineral, and phytonutrient content.

Iodine

It is the same old sad story; the wonderful microbial life and fertility of our soils get progressively depleted of all of their minerals and trace elements as they get poisoned with concentrated chemical fertilizers and pesticides of all sorts. Soil farmed in this manner is lifeless and dead. Unfortunately except for organic farms this describes the vast majority of farms in the United States today. Soil treated with those toxins cannot form humic acids and fulvic acid and consequently cannot process inorganic minerals into organic minerals and trace elements which your body can easily absorb. The humus content of the soil, which took millions of years to develop, is destroyed in a few decades, and along with it the fertility and productivity of the soil. Foods are grown that look okay but are nutritionally depleted and empty, and are lacking the fulvic acid from the soil that is so important in facilitating the human body to absorb all the nutrients it so desperately needs to function properly.

Consequently each successive generation of fruits and vegetables grown in these dead soils results in less and less mineral and trace element content. This is compounded by our modern methods of cooking and processing food, resulting in foods that are devoid of enzymes, vitamins, minerals, and most trace elements, but overflowing with high fructose corn syrup and other forms of sugar and soaked in innumerable types of toxins. This doesn't even take into account the potential environmental disaster of GMO foods, and international corporations like Monsanto and their almost total control of seeds and the resulting means of food production. Seed companies are now selling hybrid seeds that produce plants that are sterile and cannot reproduce themselves like open-pollinated seeds can. Farmers around the world are jumping on this hybrid seed bandwagon due to the promise of increasing yields, along with pest and pesticide resistance, as well as larger-sized vegetables. However, this is done at the expense of the loss of several thousand years of local plant breeding that has developed local plants, known as landraces, which are perfectly matched to the local environment as well as the local insects, soils, and weather patterns. These plants contain DNA that has many different traits and characteristics that we do not want to squander and lose forever. Once lost, these varieties of plants will be gone forever.

As a gardener and alternative medicine advocate, you have to have a seed vault of heirloom seeds that are open-pollinated and thus will produce viable seed themselves for your next season.

In the bibliography there are many books on this subject that will help teach how to do so. One fabulous source for open-pollinated heirloom varieties of fruits and vegetables is the Seed Savers Exchange. This was started in 1975 by Kent Whealy and his wife, Diane, who just wanted to save some varieties of vegetables that they ate as children that they noticed were disappearing. Gardeners of all races and ethnicities had come from all over the world to the United States, bringing with them jars of seeds from their "old countries". These seeds were grown in backyards all over the country, but were being lost by the thousands before the Seed Savers Exchange became reality.

This idea has grown into a thick catalogue of thousands of varieties of any fruit and vegetable you could imagine, and has resulted in the salvaging of an innumerable number of these plants that otherwise would have gone extinct. I highly recommend joining it and making a contribution if you have any unusual varieties.

For anyone interested in growing their own health enhancing foods and medicines it is a wonderful source of seeds at reasonable prices; currently the catalogue has over 12, 000 varieties of vegetables, herbs, and other plants. As a couple they have probably contributed more to saving the genetic diversity of our planet than any group or government.

Scientific American had a revealing article in April 2011 on the changes in nutritional content of some of the foods we grow.

From 1975 to 1997 the average calcium content in twelve fresh vegetables dropped 27 percent, iron levels 37 percent, vitamin A levels declined 21 percent and vitamin C levels dropped 30 percent! Wheat has half the protein content of one hundred years ago. We would have to eat eight of today's oranges to get the vitamin C content of one orange our grandparents ate. The calcium content of broccoli would require you to eat three heads of today's broccoli to get the same amount as one head in 1950. Alarming reports detailing the decline in nutritional content of our foods go as far back as 1935 when the Department of Agriculture began sounding the alarm, and things have gotten markedly worse since those bygone days. The quarter of the American population that eats the least fruit and vegetables has twice the cancer rate as the group that eats the most; that alone is a startling statistic.

A consequence of all of this is a drastic decline in the iodine content of soils, dropping as much as 50 percent in the last thirty years. The World Health Organization (WHO) estimates that over 2.2 billion people worldwide are at risk for iodine deficiency.

Iodine is essential for proper functioning of the thyroid gland, which in turn controls your metabolism and many other functions. Iodine, however, is not only essential for the thyroid but also is found in the thymus, breast, salivary glands, pancreas, brain, cerebrospinal fluid (the fluid that your brain and spinal cord float in), stomach, and skin.

A woman's thyroid gland is twice the size of a man's and hence she will need more iodine, especially during pregnancy and breast feeding.

The developing fetus's brain is dependent on adequate iodine (along with essential fatty acids), without which the child will be born mentally deficient (before the current political correctness was imposed on all of us, in a time when speech used to be free and not censored, these children were called cretins. Try that now and see what happens to you!). An utterly amazing fact is that just as the brain development in a fetus lacking iodine causes cretinism, the converse is that supplementing iodine during pregnancy has been shown to increase the baby's IQ by twenty points! Why we are not universally supplementing iodine in pregnant women is criminal in my opinion. One of the major reasons there is no supplementation is fear of lawsuits by money hungry lawyers. Doctors will not use anything in pregnant women for fear of litigation and that truly saddens me. That is also one of the reasons for this book, so you the health consumer can take actions into your own hands! Some of the non-thyroid side effects of iodine deficiency are easily traceable to its source in the body. In the salivary glands, dry mouth. In the brain, cretinism and slow mental development and slow brain functioning. In the skin, dry skin and a lack of sweating. In muscles and joints, fibromyalgia-type complaints of aches and pains. Iodine deficiency is also the cause of many of the cysts that develop in patients' breasts (fibrocystic breast disease) and other body organs. If you have ovarian, breast and other cysts you need to realize that you are deficient in iodine and need to start supplementing as soon as possible.

Iodine is essential to those parts of the body named above, but also its deficiency has been implicated in a large number of conditions and diseases such as ADHD, miscarriages, Multiple Sclerosis (M.S.) and Alzheimer's disease as well as Parkinson's disease and a large number of other neurological disorders.

Another major issue with getting enough iodine is a problem with competition with other halogens like fluorine, chlorine, and bromine. All of these halogens are adjacent to iodine on the periodic table of elements, and have similar structure and hence compete with iodine. With all the fluoride currently being placed in our drinking water, and all the bromine used for fire retardation and other chemical uses, this has caused a major problem. Bromine is also added to commercial breads and baked goods.

Standard laboratory tests will not pick up bromine or fluorine replacement of iodine in thyroid hormones and these hormones will be reported at levels which are wrong because they are inactive due to their replacement of iodine. Thyroid hormone without iodine that contains bromine or fluorine cannot function and is useless to the body's needs.

Lugol's solution, which is a liquid form of iodine and iodide combined, is very useful when one or two drops are placed in a small glass of water daily. Use this solution to rinse out your mouth once a day and then swallow it. This will provide enough iodine to your body and help displace any fluoride or bromide that might have displaced iodine in your thyroid and other tissues. Note: Too much iodine in a diet supposedly can lead to hypothyroidism or a slow thyroid. That being said, the Japanese have the highest intake of iodine of any population in the world, and do not have an epidemic of hypothyroidism, so as far as I am concerned, high iodine intakes have no serious adverse consequences and many benefits.

Another wonderful source for iodine is Nascent Iodine. Nascent Iodine comes as a liquid, it is iodine in its atomic or most basic form. Nascent Iodine is the form that is most readily recognized by the body and most easily absorbed. It has a high electromagnetic charge on its surface and this makes it more readily absorbed by our bodies. Because of this easy absorption, Nascent Iodine helps displace bromine, chlorine, and fluorine and also prevents their uptake, thereby helping to detoxify the body. Nascent Iodine also stimulates the thyroid to produce more thyroid hormone such as T3 and T4. Nascent is the form that was used by dentists and doctors in the pre-antibiotic era to treat infections in the mouth, topically on the skin, and internally as well. Nascent Iodine is also the best form to protect yourself from radiation exposure due to its rapid absorption in a readily usable and recognized form to the body.

Nascent Iodine also has the following benefits:

- Supports and boosts the immune system
- Helps regulate metabolism
- Boosts energy levels (especially if you have an iodine deficiency, which many of us do)
- Maintain detoxification systems and help flush the body of toxins
- Fight off infections by its antiseptic properties

The usual dose of Nascent Iodine is from one to ten drops daily depending on your situation. Keep in mind that each drop of Nascent Iodine contains approximately 400 mcg (micrograms) of iodine. I take four to five drops daily to maintain good thyroid health. It can either be taken orally mixed with fruit juice or water, or the drops can be administered directly under your tongue. I personally like it in a small glass of cold water, I also swish it around my mouth to clean my mouth of any pathogens before I swallow it. You might as well disinfect your mouth while you are at it; there is no downside to that and lots of benefits as far as prevention of tooth decay.

Many diseases gain entry into our bodies through our mouths and thus the importance of good oral hygiene, so why not use an iodine water mix to cleanse and disinfect your mouth while at same time providing yourself with a steady flow of life-sustaining iodine.

Symptoms of hypothyroidism include fatigue, cold intolerance (you always feel cold), constipation, hair loss, bags under your eyes, and if severe enough, the thyroid gland will swell (goiter)

A goiter is evident when looking at a person you will see a swollen area at the front base of their neck, below their larynx or Adam's apple. There are other more far-reaching effects of hypothyroidism including stopping of ovulation and infertility in women, increased risk of other cancers including prostate, endometrial, breast, and ovarian.

Other sources of iodine are mostly from sea vegetables like kelp, seafood, and shellfish.

Note: the iodine content of iodized salt cannot be used as a source of iodine, since the amount you would need to raise your iodine levels in your blood would be fatal.

Green Tea

There are four varieties of tea: green, white, black, and oolong. All four come from the same tea plant, Camellia Sinesis; as the Latin botanical name suggests, it is originally from China. The differences between the varieties of tea lie in how they are processed. Black tea, that is the tea most Americans drink, is fully fermented; oolong is partially fermented. White tea is made from uncured and unfermented young tea leaves and silver flower buds, and might be the most potent of the different tea types. Black tea has two to three times the caffeine content of green tea. Green tea is made from steamed, unfermented tea leaves which have many different health benefits not found in other teas.

The reason is that green tea has the highest concentration of plant compounds known as polyphenols. Polyphenols are very powerful antioxidants and thus protect you against the damaging effect of what is known as free radicals, which cause many health problems including arthritis, heart disease, and cancer. Polyphenols are able to neutralize many free radicals and therefore protect you from their damaging effects. The polyphenols in tea are classified as catechins. Green tea contains six primary catechin compounds, the most studied and active of which is known as EGCG.

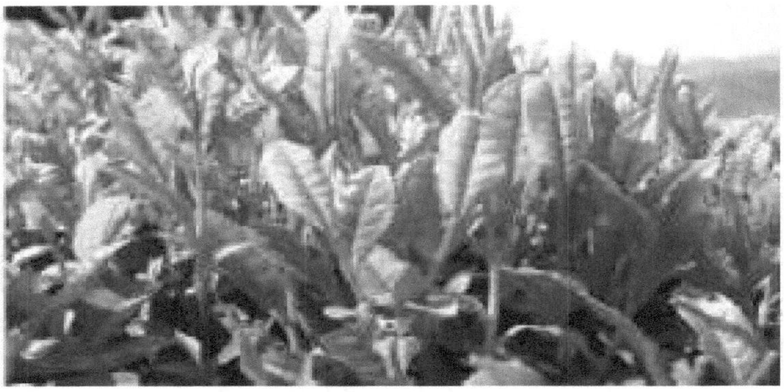

Green Tea Leaves on a Tea Plant.

Green tea also contains alkaloids like caffeine, theobromine, and theophylline. These are all responsible for the stimulating effect of green tea. Theophylline is also a medicine used to dilate the lungs and allow asthmatics to breathe easier. The average cup of green tea contains between 50-150 mg of polyphenols.

Besides the loose leaves, green tea comes in capsules and also in an extract form. Green tea should not be made with boiling water; it will destroy too many of the healthy catechins. Instead, use water between 160 and 170 degrees F. Add lemon juice to your green tea, as the vitamin C content will help the absorption of the healthful catechins, whereas dairy products like milk will do the opposite and block the absorption of catechins. The catechin content of green teas varies, the loose teas have more than canned green tea. To maintain optimal health, drink about four cups daily, two with caffeine and later in the day two without caffeine to prevent any insomnia in those of you so predisposed.

Other reported benefits of green tea:

- Weight loss: Green tea has a positive effect on your metabolism and changes your metabolism to burn more fat. The weight loss effect of green tea is increased when caffeine is present.
- Anxiety and stress: Green tea has a calming effect due to an amino acid it contains named theanine, which helps calm the body. Theanine is very useful in the treatment of anxiety, panic attacks, and depression.
- Blood pressure lowering
- Lowering of total cholesterol and elevation of good cardio protective HDL cholesterol which helps prevent atherosclerosis (hardening of the arteries)
- Stabilizes blood glucose (sugar level) in diabetics.
- Improvement of memory and brain function.

- Helps treat inflammatory bowel diseases like ulcerative colitis and Crohn's disease.
- Prevents many types of cancers including skin cancer.
- Liver disease: Green tea protects the liver from toxins including alcohol, and may slow the progression of alcohol's damage to the liver and may even be helpful in the treatment of hepatitis.
- Prevention of dental cavities.

White Tea

White tea is the most potent of the tea types and has been shown to prevent the growth of all classes of microbes (viruses, bacteria, and fungi). This antiviral, antifungal, and antibacterial effect of white tea has been utilized by toothpaste manufacturers and is currently included in many toothpastes, including Aim, Aquafresh, Colgate, Crest, and Orajel. White tea also has the most potent anticancer properties of all teas, probably due to the fact that it has the highest antioxidant levels of all the teas. White tea also boosts your metabolism and curbs your appetite and therefore helps with weight loss. Since white tea is not processed like the other teas and only steamed, it has retained almost all of its original flavanoids and other potent plant compounds. White tea is hand-picked from silver buds and young tea leaves of selected tea plants, which are allowed to wither and dry in natural sunlight. The name "white tea" is derived from the silver-white hairs on the unopened tea buds.

Currently there are four varieties of white tea: Silver needle, white peony, long life eyebrow, and tribute eyebrow. Silver needle is the highest quality, with the others descending in quality in order from left to right. Here are a few white tea tips for you:

Loose-leaf tea is better quality than tea bags, which are usually made from the bottom of the tea barrel. Just like green tea, do not boil the water but use hot water in the 160 to 170 degree F range; this will preserve most of the beneficial plant ingredients such as the polyphenols, etc. Only brew it for three to five minutes and let it steep (sit in the cup) for a few more minutes than you would with green tea to get out all the beneficial secondary plant compounds.

You can re-steep the leaves a few times to extract all the beneficial plant compounds, and this will also make it cheaper for you and stretch your supply. Drink two to four cups a day of white tea to get all the beneficial health promoting effects of the tea.

If you have the luxury of time I would suggest making a little ceremony out of drinking your tea where you relax and get a few minutes of quiet, peaceful "downtime". This will very likely become one of the most relaxing and stress-relieving times of your day. Stress relief should not be overlooked; anything that gives you some relief will go a long way to maintaining yourself in good health and peak condition.

The best types of white tea come from close to their origin in China, especially Fujian province, which is considered the heartland of white tea. Another good province for white tea is Zhejiang province. Both white and green tea are excellent for your health and if possible you should include a large supply of both of these in your natural/alternative medicine chest. I would suggest changing over your current nonalcoholic beverage of choice to one or both of these tea types, for your overall health, as well as disease and cancer prevention.

A little note about caffeine content of various tea types: All tea that is made from the tea plant Camelia Sinensis contains caffeine. Usually the less fermented or processed a tea, the more caffeine remains in it, but this is not an iron clad rule. Herbal teas (or tisanes as they area also known) are made from cinnamon, chamomile, peppermint, and other plants, and do not come from the Camelia

Sinensis plant and also do not contain caffeine. To get a decaf tea from a Camelia Sinensis tea plant requires its removal via a chemical treatment of the tea leaves.

Probiotics

Probiotics are the opposite of antibiotics; it means taking beneficial bacteria to supplement the normal bacteria that you were born with in your gut. Roughly 80 percent of the bacteria that you are now carrying in your intestines have been inherited from your mother and other family members. These good bacteria are called your intestinal flora, without which you could not live. Your flora is responsible for colonizing the entire surface of your mouth and intestines, forming a continuous colony of beneficial bacteria that occupy that area, competing with harmful bacteria and preventing their colonization. These good bacteria actually outnumber the cells in your body by a ratio of ten to one.

Probiotics were previously thought to be passive little workers that helped change inorganic minerals into organic, digestible minerals, helped digest your food, and produce vitamins for your body such as vitamins K, B12 and folic acid. Recently these good bacteria have been found to be in constant communication with your body, aiding your immune system in a symbiotic relationship, one which benefits both the bacteria and the human body. As the hosts of these bacterial guests we benefit from their assistance and they find a warm, cozy home to thrive in, protected from the outside world and continuously fed by their human host. With the recent mapping of the human genome (the DNA on our twenty-three pairs of human chromosomes), it has come to light that we have a large number of bacterial genes actually inserted among our human genes!

Talk about a close working relationship. Unfortunately, just as the beneficial microbes in our soils are being eradicated by pesticides, herbicides, fungicides, and synthetic chemical fertilizers, so is our own flora under attack by antibiotics, toxins, and chemicals we ingest and are exposed to from our environment. When this occurs it allows the pathological (disease-causing) bacteria to gain the upper hand and colonize those areas where your flora has been destroyed. This overgrowth by pathological bacteria is called dysbiosis, and is the cause of many of man's diseases. The only sensible way to combat this is by becoming a good host for your flora, by eating healthily and reducing your ingestion of processed dead foods. Eating healthy includes avoiding processed, chemical-laden foods, eating organic as much as possible and providing a healthy balance of protein, fats, and carbohydrates along with a good supply of fiber in both soluble (dissolved) and insoluble form.

You can also ingest good bacteria or probiotics in order to aid your flora as allies in their fight with the bad bacteria. You can also nurture probiotics with good nutrition or what is known as prebiotics. Whenever you take in a probiotic mix of any type you need to eat at the same time in order to provide food for those strains of bacteria. Yogurt, milk, and bananas are good meals for them, but in a pinch most foods will help. Think of it as restocking a pond in your backyard with trout fingerlings; you would not just add them to the pond without any fish food. Think of your probiotics in the same fashion. You are simply restocking your gut with beneficial bacteria that will supplement your normal healthy bacterial flora. Ironically you want the pH of your gut to be acidic, the exact opposite of your body, which you want to be more alkaline. At first this seems to be a contradiction and is counter intuitive, but upon a second look it makes perfect sense.

You see the inside of your intestines or what is known as the intestinal lumen is outside of your body. Your gut is a hollow tube running from your mouth to your anus; things inside of it have not been absorbed into your body and therefore are outside of it

Probiotics are often harmless lactic acid- producing bacteria that by doing so decrease the pH of your intestinal surface and make it more acidic. This lower or more acid pH suppresses the growth of harmful bacteria, and as such is one of the strategies these probiotics use to inhibit the growth of harmful bacteria. Acidophilus of yogurt fame is the most well-known probiotic, but there are several others that are major players, such as Bifidobacteria, which are found in the guts of breast-fed infants. Other important probiotics are Lactobacillus rhamnosus, Lactobacillus casei and Lactobacillus johnsonii, all of which are normal colonizers of human intestines. When you purchase probiotics make sure they are never in pill form but rather in a powder or a capsule, and they usually need refrigeration. The act of crushing live bacteria and compressing them into a pill with other chemical binders usually kills off the majority of these beneficial organisms. Avoidance of foods that will help harmful bacteria such as sugars and starches, artificially processed foods and fermented foods will also help control them better. Although when it comes to fermented foods, I feel they have so many other benefits that it outweighs their negatives.

Foods that benefit your good flora include rice bran, vegetables, beans, and inulin. Inulin comes from one of my favorite garden plants, the Jerusalem artichoke. All of these provide a framework of soluble and insoluble fiber that will help the probiotics form a colony. By the way, the Jerusalem artichoke has nothing to do with Jerusalem; it got its name from Italian immigrants to the United States where it is a native plant. It is in the sunflower family and hence the Italians called it Girasole (sunflower in Italian, which literally means turning to the sun) and this got bastardized by Americans hearing this name and it changed over time to Jerusalem. It is also not an artichoke. It does however have a little starch in it, but also a lot of inulin, which is a naturally occurring polysaccharide.

Plants store their carbohydrate chains, or polysaccharides, as either starch or inulin -- not both. Inulin has been shown to help beneficial bacteria flourish in the gut and inhibit harmful bacterial growth. It also decreases the inflammation found in ulcerative colitis and Crohn's disease and lowers rates of colon cancer in experimental mice. Inulin is a soluble fiber and as such has been shown to decrease total cholesterol and triglyceride levels and thus helps your cardiovascular health. Jerusalem artichoke's root tuber is the edible part; the top of the plant is just a very tall, perennial sunflower.

It is a good plant to plant around your property, it grows naturally in most of the eastern United States from Maine as far south as Florida and in Texas as well. It is a very hardy plant and can even be invasive in a garden setting. The tubers or roots of the Jerusalem artichoke are eaten like a potato, but contain no harmful starches. Inulin cannot be digested by the usual enzymes ptyalin and amylase which digest starches in the human body; instead it gets metabolized by intestinal flora. This metabolism of inulin by the intestinal flora releases carbon dioxide, hydrogen, and methane gases as a by-product and thus produces a lot of intestinal gas or farting. This lack of digestion by the body also prevents the breakdown of inulin into sugars and therefore it is a good food for diabetics, not causing any spikes in their blood sugar levels.

BENEFITS OF PROBIOTIC SUPPLEMENTATION

1. Diarrhea, especially when induced by antibiotics. Diarrhea in infants was originally cured with the administration of probiotics. I have found that most diarrheas will respond to probiotics.
2. Crohn's disease and ulcerative colitis are both helped by probiotic administration. On a personal note, I had horrific ulcerative colitis that I was able to put into remission for almost two years with the use of VSL #3, which is the most potent probiotic on the market today.
3. Eczema has been shown to improve with probiotics. Eczema is also helped by sunshine, essential fatty acids, zinc, and vitamin D.

4. Vaginal infections. Probiotic administration during antibiotic use or even eating yogurt while on antibiotics will help prevent vaginal yeast infections and thrush (oral yeast infections), and for that reason I have been advising my patients to eat yogurt when they are treated with antibiotics.
5. Blood pressure has been shown to be lowered with the use of probiotics, and that seems to be because they release a substance which is similar to ACE inhibitors (a class of hypertensive or high blood pressure medications).
6. Improve immune function by aiding the immune system and thus decrease the rate of infection.
7. Decrease inflammation in the body which is always harmful.

Fecal Transplants

As disgusting as this sounds, fecal transplantation is an ingenious use of probiotic therapy. One of the most perplexing and intangible problems for scientists studying the various members of our human probiotic family was not only the wide variability between patients but also the constant changing of the probiotic mix in the same patient over time. That was also a huge hurdle to overcome when trying to determine what to put in a probiotic mix. It has been shown that even moderate changes in your daily diet directly affect the makeup of your gut flora. The confusion was made worse by a large number of minor players in the probiotic community that occupied small niches in your intestinal lining; these also varying widely over time.

Then someone came up with the idea of just taking a large sample of stool from a healthy person and putting it directly into your colon either by a nasogastric tube going down your nose into your stomach, in a capsule, or as an enema. In effect you are taking a great mix of bacteria that has been thriving in the steamy gut of a healthy person and instilling the entire shebang right into your colon. They are readily welcomed by their buddies that are already living there and are currently losing their war with the harmful bacteria. This works great for ulcerative colitis, Crohn's disease, and especially for Clostridium difficile infections, or what is also known as C. diff, which itself is almost always caused by the use of antibiotics.

(See the section on constipation for full details on fecal transplants.)

Fungal Probiotics

There is another type of nonbacterial probiotic that comes from yeast rather than bacteria. It also has the same benefits as bacterial probiotics. Its trade name is Florastor and the yeast it contains is called Saccharomyces Boulardii, which was originally found on the skins of lychee and mangosteen fruit in Southeast Asia. A very observant physician named Boullard noticed natives chewing the skin of these fruits to prevent cholera, and was able to isolate the fungus from its surface. S. Boullardii is used to treat the same conditions as other probiotics. Since it is of tropical origins it thrives at the 96.8-degree human body temperature, it does not leave the GI tract, and readily colonizes the small and large intestines.

Florastor should not be given to immunocompromised patients because it might escape the intestines and invade their weakened bodies.

So as you have seen, there are both bacterial and fungal probiotics, and that begs the question as to the existence of viral probiotics. I think that viruses play an inordinate role in many human diseases. Viruses cannot live outside of a host cell for long and need to invade a cell and take over the cell and have it produce more viruses. They also lie dormant in cells, sometimes for years before they reemerge (think genital Herpes and Herpes Zoster or shingles). I think it is very likely that in the future we will realize that many of the bacteria that cause our problems may also be colonized in turn with viruses of various types. The flip side of that theory is the existence of good viruses that colonize intestinal flora for the benefit of both the virus and its human host. In my opinion there are probably hundreds of different probiotic viruses invading bacteria and even human host cells. We know this is true because of the presence of a large number of viral genes incorporated into our human DNA or genome! I remember the first time I ever read that fact, it blew me away. I had to reread the sentence several times; viral genes mixed onto human chromosomes, wow!

For your alternative medicine chest you should have both bacterial and fungal probiotics,. They are especially helpful with any GI problems that may arise, everything from diarrhea to colitis and have no real downside. They will boost your immune system and enhance your overall health. Practicing fermentation of foods making kefir, yogurt, vinegar, and even alcohol such as hard ciders will also enable you to have an ongoing supply of beneficial bacteria that you do not have to refrigerate. It will also supply you with healthy food and beverages that if done correctly will last for many years.

LACTOFERRIN

Lactoferrin is a protein found in both human and cow's milk, hence the lacto part of its name. The ferrin part stands for iron, and this is due to its iron- binding capacity. Medicine is beautiful that way; most names are not random and are derived either from Latin or Greek roots. Colostrum or the first milk has about seven times the lactoferrin content of regular milk. Human milk also contains more of it than cow's milk. Lactoferrin is also present in tears, nasal secretions, and saliva.

Lactoferrin is a potent antifungal and antibacterial agent. Our human bodies are amazing machines, perfectly designed by our creator. Think about it; the infant gets a huge dose of lactoferrin directly into its mouth via breast feeding from its mother. This lactoferrin binds up iron which is essential for the reproduction and growth of almost all bacteria and is present in milk, tears, saliva, and nasal secretions, therefore protecting all those surfaces from bacterial infections. Although lactoferrin binds up iron, making it unavailable to bacteria, it does at the same time make it more available to the body by increasing its rate of absorption.

Besides absorbing free iron and denying its availability to the bacteria that need it, lactoferrin has a second ingenious method of fighting bacteria; it binds to the special receptors on the cell wall of bacteria that are there to soak up iron and kills the bacteria by producing hydrogen peroxide!

Lactoferrin also prevents the attachment of Helicobacter pylorii to the stomach wall, helping to prevent ulcer formation. Could we have come up with a better system? I doubt we could have. Lactoferrin has recently been found to also be active against many types of viruses that are pathogenic (disease-causing) to man including herpes viruses, hepatitis, HIV, and others. It also has been reported to have anticancer and immune-enhancing effects

When treating a patient, the dose of Lactoferrin that I recommend using is about 300 mg a day. It comes in convenient capsule form. Another useful trick to increase iron absorption by the body is to give a small amount of red meat with your iron supplement. Iron is found in two forms in your food; it is in heme or organic iron (in red meat) and nonheme or inorganic iron (in vegetables and grains). Iron absorption is low in both forms. The nonheme iron from vegetables and grains is about 10 percent, and the absorption of heme iron from red meat is about 30 percent. The exception to this rule is Shitake mushrooms, which have an easily absorbable form of nonheme iron. The interesting fact is that iron in heme form helps increase the absorption of nonheme iron, that is why a little red meat added to the diet will enhance overall iron absorption and is probably the source of the old wives' tale that "a little red meat is good for the blood". I have found over the years that there is usually a pearl of wisdom in most old wives' tales, or they would not have persisted.

Iron absorption can also be inhibited by certain foods such as milk and dairy products, coffee, tea, soy products, and excessive calcium intake; for that reason it is best to not take any iron and calcium supplements together. Iron, on the other hand, may decrease the absorption of both zinc and thyroid supplements and thus should be taken separately from them.

Lactoferrin also has many benefits in the treatment of gastrointestinal diseases such as ulcers, Crohn's disease, and ulcerative colitis due to its beneficial effect on probiotic bacterial colonies in the flora of the gut and is probably one of the reasons it is in the colostrum, so an infant will have the mother's probiotic bacterial species to colonize its intestines and at the same time provide nourishment.

MUSHROOMS AS MEDICINE

Mushrooms as we know them are merely the above-ground fruiting part of a large underground organism known as a mycelium. Some of the oldest and largest organisms on Earth are huge mycelium that live and have spread underground for thousands of acres. Fungi do not need light to synthesize their own food and produce chemicals that dissolve the material that surround them and then simply absorb those compounds. Antibiotics are produced by fungi to kill their mortal enemy, bacteria. Bacteria and fungi are always competing for the same areas and in order to wage war on them, the fungi have developed antibiotics that they release into the immediate surroundings to kill off the competing bacteria.

Penicillin was the first antibiotic discovered and it is made by a fungus, the Penicillium fungi.

It is not surprising that mushrooms have been utilized to treat infections for thousands of years. We know this from ancient Chinese texts that refer to different medicinal mushrooms. We know they have been used just as long in Europe from the 1991 discovery of Otzi, the "Ice Man" found in the Italian Alps. Otzi was carrying a medicinal pouch at the time of his untimely death; in it were two types of mushrooms, Piptoporous Bettulinus and Fomes Fomentarius. Piptoporous B. is a fungus that grows on birch trees and is known to have antibacterial qualities. The second, Fomes F. was used as tinder to start fires. Otzi has been estimated to be over five thousand years old, living about 3,300 BCE (previously known as BC), proving the long history of medical mushroom use. Another amazing fact about Otzi is that he was found to have DNA of Borrelia Burgdorferi or Lyme disease and is thus its oldest known victim. I have a special interest in Lyme disease since I live and practice in Connecticut a short distance from where it was first discovered in Old Lyme. I have personally seen the havoc that Lyme disease can cause in patients, including my father, who was a small powerful man who came down with Lyme disease while on vacation in Europe and was unable to even carry his luggage!

Medicinal mushrooms produce substances known as beta-glucans, which are complex polysaccharides (chain of sugars, particularly of glucose molecules), similar to starch produced by plants and glycogen produced by animals. Beta-glucans are known as immune modulators, having properties that stimulate the immune system to fight infections and cancer. Various types of medicinal mushrooms produce these beta-glucans such as Reishi, Shitake, Chaga, and Maitake. Various types of grains also produce these beta-glucans in a soluble form, especially oats and bran. It has been shown that in addition to beneficial effects upon the immune system, beta-glucans also lower cholesterol.

Beta-glucans have been shown in many studies to protect against infections and to help shorten their length and severity; they have even been shown to be effective against anthrax. Anthrax is a favorite biological warfare weapon of the Soviets, and much loved by terrorists due to its lethality. While we are on the subject of terrorists, beta-glucans have also been shown to be helpful in the protection of your bone marrow after radiation exposure. Damage to the blood cell-producing bone marrow leads to many radiation-induced cancers such as leukemias; this damages the immune system and leads to death either from hemorrhage or from overwhelming infections.

For the best results medicinal mushrooms should be taken on an empty stomach. The intestinal cells will absorb them into the intestinal lymph and they will immediately interact with macrophages to activate your immune system.

Reishi Mushrooms (Ganoderma lucidum)

Reishi is a type of medicinal mushroom that has been used for thousands of years in traditional Chinese medicine. Reishi has been described as having a tough, woody taste.

As a medicine, both the mushroom which is the above- ground fruit of the fungus and the mycelium or underground fungus are utilized. Reishi has been used extensively to treat viral infections such as colds and the flu as well as bronchitis, asthma, and respiratory problems. It is also used to lower blood pressure, cholesterol, and to treat heart, liver, and kidney diseases. It has shown activity against cancer, HIV, and also helps chronic fatigue and insomnia.

Reishi use is usually free of any side effects of any significance, but it may cause some nausea and perhaps a rash. Taking vitamin C at the same time as the Reishi usually reduces its side effects by helping the absorption of Reishi. Drinking significant quantities of water will also help Reishi do its work.

Reishi comes in various colors, but only the red and the black Reishi have been shown to have health enhancing benefits. Wild Reishi is often another name given for black Reishi, which has less beta-glucan content and therefore is not as beneficial as the red Reishi. Reishi works best to prevent infections and cancer rather than to treat them. Raw Reishi is not beneficial for you, since it does not undergo a complex process of repeated high pressure boiling of the mushroom that activates the beta-glucans. This is known as hot water extraction.

Reishi is found in the wild on plum trees, but those are very rare. Fortunately, in the 1970s the Japanese developed a method of cultivation of these mushrooms Besides the numerous positive effects I have listed above, Reishi mushrooms have also been found to have analgesic properties, anti-inflammatory effects; they boost the production of interferon and therefore have antiviral effects, reduce the effects of caffeine and reduce stress as well as enhancing the production of blood cells from the bone marrow (other than red blood cells). Reishi mushrooms are excellent to have in your alternative medicine chest along with the other mushrooms listed here.

Shiitake Mushrooms (Lentinula edodes)

Shiitake is a medicinal, edible mushroom from Asia, very popular in Japan. The name "Shiitake" comes from the Japanese word "Shii", which is the name for the tree Castanopsis cuspidata on whose dead logs the mushrooms are cultivated, and the second part, "Take" means mushroom in Japanese. Americans have discovered their rich, smoky flavor and are starting to enjoy these healthy mushrooms. Long consumed in Asia for their health-promoting and longevity- promoting qualities, the Chinese have been eating them for over 6,000 years; a good track record indeed!

Just like Reishi, Shiitake mushrooms contain a large variety of beta- glucans which stimulate the immune system in two ways. First, Shiitake activates macrophages, which helps your immunity to both infections and also cancer. Secondly, Shiitake suppresses excess immune activity so it helps with autoimmune problems of disease-causing free radicals.

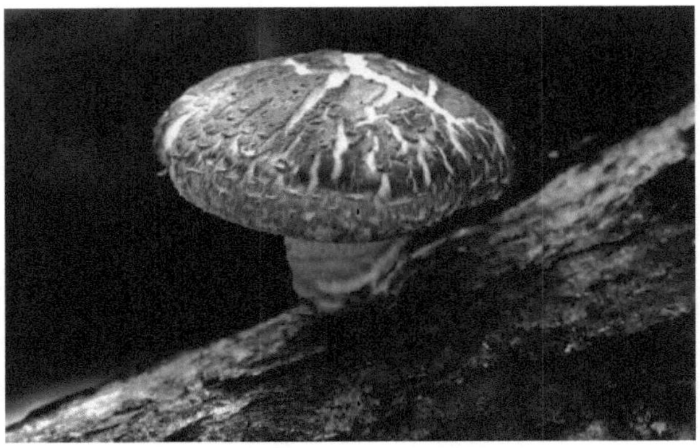

Shiitake Mushroom Flowering on a Log

Shiitake mushrooms can also be easily grown by you in a medicinal garden of your own. There are many films available on line showing you how this can be done. Shiitake can be grown on saw-dust blocks or any old hardwood logs, best done in a forest setting. This process is known as Forest Farming and has many applications for anyone interested in natural medicine and is a skill that you should acquire. Oak logs are perfect for this purpose as are most hardwood logs. You cannot use these logs for three or four weeks after they are cut; this will allow the natural fungicides (fungal killers) in the logs to disintegrate and thus not kill your spawn. You can buy wooden dowels that are inoculated with mushroom spawn, drill holes into the logs, and hammer in these inoculated dowels, cover them with wax, and let it grow! A damp spot off the ground in the shade will help; it will take from six months to two years for your crop to appear. Remember, a fungus only grows where it is wet and dark, so you need to keep these legs wet. During dry spells, water them. Another kinky fact is that you can sometimes induce their fruiting (production of mushrooms at the surface of the log) by immersing them in cold water like a pond or stream for twenty-four hours and then beating up the log with a mallet; why this works is anybody's guess.

This is a great project for you when you have some downtime; it will literally plant both some food and a medicinal source as well. Forest farming will allow you to grow medicinal herbs and mushrooms, as well as fruits of various kinds. Oyster mushrooms, which are also good for you and a good food source, can be grown on coffee grounds in a bucket with a sheet of plastic over them to keep the moisture in. As I have said before, compost when you can and save things like used coffee grounds for your garden and projects like this.

Grow your mushrooms organically without any herbicides, pesticides, or artificial chemical fertilizers. This is very important, because mushrooms absorb whatever they are grown in; that is how they eat.

So if you use any toxins they will wind up in your mushroom and subsequently in your body. Mushrooms come either raw (the best form) in which case cook them above as directed. They also come in an extract or concentrate which is made by extensive boiling of the mushrooms to extract the long chain polysaccharides and also as whole food mushroom in a powdered pill. This is better for you than the extract form. Take as directed on the bottle.

An excellent source for all information about mushrooms is a website called Fungi Perfecti.com: they sell a wide variety of mushroom spawn kits of various species and provide good growing information. Forest farming is easily done and is a lot of fun. If you have an unused piece of forest I would look into growing ginseng, huckleberries, and other types of shade-tolerant berries, medicinal herbs, and mushrooms. It is very easy to do and could save your life in the right situation. Ginseng growing is a lot of fun and can be quite profitable; the price of ginseng fluctuates like any commodity but always brings a pretty penny due to the demand from Asia. A good website with all the information you need to grow your own ginseng is Wildgrown.com. There are also many books on the subject; see the bibliography at the end of this book for some excellent sources.

All mushrooms readily absorb water, so cleaning them should not be done under running water or by soaking them; instead, wipe them down with a wet towel. Overcooking mushrooms destroys all the healthy benefits of them; instead, simmer them in a sauce pan or skillet. First add some broth and then once that is heated and starts to steam add the mushrooms and stir continuously. Do not cook them for longer than seven minutes. Onions and garlic can be added for more flavor and even more healthy benefits. Adding these sautéed mushrooms to your diet is the best way to get all of their benefits.

Weird fact: You can dramatically increase the vitamin D level of your mushrooms by placing them in the sun where just like the skin of mammals, exposure to sunlight will convert vitamin D precursors to vitamin D. Even cut up mushrooms will soak up sunlight and convert it to vitamin D. This is best done with the mushrooms upside down; that is, gills facing skyward, and takes about six hours a day of sunlight during the June to September window here in the United States. Do this for two consecutive days, covering the mushrooms with cardboard at night to keep them dry. After two days place them in a food dehydrator or just dry them out naturally and then place them in a glass jar or sealed container for storage with a tablespoon of rice to absorb moisture. The increased vitamin D levels will last an incredible year! Dried, pulverized mushrooms will also be very efficient at absorbing Ultraviolet B light from a lamp and converting that to vitamin D. In fact, six times as much vitamin D is produced by this method as compared to natural sunlight; it also sterilizes the surface of the mushrooms.

One word of caution; when using these UVB light lamps be careful not to expose your eyes or your skin, due to their harmful effects. Please refer to the Fungi Perfecti site for very detailed instructions, and with their excellent product line for all things needed to grow mushrooms, I am sure you will find them an excellent resource.

As practitioners of natural and alternative health, the more versatility we have the greater our chances of not just surviving, but thriving in robust health, and that is the underlying premise of this book, to teach you all the varied methods of maintaining your health and vigor.

Chaga Mushrooms (Inonotus obliquus)

Unlike most mushrooms, Chaga mushrooms are not soft, but are hard as wood and almost black in color due to its very high melanin content (the same pigment that is responsible for human skin color). Chaga only grows on birch trees (sometimes on alder, chestnut, and hornbeam trees but infrequently) mostly in Siberia and northern Japan, the United States as far south as North Carolina, usually in very harsh climates where the fungus has to produce many compounds to help it survive, as well as helping its tree host. Eventually it will kill off the host and fungus-eating insects and the wind will help spread its spores to another host plant.

Fungi seem to do this a lot; think of the mycorrhizal fungi that are symbiotic (their growth not only benefits themselves, but also their host, nature's win-win so to speak) with plant roots, providing them with water and minerals converted to an organic form the plant can use in return for sugars from the plant to help the fungus survive. Chaga, in its effort to both survive and nourish its tree host, will produce a large number of phytochemicals (phyto means from plants).Those same phytochemicals are what gives Chaga such strong, health- giving properties and have led to its Chinese name, the "king of plants", which is impressive, considering the long history the Chinese have of using medicinal herbs and plants of all kinds going back about six thousand years! The Siberians, who are not a bunch of wimps by any standards, refer to Chaga as "a gift from God" and the "mushroom of immortality".

You get the idea; this mushroom has some outstanding benefits. Let's take a look at some of them. Chaga contains large concentrations of B vitamins, minerals, enzymes, phenols, and flavonoids, all of which are health-enhancing. Chaga is a very potent antioxidant due to its large concentration of the enzyme SOD (superoxide dismutase); in fact, it has the highest concentration found anywhere in nature. The Russians did a lot of research on plants to see which ones helped with promoting strength and vigor and warding off diseases -- they named those plants adaptogens and they found Chaga to be the most potent adaptogen known. In Japan ,Korea, and China. Chaga is known for producing longevity by fighting stress and increasing vigor, and so is widely used in those countries.

The extraction of the active phytonutrients from Chaga needs to be done in order to get their full benefit. Most of these phytochemicals or phytonutrients are encased in a chitin wall for which humans lack the necessary digestive enzymes. The most common extraction method is to make a tea using ground up Chaga.

This will release all of the water soluble phytonutrients, but none of the fat soluble ones. Then the Chaga is exposed to ethanol (the kind of alcohol we drink for fun); this gets out the fat soluble phytonutrients. Some people ferment the Chaga, but this is complicated and produces varied results.

The best results come from the combination of hot water or room temperature water and ethanol extraction.Many people take Chaga in its various forms, such as a tea, beverage, syrup, emulsified drops, and also in supplement form. You will find it invigorating, and it will give you increased strength and vigor; that is why the Russians mandated its use in their Olympic athletes and their astronauts. For our purposes it is a very useful nutrient to use for maintaining health and vigor as well as helping your body ward off infections. It has been touted as a cancer treatment, and studies have shown that it is very effective against flu and other viruses.

Maitake Mushroom (Grifola frundosa)

Maitake mushrooms are also known as Hen of the Woods, ram's head, sheep's head and, among Italian-American communities in the northeastern United States, as "signorina". Maitake typically grows in large clusters at the base of trees, especially oak species. Maitake is a perennial fungus and will therefore grow for years on the base of trees; in the United States it will grow from the northeast as far west as Idaho. In Japan it sometimes grows as large as 50 pounds, and is widely used for cooking and medicinal purposes. Maitake is very rich in minerals, B vitamins, fiber, and amino acids (the building blocks of proteins). As with all medicinal mushrooms, maitake are high in beta-glucans which help boost the immune system and treat inflammation as well as infections. Maitake is purported to have strong anticancer effects; it also helps control blood glucose levels and therefore diabetics should use it with caution since it might lower their blood sugar or glucose levels too much. Maitake also lowers cholesterol and triglyceride levels and has been used to treat cancer as well as help patients deal with the side effects of chemotherapy. It has been used to treat HIV, hepatitis, polycystic ovarian syndrome, hay fever, chronic fatigue, and hypertension.

As a food, Maitake is 25 percent protein, 28 percent fiber, has no cholesterol (cholesterol is only contained in animal products), and it is high in potassium, minerals, B vitamins, and enzymes. It is 60 percent carbohydrate and the vast majority of those are complex carbohydrates. Maitake is a wonderful, health-promoting food as well as being a useful medicinal plant to acquaint yourself with, and should be part of your Alternative medicine chest as well as your forest farm, where it can serve as a good emergency food stash.

WHAT TO DO IF YOU THINK YOU ARE COMING DOWN WITH AN INFECTION

You have to act fast; in addition to all the ways you can boost your immune system listed above, you now have to send in the Marines. Here are some excellent ways to stave off an impending infection or treat one that is starting to take hold.

Hydrogen Peroxide (H2O2)

Hydrogen peroxide is a wonderful way to treat infections anywhere, but especially in areas to which you can apply it directly, such as your skin and mouth, etc. Hydrogen peroxide is inexpensive and readily available. I would purchase the food grade peroxide and dilute it down to the 3.5 percent you need. Never use the full 35 percent strength of hydrogen peroxide; it is too strong and will burn your skin, and certainly never take it internally where it will cause serious harm. These formulations are mostly free of any toxic metal contaminants that may or may not be present in the store-bought variety. If you are using it topically it doesn't really matter which one you choose, but the 35 percent strength is dangerous and can never, ever be used undiluted, whether externally or internally. It will cause serious burns to your skin and will be like drinking acid if you take it orally, causing serious damage to your mouth and throat. Hydrogen peroxide is essentially what your body's white blood cells release to kill microbial invaders. Hydrogen peroxide foams up when you put it on a cut or open sore because of the presence inside of cells of an enzyme called catalase. Catalase converts hydrogen peroxide into its water and oxygen parts at an amazing rate of 200,000 molecules per second, and it is that production of oxygen that causes the foaming. That is the same reason why when you put hydrogen peroxide on the skin's surface there is no foaming, because there is no catalase present on the surface, it is inside the cell. I should say that there sometimes is foaming on the surface of the body, but this comes from hydrogen peroxide's contact with bacteria and is slight. Hydrogen peroxide is easily destroyed by light, so must be stored in dark bottles to keep it from breaking down, which also limits the time it can work on the surface of your skin. For that reason it is best to apply peroxide and then cover the area with an opaque dressing (one that you cannot see through). Hydrogen peroxide's chemical formula is H2O2, which is essentially H20 or water and an extra oxygen atom. Hydrogen peroxide gets its medicinal powers from its ability to oxidize, or donate that extra oxygen atom upon demand, leaving pure water behind as a by-product. Here is the interesting part; most diseases and cancers thrive in an anaerobic (without oxygen) environment, so by hydrogen peroxide donating oxygen molecules it is capable of killing many microbes and infections.

Many people think for the same reason it can be useful against cancer, but that is another book's worth of debates. If you suspect you have a mouth or throat infection or simply an infected tooth, then use some of your diluted hydrogen peroxide mix (3.5 percent); mix it in a glass half-filled with water or use it straight without any further dilution.

Swish it around your mouth vigorously and then gargle it and allow it to remain in your throat as long as you can, and then expectorate it (spit it out). Repeat the above process up to four times a day until the infection resolves.

How To Dilute 35 Percent Food Grade Hydrogen Peroxide To 3.5 Percent Hydrogen Peroxide

The simplest way is to mix nine parts of water with one part of the 35 percent hydrogen peroxide. To use a simple example, mix 1 ounce of 35 percent hydrogen peroxide with 9 ounces of water. If you are comfortable with the metric system you can mix 100 ml of the 35 percent hydrogen peroxide with 900 ml of water to get a liter of 3.5 percent hydrogen peroxide. Any amount will work on one side of the formula as long as there is nine times as much water on the opposite side.

WARNING: Never use undiluted 35 percent hydrogen peroxide anywhere in or on your body; IT WILL SEVERELY BURN YOU. It needs to always be diluted to a less potent dilution. See the photo below of the effects of a very brief exposure of some fingers to 35 percent hydrogen peroxide.

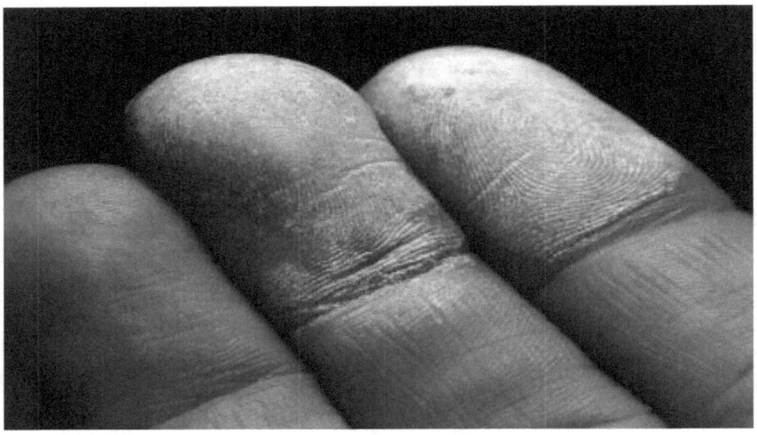

MMS Or Master Mineral Solution (Formerly Known As Miracle Mineral Supplement)

This is a very effective antimicrobial substance to have in your medicine chest to treat most infections that may rear their ugly heads. However, its use is very controversial. I am not recommending its use; I am just providing information on how it works and how it has been used in the past. There are reports of its toxicity by the governments of the United States and Canada, however, many people have used it for many years without any problems, at least according to anecdotal reports all over the Internet.

Here is the basic science behind this powerful medicine. MMS is chlorine dioxide. It is produced by mixing sodium chlorite with equal parts of 50 percent citric acid as an activator. Mixing these two produces the chlorine dioxide that is the active ingredient, which is then mixed with water, and drank. The taste takes some getting used to and it smells similar to bleach; in fact it often causes nausea due to its strong odor.

There are newer alternative methods of producing chlorine dioxide using some simple chemical tubing and beakers. There are films on Youtube about how to produce this CDS or Chlorine Dioxide solution, but that is beyond the scope of this book.

How does MMS work? It is a very potent oxidizer, just as we discussed with hydrogen peroxide. This means it donates oxygen to kill off pathogens of many types including bacteria, viruses, molds, yeast, fungus, and biofilms. Biofilms are what many bacteria produce in order to protect themselves from the body's defenses. Biofilms are essentially domes of biological material that the bacteria produce to cover themselves and produce a powerful shield from the body's defenses, thus making eradication of these infections very difficult. Chlorine has been used for over a hundred years to purify water by water companies, and is still in use by the majority of them today. If used properly it is safe and very effective.

Chlorine does lead to the production of some carcinogens and has been phased out in favor of chlorine dioxide (MMS), which does not.

A clarification of how MMS actually oxidizes pathogens (disease- causing organisms like bacteria, fungi, and viruses) is not actually from the donation of the oxygen atom that it has on its surface, but rather by using the power of this oxygen atom to pull off other atoms from the microbe and tear it apart. It is important to remember that chlorine dioxide does not chlorinate pathogens to kill them, chlorination involves the donation of a chlorine atom that combines with the target molecule and forms new chemical compounds that sometimes are carcinogenic (cancer-causing). MMS as well as oxygen itself are powerful oxidizers against invading microbes but do not damage healthy cells because of their voltage. Chlorine dioxide has a oxidation potential of 0.95 volts and pure oxygen only of 1.28 volts (The two remaining oxidizers that can be used inside of the body are hydrogen peroxide at 1.8 volts, and ozone, the strongest oxidizer of all, at 2.07 volts). None of these voltages are strong enough to overcome the opposing voltages of healthy cells and tissues, therefore they have no effect upon them in any way, and that is very good news.

How To Properly Mix MMS

First of all, the mix depends on the strength of the citric acid activator you use. If you have 50 percent citric acid then you mix it one-to-one with the MMS. If you are using 10 percent citric acid, then you need five drops mixed with every drop of MMS. So, the first thing you should do is check the percentage of the citric acid activator you have.

The first time you use MMS you need to take only a few drops as a test solution to insure that it does not upset your stomach.

The chemical reaction between the MMS and the citric acid activator solution takes one minute at the 50 percent strength and three minutes for the 10 percent strength. You will smell a strong bleach-like odor from the glass, this is normal.

Now pour the new mixture into a glass of water. Don't be concerned about diluting it, it doesn't matter how much water you mix it with, the potency of the MMS will not be altered. You can also use apple juice for flavor; the mix does not taste very good.

Note: Do not mix it with any vitamin C-containing juices like orange juice or other juices with vitamin C added to them, vitamin C will react with the MMS and reduce its effectiveness. You can slowly build up your dose of MMS as tolerated. In the beginning you may feel ill for a short time with some stomach upset, this is especially true if you have a serious infection with bacteria, viruses, or fungi, due to the killing off of these organisms and the release of all the toxins involved with their death.

This is usually a short-term phenomenon and will not last very long; the length of time depends on the patient as well as their tolerance and the extent of their microbial infection. Once you feel okay then slowly titrate up the dose until you reach a maximum of fifteen drops of MMS daily. It is best given in divided doses, and is better tolerated at bedtime. Most conditions will improve before you reach the maximum dose of fifteen drops daily. MMS can be taken to treat infections or can be used daily to rid the body of pathogens. The beautiful part about taking MMS is that it is selective for pathogens only and will not harm normal cells or the beneficial bacteria that live within our bodies.

Note: MMS is very controversial, and is banned for human use in the United States and recently, in Canada, where it has been seized and removed from store shelves. The governments of both countries warn of its toxicity and for that reason have banned it.

I AM NOT RECOMMENDING ITS USE HERE, I am only describing to you how it works and how some people take it. This should not be construed as medical advice and is only for informational purposes.

Zinc Supplementation

Zinc is an essential mineral that also has other health-enhancing and immune-enhancing properties as well as being essential for over a hundred enzyme reactions in the human body. Zinc is also involved in wound and tissue healing as well as normal growth. I routinely use zinc for canker sores in the mouth or what are known as apthous ulcers. Using zinc lozenges for this has worked every time for me in over twenty-five years of medical practice. Zinc promotes healing by playing an essential role in protein synthesis, immune function, DNA synthesis, and cellular reproduction. As with most minerals and trace elements, zinc is sorely lacking in our current diets. This lack of zinc in our foods is due to the use of chemical fertilizers, herbicides, pesticides, and fungicides, destroying the microbial life of soils and thus their conversion of inorganic minerals to usable organic forms, exhausting soils of their zinc. The processing of foods during preparation also strips out much of the zinc.

Unlike many nutrients, the body has no way to store zinc for future use and must get a constant supply of it in our daily diets. Vegetarians, alcoholics, and patients with chronic digestive problems and low stomach acid (especially caused by taking medications to reduce stomach acid such as Prilosec, Prevacid, Zantac, Pepcid, and others) all will have problems with zinc deficiency.

Some of the early signs of zinc deficiency are white flecks in your fingernails, slow wound healing, increasing allergies, and when it is severe, there will develop a lack of the ability to taste foods. Zinc is involved in many bodily processes and its deficiency will lead to low libido (low sex drive) and also can cause infertility in both women and men. Zinc works against all types of infections by its positive effect on all lines of white blood cells, boosting their function and enabling them to fight off microbial invaders of all types. Zinc also plays a very important role in fighting off viral infections of all types, famously used for the common cold in various preparations. Zinc is a powerful antioxidant and also plays a role in decreasing inflammation.

If you have a child with ADD or ADHD, zinc supplementation is also very helpful (along with B complex, magnesium, and omega-3 fatty acids or fish oils). The mechanism by which zinc helps in these children is by its essential role in neurotransmitter function (these are the chemicals that control the way the brain communicates and performs its various functions), as well as its break down and utilization of fatty acids that are essential for proper brain function. Zinc given to children with ADD and ADHD at a dose of 150 mg of zinc sulfate a day showed marked improvement in their behavior and their hyperactivity. Zinc has also been shown to elevate mood and help depression. Zinc also plays a role in the detoxification of heavy metals from the body, especially the brain.

Zinc is also essential for the metabolism of melatonin and most hormones in the body and is also necessary for the production and function of insulin and therefore plays a large role in diabetic patients. Zinc also plays an important role in eye health and is used in cases of macular degeneration, night blindness, and cataracts. Zinc is also essential for skin health and is useful in eczema, psoriasis, acne, and other skin conditions; you can apply it topically as zinc oxide. That is the same stuff you saw the lifeguards using over their noses and cheek bones, it works well to protect against sun damage to the skin. In the section on burns I explain how to make your own sunblock with non-nano zinc oxide.

The daily dose of zinc for men is 11 mg and for women is8 mg daily. Men need more due to its use in the production of the male hormone testosterone. In fact, testosterone levels can be increased significantly with zinc supplementation (The trace element boron also helps significantly raise testosterone, lower estrogen and C-reactive protein levels, raise DHEA, decrease inflammation, and build rock hard bones. The dose of boron daily should be about 3 mg.), and this is much less expensive than using testosterone supplements. Zinc is absolutely essential for male sexual health and adequate sperm production and motility (how well the little bastards swim towards that egg), approximately 5 mg of zinc is lost in each ejaculation!

Knowing that figure, it is surprising that all high school boys are not deficient!

Zinc is also involved with a healthy prostate gland and in fact, other than bone, the prostate contains a higher concentration of zinc than any other of the body's tissues. For that reason, zinc deficiencies may lead to BPH (benign prostatic hyperplasia) and inflammation of the prostate, or prostatitis. Zinc toxicity can easily develop and for that reason you should not exceed 20 mg of zinc daily.

Caution: Long-term supplementation with zinc may lead to a copper deficiency. You should take a 1 mg copper supplement along with zinc if you are using it for any length of time.

ESSENTIAL OILS AND THEIR EFFECT UPON YOUR IMMUNITY AND INFECTIONS

In the days before antibiotics, essential oils were one of the primary ways to treat infections, and were very useful and surprisingly potent in the eradication of bacterial infections of many kinds as well as fungal and parasitic infections. Currently there is a great need for healers who are knowledgeable in the production and use of essential oils. The use of essential oils as medicine is known as Aromatherapy. I personally do not like that name very much; it sounds like you are treating illnesses with certain smells or aromas, and nothing could be further from the truth. Many scientific studies at major universities worldwide have shown the effectiveness of essential oils in eradicating even serious infections such as MRSA (Methicillin-resistant staphylococcus aureus) and VRE (Vancomycin-resistant enterococcus).

The knowledge of how to make these oils as well as tinctures and other preparations, it is beyond the scope of this book. There are several good books on the market and you can easily find them on Amazon or even eBay if you are lucky. One of my favorites is by Kurt Schnaubelt, called *The Healing Intelligence of Essential Oils*. It is an easy read for someone with little or no medical training and contains a wealth of information.

Life originated in the oceans of the earth and eventually those simple, Single-celled life-forms became more complex and eventually developed into sea creatures. These sea creatures eventually left the world's oceans and evolved on land. As plant life developed on land, it too became more complex, and eventually started producing what are known as secondary plant metabolites. These secondary plant metabolites perform all of the specialized functions for the plant, such as repelling certain animals from eating them as well as communication between plants and their environment. As animals coevolved with plants they had to develop systems to handle these complex chemicals that they were ingesting from plants without being poisoned by them. Animals eventually developed the cytochrome P450 system of enzymes in their livers to break down these secondary plant metabolites that include essential oils, and make them harmless to the animal, but at the same time keeping their beneficial effects.

Iron is one of the minerals that is essential for this cytochrome P450 system to function; just thought I would mention that since we just covered the importance of iron for your health. In fact, we have enzyme systems in our bodies that have evolved specifically for the removal of essential oils that were previously considered to be toxic. For that reason most essential oils are not harmful to humans when used properly and real toxicity from essential oils is quite rare.

The secondary metabolites made by plants usually target proteins that are common to many types of microorganisms and are not species specific. This nonselective targeting of proteins by these secondary metabolites makes the development of resistance practically impossible; hence these essential oils have not become obsolete over time. Microorganisms may be able to resist an attack on one of their proteins, but not on several proteins at once. This nonspecific targeting also is the reason for the broad spectrum of activity by most essential oils against numerous types of bacteria. The flip side of this is one of the reasons for physicians to not feel comfortable with the use of essential oils for a specific type of infection. Modern medicine likes reductionism, where one medicine is used specifically for one type of infection: the proverbial magic bullet.

I will teach you the best essential oils to use for the treatment of infections both on your skin as well as internal infections. A few words of caution, many of the topical oils used to treat skin infections will need to be diluted or they will irritate the skin. The dilution of these essential oils for topical use is usually done with a carrier oil that will also help penetrate the skin. The final word of caution; do not use essential oils if you are pregnant or breast feeding.

Lavender Oil (Lavandula augustifolia)

Lavender oil has been used medicinally since before ancient Rome. It was renowned for its healing of both wounds and burns and its antiseptic properties. It also works very well as an insect repellent. It is very useful to wash and clean out wounds and had been used for that purpose right up until WWII. Lavender oil is very mild and is the only essential oil that does not need to be diluted with a carrier oil. Lavender can also be made into a tea, by using the fresh or dried flowers that is useful for internal use. The recommended dose is about one and a half teaspoons of dried flowers in an 8-ounce glass of water. Lavender oil is made by steam distillation of the plant's flowers. It is easy to make and even easier to grow. You should not use lavender oil internally on your cats or dogs; it may cause liver and kidney damage; it is not a problem in humans. In young boys lavender oil and tea tree oil have been linked with gynecomastia, which essentially means the boys developed some big boobs, so use it with caution with them. No father really likes hearing, "good looking boy you have there, that's quite a rack on him". The good news is that the gynecomastia in these boys disappeared when they stopped using the lavender oil. Life is stressful enough for teenage boys these days without them having to deal with breasts!

Medically, lavender oil has many uses such as an excellent topical antiseptic as well as a mild anesthetic (pain reliever), so it is very useful for cuts, burns, scrapes, insect bites, bee stings, sunburn, eczema, psoriasis, poison ivy oak and sumac, and skin infections. Lavender is said to be useful for head lice either as a hair rinse or applying it to a comb to comb out the nits. Lavender oil works as a bronchodilator (it opens up your large airways) and a few drops can be added to a vaporizer, or it can be rubbed directly on a patient's chest. Lavender oil is also reported to help with anxiety and stress and is used frequently for that in Germany, where they are light years ahead of us in the use of medicinal plants and oils.

Lavender tea has been found to be useful against internal pathogens and works very well for Candida infections. Lavender oil will also help infections including strep throat, pneumonia, bronchitis, diphtheria, laryngitis, and even toothaches. The tea can be drunk up to four times daily. For children with ear infections, put a few drops of lavender oil, undiluted, into their ear canals and have them tilt their head so it will go in further. Instead of making a tea, a few drops of lavender oil can be placed in a glass of water to gargle for a sore throat. Lavender oil also normalizes blood sugar output from the liver. Lavender oil also has a benefit with appetite control; a few drops under your tongue will decrease your hunger in about fifteen minutes. Hunger control is a useful benefit of lavender oil if you are trying to lose weight, and how many of us are not looking to shed a few unwanted pounds.

Lavender oil is oftentimes combined with geranium oil. The two together seem to have a synergistic effect and are very potent.

Geranium oil (Pelargonium odorantissimum)

Geranium oil is made from a Pelagaronium species of geranium from South Africa, not the garden variety you are used to, which is a European geranium. Since the seventeenth century it has been grown extensively in France, Italy, Spain, Egypt, Morocco, and Madagascar. The best geranium oil in the world comes from Madagascar and Egypt. In those countries it is grown in hedge rows of about three feet in height. The oil is steam-distilled from the aromatic green leaves before the plant flowers. It takes a lot of leaves to make the oil and for that reason it is a rather expensive oil, and there are many adulterated oils for sale. Geranium oil comes in a variety of colors ranging from brownish yellow to light green; this is due to the different distillation methods used in various countries. The medicinal uses of Geranium oil are many, including as an antiseptic, antibiotic, diuretic (makes you urinate), haemostatic (stops bleeding) and an antispasmodic (prevents muscle spasm). It also has been used to treat depression. It is very useful for skin conditions ranging from eczema, poison ivy, cuts, scrapes, burns, athlete's foot, and even frostbite. To prevent wound infections apply it to a wound (diluted by at least half with a carrier oil) and cover it with a gauze and then reapply and change gauze daily.

Geranium oil is also an astringent (it will shrink something); that quality along with its haemostatic effects will work nicely to shrink hemorrhoids and control their bleeding.

When used for hemorrhoids it has to be mixed in a carrier oil to dilute it and also to allow deeper penetration. The carrier oils can be wheat germ oil, for example, at a mixture of one drop of geranium oil to one teaspoon or 5 ml of wheat germ oil and cover it with gauze. There are many carrier oils that can be used such as coconut oil, avocado oil, black seed oil, jojoba oil, and others. One of geranium oil's greatest effects is its antimicrobial effect. It will prevent bacteria and other microbes from growing in a wound and is excellent as a wound wash, in addition to which, it boosts the immune system. Geranium oil also prevents scar formation and is thus useful after surgery to promote healing without excessive scar formation and skin discoloration. It will help prevent and treat lesions such as boils and acne.

Geranium oil helps wounds keep from bleeding excessively by two methods. First, it causes the blood vessels to contract and secondly, it assists in the clotting process, helping to plug the hole in you that is bleeding. It is very effective in doing both of these things and that why it is so useful for wounds and even hemorrhoids. Geranium oil also promotes and accelerates the healing of wounds.

Another benefit of geranium oil is its effect upon parasites such as intestinal worms. This is especially helpful in children; it will rid their body of parasitic worms. Geranium oil is also helpful for acne, eczema, and other skin conditions; it can also be used for infections of the nose and throat.

Geranium oil contains a large amount of esters and for this reason it is very active against fungal infections of all types including Candida Albicans. It also works on women suffering with mastalgia (breast pain) that often accompanies menstruation. When using it on a woman's breast, mix it in a ratio of 10:1 of carrier oil to geranium oil, so for those of you who are math-challenged, this means 100 ml of carrier oil mixed with 10 ml of geranium oil. It is a sad commentary on our schools that most people cannot carry out such simple calculations.

Tea Tree Oil (Melaleuca alternifolia)

This wonderful oil from Australia got its name from Captain Cook, who upon landing in Australia made a tea from its leaves. Tea tree oil is renowned for its exceptional antimicrobial properties, and was even put in first aid kits for Australian troops fighting in WWII. Tea tree oil contains a large amount of terpenes, and this is what gives tea tree oil its strong pine scent. Tea tree oil is distilled from its leaves and terminal branches, and this distillation produces a clear to pale yellow oil with a strong musk-like smell.

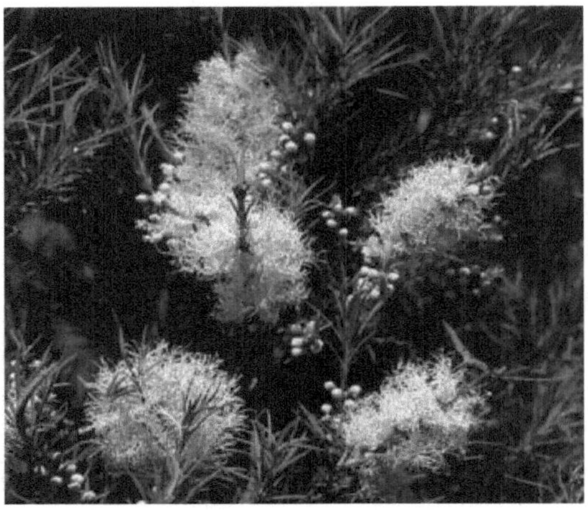

A Tea Tree in Flower

Tea tree oil's outstanding antimicrobial activity works against bacteria, fungi, and viruses. In tests done by the Australians it was able to dissolve pus and other wound debris and get down to the wound itself where it was an excellent antimicrobial. Tea tree oil also seems to promote wound healing; it is used quite extensively for wounds as well as burns and for all types of skin infections and ailments.

The good news is that tea tree oil does not harm healthy tissue, for all those reasons it is an essential ingredient for your natural/alternative medicine chest.

Tea tree oil is very potent as an antiseptic to clean surfaces such as a cutting board for meat or any surface you want to disinfect. Using a ratio of 4 parts of tea tree oil to 1000 parts of water, it made an outstanding antiseptic, wiping out both Staphyloccocus Aureus and Candida Albicans for up to thirty-five days after its application.

Tea tree oil can also be used for vaginal infections such as Trichomonas as well as others. It can be inhaled in a vaporized form and made into a mouth wash for mouth and throat infections. Tea tree oil also works very well for acne, naturally applied topically. A word of caution: Tea tree oil is a very potent germ killer, however, if diluted too far and weakened, it can result in the development of bacterial resistance. This only occurs when it is mistakenly used over-diluted with too much carrier oil. Tea tree oil, just like lavender oil, has been known to cause young males to develop gynecomastia (breasts).

Thyme oil (Thymus labiatae)

Thyme oil comes from over 300 species of plants that grow primarily in the Mediterranean region. Due to its popularity it has spread all over the world, and is now grown as far north as Iceland, however the strongest oils are made from those plants grown in its original Mediterranean climate. The name "thyme" derives from the Greek work thumos or smell, and is so named for its very aromatic leaves. Thyme oil is steam-distilled from the leaves and flower tops, and can be either white or red in color. Thyme oil contains several substances that have strong antimicrobial activity and has been used as an antimicrobial agent as far back as the ancient Egyptians.

It has one of the strongest killing powers against MRSA and VRE infections and even has been reported to work on anthrax, tuberculosis, typhoid, and meningococcal infections. Like tea tree oil, thyme is a strong disinfectant and will kill germs on most surfaces, including E. coli. Thyme also works for fungal infections topically and Candida Albicans internally. Thyme oil will also work for aches and pains when about fifteen drops are infused into a bath mixed with two tablespoons of baking soda. Thyme oil can also be used topically for acne; boil a pinch of thyme in two cups of water for fifteen minutes, allow it to steep for five minutes, and then mix in some lemon juice and apply it to the acne several times a day. Thyme oil can be used by mouth for respiratory infections such as bronchitis, sinus, and ear infections. It also works for intestinal and stomach infections and disorders such as diarrhea. It also works on infections from parasites such as worms, urinary tract infections, and skin disorders. It can be applied topically to ear infections and also to the larynx for hoarseness. Thyme can be made into a mouth rinse for mouth and throat infections, including dental infections and abscesses.

Oregano Oil (Oreganum vulgare)

Oregano oil is not made from the oregano used for cooking, but rather a rare wild herb from the eastern part of the Mediterranean called Oreganum Vulgare. It is famous for its very potent antiseptic and antimicrobial effects against bacteria, viruses, intestinal parasites, fungi, yeasts, and molds. It not only is bactericidal (kills bacteria) but also prevents their regrowth for some time. If that wasn't good enough, oregano oil is also a powerful antioxidant, helping to protect your body from toxins and cancer. Oregano oil is made by steam distillation of its leaves.

Oregano oil works wonders for sore throats and mouth infections, and can also be inhaled via a vaporizer for coughs, croup, asthma, and lung infections. It can be used topically but be careful on broken skin where it can be very irritating.

Oregano oil is very strong and cannot be used without a carrier oil. A good general formula is one part oregano oil to three parts carrier oil. When using it on the skin, mix ten to twelve drops of oregano oil per ounce of a carrier oil such as jojoba, sweet almond, olive, or grapeseed. The same mix can be rubbed into sore, tired muscles to help rejuvenate them. It is antifungal, so it will also work when applied to athlete's foot, jock itch, ringworm, and other topical fungal infections.

Orally it works against Candida Albicans and other internal fungal infections. Adding a few drops of oregano oil to juice or water and then gargling it and swallowing it will work to treat a sore throat. Be prepared for a very strong bad taste; oregano oil is so much more concentrated than oregano, that it has a very potent flavor. One of the compounds that oregano oil contains is Carvacrol, which acts as a natural insect repellent which is also present in mint and thyme.

A little interesting tidbit about mint that I always found fascinating -- it is the only plant with a square stem. Okay, so I admit I am a nerd. Odd facts excite me, That is probably why my wife, Lynne, calls me the King of Useless Knowledge.

Oregano oil also helps with digestion by increasing the flow of bile, which is used to emulsify and digest fats and oils. It also works against intestinal infections and parasites, including intestinal worms. Most infections that are being treated with oregano oil can be eradicated using four to six drops of oil for seven to ten days. Oregano oil is too strong for infants and small children and naturally, like almost everything, it cannot be used in pregnant or breast-feeding women.

Mountain Savory Oil (Satureja Montana)

Mountain savory oil is made from the plant of the same name; it is also sometimes referred to as winter savory. Mountain savory oil has been used as early as Roman times. The Romans referred to it as Satyr's herb because of its reported sexual stimulation and enhancing effects; in other words they believed it was an aphrodisiac.

A satyr, for my readers who do not know Greek or Roman mythology, is a woodlands god who is typically depicted as half-man and either half-goat (Roman) or half-horse (Greek), who is often drunk and always horny. Mountain savory also has strong antibacterial, antifungal, antiviral, and anti-parasitic effects, as well as being a stimulant of the immune system. Mountain savory is also a strong antioxidant, helping nullify the harmful effects of free radicals. In aromatherapy it is also used as a strong mental stimulator and a motivator.

Mountain savory is made by steam distillation of the entire herb and usually is golden to pale yellow in color. It is primarily produced in Hungary, Spain, and France, and originates from the southern Mediterranean region. Mountain savory oil, like most essential oils other than lavender oil, has to be diluted with a carrier oil before it is applied to the skin. Mountain oil should not be used in children younger than eighteen months and should not be used in pregnant or breast-feeding women. Mountain savory may also be toxic to the liver if used long-term, but there have been no definitive studies on this. Mountain savory can also be an irritant to the mucous membranes lining your mouth and should be used with caution, hence the importance of dilution with a carrier liquid.

Mountain savory oil should be diluted with a carrier oil at a 1:4 ratio, meaning one part of mountain savory oil to four parts of a carrier oil.

It can also be used topically to treat burns, bacterial and fungal infections. It can be used internally to treat a large number of infections and conditions including digestive disorders. Mountain savory oil can also be put in a vaporizer and inhaled to treat upper and lower respiratory tract infections and cough.

When taken internally it can be mixed with rice or soy milk or another liquid at a rate of one drop of mountain savory oil per 4 ounces of carrier liquid. Mountain savory is very useful for gastrointestinal (GI) infections as well as genital infections in both men and women. Mountain savory can also be mixed with honey at a rate of one drop of mountain savory oil per two teaspoons of honey.

Lemongrass Oil (Cymbopagon Flexuosus)

Lemongrass oil is made from a grass species which has a distinctive scent of lemon. Lemongrass oil has been known to have antibacterial, antifungal, anti- inflammatory, and antiseptic qualities, as well as being a vasodilator (enlarges blood vessels) and a stimulant to lymphatic flow -- and if that wasn't enough, it also improves circulation. This improvement in blood circulation and lymphatic flow both help it to improve edema (swelling) in the legs.

Lemongrass oil, like almost all essential oils, needs to be diluted in a carrier oil; the usual ratio is one part of lemon oil to four parts of carrier oil. Lemongrass oil is very useful for the repair of connective tissue, therefore it is very useful in joint, rib, tendon, and ligament injuries and can be applied as a liniment. It also repels insects and soothes the skin and is in the same family as citronella, just like those citronella candles your parents lit in the backyard to ward off those swarms of insects during your summer barbecues.

Lemon Myrtle Oil (Backhousia citriodora)

Lemon myrtle oil is made from the steam distillation of the leaves of an Australian tree of the same name. Lemon myrtle oil is an antibacterial, antifungal, antiviral agent as well as being a strong antiseptic. It is frequently used in atomizers or vaporizers to disinfect an entire household. It has very potent germicidal properties and eradicates many types of household germs on contact. Lemon myrtle derives its name from the strong lemon scent of its crushed leaves; it has a golden yellow color.

It is also very useful in a household if one member of the family is sick and you are trying to keep the others from becoming infected. Placing a few drops in a pan of water on a wood stove will also work just fine.

Lemon myrtle oil has also been used for skin infections and especially for treating acne. For acne, a drop of lemon myrtle oil can be added to a cotton ball that has been soaked in distilled water, and dabbed directly on the involved skin. Lemon myrtle oil cannot be used on broken skin due to its potential to irritate skin; of all of the essential oils, it is the most irritating. Lemon myrtle oil also cannot be used in pregnant or nursing women.

CHAPTER TWO

SOIL TO SELF: THE KEY TO VIGOROUS GOOD HEALTH

INTRODUCTION

TABLE OF CONTENTS:

I am a true believer in the concept of maintaining your body's natural state of health and vigor by several methods that I will outline in this discussion. Think of your body as a plant; for example, a plant grown in good healthy soil and given all the nutrients and minerals and trace elements it needs, will develop into a rigorous, healthy strong plant. This plant will not require pesticides and fertilizers and antifungal sprays to keep it healthy, its cells are healthy and therefore the entire plant is healthy. Only weak, malfunctioning cells become infected, since they are easy targets for microorganisms that want to infect them. When a plant or human cell is healthy, it has the right pH and the correct nutrients for all its needs, is able to get rid of waste, it is able to mount a vigorous defense and is vibrating at the right frequencies, it is impregnable and cannot become infected. Nature is no fool. Nothing your body does or contains is without a reason. Millions of years of evolution have molded and transformed us into the human beings we are today. Nothing was by chance. As Albert Einstein was fond of saying, "god does not play dice with the universe". Neither does mother nature; everything in this world is by design. I feel it is the hand of God, you may disagree.

Either way, the human body is an incredibly well designed system that only needs the right building blocks in the form of minerals, trace elements, phytonutrients, enzymes, vitamins, essential amino acids, and essential fatty acids in order to construct a strong body and immune system that will resist all diseases. When those proper ingredients and conditions are not available, the cell's pH becomes more acidic, its oxygen levels drop, it vibrates at a different frequency, waste builds up, its immunity weakens, all the processes that take place within the cell begin to malfunction and it becomes susceptible to infection. It is easier if you think of the cell as a small fort. The fort's soldiers make up your immunity; the more of them, the stronger your immunity. When you are weak you have hardly anyone guarding the wall and soon there are foreign soldiers making it over the wall into the fort, and you are infected. The best way to avoid infection is to build a higher wall and man it with Special Forces; no foreign soldiers will even make it close to the wall, much less over it and into the fort (your cell). As patients who want to take their health into their own hands, that is what we need to do; we need to become the people who do not get infected, and I will teach you the building blocks to construct that fort.

Think about it; every day you are exposed to an entire host of germs from viruses, bacteria, and fungal organisms, yet you do not catch any of these infections. No epidemic in history has infected 100 percent of humans exposed to it; there are always people who, despite the same conditions as everyone else, Remain stubbornly immune.

Why some people get infected and others don't is not a question that is usually asked by physicians. Physicians are trained to attack problems, they usually do not concern themselves with prevention; they are concerned with how to wipe out the flu or whatever other infection they find themselves treating.

Physicians and most other scientists obsess over what organism causes which disease, not why those cells became infected. I think we need to take it back one more step and find out why cells become infected. Once we do that we will not need all the other treatments.

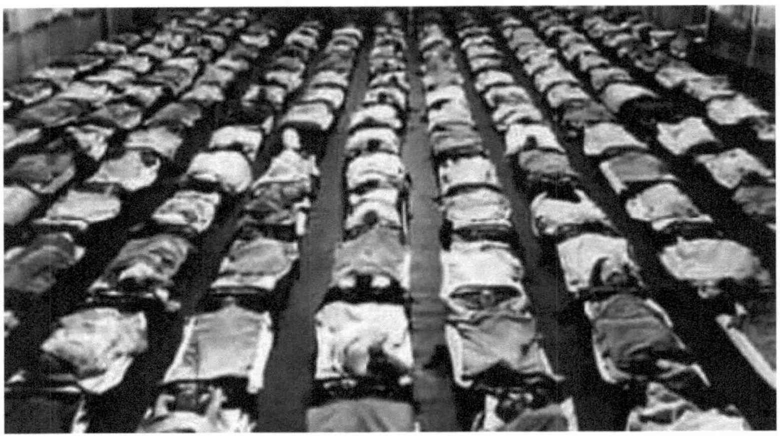

Hospital Ward During The Spanish Flu Epidemic of 1918

A LOOK AT SOME OF THE MOST DEADLY DISEASES IN HISTORY

The Black Death, or Plague, at its peak killed about 60 percent of the population; we don't know how many were infected and survived. All attempts to control it, including quarantine, did not work. The word quarantine is from the Italian quarentina meaning forty days. There was no scientific basis to that number. It was based on the Bible's description of the time Christ spent in the wilderness. Ships suspected of being contaminated were quarantined in port for forty days, families of the sick and healthy together were actually sealed in their homes and left to starve to death in an attempt to control the disease, all to no avail. The disease is carried by fleas that infect rats.

The rats simply climbed down the mooring ropes or scurried out of the homes of infected patients and went on their merry way infecting new victims. Infected rats became progressively more sick and weak until they died, at which point the fleas would leave them and look for another warm-blooded host, like the nearest human. Considering their size, fleas are the greatest Olympic long jumpers ever; they could jump an incredible six feet looking for another host! Hence, the plague spread across Asia and Europe, killing millions in its deadly wake, but not everyone.

The Spanish Flu of 1918 was airborne and incredibly virulent; it spread rapidly among large groups of people, like soldiers, and killed so many of them that it effectively put a halt to World War I.

We now know that it was the first instance of the deadly H1N1 flu virus. It infected one third of the world's population and killed 20 percent of those infected! At one point there were so many sick and dying people that it became difficult to dispose of the dead bodies. Think about those numbers; they are staggering. The United States currently has a population of roughly 300 million. That would mean 100 million infected Americans with 20 million of them dying!

The current Ebola outbreak in Africa (and likely coming to the United States soon) has a mortality rate of between 25 and 90 percent, with an average mortality of approximately 50 percent. The mortality rates vary from country to country. There are persistent, disturbing reports of airborne transmission; if that is the case you can expect this to possibly become a pandemic, spreading over the entire world. Ebola is a virus on the move; the first known cases were in 1976. The current outbreak, which began in March 2014, already has more cases and deaths than all the other outbreaks combined, and it is not even close to becoming controlled.

As you can see from history, no epidemic infects everyone or kills all of its hosts, for two reasons. The first reason is from an evolutionary point of view; it is a dead end for a disease-causing virus, for example, to kill all of its hosts within a short time. Like all life-forms, the virus's entire reason for existence is to reproduce and spread; this guarantees its survival. If a virus makes you so sick so quickly that you immediately wind up in bed and then die, it will not allow enough time for the virus to spread to its next victim.

Ideally, a virus will incubate for several days in the host, taking over its cellular machinery, and then reach critical mass and explode out of the infected cells, spewing out millions of viral particles ready to infect the first person they reach whose immune system is not able to kill it. They now gain entry into the new host's cells and the deadly process repeats itself.

That defense by the immune system and healthy cells is the second reason (and I think the more important of the two), why viruses do not infect everyone they come in contact with. Now we need to figure out how to keep our cells so vibrantly healthy that they will naturally resist most if not all infections. The answer lies right below your feet, it is your soil.

THE "DIRTY" SECRET TO GOOD HEALTH

If you are interested in building a vibrantly healthy body that is impervious to disease then you need to build strong bodies literally from the ground up. This is the only way we can guarantee ourselves good, long-lasting, disease free bodies that will resist the inevitable waves of viral, bacterial and fungal diseases that spread through our communities. It is also the only way we will be able to bear children who are healthy both mentally and physically, and who are better able to survive in this ever more toxic world.

When I say from the ground up I mean it literally, the "dirty" secret to good health lies in the dirt or soil of our gardens, fields, and orchards. It is the only way to build healthy bodies and immune systems that will be able to resist everything thrown at them.

Our bodies are incredible machines that will build remarkably strong bodies if provided with the proper environment or terrain and all the building blocks they need. In the above paragraphs I alluded to the mistake that modern medicine is making by attacking the organisms that they feel are causing diseases. This idea of one germ causing one disease state is known as Germ Theory. Don't mistake what I am saying. Germ Theory has served us well, but in my opinion its time has come and gone. The endless war we have waged against germs has been lost. We have to face facts, antibiotics worked for years but now the bacteria have outsmarted us and resistance is spreading faster than new, novel antibiotics can be developed. It has been an arms race of sorts since the 1940s and we are losing it. That leaves us with two options, double down and try as hard as we can to come up with new antibiotics, or try option two build healthier cells and immerse them in a healthier environment that will be able to handily resist infections.

Louis Pasteur was the father of Germ Theory, but by the time of his death he saw its futility and on his deathbed he recanted and proclaimed, "It is the terrain that is most important." The terrain is the area between cells and all around them it is also known as the ECM or extracellular matrix. This is not a dead zone at all; it is the way cells get their nutrients by diffusion of nutrients between cells. Oxygen is also delivered through the terrain, waste products are removed, and cells communicate with each other through it.

Cells send messages to each other through the terrain, which also provides a structure to embed the cells into and allows the cells to adhere or stick to each other. Growth factors that control cell behavior such as hormones and other protein molecules lie within the terrain and await activation so they can control cell functions. As you can see, this is not a glue merely holding cells together but rather it is the key to controlling cell health and in turn human health.

To ignore its importance in favor of finding new ways to attack germs is utter madness. Why do we continuously try to reinvent the wheel?

The idea that the environment or "the Terrain" the cells are immersed in predisposes cells to become sick or diseased was abandoned in favor of Germ Theory almost a hundred years ago by modern medicine and unfortunately new theories take a long time to become accepted as truths. Modern medicine is still on the attack, embracing germ theory to the exclusion of evidence to the contrary and its continual failure to permanently conquer germs with ever more toxic antibiotics. Even recent progress that has been made in studying and identifying the human microbiome (the beneficial bacteria and fungi that live and breed in our intestines) and its incredible contribution to our health and our immunity has been ignored in favor of ever stronger antibiotics that devastate these wonderful probiotics.

The evidence continues to mount in favor of the terrain, yet it is continually ignored or played down. Healthy cells produce healthy tissues and organs and healthy bodies, plain and simple. These cells require all the building blocks I mentioned above, plus the right pH (slightly alkaline), and plentiful oxygen provided by good blood flow (which also removes waste products that are acidic). These healthy cells actually vibrate at certain frequencies, "buzzing" together, having the correct pH, well oxygenated and also the correct electrical voltage all adding up to vibrantly healthy tissue. These cells will never become infected by any germ that tries to attack them. The germs will be repelled by the electric charge and will not find a receptive environment due to the alkaline pH and will not be able to penetrate the cell membrane that is strong and healthy, in good repair, and strongly vibrating, and fully capable of resisting any germ assaults.

Germs cannot overcome this collective electric charge of healthy cells which repels them, they cannot survive in an alkaline pH, and they cannot gain entry into cells that are strong and healthy. Germs need low oxygen, acidic environments to grow and reproduce and be able to spread. They need a certain frequency of vibration to be able to enter a cell. Think of it like an FM radio dial ....if you want to listen to a certain channel, you can only gain entry to that channel at the correct frequency. The wrong frequency number on the dial and you get static and you can never pick up or enter that station.

It is the same for germs; these microorganisms are alive and as living organisms they too vibrate at a certain frequency, they need cells which are "sick" and whose electrical charge and vibratory frequency are compromised enough to allow them to enter; if not, it is like searching for an FM station at the wrong frequency.

The blueprint for perfect, healthy, disease-resistant bodies is already encoded in our DNA. We have recently discovered epigenetic (literally meaning around or outside the genes) mechanisms that in turn are the on and off signals for our genes. Many of these epigenetic influences are negative and disease- promoting, but not all. We are rapidly learning how to better control negative epigenetic influences, and the good news is that they can be overcome. The messengers for this epigenetic control come in the form of microRNA. We can provide our bodies with all the proper building blocks to construct the perfect body but this needs to be done in the context of the right terrain with the proper pH and also by providing microRNA to send the correct signals to our genes so they can correctly choreograph this amazing construction project.

In order to build healthy cells as I described above, you need to start in your dirt or soil; that is the "dirty" secret to good health. Healthy soils will grow healthy plants, animals grazing on healthy plants will build healthy, strong bodies and humans eating these plants and animals will in turn become strong, robust, and very disease resistant. In effect, to develop our own healthy terrain we need to start with healthy terrains in our gardens, fields, orchards, lakes, rivers, and pastures.

HOW TO BUILD HEALTHY SOIL

Bear with me here. Before you start to think you mistakenly bought a gardening manual, know this; you and your family's destiny depends on your soil. If you want to not only survive but to be healthy, free of chronic diseases, infections, and reproduce sane robustly healthy children then you better pay attention to what I have to say. Your health begins in your gardens dirt or soil.

Your soil, if properly nourished and maintained, will prove to be the "goose that laid the golden egg", and will feed you through its plants with an unending stream of essential amino acids, essential fatty acids, protein, healthy carbohydrates, vitamins, enzymes, minerals, trace elements, and phyto-nutrients. God made it possible, our job is to take all of his blessings and utilize them as they were intended for us, return to the garden.

First of all this entire process by necessity needs to be organic, meaning no artificial fertilizers, herbicides, pesticides, or fungicides of any type.

No man-made chemicals are to be added to the soil at any time, recognizing that these are poisons and will kill the extensive web of life contained in the soil. A soil devoid of life is worthless for nutritional purposes. In lifeless soils it is impossible to grow healthy plants.

Soil Life

Healthy soil is alive and teeming with life of all kinds. Healthy soils contain large amounts of bacteria and fungi that help convert inorganic minerals (which plants cannot utilize) into organically chelated minerals that plants can readily uptake. That is an important distinction to understand; plants and animals (including us humans) cannot absorb inorganic minerals, except for a very small amount that can be made by the intestinal bacteria. We can, however, readily absorb organic materials, since they are usually wrapped in proteins that we can absorb; that process of enclosing the mineral in a protein or humic acid matrix is called chelation.

We absorb organic minerals and other organic compounds by eating plants that have absorbed those organic minerals and trace elements from the soil. If soils are deficient in any mineral or trace element, then it is impossible for the plants to obtain them for their needs, and in turn the animals that eat the plants, including us humans, will not be able to get the minerals and trace elements that we need to correctly construct our complex bodies.

Organic Matter And Soil Ph

The bacteria and fungi in the soils live by virtue of the organic content of the soil; in other words they live by eating the decomposing organic matter in the soil such as decomposing plants and animals and other microorganisms. If the bacteria and fungi did not do this we would have mountains of dead and decaying plant materials. You need to supply lots of organic material to help these microorganisms flourish. Other living organisms in the soil such as nematodes, protozoa, mites, springtails, and earthworms also need this organic material to flourish and add to the goodness of the soil.

Some excellent sources of organic matter can readily be made by composting. We should try to never waste any materials, including food that we do not consume, or parts of food discarded from food preparation. All the vegetable matter should be put in a compost bin or compost pile. These do not have to be elaborate store-bought contraptions. You can easily make a compost bin as I have done with a handful of old wooden pallets and some wire.

Learn to improvise, learn to think outside of the box and you can come up with some wonderful, simple solutions for not only composting but many of the problems that life will inevitably throw at you.

Another easy way to increase the organic content, especially the carbon content of soil, is by making Biochar. Biochar is made by partially burning vegetable matter of any type then putting out the fire when it is only partially carbonized (looking like coal). This is an ancient method of fertilizing soil that was used by Native Americans to increase the fertility of their soil. It creates a finely grained, porous charcoal that is home to many soil microbes and increases both fertility and water retention capacities of soils. It is a wonderful way to convert garden and woodland waste into a valuable soil amendment.

Biochar is made when wood, bones, leaves, or manure (or any vegetable matter) is heated or burned at low temperatures in a kiln, this is done by limiting oxygen to the process and keeping the temperature below 700 F. The resulting half-burned charcoal-looking material is biochar, and is ready to be added to your soil. Biochar like wood ash is alkaline and works best when used as a soil amendment on acidic soils. Mixing biochar with compost works best by helping to properly age the biochar and add the fertility boosting effects of compost.

As with any composting system, you cannot use meat, fats, or dairy products, which will ruin the compost and attract insects and mice and other vermin as well as stinking up your house. You can use newspaper, cardboard, fruit, vegetable matter, bread, teabags, and coffee grounds.

Soil can be improved by using a variety of readily available organic materials. As mentioned above, composting is a wonderful idea and will provide you with a steady supply of "black gold" for your garden.

Other sources of organic materials are coffee grounds (I go to my local Starbucks and they are very nice about providing buckets of their coffee grounds); cover crops such as legumes, buckwheat, and cereal rye can be grown and then gently turned under and buried in the top layer of soil (it is a good policy never to leave your soil bare and open to the elements); dried manure (you cannot use fresh manure, it will burn your plants). Peat moss, wood chips, sawdust, grass clippings, leaf mold, and shredded and composted leaves are all wonderful sources of organic material for your garden; these all will lower your pH and make your garden more acidic.

You can raise your pH by the addition of crushed rocks (rock dust), ashes from your fireplace or any wood burning, bone meal, and crushed oyster shells .If you live near the ocean, lakes or any body of water that can be used for fishing you can use dead fish to improve your garden soils. Salt water fish are better than fresh water but both will suffice.

Bury any fish or fish parts that you are not eating into your garden; they are wonderful sources for many minerals and trace elements and have been used for centuries to enhance garden soils. Dried seaweed such as kelp is also an excellent source of minerals, nutrients, and phytonutrients such as growth hormones.

The ideal pH of your garden should be between 6.5 and 6.8, which is very mildly acidic. That pH range has been found to be optimal for plants to be able to uptake minerals and other charged particles from the soil. Lower or higher pH levels result in a binding of the nutrients and results in them being unavailable for uptake by your garden plants. Simple soil pH kits are available in any garden center and I would buy several of them to have on hand. Growing plants in the wrong pH will result in disaster. Most soils found east of the Mississippi river are slightly acidic in nature.

Soils that are too acidic can be sweetened by the addition of powdered limestone (lime), which is alkaline and will raise the pH into your target range of 6.5 to 6.8. You can also use wood ashes from your fireplace if no lime is available, which also contains potassium and many trace elements. Do not use more than 2 pounds of ashes per hundred square feet of garden (for those of you who are math-challenged, this means a ten foot by ten foot garden space, or twenty feet by five feet, etc.). Another formula to use to sweeten your soil is to add 4 pounds of lime per one hundred square feet for every one point of pH below 6.5.

If you have alkaline soils (which are much less common) you can use sulphur on it to make it more acidic and you can also use pine needles or other acidic materials. The formula for the addition of sulphur to alkaline soils is 1 pound of Sulphur per one hundred square feet (for each point of pH above 7.5.

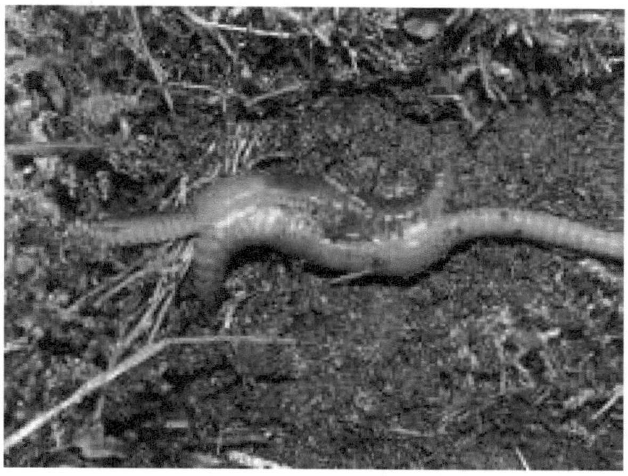

Earthworm Porn: Photo of Two Earthworms Copulating

Earthworms

Earthworms are one of the most important contributors to soil fertility, they add their "castings" (their feces) to the soil, which is loved by all plants and makes them flourish. They also create tons of castings annually and aerate the soil and help bring organic matter from the upper layers, mixing it with the lower soil layers with their digging. If you have 500,000 earthworms living in an acre of soil they will create an incredible fifty tons of castings! The burrowing and digging done by the same 500,000 earthworms will create a drainage system equivalent to 2,000 feet of six-inch pipe! Worms actively convert large pieces of organic matter into humus, also helping to build soils. Earthworms need lots of nitrogen-rich organic material to eat, but adding nitrogen-rich fertilizers will not work and in fact will drive away earthworms that tend to get burnt by these man-made chemical fertilizers.

Vermiculture, or the raising of earthworms, is a very good idea for anyone interested in becoming healthy through sustainable, organic gardening.. It is very easy to do, and is done basically with a composting bin and will provide you with compost that is very rich in worm castings. Each worm will defecate their body weight daily in these rich organic castings. Kept in a cool dark place like your basement and kept moist, it will work not only to compost your vegetable waste from your kitchen but will also be a great source of earthworms for your garden. Many of the commercial bins made for vermiculture have a catch basin system on the bottom of the bins with spigots that can be used to dispense "worm tea" that is a wonderful natural fertilizer for your garden plants, and should never be wasted.

Humus

Humus is the brown/black material without any trace of plant cells left in it. It is made by bacterial and fungal action upon decaying plant materials; you can make it by composting. It is the life force of the soil and feeds much of the soil life. Humus does not decay, and permanently adds to the fertility and the water retention capacities of the soil. Humus is made of organic material that is wrapped in soil minerals and particles protecting it from further decomposition. Humus is capable of retaining moisture in soils since it will hold approximately 90 percent of its own weight in water.

Humus is the lifeblood of the soil and is vital to any soil's health and slowly increases from the activity of microorganisms in the soil upon the decaying organic material in the soil.

These microorganisms take the minerals in the soil and add humic acid and proteins (amino acids) and chelate or wrap these minerals in these materials to make them accessible to plants. Without the presence of these bacteria and fungi there would not be any organic or chelated minerals available to plants, so you can see the importance of keeping your soil alive. These microorganisms supply all kinds of nutrients -- proteins, hormones, vitamins, minerals, and trace elements - to the roots of the plants and in return the plant roots exude sugars as a food source for these soil microorganisms.

Mycorrhizal Fungi

The roots of most plants also live in a symbiotic relationship with soil fungi known as mycorrhizal fungi that began more than 400 million years ago. These mycorrhizal fungi are the "godfathers" of the soil. They attach themselves to plant roots and "make them an offer they can't refuse". Each plant root has an entire network of fungal tendons called hyphae that reach out into the surrounding soil, vastly increasing the surface area of each root, helping to absorb water, minerals, and other nutrients from the soil and supplying them all to the plant's hungry roots. The hyphae are much smaller than the smallest plant roots and extend deeply into the surrounding soil. The hyphae release organic acids that dissolve minerals and trace elements in the soil and then chelate them and absorb them and pass them on to the plant. In turn the plant gives sugars for the fungus to live upon, a really beautiful symbiotic relationship that is used by most plants of the world.

The only plants that do not like mycorrhizal fungi are the brassicas, which are members of the mustard family, including turnips and radishes. The extended surface area of hyphae also helps fuel growth and also confers greater resistance to drought and disease. The mycorrhizal fungi also improve the soil; they help make clumps of soil that hold water and air and make them available to plant roots on demand. The fungal hyphae do this by secreting a form of sticky carbon particles, known as glomalin, which acts like a sticky glue holding soil together, giving structure to the soil, helping to resist erosion and loss of nutrients.

You can buy mycorrhizal fungi online or in your local garden supply store. I always sprinkle them onto the roots of all my plants They help to jump-start growth and spread through soils making their nutrients much more accessible. You have to make sure they come in direct contact with the roots of the plant you are inoculating.

There are several things you can do to help foster the growth of mycorrhizia in your garden soil.

First, dig and/or rototill as little as possible. This snaps off the hyphae and inhibits their spread in the soil. Keep as diverse a group of plants as you can in your garden, since mycorrhizae need live plant roots to develop. Rotation of crops helps this goal, but make sure you don't use the brassicas (plants in the mustard family and cabbage). Rotating crops also helps because it provides a variety of different types of plant roots, which is important because different types of plant roots support diverse types of mycorrhizae subspecies. Avoid high phosphorus fertilizers like manures, because high phosphorus levels prevent the association of the mycorrhizae with plant roots. Leave some weeds in your garden since weed roots also support diverse colonies of mycorrhizae. The last recommendation is to mulch your garden in the winter and plant a cover crop that will provide live plant roots as food for your mycorrhizae.

Minerals and Trace Elements

Now that we have built a soil with the correct pH, full of organic matter, teeming with microorganisms of all types, full of earthworms and loaded with humus, we need to insure that it is full of the entire spectrum of minerals and trace elements that our bodies so desperately need. By supplementing our soil with the full spectrum of these minerals, we are in effect feeding the microorganisms in our soil that will hungrily devour these minerals and chelate them from their present inorganic state by binding them with humic acids and proteins and thus rendering them organic and thus able for the plants to also utilize for their nutritional needs. Inorganic minerals are not taken up by plants and cannot be used by them.

Keep in mind that human blood has all the minerals and trace elements that are found in the world's oceans.

The reason for that is quite simple, it is where we evolved from. Our blood is incredibly close to ocean water in its composition. The only difference is the world's oceans currently are moderately more salty than our blood. However, when life first developed in the sea its salt content was identical to ours; over the centuries mineral salts have leached out of land, carried by fresh water to the world's oceans, slowly increasing their salinity.

I have studied the human body my entire adult life and its beauty and complexity never cease to amaze me. One thing I have noticed is, nothing is done by accident. If there is a chemical substance created by the body it is for a predetermined function or a series of functions. All the minerals and trace elements are in our blood because each has a definite purpose and function.

Science has consistently supported this theory by continuously discovering new functions for these little known trace elements.

The only way we can guarantee their presence in our bodies is to make sure they are present in our food, and this can only be done by supplementing them in our soil.

Mineralization of your garden is the only way to guarantee the presence of the full complement of minerals and trace elements; extra will not hurt, a deficiency eventually could be devastating for your health. There are many options for mineralizing your soils. In the 1950s several different scientist/ authors wrote books on the amazing benefits of using sea solids (minerals, trace elements, and other factors removed from sea water) to fertilize crops. Their results were amazing, growing bumper crops of large, healthy vegetables that were chock-full of minerals of all types and trace elements. I have listed several of the books in the bibliography at the end of this text; they make for fascinating reading and can easily be found online. For our purposes it will very likely not be practical to utilize sea solids for our garden needs, but fortunately we have several other viable options.

Utilizing the same theme of using sea solids brings us to a wonderful product mined from an ancient seabed in Utah called Azomite. Azomite is an acronym for A to Z Of Minerals Including Trace Elements. Azomite contains over seventy minerals and trace elements. Scientists have determined that thirty million years ago a local volcano erupted and deposited all these minerals directly into an ancient sea where it combined with the seawater and settled to the bottom over years and collected in these unique deposits. Azomite also contains many rare earth elements that have become depleted in soils worldwide. Adding this fine powder to your soil will guarantee the full complement of minerals for your plants' needs. For plants to achieve their full potential and be strong and disease resistant they need the full complement of minerals and trace elements.

I add it to my garden soil annually, since I want to progressively build up the minerals and trace elements sequestered (stored) there for later use by the plants. The addition of Azomite to soils will produce larger fruit and vegetables that are tastier and more disease and pest resistant. Many fruit trees that are old and starting to wane in production will come alive the year after treatment with Azomite, and produce much larger bumper crops of tasty fruit.

Azomite is safe for humans and animals and many people take a teaspoon of the powder daily in a large glass of water to guarantee they get all the minerals and trace elements they need directly. This will provide some, but I do not recommend it because Azomite is inorganic and needs to be chelated to organic form by soil microbes so you can assimilate it properly.

Feed it to your soil through which it will be chelated for your plants, then you eat the plants that are chock-full of all the minerals they assimilated from your mineral rich soil.

Note, each plant will only take up a certain number of minerals and trace elements they specifically need, but eating a diverse group of garden plants grown in such soils will eventually get you all you need.

You can also take Supreme Fulvic orally to get your mineral and trace elements. Supreme Fulvic is fully explained in chapter 3. It is a wonderful mineral and trace element supplement along with many other nutrients. It can be found on line at www.supremefulvic.com.

Azomite is often added to animal feed up to 2 percent and results in larger, healthier, and tastier animals. You can find it online from the company, that lists all their dealers of it nationwide, or buy it on Amazon or eBay.

Azomite comes in three forms: Micronized, which is a fine powder; a more affordable type known as field grade; and finally, a granulated form that can be applied using a spreader. You can mix Azomite with compost and spread it on your soil, which sometimes is easier since it is such a fine powder.

There are other products on the market that work very well to remineralize your garden, pasture, and orchard soils. Rock dust is one and comes either from quarries from pulverized rock powder or is mined from glacial deposits. The difference between Azomite and rock dust is that Azomite is volcanic in origin then combined with sea water, whereas rock dusts are primarily glacial deposits formed by the actions of ancient glaciers slowly grinding rock down as these huge masses of ice passed over them. Rock dust is used in the same way as Azomite.

DIRECT MINERALIZATION OF YOUR BODY

The best way to feed and maintain your body's extracellular fluid (terrain) as well as its microbial populations (microbiome) is to get back to evolutionary basics. We humans began our journey to our present state from very humble beginnings in the seas and oceans of Earth. At the time that the first unicellular (one cell) organisms developed, they did so in a sea almost identical to our present blood plasma and extracellular fluids (the fluid of our body's terrain). That primordial sea was chock-full of minerals, trace elements, and amino acids (building blocks to proteins) in a perfect pH solution thus maximizing nutrient absorption and uptake.

As evolution took place over millions of years, a full complement of sea creatures developed. Eventually these creatures left the sea behind for a land- based existence. They now had self-enclosed bodies that were no longer bathed in seawater's primordial soup of nutrients, minerals, and trace elements that they previously enjoyed.

However, inside these self-enclosed bodies each cell swam in a sea of the same composition. Clearly this internal sea, or extracellular fluid, and blood plasma have the same composition for a reason. Remember me saying that nature does not do anything without a reason. Your body, in order to properly function, needs every one of those minerals and trace elements, without which the chain of health is broken and the body is unable to produce the enzymes, proteins, and hormones, or activate the vitamins it needs to fully thrive.

Fortunately for mankind, a French scientist named Rene Quinton in the late 1800s became obsessed with this idea of the sea acting as an incubator for life and providing all sea life with not only the proper mix of minerals and trace elements, but also in the right ratios and in an organic form for life to thrive. He did extensive research and discovered that at any given time there were approximately seven huge vortices in the oceans. These vortices (think huge twisters in the ocean) extend with their narrow end on the ocean bottom and their mouths hundreds of miles wide at the surface. The spinning action of these vortices scooped up large amounts of minerals and trace elements and organic materials from the oceans' floors and sent them up in giant, nutrient-rich spirals towards the surface of the ocean. Inside of this, phytoplankton (plant plankton) thrives and reproduce in huge schools; these in turn are fed upon by zooplankton (animal plankton). These zooplankton release large amounts of nutrients from their digestion of the phytoplankton. This results in a soup chock-full of nutrients including DNA, RNA, organic proteins and carbohydrates, as well as all minerals and trace elements. This "plankton milk", as it is called, is the source of much of the life in our oceans. Sea creatures of all sizes ranging from microscopic to whales come into these vortices to feed on this nutritious substance.

Dr. Quinton made a way to cold-filter and process this water to remove the plankton, leaving just the nutritious soup.

He named this Quinton's Marine Plasma, and he formed hundreds of free clinics to treat the poor and destitute all over Europe. He was a huge success in treating all types of diseases and afflictions suffered by his patients. The company still exists to this day and is currently in Spain. You can order online or through participating health care practitioners. It comes in two forms, an isotonic form and a hypertonic form. I recommend the isotonic form as best for most patients' needs. It is a clear, salty-tasting drink, and 1 ounce a day should suffice over time to completely rebuild your terrain and restock it and recharge it with the beneficial substances your body desperately needs. This will probably take several months. Quinton's Marine Plasma will also serve as a wonderful prebiotic for your body's probiotic bacteria, feeding them and nurturing them. You can purchase it at www.purative.com.

Other than Quinton's Marine Plasma there are several other options. You can mix a teaspoon of Azomite in a large glass of water and drink that daily, but as I stated earlier, since it is inorganic I am not sure about the wisdom of going this route. However, there is no denying that giving it in animal feed produced larger, healthier animals. In a pinch if I had no other mult-mineral and trace element source, I would try using the Azomite.

There are also several other mineral and trace element drinks on the market. You should look for a colloidal mineral mix. A colloid is a mixture in which, due to their electrical charges, the substances contained in it are in permanent suspension and cannot settle out of the mixture. Think Jell-O; it never settles or comes out of mixture. Milk is another example, but that will eventually develop into cheese. Most plants produce their proteins and fats along with their minerals as colloids. Colloids are easily digested and assimilated by the human body and do not require extensive transformations like non-colloids. For several years I was sending my patients to GNC. Up until recently they had a wonderful Colloidal Mineral drink that is no longer in production.

One pioneer of good health and a healthy terrain is Dr. Wallach. He produced a very popular book and audiotape called Dead Doctors Don't Lie. As much as I hate the title and the premise, it is an excellent book and will give you some valuable insight into the necessity of having proper minerals and trace elements for good health. He grew up on a farm and was first a veterinarian and then trained as a medical doctor. He witnessed firsthand what the lack of soil nutrients did for his herds and how supplying those nutrients prevented miscarriages and diseases in his animals. Once he trained as a physician, he applied the same principles of nutrition and healing through minerals and trace elements to his fortunate patients. He too has a line of mineral drinks that I highly recommend.

You can get them through a company called Youngevity. They have powders and colloidal mineral drinks like Majestic Earth Plant Derived Minerals

As I said, it also comes in a powdered form which has the advantage of being much easier to store and carry. Either one is fine for our needs. Another source of the same product is T.J. Clark's Original Colloidal Trace Minerals. You can easily find either one on the web and order it from them. They both will supply all of the minerals and trace elements we need to properly function. Note: In order to maintain your body's terrain you will need fresh, clean water and proper nutrition to supply the necessary proteins (and their constituent amino acids, many of which are essential for health), fats, and carbohydrates. Presently our diets are full of carbohydrates and bad fats and lacking in proteins (especially those with a broad spectrum of amino acids).

We need fats -- they are essential to our health. They have gotten a bad name over the last few decades and most Americans are fat-phobic. We need good fats in the form of omega-3 fatty acids; presently our diets are out of balance with too many omega-6 fatty acids and too few of the omega-3s. Omega-3 fatty acids are anti-inflammatory and health- promoting and should be consumed in adequate quantities to provide your body with the essential fats we need. They come in various forms such as fish oil, krill oil, flaxseed oil, and walnut oils. All of these are beneficial and contain different ratios of good fats in various forms.

WHAT DOES YOUR BODY ACTUALLY NEED?

Your body needs about forty-five known essential nutrients plus enzymes. The breakdown is as follows:

10 ESSENTIAL AMINO ACIDS

The ten essential amino acids are arginine, histidine, isoleucine, leucine, lysine, methionine, phenylalanine, threonine, tryptophan and valine.

Humans can make the other amino acids, but do not have the enzymes necessary to produce these; that is why they are considered essential and must therefore be included in your diet. Failure to provide all of these will result in the failure of your body to construct proteins it needs for its various functions. Almost all of the body's functions are controlled by proteins .Food sources of these essential amino acids include eggs (which contains all of them), soy protein, seeds of various types, tofu, peanuts, parmesan cheese, beef, sesame seeds, winged beans, whitefish, and pork.

The Three Sisters

An easier way, if you are planting a garden, is to follow what our Native American tribes utilized for agriculture to obtain all their essential amino acids, called the three sisters method of agriculture.

Native American tribes out of necessity developed an agricultural system that they referred to as the three sisters. It was utilized all over the continent with some minor variations.

It encompassed the use of three main agricultural crops: squash, maize (corn), and climbing beans (typically tepary beans or common beans). They used what became known as companion planting to maximize their crop outputs and to minimize their work input.

They made flat-topped mounds of soil about a foot high and twenty inches wide. Several maize seeds were planted close to each other in the center of the mound. In the Northeastern United States the tribes added rotten fish or eels to help increase the fertility of the soil. When the corn or maize reached a height of six inches tall, beans and squash were planted in an alternating pattern.

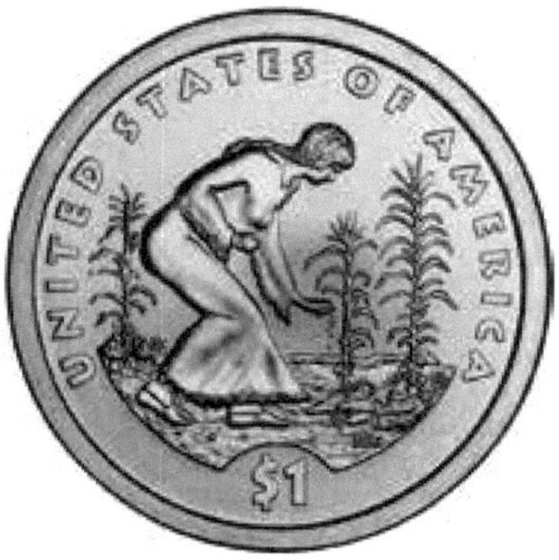

2009 Native American Dollar Coin

The idea was simple and ingenious. The corn grew tall and acted as a rigid structure for the climbing beans to grow upon, the squash shaded both the base of the corn and the beans and prevented weed growth and kept the soil cool and moist, creating a perfect microclimate. The squash also had prickly hairs on the stem which prevented insect pests from climbing upon the plants. Together all three of these agricultural crops provided all the essential amino acids humans require.

I would suggest mimicking the three sisters as a minimum in your family garden, that way you are getting all the essential amino acids. The remaining crops you plant can be according to your diet and tastes without worries over their amino acid content. One variation of the three sisters agriculture was in the southwestern Unites States where indigenous tribes used a fourth sister known as the "rocky mountain bee plant" (Cleome serrulata), which attracts bees to help pollinate the crops.

Two Types of Fat

The two types of fat required in your diet are also called essential because, just like the above amino acids, your body cannot construct them and must get them in its diet. The two essential fatty acids are: alpha-Linolenic acid (an omega-3 fatty acid) and Linoleic acid (an omega-6 fatty acid). Some of the foods that contain these essential fatty acids are: fish oil, krill oil, shellfish, fish, canola oil, hemp seed oil, green leafy vegetables, seeds (chia, pumpkin and sunflower seeds), soya oil (from soy sauce, soybeans, natto, etc.) and walnuts.

Thirteen Vitamins, Nineteen Minerals, and Carbohydrates

Your body needs all the known vitamins, both fat and water soluble. They have to be in the foods you eat, although some can be manufactured by your gut bacteria and vitamin D can be obtained by exposing your skin to sunlight. Most of the minerals can be obtained by mineralization of the soil or taking a mineral supplement directly. Carbohydrates are needed for fuel production and energy needs and are easily met by fruits and vegetables in our diet. Those natural carbohydrates are much better for you than man-made carbs because they are packaged with significant quantities of soluble and insoluble fiber as well as vitamins, enzymes, minerals, and those all-important phytonutrients. Unlike proteins and fats there are no essential carbohydrates, since your body is able to manufacture carbs from proteins and fats.

Water, Fresh Air, Enzymes and Exercise

This list does not include water (fresh and mineralized is best), all the trace elements, and as many enzymes from plant sources as you can get in your diet. This means raw fruits and vegetables since cooking at above 120F destroys the enzyme content of foods. All raw foods are supplied with all the enzymes you require to digest them, but no extra enzymes. Therefore it is important to supplement your body's enzymes with oral enzymes when eating cooked or processed foods. Contrary to prevailing opinion, enzymes are not destroyed in the stomach and are absorbed in the small intestine. Your body has an enzyme potential, and drawing down on that leads to poor health and chronic diseases. Humans and our unfortunate pets are the only animals on Earth that eat cooked foods.

Fermented foods are good for you because they are loaded with enzymes from the fermentation process. Vinegar has hundreds of wonderful uses and is very good for your health. Other health giving fermented foods are sauerkraut, kimchi, yogurt, soy sauce, natto, kefir, and pickled foods.

Exercise is a very important component of maintaining excellent health. We have become a very sedentary society and it shows. Obesity has become a major problem, not only in the United States but worldwide. Our children no longer go out and play like we did. Most of us stayed outside playing until it got dark every night or we had to come in for dinner. We ran, swam, and biked for hours every day. In addition to which, we had gym class for an hour a day in school. Gym is essential in our schools and has been thumbed down and/or eliminated over the years.

We would not have the astronomical levels of Attention Deficit Disorder and hyperactivity, especially among our boys, if they had an hour of gym every morning to burn up that energy (along with less sugar and chemicals in their diet and more of the essential nutrients and trace elements, etc. listed above).

I would highly recommend daily exercises to maintain muscle tone and strength, which you will eventually need. A simple routine of stretching first for a few minutes (watch your dog or cat, no animal gets up and starts exercising, they always stretch to limber up their muscles.). Follow your stretching with a routine of knee bends, sit-ups, and the most important, push-ups. Push-ups, if done correctly, tone your entire body. Push-ups should be done slowly, exhaling as you push up and making sure your head is up looking straight ahead and your chest touches the floor. You will be amazed how this tightens up your chest, abdomen, back, neck, and legs. You will also be amazed at how fast your strength grows and the number you do keeps going slowly up. Psychologically, this will also help you by releasing endorphins and helping your mood.

CHAPTER THREE

VITAMINS AND YOUR NUTRITION

INTRODUCTION

TABLE OF CONTENTS:

First of all let me say how even after twenty-five years in private practice, I am continuously astounded by the lack of understanding of vitamins among the general public and even my fellow physicians. Countless patients have told me they know everything about vitamins and yet for years and sometimes decades they were taking them wrong and not absorbing them. That amounts to some very expensive urine and stool, with none of the potential benefits.

VITAMIN BASICS: FAT AND WATER SOLUBLE VITAMINS

What Does Soluble Mean?

Vitamins come in two types: Fat soluble and water soluble. Soluble means what they dissolve in. Remember this: If they don't dissolve they cannot be absorbed by your body and will pass through you as if you never took them. As the names suggest, fat soluble vitamins will only dissolve in fat.

Water soluble vitamins dissolve only in water. Since your body is largely composed of water, you can take these on an empty stomach and still absorb them. The fat soluble vitamins must be taken with fat, i.e. with a meal that has fat-containing foods. Most of the foods in our diet contain fat, the more the better for absorption purposes.

Fat free yogurt or ice cream or skim milk will not work. A salad will work only if you put a lot of olive oil on it. For that matter, any oil will work; you can use walnut oil, flaxseed, or even hemp oil. Oils are liquid fats at room temperature. There are all kinds of wonderful oils that enhance your health. See the sections later in this book on Seed Oils and Essential Oils.

MILK

Unfortunately, we were all taught as kids to take our vitamins with breakfast. In those days, that consisted of whole milk (Whoever drank 1 or 2 percent milk or skim milk in those days?) on our cereal and maybe some toast with butter. That was enough to absorb your fat soluble vitamins.

Whole milk has about a 4 percent fat content. Everyone seems to think that 2 percent milk has 98 percent of the fat removed; wrong, it is 50 percent fat free, 1 percent is 75 percent fat free. Many adults become lactose intolerant to varying degrees as they age, some more than others. You might notice that milk gives you gas, bloating and diarrhea, or if you eat a meal heavy with cheese; these are signs that you are developing some lactose intolerance.

You have the option of taking Lactaid tablets to help digest the lactose in milk thereby neutralizing your lactose intolerance.

Sometimes it is difficult to distinguish lactose intolerance from Irritable Bowel Syndrome (IBS). This usually involves diarrhea alternating with constipation, with or without accompanying abdominal discomfort. Other times a full-blown milk allergy might be the culprit. This is usually to the proteins in milk such as whey and casein. This is very common in children even under the age of one. Milk allergy is much more severe than lactose intolerance, since it involves the immune system, whereas lactose intolerance is merely an enzyme deficiency. Milk allergy can result in hives, congestion, wheezing, itching, and even full-blown anaphylaxis and death. In milk allergy complete avoidance of all milk and milk products is necessary. If you or one of your children has a milk allergy they might outgrow it in time, but in the interim you need to be vigilant and have an EpiPen ready; it could save your child's life.

If you can find it, the absolute best milk for you nutritionally is raw milk. Raw milk will not only help your children grow, but it will boost their immunity and the fats in it will help their brains. Raw milk is quite safe it comes from cows grazed in pastures, free to roam and not kept in industrial barns standing in their own feces and fed copious amounts of antibiotics. Pasteurization destroys much of the best parts of milk. The heat denatures proteins and the homogenization explodes the fat droplets, severely altering milk. In raw milk each droplet of fat is enclosed in a phospholipid membrane, similar to our cells. In this form, the intestinal lining recognizes the proteins and phospholipids on the surface of milk as it is absorbed, not triggering any allergic reactions and not causing the gallbladder to secrete bile to digest the fat. Processed milk contains less protein, less minerals and trace elements, and is more difficult to digest and much more allergenic (allergy-causing). Many states have archaic laws on the books against raw milk, so its availability depends on how enlightened your state is. Here in Connecticut it is legal.

Nutritional Content of Milk

Milk is about 85 percent water and as such is a wonderful thirst quencher. Milk also contains many other nutrients; the milk we currently get in stores is usually vitamin D-enriched. If you have the land and are so inclined then keeping a goat or a dairy cow is a good source of ongoing nutrition, especially for its colostrum. There is an entire explanation of the benefits of colostrum under the first chapter on Health Essentials. Milk also contains the following healthy ingredients:

Protein

Vitamins A, B6 and B12, riboflavin, folate, and niacin Thiamine Pantothenic acid (which helps convert food into energy and build tissues)

The minerals calcium, magnesium, zinc, selenium, potassium, and phosphorus.

THE WATER SOLUBLE VITAMINS: B COMPLEX AND VITAMIN C

The water soluble vitamins are vitamins B and C. There are many subtypes of B vitamins and the group as a whole is called B complex. B complex is all the B vitamins together in one pill. It is important to take them as a group or complex because of their different functions and the importance of keeping them in their proper balance.

Also, remember multivitamins need to be taken with fat, since they contain both fat and water soluble vitamins and therefore will not be absorbed without fat. There is always water in your stomach to absorb the water soluble vitamins. That is also the reason that taking vitamins on an empty stomach sometimes makes you nauseous.

THE FAT SOLUBLE VITAMINS: A, D, E, AND K

The fat soluble vitamins dissolve on the surface of fats, leave your stomach, and enter the duodenum where they are acted upon by bile released from the gallbladder. It is then absorbed by your intestines and sent to the liver. Without the presence of fats there is nothing to dissolve the fat soluble vitamins and no bile released to digest them and for this reason you may become nauseous.

ALPHA LIPOIC ACID

There is one exception to the fat or water soluble vitamin rule, and that is alpha lipoic acid (ALA). ALA is one of the only substances known that is both fat and water soluble. Since ALA has such dual capability, it enables it to readily cross all the barriers of the body, including the cell wall and blood-brain barrier, thus entering every cell in the body.

ALA is also the keystone in the antioxidant cascade, regenerating both the fat and water soluble arms of that cascade, supercharging the immune system and squelching inflammation. I will get more into the immune cascade later on in this book.

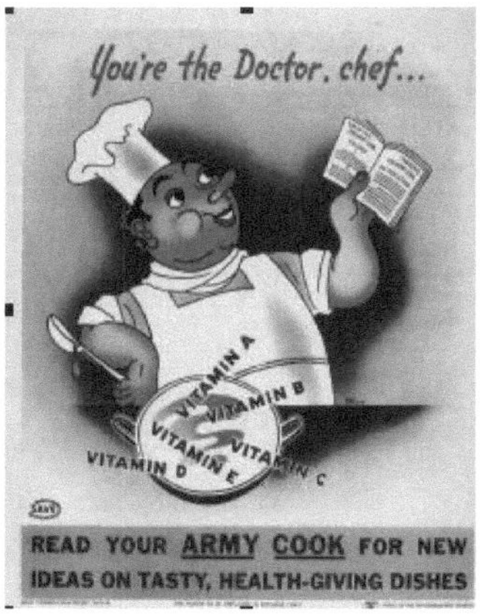
You're the Doctor, chef...
VITAMIN A
VITAMIN B
VITAMIN C
VITAMIN D
VITAMIN E
READ YOUR ARMY COOK FOR NEW
IDEAS ON TASTY, HEALTH-GIVING DISHES

VITAMIN QUALITY AND GENE EXPRESSION

However, the best vitamins by far are those made from whole foods, extracts of animal organs, and those made from nutritional yeast which is grown in nutrients that are enhanced with vitamins and minerals. When you have vitamins made of whole foods that are natural and derived from plants, animals, or even bacteria, they will contain microRNAs that are able to communicate with your own cells' DNA and control gene expression.

Genes are able to exert their influence by direct communication with the cells of your body; this process is known as gene expression. As it turns out, they appear to be in continual contact with an ongoing dialogue. Gene expression in turn is controlled by the microRNAs found in whole, nutritious natural foods such as raw foods, organs, glands, and other animal and plant material. Supplements such as brewer's yeast and other whole food supplements that are made of organic, chemical-free plant and animal material is chock-full of microRNAs that send the right nucleic acid messengers to your genes telling them to turn on certain genes and inhibit or shut off others. In addition to which, these are not "generalists" having general effects on the genes and in turn the body, but rather these microRNAs have specific targets such as the thyroid or the liver, etc.

Vitamins made in this manner with whole foods containing loads of microRNAs are recognized by your body as a food and are easily assimilated and enter your cells where they then can communicate with the cell's nucleus and exert their effect upon gene expression. These vitamins are infinitely more powerful than the inorganic, synthetic man-made vitamins that are offered in most stores.

Eating a diet full of whole foods will not require any vitamin supplements, but may require minerals and trace element supplementation depending on the quality of the soils the foods were grown on and the animals were grazed upon. However, we have to be practical as consumers, and many times the only vitamins we will have available will be the store-bought variety.

The quality of vitamin supplements varies widely among manufacturers. Unfortunately many manufacturers have no quality control and their vitamins' composition does not match their labels. The larger brands such as GNC (the General Nutrition Centers or vitamin stores found in most malls) and other national brands are usually of better quality than the smaller, lesser known companies. I personally like both GNC's and Life Extension Foundation's line of products. If you buy vitamins from other manufacturers, try to stick to name brands and large manufacturers; avoid fly-by-night companies that may be selling you empty promises. Buy the best vitamins you can afford. Keep all your vitamins in a cool, dry, dark area out of direct sunlight. Water will damage most vitamins and that is the reason that vitamin bottles frequently have a cotton ball or sachet of chemicals for absorption of any excess moisture.

EXPIRATION DATES

Expiration dates on most pharmaceuticals and vitamins are a lot of baloney. I have taken prescription drugs that have expired ten years ago and they work as well as when they were "fresh". As long as you store them in a cool place and out of sunlight and moisture they will hold up nicely. If you get them wet or expose them to sunlight they will rapidly deteriorate. So, don't throw away your old medications or vitamins just because they are beyond their expiration dates. There may be some drop off in potency, but it is still better than nothing and most will work just fine.

The Essential Quartet of Vitamins, Minerals, Enzymes and Phytonutrients

Another important fact about vitamins and enzymes is that they require minerals to activate them. Everything works in concert, nothing alone. We are constantly trying to strip out the one key ingredient or chemical that heals this or that, when in reality it is an entire host of vitamins, enzymes, minerals, and phytonutrients that work together. One isolated chemical may have some properties that are good for you, but kept whole, the entire plant has been designed by nature to provide all you need, not to be torn apart.

As a golden rule you should always watch nature and learn from her. She never does things without a reason. Plants and their fruits are designed with a specific purpose in mind; their secondary plant metabolites are specifically designed to work on their target insects and animals.

Natural foods such as fruits and vegetables are made to attract animals to eat them and then to defecate their seeds.

The offering of pollen, nectar, berries, fruit, and vegetables of all types by plants is simply a very shrewd reproductive strategy; its entire purpose being seed dispersal. Think about it. If you are a plant and cannot move, dropping seeds on the ground next to you will certainly work in the short run, but eventually those small plants that have sprouted will crowd out each other or the mother plant without spreading itself very far. Once plants developed flowers it was simply to attract pollinators such as bees and other insects. These pollinators then spread the pollen to another plant and cross-pollinate it, thus spreading the original plant's genes as well as cross-breeding plants of the same species with nearby neighbors who may have different qualities. Once the flower is pollinated it often will develop into a fruit or berry of some kind, which is just a snack for passing animals that is filled with sugar, vitamins, minerals, enzymes, other nutrients, and most importantly, seeds.

This passage through the GI (gastrointestinal) tract of animals enables them to absorb the nutrients they need and the acid bath of their stomachs helps remove the outer coating of many seeds which prepares them for germination. The seeds are then defecated in a pile of feces which acts as its own fertilizer and hence the plant is able to send seeds far from the mother plant (so as not to compete with her, yet still propagate the species).

Mother Nature doesn't produce foods like we humans do, which are processed chemical- and toxin-laden, enzyme poor, full of sugar and or salt, lacking fiber, lacking minerals and trace elements, and devoid of most of the life- enhancing properties of natural foods such as the all-important phytonutrients (phyto means plant-derived), essential oils, microRNAs, and other secondary plant metabolites the importance of which we are just now beginning to discover. We need to eat foods that are packaged chock-full of their minerals, trace elements, fiber, enzymes, phytonutrients, and vitamins. We should not attempt to fractionate them into their individual parts; this strategy for health never works and never will. It causes havoc with our bodies by starving them of the nutrients they need, not sending the microRNA messengers they need to control their genes and then poisoning them with toxins. Is it any wonder that we American's are all suffering with chronic debilitating diseases like hypertension, diabetes, and autoimmune diseases?

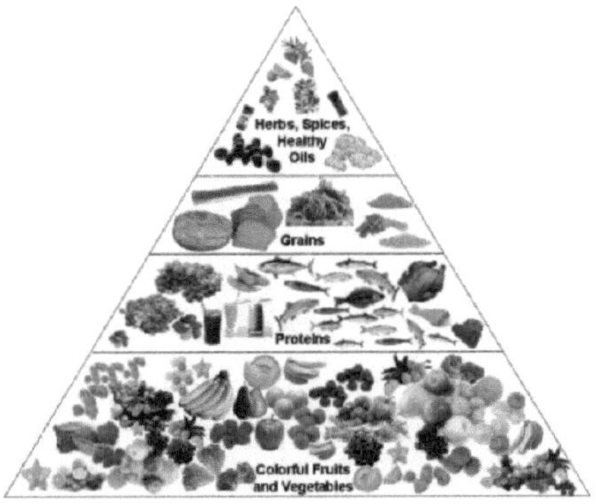

The Healthy Food Pyramid Based on
7-9 Servings of Fruits and Vegetables Daily

Phytonutrients

Phytonutrients are also known as phytochemicals. Scientists so far have found more than 25,000 different types of phytonutrients produced by plants. Plants are amazing biochemists, producing these phytonutrients for their protection from insects and other predators, to attract pollinators, to ward off diseases from bacteria, viruses, and fungi, to communicate with other plants and countless other reasons.

Phytonutrients are not currently considered to be essential, as are vitamins, minerals, fats, and amino acids, but I think in the future that will change. Phytonutrients are very important for maintaining vigorous good health and also for disease and cancer prevention. We are also finding out the importance of epigenetic mechanisms for the control of gene expression that work through the microRNA content of many plants -- quite simply, plants can control your genetic destiny.

THE VITAMIN / MINERAL CONNECTION

Very few nutrients work in the body in isolation. Vitamins will not work without the presence of minerals and trace elements to activate them and vice versa; they need each other to function. Calcium will not be absorbed without vitamin D, for example. Vitamin C helps increase the absorption of iron. Vitamin B 12 will not work without cobalt, etc.

Vitamins are organic nutrients and minerals are inorganic. Since vitamins are organic they can be broken down by heat, acids, and air; minerals are inorganic and their structure cannot be broken down any further. Minerals have to be chelated or bound to a protein/amino acids to be absorbed by the body. This is done by microorganisms in the soil and taken up by plants which make them available to humans to absorb. Some chelating can occur in the intestines by its bacterial inhabitants or micro flora, but this is only a small percentage. That is why you cannot get nutrients from chewing rocks. Those inorganic minerals are just not available to your body for absorption. Inorganic vitamins and minerals are poorly absorbed by the body and are not recognized by the body as food or as essential nutrients, and therefore do not communicate with the body like whole, organic foods.

The Magical Role of Humic and Fulvic Acids

Soil microorganisms partially decompose plant and animal matter in the soil and create humic and fulvic acids.

Humic acids create humus, the black, fertile, water-holding part of the soil that gives soil its amazing fertility. Humic acids actively exchange mineral ions and trace elements with the clay portion of soil in an active ion exchange that is based on their electrical charges. Ions with a positive electric charge are known as cations, ions with a negative charge are known as anions. If the soil is formed from limestone, then calcium will be the major cation in this ion exchange. In other types of soils there are other cations such as magnesium, potassium, sodium, and many others along with trace elements.

Fulvic acids are a type of humic acid of lower molecular weight and higher oxygen content. Fulvic acid is not tightly bound to the soil like humic acids and so it is taken up by plants. Fulvic acid is a very important substance with many roles, the most important of which is to increase the permeability of cells. This allows vitamins, minerals, trace elements, and phytonutrients to be better absorbed. Fulvic acid is a type of colloid that is capable of crossing all the barriers in the body with complete access to every cell.

Healthy, mineral-rich fertile soils are priceless to the future of the every country, and as health conscious people we have to grow our foods on the same type of soil. Man is so incredibly wasteful, when the pilgrims first arrived in the New World the average depth of the black top soil was 3 feet, it is currently about six inches!

Natural Mineral Deposits: Azomite and Supreme Fulvic

Natural soil colloids carry a negative charge and therefore easily attract the positive-charged (remember, like charges repel and opposites attract). Over thousands of years many soil colloids along with their minerals and trace elements will settle out, especially when inundated by water for years as in ancient sea beds as well as ancient forests and jungles, eventually forming thick deposits. Ancient colloidal beds like these are in the western part of the United States in places like Utah, and this is where these colloids are being mined today and sold as soil amendments such as Azomite.

Azomite and other colloidal mixes contain ninety-two minerals and trace and rare elements in total. The name Azomite stands for A to Z of minerals and trace elements. I recommend my patients take these colloidal mixes to improve their health by providing all the minerals and trace elements in the proper balance for your body. Remember, since our bodies evolved in the ancient seas our blood contains all of the same ninety-two minerals and trace elements found in sea water; in fact, in the same proportions.

For that reason I feel that since it is impossible to obtain all of these ninety- two minerals and trace elements from our depleted soils and since they are so vital for maintenance of perfect health, then we must supplement with one of these mixes.

A few of my personal favorites include Supreme Fulvic, which is mined from similar ancient lake beds. It is not colloidal but still contains the full complement of minerals, amino acids, and trace elements. Since it is not colloidal it is not permanently in suspension and needs to be shaken to properly mix it. Other sources are pulverized rock dust. This, depending on the rock crushed, has a variety of minerals and trace elements and does very nicely to feed depleted soils and make them very productive once again. Another is Quinton's Marine Plasma, which comes directly from pure, open oceanic vortices. See the chapter entitled Soil to Self for full details on Quinton's Marine Plasma.

Enzymes

Enzymes are the third leg of this very important triad that also includes vitamins and minerals (and trace elements). Enzymes are proteins that are catalysts that encourage and greatly accelerate chemical and biological reactions within our bodies. Many enzymes are made by plants and others are made by our bodies. Enzymes themselves need to be activated by minerals and trace elements. For example, thyroid hormones can only be converted from their inactive T4 form to their active T3 form by enzymes that are totally dependent on the presence of selenium. There are many enzymes that are dependent solely upon selenium, 300 other enzymes are dependent on magnesium to properly function, and hundreds more are dependent upon zinc, to name but a few. You get the picture. One of the best descriptions I have ever read on the interaction of these elements was written by Dr. Howard F. Loomis, Jr., in his outstanding book, Enzymes the Key to Health. He writes:

> *"Enzymes are the construction workers of the body. They use the vitamins and minerals as building materials to put up the latest architectural marvel - your body. At times there is an ample supply of building material but not enough workers to complete the job. The building materials will remain unused until enough workers show up at the job site."*

When you eat plant-based foods you get the whole package and therefore it is always preferable to taking man-made vitamins. Our bodies are wonderfully designed to digest these plant-based foods which in turn nurture us in so many wonderful ways. If they are raw plants, or cooked for less than twenty minutes at 125 degrees F, they will retain their enzymes that help us digest these foods. Once they are cooked and processed, then they are devoid of these life-giving enzymes. That is one of the reasons why raw fruits and vegetables are so vital for your health. Raw and fermented foods are chock-full of wonderful enzymes, maintain many of their minerals and trace elements, are packed with soluble and insoluble fiber as well as phytonutrients, vitamins, essential oils, microRNAs, and other wonderful, secondary plant metabolites that we are just beginning to discover.

THE OBESITY/INSULIN CONNECTION

Do not be afraid of taking vitamins with fat because of weight gain, etc. You cannot gain weight from vitamins of any type, nor could you survive on them without food. Fat is also an essential element of our diets, hence the essential fatty acids. Americans have been obsessed with their fat intake for the last thirty years and have avoided fats at every turn. Guess what all of this fat obsession has gotten them….nowhere….in fact we are significantly more obese than we were when this fat free craze began. Remember this…. generally speaking, fat intake is not what makes you obese, carbohydrate intake is the culprit. The reason for carbs being so bad for you is that they cause insulin levels to rise. INSULIN IS A FAT-PRODUCING HORMONE. Insulin takes all those extra calories from carbs and stores them as fat. It also protects the fat you already have from breaking down, while using muscle tissue for energy. What that means is high insulin levels not only increase your fat deposits making you obese, it also preferentially burns up muscle for fuel, making your muscles smaller. That is a double whammy, giving you a tire around your waist, a big butt, and shrinking your arms and shoulders. Not a pretty picture. Whole natural foods do not cause these insulin spikes because they frequently have soluble or insoluble fiber, or both. Soluble fiber dissolves in water and forms a gel-like mass in your intestines, absorbing toxins and fats and cleansing your intestines while at the same time feeding your good bacteria, or probiotics. The insoluble fiber does not dissolve and instead acts like a sponge, absorbing water and keeping your stools soft and pliable. Fiber slows the release of sugar into the blood, thus avoiding spikes in blood glucose levels that will in turn spike your insulin levels.

One of my specialties is bariatrics (weight loss), what all bariatric physicians know is that fats are essential in your diet.

Fat free foods make you gain weight because they usually are made with either sugar or salt to replace the fat, otherwise they would have less flavor than they already have.

ORGANIC FOODS

Organic foods are also better for you than nonorganic foods. Do you really want to eat food that is grown in a field soaked with inorganic fertilizers, herbicides, and pesticides? On the one hand there are farmers spraying the food you are going to eat with Hazmat suits on with skull and crossbones symbols, clearly warning us about their toxicity. On the other hand, here we are in our homes and restaurants eating this same food, ingesting countless toxins that our body must either detoxify or, if that is not possible, then they need to be stored somewhere safe...guess where that is...it is stored as fat! Toxin exposure in our diets leads to obesity!

A weak, sick plant that has not gotten the proper nutrition it needs from the soil has a weakened immune system and is readily attacked by insects, fungi, viruses, and other plant pathogens, hence the ever-growing need for more powerful (and toxic) pesticides, herbicides, and fungicides. It is an endless arms race of ever larger doses of these poisons on a soil that is rapidly becoming dead and lifeless.

I will give you a great example of my own experience with an organic permaculture orchard I designed. I use no chemicals on my trees; I feed the soil and the soil feeds the plants. Permaculture stands for permanent agriculture. Permaculture was started in Australia by a fellow named Bill Mollison in the 1970s and is a system of working with nature without chemicals or outside input once it is established. I started with forest soil and I supplement it with organic materials, minerals, trace elements, and mycorrhizal fungi. Here in New England most of the soils that are now in forests were formerly farms that were no longer farmed due to the rocky, depleted soils, and became forest once again. The organic material I added was from peat moss and compost and manure. I also add mycorrhizal fungi when I plant anything. Mycorrhizal fungi have a wonderful symbiotic relationship with plant roots. They attach themselves to the roots and extend their filaments into the soil; this vastly increases the surface area the roots can draw upon. They also chelate minerals with amino acids which make them water soluble and they are taken up by the plant root along with trace elements and fulvic acid. My fruit trees and bushes grow at an incredible rate and are robust and healthy, bearing such large loads of fruit that I have to heavily thin them out or I fear the branches will snap under the weight. Native insects, native bees, butterflies, and humming birds abound. The soil is full of earthworms and has a wonderful smell to it. The fruit is delicious and nutritious and chemical free.

Just like sickly people catch everything that they are exposed to, so do sick plants. The toxic farming methods that modern farmers are using on their soil are having dire consequences for all of our health. It is unsustainable and inevitably will lead to disaster.

When it comes to growing your own food, diversity is key. Diversity provides a continuous supply of nectar for pollinators and also ensures that your garden will not depend on a single crop or two, but is broad-based on an entire array of different fruits and vegetables as well as fish and livestock. Diversity also provides you with a varied source of foods and their all-essential phytonutrients.

The Standard American Diet

In my practice I see the consequences of our SAD (Standard American Diet) and how it ravages our health. SAD is typically 50 percent carbohydrate, 35 percent fat and only 15 percent protein. It is very processed and very low in both soluble and insoluble fiber, and full of man-made chemical toxins such as dyes, pesticide residues, and other chemicals.

A good practice overall is to avoid man-made or processed foods. Try to stick as close to the natural source as possible. A good example I always use are apples. An apple is better for you than apple sauce and apple sauce is better for you than apple juice. As man processes the original healthy apple, he eliminates more and more nutrients and fiber at each stage. Fiber is important not only for your digestion and the prevention of constipation, but also to allow a slow, steady supply of sugar from the apple into your blood, avoiding spiking your blood glucose levels. Remember the point I made earlier about insulin spiking and all its dire consequences, especially with weight gain. An even better choice is an organically grown apple which does not contain all the herbicides, pesticides, and toxic fertilizers.

Fruits and vegetables organically grown on mineral-rich soils will have the full complement of minerals and trace elements available to them and they will utilize these on an as-needed basis as they grow this results in them being much tastier, as well. One point to note, organic foods will not necessarily have a high mineral and trace element content, that depends on the soil they are grown in, growing organic by itself will not create minerals that do not exist in the soil, that requires soil remineralization as well as increasing its organic content by using biochar, compost, organic fertilizers, and other organic soil amendments.

The Importance of Food Preparation and Enzymes

Preparation of food is also critical in helping you absorb their nutrients better.

One of the main reasons for that is due to their enzyme content. If you cook food to above 120 F for more than a half an hour you will destroy its enzymes.

Enzymes are proteins that plants and animals make. They are essential for good health. I will go into this in greater detail later. This is why raw foods are much healthier for you than cooked foods. Enzymes help you digest your foods and properly assimilate them into your body. Remember, vitamins cannot be activated without enzymes and minerals and trace elements, all of which are in natural foods properly grown in mineral-rich soils, but not in processed foods.

Dr Pottenger did a famous experiment with cats early last century, showing the effects of eating denatured (cooked foods) enzyme-free foods. What he found was astounding....after two or three generations the cats fed the denatured man-made foods without enzymes resulted in having all of the diseases of modern man....diabetes, heart problems, arthritis....all the degenerative diseases that Americans are developing more and more. They also became infertile, having miscarriages, or were bearing deformed, sickly kittens. When he put them back on raw, enzyme-rich foods, all of these problems were reversed.

Infertility is a growing epidemic among American and European women and is growing every year. Part of that is deferring childbearing to a later age, but the vast majority of the problem is nutritional. Our diets have become primarily processed, denatured, enzyme and mineral poor, empty dead foods that make us fat and full but do not nurture us with the essential fatty acids, essential amino acids, enzymes, phytonutrients, minerals and trace elements we need for good health. We have to commit ourselves to growing our own organic foods on enhanced, mineral-rich, healthy soils, filled with earthworms and with a teeming microbial community that will convert the minerals to organic forms and will fill the soil with health-enhancing humic and fulvic acids. Once we are eating those foods and drinking fresh water and breathing clean air, then we will have robust health and our resistance to infectious diseases as well as degenerative diseases will skyrocket. Eating such a diet, we will become just like the plants that we grow in those rich organic soils, we will be strong and healthy and resistant to disease. There will be another benefit; we will be smarter, and that is always a good thing.

CHAPTER FOUR

SEED OILS AND THEIR NUMEROUS HEALTH BENEFITS

INTRODUCTION

TABLE OF CONTENTS:

Seed oils are wonderful medicinal and nutritional oils that you and your family can use to maintain good health and vigor. Seed oils are different from essential oils in several important ways. Seed oils are usually pressed from a plant's seeds and are mainly fatty acids or fats. They are much larger in size than essential oils and therefore usually cannot cross the skin. They are also not volatile like essential oils so they will not evaporate and usually have less of a smell. Greasy in nature, they will go rancid if left unrefrigerated after opening them. There are many types of seed oils that will certainly be an important part of your alternative medicine chest. Some very good and healthful seed oils are hemp, black seed, walnut, olive, flax, almond, amaranth, and soybean. Let's take a look at several of the most potent and useful seed oils for our medicinal needs.

HEMP OIL

Hemp oil is made from the Cannabis sativa, a name you might better recognize as marijuana; however, its Latin name means "useful hemp". The sativa designation with any plant name truly speaks to a plant's usefulness, and Cannabis sativa is no exception. As a point of fact marijuana comes in two basic botanical varieties, Cannabis sativa and Cannabis indica, as well as endless hybrid mixes of the two.

Hemp oil is usually made from a type of Cannabis sativa plant that has a very low THC or Tetrahydrocannabinol level. THC is the substance in marijuana that makes you high. You cannot get high from hemp oil due to this very low THC content. The THC produced by marijuana comes from the resin produced in the flowering tops of the female plant's flower buds. Hemp oil is cold-pressed from the seeds, thus it does not have the THC to make you high. Many college students who, like me, went to college in the seventies might not know much about botany but they do know how to grow and harvest pot. Many of the current books on growing marijuana are from these old hippies, many of whom have become millionaires growing medicinal marijuana.

There is also a second oil made from the Cannabis sativa plant that is not hemp oil and is not made from hemp seeds but rather is harvested from the entire plant. This is called CBD oil or Cannabadiol. Cannabadiol is a very abundant fatty substance and is a major constituent of the hemp plant and is also purported to have several medicinal qualities.

Cannabadiol is not a psychoactive substance and will not get you high. But, since this chapter is about seed oils I will not go any further into CBD oil which is not made from the seeds of the hemp plant.

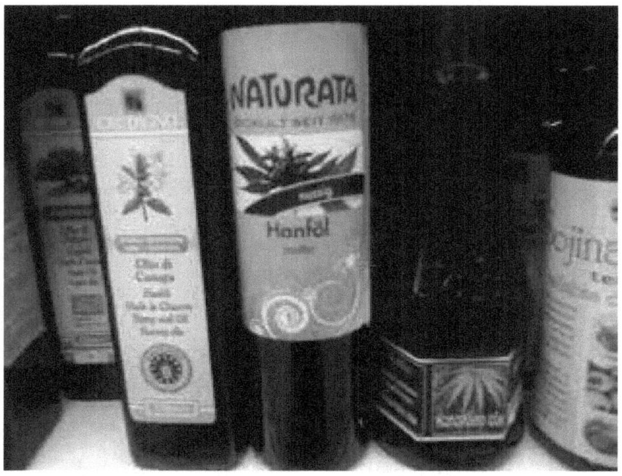

(Photo by Irena.barlic)

Hemp was commonly used to make rope and cord and is still used so today. In fact the word "canvas" comes from Cannabis sativa, since even today most canvases are made from hemp. Most of the hemp oil consumed in the United States currently comes from Canada.

Hemp Oil The Perfect Food

Hemp seed and hemp oil have been called the perfect food for humanity. The reason for this is that hemp oil contains all the essential fatty acids and essential amino acids your body needs. You remember essential means that they cannot be manufactured by your body and therefore are essential to get in your diet to maintain good health and functioning of your body. In the case of hemp oil it has them all, all the fats and all twenty of the amino acids your body needs to make proteins of all types.

Hemp oil contains the perfect balance of fatty acids, with a 3:1 ratio of omega-6 to omega-3 fatty acids and is the only seed that contains this perfect balance. Fish oil also contains many essential fatty acids but frequently is contaminated with mercury and other toxins that have polluted the world's oceans, unless you get a pharmaceutical grade fish oil such as Lovaza or Vascepa, both of which are only available by prescription. Hemp oil also contains a very rare protein called globule edestins that is very similar to the globulin protein found in human blood plasma, which is known to help digestion. Hemp oil also contains albumin, which is the same protein found in egg whites. The proteins in hemp are more easily digested than meat, eggs, cheeses, milk, or just about any other protein source, including soy .Hemp seeds and oil also contain GLA or gamma linolenic acid, which is very rare, and helps with breast pain and skin problems like eczema.

In fact, hemp seeds are the most nutritious seeds in the world. In addition to the above-mentioned ingredients, hemp seeds also contain vitamins such as vitamins D and E, enzymes, and a relative lack of sugars, starches, and saturated fats, and has the highest content of unsaturated (the good ones) fatty acids found in the entire plant kingdom. For this reason many people consider hemp seeds and hemp oil to be an ideal food for your body or a Super Food by some nutritionists.

Sun And Seed Oil

Several courageous physicians have used high dose essential fatty acids to treat a variety of conditions including heart attacks, cancer, arthritis, and other chronic degenerative diseases with great success. Dr. Johana Budwig was a pioneer in essential fatty acids and was the discoverer of omega-3 fatty acids. She also has been nominated for a Nobel prize seven times and clearly is no renegade snake oil saleswoman. Dr. Budwig believes that these seed oils are very healthy for humans due to their highly unsaturated nature and their electron-rich nature. She feels many of our current health problems are due to a combination of lack of adequate sun exposure and lack of these essential fatty acids that are so important, especially because they are able to counteract the trans fats and saturated fats that are so prevalent in our diets. Dr. Budwig successfully treated many of her very sick patients with a diet high in essential fatty acids combined with sun bathing to absorb the sun's radiant energy through its flow of photons directly to the human body. Dr. Budwig is adamant that you cannot be healthy with just the sun or just the seed oils, your body needs both.

Why Your Hemp Oil Needs To Come From Outside The U.S.A.

In the United States hemp oil cannot be processed unless the seed is killed with high temperatures. The problem with that is that high temperature destroy the essential fatty acids by changing their composition and accelerating the destruction of the beneficial properties of hemp oil. For that reason you should look for cold-pressed oil which will by necessity have to come from outside the United States. This is also the reason why Canada produces most of the cold-pressed hemp oil consumed in the United States. By the way, the heat destruction of the essential fatty acids in hemp and other seed oils is the reason you should not use them for frying.

Also seed oils will become rancid if left exposed and not refrigerated, so always store them in your refrigerator to vastly increase their shelf life. When you buy any seed oils always look for cold-pressed, which produces the highest quality oils while retaining most of their beneficial qualities.

What Health Benefits Are Associated With The Use Of Hemp Oil?

Hemp oil has many health-enhancing qualities due to the many healthy substances it contains. As I said earlier, the most important of the healthy substances contained in hemp oil are the essential fatty acids. Many people are confused by the health benefits of fats and think all fats are unhealthy, but nothing could be further from the truth. Without essential fatty acids life would be impossible. Your body needs fats to produce many of its structures, including most notably your brain, as well as other important substances like prostaglandins.

Prostaglandins are a group of hormone-like lipid (fat) compounds that are made from the action of enzymes on essential fatty acids. Now that I have made your eyes glassy and have you yawning with that explanation, allow me to explain why prostaglandins are so very important for your health. Prostaglandins are produced by every cell in the body except red blood cells, which speaks volumes about their importance. They control inflammation, blood pressure, platelet aggregation, mediate pain in the spinal nerves, control fever, regulate kidney function, regulate intraocular (inside your eyeball) pressure, control labor, cell growth regulation, and acid secretion by the stomach.

If you have a lack of essential fatty acids which are needed to make prostaglandins, you will naturally have low levels of them and will lack their positive effects in your body and consequently suffer with a large number of conditions. That is why hemp oil has been reported to have so many different positive effects such as:

1. Significantly decrease inflammation in joints and muscles, thereby helping arthritis, muscle aches, fibromyalgia. Lower blood pressure by relaxing blood vessels.
2. Prevent platelet aggregation, which prevents clot formation and thereby strokes and heart attacks.
3. Helps control pain. Control fevers.
4. Help glaucoma.
5. Help labor pain.
6. Helps asthma by relaxation of airways.
7. Improve circulation by relaxing the blood vessels and allowing greater blood flow.
8. Improving immunity and thereby helping reduce infections of all types as well as cancer.
9. Helping with skin problems like eczema, psoriasis, and acne.
10. GI problems like ulcers, irritable bowel syndrome, abdominal cramping, and constipation.

How To Take Hemp Oil

Hemp oil is best taken without heating it, such as added to salads or other vegetables as a condiment. It can be added to vinegar, replacing olive oil and making a wonderful salad dressing that is quite tasty.

It has a nutty flavor and can be taken orally without mixing it in anything, or can be added to organic yogurt or to any food you might prefer. Depending on the severity of your medical issues, you can take up to five tablespoons a day, but I would normally recommend taking two tablespoons a day for general health maintenance. If you are eating the shelled hemp seeds, you need to take about four heaping teaspoons daily.

Hemp oil can also be applied topically if you have a skin condition of any type by rubbing it into the skin several times a day until the issue resolves. Hemp oil is a natural moisturizer and is also useful as a sunblock.

Does Hemp Oil Have Any Side Effects?

Any substance can cause side effects if ingested, since different people react in different ways. That being said, hemp oil is very well tolerated. There could be a little diarrhea or loose stools or abdominal cramping. Since it may affect the clotting ability of platelets, it may cause bleeding or bruising problems in patients already on Coumadin (warfarin) or other blood thinners.

Other Uses Of Hemp Oil

Hemp oil can be used mixed with lemon oil as a wonderful varnish to finish wood.

Hemp oil can be used to make candles.

Hemp oil can be used as a lubricant for bicycle chains and chainsaws, etc.

Hemp oil can be used as a biodiesel fuel this alone may prove to be one of its greatest uses, since marijuana is so easy to grow (hence its nickname "weed").

Growing an ample supply for medicinal and biodiesel fuel use will probably become widespread. Those above-named benefits of hemp oil are primarily from its high content of essential fatty acids.

From an alternative medicine viewpoint hemp oil answers all of our problems as far as nutrition is concerned, because here in one seed oil we are able to give our bodies all twenty of the amino acids including the nine essential amino acids that we cannot produce ourselves, in addition to which we can get all the essential fatty acids and a host of other vitamins, minerals, and enzymes. Due to its high nutritional content it indeed qualifies as a Super Food for our needs. Cannabis sativa is also very easy to grow, does not require any special soils, does not need pesticides or even fertilizer and has no natural enemies that ravage it.

In short, Cannabis is a weed and is very easy to grow and provides us with complete nutrition as well as a useful medicine, and, if you are so inclined, a psychoactive substance (it will get you high).

BLACK SEED OIL

Black seed comes from the annual plant Nigella sativa, which is a member of the buttercup family, and is native to the Middle East and countries surrounding the Mediterranean. Remember from the preceding section that the Latin name "sativa" means useful. This should always get your attention as a plant that has many and varied uses and usually will mean it is wonderful for our needs. It has various other names including blessed seed, black cumin, Roman coriander, black caraway, onion seed, and black sesame, they are all the same plant.

The name black seed is a very apt physical description of the seeds, which are large and black. The use of black seed oil dates back to the ancient Egyptians and some black seed oil was found in the tomb of King Tut. In Islam the prophet Mohammed supposedly said that "black seed is a remedy for all diseases except death." Black seed had and still has widespread use as a medicinal and health-enhancing agent in most of the Middle Eastern countries as well as parts of Africa and Asia.

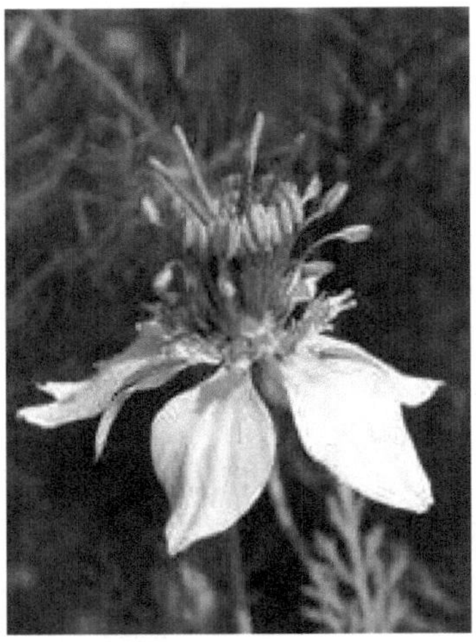

Photo of Nigella sativa plant in flower

Nutrients in Black Seed

Black seed oil is endowed with a very rich, diverse chemical composition.

Black seed oil is very rich in antioxidants, amino acids, whole proteins, fixed and volatile oils, alkaloids, saponins, and important phytochemicals (plant based chemicals) such as thymoquinone and crystalline nigellone. Thymoquinone is found only in black seed and is a powerful antioxidant and anti-inflammatory compound. Nigellone has antihistamine and bronchodilator effects and so helps allergies and asthma. Black seed oil is also very rich in many minerals including calcium, iron, potassium, phosphorus, sodium, and zinc as well as many components that have yet to be identified. It is also a wonderful source of essential fatty acids, remember anything "essential" cannot be made by the body and must be obtained from your diet. As with most oils, the beneficial components are best extracted by "cold-pressing" rather than by heat or chemical extraction methods. Cold-pressing preserves almost all of the beneficial ingredients from the original seed.

There have been over four hundred peer-reviewed medical studies on the health benefits and medicinal uses of black seed oil dating back to the 1950s and continuing to this day.

Health Benefits of Black Seed Oil

1. Antimicrobial…it works against bacterial, fungal, and viral infections.
2. Antioxidant as well as having anti-inflammatory effects.
3. Antispasmodic
4. Bronchodilator, which means it opens up and enlarges your airways, making breathing easy, and helps asthma.

5. Lowers blood pressure.
6. Protects both the liver and kidneys.
7. Helps diabetes by making insulin work better.
8. Helps eradicate Helicobacter pylori infections in the stomach which oftentimes lead to ulcers.
9. Seizures: The frequency and severity were both lessened with the use of black seed oil.
10. Chemical weapons exposure side effects were markedly reduced with the use of black seed oil.
11. Opioid drug addiction (heroin, morphine, and related narcotic painkillers or analgesics): Black seed oil was found to lessen the symptoms of withdrawal.
12. Radiation damage: The active compound contained in black seed oil is thymoquinone, this has been shown to help protect brain tissue from radiation- induced damage. Parkinson's disease: The same ingredient, thymoquinone, helps protect the brain tissue and helps prevent the progression of Parkinson's disease.
13. MRSA: Black seed oil helps eradicate persistent MRSA infections.
14. Psoriasis: Applied topically it will help heal psoriasis lesions.
15. Anti-parasitic, meaning it kills parasites.
16. Acne
17. Migraine headaches
18. Helps digestion.
19. Supports metabolism.
20. Supports immunity and boosts your immune system.
21. Soothes upset stomachs and calms inflamed intestines.
22. Black seed is also an opioid agonist, which means it will strengthen the effect of narcotic painkillers. Increasing milk production in breast-feeding women: I might just mention that breast milk is far superior to cow's milk for a number of reasons. Personally, I think they did an outstanding job with the packaging, but that is just my humble opinion.
23. And finally, the most convincing evidence I have heard yet is that Nigella sativa is eaten by elephants to aid in their digestion! I don't know about you, but I wasn't quite sure if that was a good thing, because when you think about it elephants must eat all kinds of stuff; after all, look at the size of them. But in the spirit of full disclosure I thought I would just mention that.

What Is The Difference Between Black Seed And Black Seed Oil?

The major difference is that the oil is a more concentrated form. It contains the same beneficial components but with more of the essential fatty acids. Beware of products coming from the Middle East which many times are heat-extracted or chemically extracted using a petroleum-based chemical called hexane which is a solvent and is used as such to extract the oil from its seed. That is why I always recommend using cold-pressed oils that are unadulterated. Hexane is one of the components of gasoline. Given a choice, who in their right mind would ingest hexane?

What Is Cold-Pressing?

Cold-pressing is the process by which seeds or fruits are crushed and ground down using either large, heavy granite millstones or stainless steel presses. Although the pressing and grinding will produce heat through fiction, the temperature must not exceed 120 degrees F (49 C) to be called cold-pressed. The cold-pressing process produces oils that retain all of their aromas, flavors, and most importantly, their original nutritional content, and that is why I always recommend buying cold-pressed oils.

How to Take Black Seed

If you have the raw seed, you can heat it in an oven at a low temperature. They will sometimes make a popping noise; this is normal. Think popcorn. Raw black seeds have a very harsh, bitter taste and are rough on your stomach and therefore are better eaten after heating. Stir them frequently and keep tasting them. Once they have become bland, you can stop heating them and allow them to cool. Take them and grind them to a fine powder either using a coffee grinder or alternatively with a grinding stone.The traditional method for taking black seeds is with honey. How this mix is made is by taking a jar and filling it a quarter way with honey and then add another quarter of very finely ground black seed, stir and then repeat the layering of the honey and black seed until the jar is full. You can add ground ginger or ground nuts for flavoring if you so desire.

The usual dose is one teaspoon of this honey/black seed mix daily for health maintenance. If you are using black seed to treat a condition such as allergies, acne, migraine headaches, respiratory problems, etc., then double the dose to two teaspoons daily. I have to tell you, in my humble opinion the flavor of black seed oil is horrible and I can only tolerate it when mixed with honey or some other ingredient in order to mask its flavor. That being said, who knows, you may very well like it; hey, my son, Marcus, eats ghost chilies and thinks they are wonderful!

One thing to keep in mind is that more is not necessarily better when taking black seed or black seed oil. The reason for this is that at high doses black seed is toxic and for that reason you should not exceed 25 grams a day of black seed.

Black seed in the oil form can be taken orally as well as used topically (applied directly to the skin) for problems such as acne, eczema, and psoriasis.

Black seed oil can also be mixed with green tea, for example, and taken orally. The usual dosing is one teaspoon of oil per cup of tea. This has also been shown to help anxiety and fatigue. It can also be mixed with orange or any juice at about one tablespoon per glass. This will also provide energy and invigorate you for most of the day. Black seed oil taken with a hot drink will also promote cardiovascular health by lowering your blood pressure and helping to relax your arteries and dilate your blood vessels. This is one of the reasons that there is a precaution on using black seed, due to its effect on your blood pressure.

Another method is to take two cups of water and boil it and then add one tablespoon of black seed oil, put your face over the pot containing this mix, put a towel over your head enclosing the entire sink and the pot and you, and inhale the steam deeply.

This will help alleviate colds, bronchitis, coughs, sore throats, and sinus problems. Black seed also comes in capsule form and can be taken this way. The dose of black seed oil in capsular form is two capsules daily before breakfast; this is 1,000 mg. Once again, the two capsules daily dose is for health maintenance; if you are sick, double that dose. Some patients have been having success treating cancer with black seed. In these cases the dose is much higher and usually three or more times daily.

FLAXSEED OIL

Flaxseed oil is made from the flax plant, known botanically as Linum usitatissimum. The Latin name linum means linen and this is because of flaxseed's earlier role as the source of linen for over 3,000 years. The usitatissimum part in Latin means "of greatest use" and this is due to its many uses beyond just food and linen. Flaxseed was used to make ship sails, bowstrings, and even body armor!

Flaxseed is also known as common flax or linseed, and the oil is also known as linseed oil or flaxseed oil. Linseed oil is a drying oil which means that it dries to a hard shell-like coating. For this reason it has been used alone and in combination with a variety of substances as a varnish for wood. The way linseed oil is extracted makes it unfit for human consumption. Flaxseed oil, on the other hand, comes in a food grade variety that can be used as either a food or a medicinal agent.

Flaxseed and flaxseed oil has a very long history as a medicinal agent and was used over 3,000 years ago in ancient Babylon. It was also much beloved by King Charlemagne in the eighth century, who was so convinced of its health benefits that he passed laws requiring his subjects to use it. Its usage in modern times and its popularity has been growing annually. Hundreds of products are introduced each year that contain flaxseed products in its various forms. Currently it is even used for chicken feed to get chickens to produce eggs that are high in omega-3 fatty acids and it is also used in feed for cows to raise the omega-3 fatty acid content of their beef.

Flaxseed and flaxseed oil has a very long history as a medicinal agent and was used over 3,000 years ago in ancient Babylon. It was also much beloved by King Charlemagne in the eighth century, who was so convinced of its health benefits that he passed laws requiring his subjects to use it. Its usage in modern times and its popularity has been growing annually. Hundreds of products are introduced each year that contain flaxseed products in its various forms. Currently it is even used for chicken feed to get chickens to produce eggs that are high in omega-3 fatty acids and it is also used in feed for cows to raise the omega-3 fatty acid content of their beef.

Types of Flax Seed

Flaxseed comes in two varieties, brown flax and golden flax (sometimes called yellow). Both types have the same nutritional content. There is one type of golden flax that food scientists have made into a cooking oil called Solin (also known as Linola oil as its trade name). This has a much lower nutritional content (1/10th of the ALA content) than the other two types and should not be used for medicinal purposes. You should also note that New Zealand Flax is not the same plant and although it has a high fiber content, it does not contain the other healthy ingredients as flaxseed does. Flaxseed oil can come as a liquid or in soft gel capsules. The best flaxseed oil is made by cold-pressing and due to its extreme sensitivity to light and oxygen; it should be kept in an airtight, dark bottle.

Nutrients Contained In Flaxseed

Omega-3 fatty acids - Each tablespoon of flaxseed contains 1.8 grams of plant-based omega-3s, which are very heart-healthy, as well as excellent brain food. One of its components is ALA or alpha linolenic acid, which has been shown to be a strong anti-inflammatory agent; hence the use of flaxseed oil in the treatment of arthritis forms such as osteoarthritis and rheumatoid arthritis.

Lignans are unique fiber-related polyphenols which contain plant- based estrogens as well as being a strong antioxidant. Flaxseed has up to 800 times more lignans than other plant foods, completely blowing away its closest competitor, sesame seeds, by seven times the lignan content. It seems odd that an oil like flaxseed oil would have a strong antioxidant role, but it does. This is because polyphenols are very strong antioxidants; in fact, flaxseed is a stronger antioxidant than blueberries or even olives.

Flaxseed has both soluble and insoluble fiber that your body needs to maintain its health. The water soluble fiber in flaxseed is a mucilage. A mucilage is a gum which is water soluble and forms a gel that acts to slow down the emptying of the stomach and the intestinal transit time (the amount of time food remains in the intestines), so slowing it down allows the food to remain in the intestines for a longer period of time therefore increasing the absorption of its nutrients. The slowing of food moving through your GI system also contributes to the feeling of "fullness", so you eat less and lose weight.

Flaxseed also has a high mineral content, especially magnesium, zinc, manganese, and potassium. (Flaxseed has seven times the potassium of bananas.) It is also very high in B vitamins. Flaxseed oil is higher in the omega-3 fatty acids than the ground form, but the oil does not contain the lignans, fiber, and proteins of the ground flaxseed (meal).

Health Benefits of Flaxseed

All seeds are healthy and provide significant nutritional and health benefits, but flaxseed has health benefits not found in other seeds and is nutritionally unique due to its high content of omega-3 fatty acids, lignans, and fiber such as mucilage. Technically, flaxseed is not a grain but has a very similar nutritional profile. Where it differs is in its high fiber, lignin, and omega-3 fatty acid levels, and unlike grains, flaxseed is very low in carbohydrates so it is great for weight loss.

Flaxseed has reported health benefits for cancer prevention, maintaining cardiovascular (heart and blood vessel) health, as well as helping with lung diseases. Many of these health benefits are from the ALA or alpha linolenic acid that flaxseed contains in very high quantities. The good news is that ALA is not destroyed by cooking it for even several hours at 300 F, therefore flaxseed can be incorporated in many foods you make such as bread, muffins, even cookies. Only the ground up flaxseed can be used for cooking, flaxseed oil is easily oxidized and ruined by cooking.

ALA works as an anti-inflammatory agent helping to prevent or reduce the inflammation of blood vessels; in this role it is helped by other omega-3 fatty acids contained in flaxseed such as EPA and DPA (I won't dare try to give you their full names, which are real tongue twisters). The incredibly high lignan content of flaxseeds also helps reduce inflammation along with the omega-3 fatty acids. Those same lignans also contain significant amounts of the mineral manganese which also functions as an anti-inflammatory agent. Decreased inflammation along with decreased oxidative stress both translate to lower blood pressure and reduced heart disease and also decreased cancer rates. The decreased cancer rates are presumably due to the same decrease in both inflammation and oxidative stress which are both risk factors for cancer.

Several of the lignans in flaxseed are converted by the bacteria in our guts to enterolactone (ENL) and enterodiol (END). Both END and ENL work to balance hormones and by this effect directly reduce the rates of hormone-related cancers such as breast and prostate cancer. Another reason that flaxseed may help in cancer prevention is due to its stimulating effect on the detoxification enzymes in the liver, allowing the liver to detoxify many more toxins.

Other Health Benefits Of Flaxseed and Flaxseed Oil

1. Lower colon cancer rates.
2. Weight loss
3. Decrease of Insulin Resistance (which is the major cause of type 2 diabetes).

4. Hot flashes and Menopausal problems
5. Lowering of cholesterol, especially the bad LDL cholesterol, Relieve constipation. Sjogren's Syndrome: At 1 to 2 grams a day will help decrease the dry eyes associated with this.
6. Protects the skin from damage.

How to Prepare and Store Your Flaxseed

Flaxseed can be purchased as whole seeds (in bulk if you want to stockpile it), ground seeds, or as an oil. Keep in mind that once the seeds are ground into meal they will need to be refrigerated to prolong their storage life. Flaxseed oil also needs to be refrigerated or kept in a very cold, dark corner of your basement. Flaxseeds, unlike many other seeds, are difficult to chew and are difficult to digest when not ground up properly. This is due to their hard outer shell which prevents their proper digestion unless ground up well.

Whole flaxseeds can be stored for one to two years if refrigerated; if kept out of direct light and kept in a cool dark area; they can last up to a year. Once ground, their shelf life rapidly diminishes if refrigerated to about four months maximum. If refrigerated, flaxseed should be kept in an airtight container, preferably dark to reduce light exposure, which will shorten their freshness. The whole flaxseeds can be ground up with a spice or coffee grinder, and it is best to grind them up as needed, because once ground up, flaxseeds are easily oxidized and will turn rancid.

How to Take Flaxseed

One of the easiest ways to take ground flaxseed is to sprinkle it on cereal, salads, and even fresh fruit. Ground flaxseed can also be added to fruit or breakfast smoothies. Ground flaxseed can also be added to cookie, muffin, or bread mixes and eaten that way. A teaspoon of ground flaxseed can be added to mustard or mayonnaise when making a sandwich, or can be added to yogurt or ice cream. Due to flaxseed's high fiber content, you should always make sure you drink a lot of water any time you take it. The oil can be added to salads or drank by the tablespoon. In the form of gel capsules it can be taken orally as a dietary supplement. Neither flaxseed meal (ground flaxseed) nor the oil has a recommended daily dosage. I would recommend taking one or two capsules or one or two tablespoons daily of either the oil or the ground flax meal, but please remember to drink a lot of water with this due to its very high fiber content or you will get constipated.

You should also not take flaxseed with oral medications due to its ability to "soak up" many medications due to its high fiber content.

Flaxseed contains large amounts of ALA and sometimes the body cannot efficiently convert ALA to DHA and EPA (two other forms of omega-3 fatty acids contained in fish oil), therefore if you want to increase your levels of DHA and EPA you should take fish oil.

OLIVE OIL

Olive trees originated in the Mediterranean basin, probably in Crete or Syria, around 5,000 years ago and slowly spread around the middle east and north Africa as well as southern Europe. Spanish explorers introduced olives to the new world and started growing them in Mexico and southern California. Olives have been used as a food as well as a medicine in those countries where they were grown. Today Spain, Italy, and Greece are still among the largest producers of olives, recently joined by Chile and Australia.

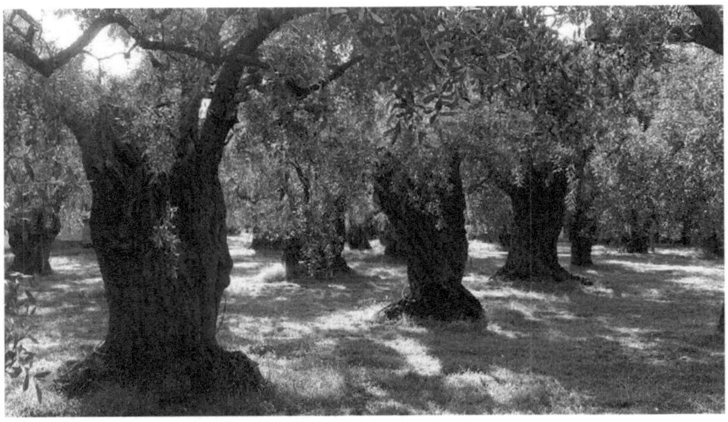

Photo Of Old Olive Trees in Greece (Photo courtesy of Petr Pakandl)

Types of Olive Oil

Extra virgin olive oil is simply the first pressing of the olives; however it does contain beneficial chemicals not found in the subsequent pressings. Extra virgin is made by cold-pressing of the olives without any heat or chemical solvents or radiation, etc. Virgin olive oil is also from the first pressing but is not as good a quality as extra virgin and has a greater acidity and a less delicate flavor and less of those wonderful phytonutrients (phyto means derived from plants).

The term "virgin" means it is done by mechanical means only, usually by grinding the olives with a millstone and then putting the extract into a

centrifuge, but without any chemicals or other solvents or methods used. One theme that seems to recur is that "cold-pressing" of any oil seems to be the preferred method for retention of the greatest amount of nutrients, vitamins, minerals, and especially, phytonutrients. I have not run across any exceptions to that rule so far, so you can "hang your hat" on that one.

Nutrients In Olive Oil

Olive oil is a unique plant oil in terms of its fat composition. Unlike other plant oils, olive oil contains about 75 percent of its fat content in the form of oleic acid, which is a monounsaturated omega-9 fatty acid. Remember, saturated fatty acids are bad for you and unsaturated fatty acids, both mono- and poly- types, are good for you. Mono is Latin for one and poly for many, so don't get intimidated by the names, just methodically take them apart; science is so beautiful in that regard. Olive oil is also an excellent source of vitamins E and K as well as antioxidants such as beta carotene and squalene, which makes it so useful for skin health. I go further into the properties of squalene under the amaranth section below.

Phenols Are Your Friend

Olive oil is also chock-full of a wide variety of phenols. As we have seen in flaxseed and other oils, phenols are wonderful for us in an entire spectrum of ways. Phenols are produced by plants or even microorganisms when they are under attack, wounded, or are trying to prevent invasion by another type of infecting agent such as a virus or a fungus....and guess what....they have turned out to be wonderful for humans, with germicidal and antibacterial properties....always a good thing to have on board, since they do not appear to damage normal intestinal bacteria or flora as well. Phenols are also powerful antioxidants, anti-inflammatory, cancer-preventing, and detoxifying to the human body… as far as science can determine they have no down side for humans.

For people interested in alternative/natural medicines; finding nourishing, nutritional, storable foods is of the utmost importance and foods/medicinal agents such as olive oil, hemp, blackseed, and flaxseed oils are all wise things to stockpile in a cool dry place, out of the sun; a root cellar would be ideal, or a cool dark corner of your basement. Even better is having something that is so good for you taste so wonderful.

One of the things I love doing in a nice Italian restaurant is to get some good crusty, warm bread and cover it with roasted garlic then soaking it in olive oil….add a touch of sea salt and voila….oh baby, is that good stuff!

Health Benefits of Olive Oil

The Mediterranean diet is famous for its health benefits, especially cardiovascular health, and olive oil is a major contributor to those benefits. Some of the reported benefits of olive oil are:

1. Helping lower your cholesterol.
2. Lower blood pressure. Lower cardiovascular risk by improving heart health.
3. Help normalize blood clotting.
4. Help control blood glucose levels and thus diabetes.
5. Improving the actions of insulin.
6. Boost your immune system and attack viruses.
7. High in antioxidants.
8. Helps osteoporosis .Excellent for dry skin and overall skin health, primarily due to squalene, which helps prevent skin damage and helps to moisturize the skin. Roman women used this for centuries to keep their skin supple and beautiful; think of Sophia Loren, probably one of the most beautiful women who ever lived!
9. Treatment of arthritis pain via its anti-inflammatory properties. Prevention of strokes and dementia and even improves depression. Will make your penis much larger….only kidding, just checking to see if you skimmed over the list or really read it. The penis thing always gets men's attention, sorry ladies.

Olive oil has been reported to even help obesity…although you always have to be careful with oils, remember they are fats liquid at room temperature and are high in calories. Fat has over twice the calories of proteins or carbohydrates. So, to help obesity, apparently there have been studies showing weight loss, but keep in mind that these diets mostly replace butter and margarines with olive oil, not adding them to it, which would be disastrous for your weight.

How Much Olive Oil Should I Take?

There are no set doses of olive oil….it is just one of those things that provides many benefits and for that reason should be incorporated into your diet in place of butters and margarines.

Margarines should never be anywhere in your diet; they are full of trans fats that stiffen your cells and your blood vessels and are unnatural and wreak havoc with your health. That is why there is such a big push to get them out of our diets. I like to use olive oil in place of butter as I described above, as well as adding it to salads with apple cider vinegars that are also chock-full of "benes" for us. Listen, I went to medical school in Italy and lived there for eight years, I love Italian food and olive oil is an integral part of that for me, so I have no need to incorporate it into my diet. Once you try it you will love it and I am of the opinion that taking whole natural foods instead of synthetic vitamins is the way to go, and organic is always better than inorganic. Your body knows how to detoxify and rid itself of organic molecules, usually without too much harm. The easiest way to get these health-giving oils and minerals and vitamins into your diet is to switch them out for the unhealthy stuff. One of the easiest switches is with olive oil. Another is with table salt for sea salt and change your fruits and vegetables when possible to organic, free-range, non GMO and non-man made foods.

If you just want to take olive oil you can take two tablespoons of extra virgin olive oil daily to provide yourself with those wonderful phenols, fatty acids, vitamins, and other phytonutrients.

WALNUT OIL

Walnut oil is another oil that is both quite tasty and very beneficial for you. At this point do I insult your intelligence with a stupid sentence like ... "Walnut oil comes from walnuts."... as with all oils the best walnut oils are cold-pressed . It is usually topaz in color and has a limited shelf life of six to twelve months.

Nutrients In Walnut Oil

Walnut oil is full of our phenol friends as well as a wonderful form of vitamin E. Vitamin E is found in two forms, alpha-tocopherol and gamma- tocopherol. It's the gamma form that gives vitamin E many of its heart-healthy benefits, and walnut oil has a lot of the gamma-tocopherols. Walnuts are a great source of magnesium, selenium, zinc, iron, phosphorus, calcium, fiber, and potassium, as well as being low in sodium. Natural foods such as fruits and vegetables are usually high in potassium and low in sodium, and that combination is always good for you; they are also very alkaline as well, which is also good for you.

Walnuts are wonderful sources of vitamins, minerals, and antioxidants; they also contain many phytonutrients, including one almost unique to walnuts called juglone. The phytonutrients act to decrease inflammation and reduce oxidation and thus have anticancer as well as anti-arthritic properties and are health-promoting in many ways. Juglone is a chemical produced by all parts of the walnut tree, but the variety with the highest content is the black walnut. This chemical affects the growth of other plants and prevents many plants from growing beneath a walnut tree. One of the antioxidants found in walnut oil is ellagic acid, which has been shown to help detoxify many of the chemical toxins that lead to cancer, in addition to which it helps prevent the replication of cancer cells.

Health Benefits of Walnut Oil

Oddly enough, walnut oil is also rich in melatonin, which is a natural sleep aid, the production of which declines as you age, hence the many problems with insomnia that increase as we become old geezers. Cherries also contain significant amounts of melatonin. Melatonin actually works more like a hormone, helping to regulate the sleep/awake cycle (circadian rhythms) and light/dark adjustments among other actions.

Walnut oil is also naturally rich in omega-3,-6 and -9 fatty acids as well as ALA (alpha linolenic acid, just like flaxseed oil) which helps reduce inflammation and helps keep your blood vessels healthy, thus improving cardiovascular health. In fact, for those of you who do not like fish oil, walnut oil is an excellent source of omega-3 fatty acids.

Walnut oil contains a wonderful assortment of nutrients that help keep your skin healthy including phytonutrients, B vitamins, omega-3 fatty acids, and vitamin E, all of which work synergistically (work together) to keep your skin beautiful and well nourished, helping with conditions such as eczema and psoriasis. The abundance of antioxidants in walnut oil also prevent skin damage and keeps it healthy by neutralizing the free radicals that damage skin. Tip: If you are eating whole walnuts (which I encourage you to do for their many health benefits) you should be aware that 90 percent of our friends the phenols are contained in the walnut skin. The skin is not the shell, but rather the white/yellow waxy material that surrounds the nut. It sometimes has a bitter taste and this is from the phenols. As I have mentioned previously, phenols are wonderful for detoxification (destroying toxins), are antibacterial, antiviral, antifungal, and are strong antioxidants and are strongly anti-inflammatory.

In point of fact the entire family of tree nuts has similar health enhancing properties; these include Brazil nuts, pine nuts, pecans, pistachios, cashews, walnuts, hazelnuts (also known as filberts) and macadamia nuts. If you are eating raw walnuts, approximately seven shelled walnuts daily will give you all of the health benefits without too many calories. Remember: all nuts are very nutrient-rich and therefore are very high in calories.

In ancient times, the Romans used walnuts like Viagra, giving them to newlyweds to help enhance their sexuality as well as their fertility. Sorry guys, there are no modern studies on walnut oil or walnuts and sexual performance, you are going to have to do your own study!

Dose of Walnut Oil

There is no recommended dose of walnut oil or daily intake recommendations. If you are trying to stretch your food supply and have a lot of vegetables, then I would recommend adding any of the seed oils to your veggies. This will enhance their flavor as well as provide you with fat calories that will keep your hunger at bay for much longer than just vegetables alone.

AMARANTH OIL

The Amaranth plant was cultivated by the Aztecs for over 8,000 years and still is a very important crop in Peru. The botanical name is Amaranthus. It is not a grain but is used like one; it is in fact a seed, each plant producing up to 60,000 seeds. The name comes from the Greek amaranthos which means "one does not wither". This is due to the red flower buds which do not wilt even with drying. The plant itself grows to over six feet tall and has twice the protein content of rice, no gluten, and is chock-full of other important nutrients like the amino acid lysine. It is higher in minerals than almost all other vegetables. By the way, L-lysine is what you need to treat any Herpes family infection such as Herpes Genitalis (genital herpes), H. Labialis (cold sores on your lips), chickenpox, and Herpes Zoster (shingles). L-lysine is helpful because its chemical structure is very similar to another amino acid, arginine. Arginine is required for the herpes virus to reproduce, so if you flood your arginine receptors with L-lysine, that will prevent the uptake of arginine and the outbreak will subside. I have also found that it helps prevent the painful condition known as PHN or post herpetic neuralgia that frequently comes after shingles, keeping the nerves in pain for years.

Nutrients In Amaranth

The protein content of amaranth is also excellent due to it containing all of the essential amino acids that our bodies need. Essential amino acids are those amino acids that cannot be made by the body and therefore have to be obtained in our diets. Amaranth also is full of iron, low in carbohydrates, has a nice supply of fiber, and is full of minerals like calcium, manganese, magnesium, phosphorus, and potassium. Amaranth is also about 6 to 10 percent oil; not just any oil, but primarily unsaturated fatty acids (which are good for you), including linoleic acid. Amaranth is also the only grain (technically it is considered a pseudo grain or false grain) with a significant content of vitamin C. Amaranth seeds are also reported to have a high content of rutin and nicotiflorin, both of which help lower blood pressure and the incidences of cancer. Amaranth can be cooked like rice, popped like popcorn, or made into a pasta or ground into a flour.

The leaves of amaranth are also used by Greeks and other cultures as a green, leafy vegetable, like lettuce or chicory or endive, and was found to have high levels of beta-carotene and lutein. Amaranth also has been shown to contain very high levels of phytosterols which help lower cholesterol levels (both total cholesterol and LDL or bad cholesterol). The protein content of amaranth is so high it is considered on a par with animal-based proteins like cheese, which is great news for we natural food lovers; it gives us a food source that is easy to grow anywhere in a temperate climate (most of the United States) as long as it has well drained soil and plenty of sun. It prefers a high elevation, but this is not absolutely necessary. The entire plant is edible; as I mentioned, the most well- known part are the seeds, but you can also eat the leaves in a salad or added to a soup or even stir fried.

Amaranth Oil And Squalene

Amaranth oil is made from cold-pressing the small amaranth seeds, which are just slightly larger than a poppy seed. Amaranth oil is high in unsaturated fatty acids and many other wonderful nutritional phytochemicals, including squalene. Squalene is a compound originally discovered in the livers of sharks, thus the name. Amaranth oil contains approximately ten times the squalene content of shark liver oil and is the greatest source of squalene found anywhere in nature. Squalene is a precursor (from which other substances are manufactured by the body) of cholesterol and many steroid hormones.

Squalene is also included in many vaccines due to its effect upon stimulation of the immune system. This part gets a little confusing…squalene is wonderful for you and is naturally made by your skin, nasal mucosa, and other parts of your body.

Supplementing it orally is also wonderful for you for a host of reasons I will get into shortly, but when it is included in vaccines (injected), it overstimulates your immune system and results in its attacking all the good squalene in your body, thus possibly triggering such things as the Gulf War Syndrome in veterans who received vaccines with Squalene. As you remember Squalene is also contained in olive oil and enhances its health benefits just like it does with amaranth oil, so the take-home message here is the importance of the way Squalene is administered. Orally is excellent, injecting it in a vaccine is a terrible.

Squalene And Radiation

Squalene also is very important due to its role in the protection of the body from radiation of all types. Using olive oil or amaranth oil topically protects the skin from ultraviolet and ionizing radiations that damage the skin. Squalene is a strong natural antioxidant and is actively secreted by the sebaceous glands in our skin. This squalene prevents ultraviolet B and ionizing radiation damage to your skin. Ionizing radiation gets its name from its actions upon the body's tissues, where it ionizes them or tears away electrons from the body's molecules, thus damaging them. The shorter the wavelengths of radiation, the more energy the waves carry and thus the more penetrating or harmful the radiation is to the human body.

Ionizing radiation comes from cosmic sources (outer space), medical testing, and nuclear fallout and accidents. Ionizing radiation penetrates the human body and wreaks havoc on our cells; how Squalene actually protects us from this radiation is not completely clear, but probably is due to several effects. The most prominent effect of Squalene for protection of the human body is by its antioxidant role, another is its ability to protect and help repair the cell membrane, and finally its stimulation of the immune system. Squalene is most prominent in human skin but is also present in the lungs, kidneys, spleen, and brain, and in all of these areas the Squalene is depleted by exposure to radiation and needs to be renewed in order to protect those tissues from further radiation exposure. Surprisingly, Squalene is also contained in large quantities in fatty tissue, the reason for which is not entirely clear but its presence might be due to its ability to detoxify or rid the tissues of toxins, and toxins are readily stored in fatty tissue and might be the driving force behind some obesity. The anti-cancer properties of squalene might very well also be secondary to its ability to aid in detoxification, stimulation of the immune system, and a directly toxic effect on cancer cells as well as squalene's ability to block the cancer tissue from producing new blood vessels so the cancer can feed itself.

Sunlight has three primary components to it: visible light, Ultraviolet light types A, B, and C, Infrared light (this carries the heat from the sun).

It is primarily UVB or the ultraviolet B component of sunlight that does the most damage to your skin (think B for burn), and the good news is that this is neutralized by squalene in the skin. Squalene applied either topically or taken internally will help protect skin from this UVB damage as well as ionizing radiation that is present all around us and increasing annually.

Other Benefits of Squalene

Squalene also has antimicrobial effects, killing bacteria, fungi, and viruses. Squalene is particularly effective against candidiasis and other fungal infections. This antimicrobial ability of Squalene might be due to several factors including antioxidant effect, stimulating the immune system to fight off these infections, and also squalene's unique ability to deliver oxygen to the cells.

Oxygen kills all infections, which prefer an anaerobic (without oxygen) environment. Oxygen also kills cancer cells, and this might be part of the mechanism of Squalene's anticancer abilities. This same ability to provide oxygen to the body's cells might be the reason that dogfish (a type of shark that lives in large numbers deep in the ocean in an oxygen poor environment) livers produce so much Squalene. Squalene's ability to provide oxygen to the cells is probably a major part of its remarkable ability to stimulate the immune system.

A Short List of Squalene's Benefits:

1. Protection of the intestinal lining and the stomach lining, preventing ulcers.
2. Protection against all infections including colds and the flu.
3. Squalene is a source for vitamin D production by the body after exposure to sunlight (UVB to be exact; that is the good side of UVB).

4. Squalene lowers total cholesterol and LDL cholesterol (both of which are bad for you) and raise HDL or your good cholesterol, thus promoting heart and blood vessel health.
5. Healthy hormone production: Since squalene acts as a basic building block for cholesterol as well as steroid hormones like estrogen, testosterone, vitamin D, and progesterone, it helps keep a good hormone balance in the body.
6. Squalene helps energize your body, probably also by its effect on promotion of oxygen delivery to the cells.
7. Amaranth oil also contains large quantities of folic acid, other vitamins, minerals, essential amino acids, and essential fatty acids (remember essential means the body cannot product it and thus it must be obtained in your diet) and our friend the phenols. This folic acid content will prevent many birth defects and miscarriages in women as well as preventing ovarian cancer.
8. Helps respiratory disorders such as asthma, COPD, chronic bronchitis and tuberculosis (TB).
9. Increases energy and helps fatigue and even increases memory.
10. Helps decrease inflammation in the body's tissues, thus helping arthritis.
11. Helps treat burns of all severities.
12. Helps treat skin conditions such as dry skin, acne, eczema, and psoriasis, as well as moisturize skin and prevent and reduce wrinkles
13. Helps treat inflammatory bowel problems like Crohn's disease and ulcerative colitis as well as helping gastric and duodenal ulcers (duodenum is the first section of the small intestine).

Dose of Squalene or Amaranth Oil

Once again, this is difficult to answer with any precision since there are no recommendations. Squalene, whether it is from amaranth oil or fish oil, should be cold-pressed without the use of any solvents like hexane and should be 99 percent pure. Squalene can also be found in capsules. If it is in capsule form, then two of the 450 mg capsules daily should work well for maintenance. If you are ill, triple that to six capsules a day. For children one capsule daily and if ill double it to two. Squalene is also safe in pregnancy.

As far as Amaranth oil there is no set dose; if the manufacturer does not recommend a dose on the bottle then I would take about 18 ml daily; since one teaspoon is about 5 ml then about 3 ½ teaspoons daily should suffice. Naturally if you become ill then you should double that dose.

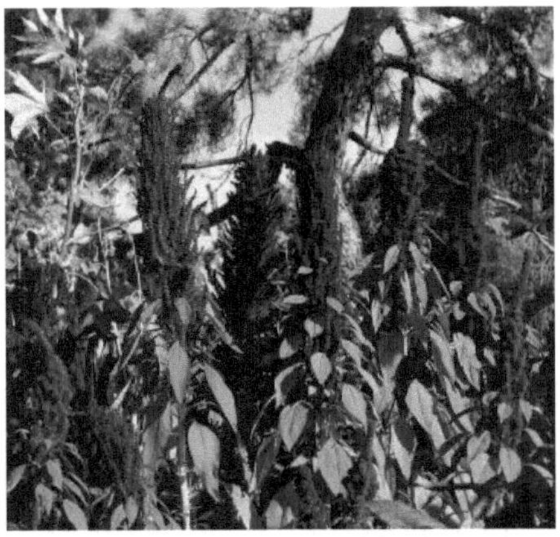

Amaranth and Your Garden

Amaranth is easy to grow just about anywhere in the continental United States.

It is basically a hardy, nutritious weed and will grow even in poor soils, it is relatively drought resistant once the seedlings are established, and does not require much care. All of these attributes of amaranth along with nutritional content and its ability to be converted into oil form make it a very wise choice for any medicinal gardens.

One thing to keep in mind is that amaranth is a thermophilous plant, meaning that it needs higher soil temperatures for the seeds to germinate, so if you want to have an early germination it will have to be done in a greenhouse, hot house, or on seed trays heated from the bottom. Amaranth seed heads do not all mature at the same time; harvesting should be done after the first frost on a dry day when two-thirds of the seeds in a given head are already ripe.

Both the seed heads and the leaves of amaranth are edible and quite nutritious. Amaranth leaves are similar to Swiss chard or spinach; however they are nutritionally far superior with 3x the calcium, iron, and niacin than spinach and twenty times more than lettuce. Do not pass up these nutritionally packed leaves; there are many recipes online for preparing these leaves, but essentially it is no different than cooking spinach. The seed heads of amaranth are where the true gold lies... the oil of amaranth cold-pressed from its seeds. However, there are other ways to enjoy these nutritional powerhouses...you can pop them, toast them on a skillet, sprout them, eat whole, and last but not least, grind them into a wonderfully nutritious flour. Eating them whole is easy; you just add an equal volume of water and simmer them for ten minutes.

The best varieties of amaranth for your survival garden needs are as follows:

Amaranthus caudatus
Amaranthus cruentus (this variety also has the best leaves)
Amaranthus hypochondriacus
Amaranth retroflexus.

A wise move is to stockpile some seeds of these varieties, as well as growing them in your medicinal garden.

CHAPTER FIVE

FERMENTATION AND FERMENTED FOODS

INTRODUCTION

TABLE OF CONTENTS:

Fermentation of foods is primarily done by yeasts and bacteria. These hungry little microorganisms are able to thrive without oxygen and convert foods into a variety of substances we know and love such as alcoholic beverages, sauerkraut, cheese, yogurt, etc. Fermented foods are super foods...they are able to provide an entire portfolio of benefits for our bodies. The added benefit is that fermentation is easy to learn and fun and provides your survival group with everything from booze of all types including beer, wine, and my personal favorite hard ciders, to vegetables, pickles, kefir, yogurts, and many others.

HOW DOES FERMENTATION WORK?

Fermentation is done by either yeast or bacteria (or both) that convert the carbohydrates (sugars) in foods to a variety of substances such as alcohols, fatty acids, amino acids, carbon dioxide, and organic acids. The fermentation process is done anaerobically, which means without oxygen. How is this done, you naively ask?....By keeping the material you are fermenting in a closed container sealed away from the intrusion of any of the surrounding air's oxygen. Now don't you feel silly for not figuring that out yourself…an author giving you, the reader, a hard time… I think I drank too much of that hard apple cider…LOL.

When the fermentation process produces ethanol from the sugars in foods, we produce wine, beer, and hard ciders. This is quite easily done at home with home brewing kits of various types. In many communities there are stores selling these items and they can also be bought online. Mankind has been brewing alcohol since Neolithic times and let's face it, most people like to have a drink, some more than others, and the harder the times the more folks like to "tip a bottle". I for one love an occasional drink but find as I get older I seem to get severe headaches from hard liquor like vodka, but I do tolerate fermented drinks like beer and cider much better.

LEAVENING OF BREAD

The leavening of bread is another wonderful use of fermentation. The leavening of bread was discovered in ancient times. What the ancients found out was that if you took some flour and mixed it with water and left it in a cool, covered area, the dough would rise. They also soon discovered that if you took a little of that dough and added it to the next batch, you would speed up the process. What they essentially discovered was the leavening of bread.

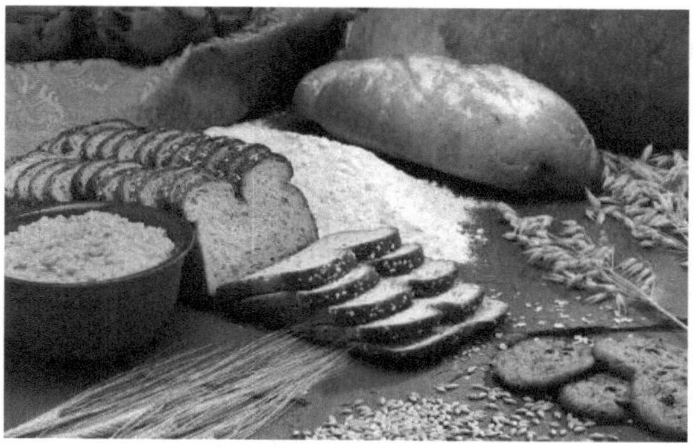

Leaven is really another word for wild yeasts. Some of these are better than other, and what men soon discovered was that if they had a particularly good batch, then they should save a little and use that as "starter" for subsequent batches. That worked much better than relying on just any wild yeast to be the leavening agent. Like bacteria and many viruses, yeasts are everywhere; they readily colonize areas that provide them with the perfect storm of dark, wet, and especially, anaerobic (without oxygen) conditions. Some strains that mankind has found especially useful have traveled with us thousands of years and are still being propagated in vast quantities for our culinary needs. Unleavened bread (most flat breads and matzoh, etc.) is made by mixing flour and water and then immediately baking it before the yeast can colonize the dough. When there is no fermentation there will be no carbon dioxide produced and no rising of the dough, hence the flat bread and crackers, etc. Historically, the reasons Jews eat matzoh or flattened, unleavened bread, for Passover is that they had to flee Egypt for their lives and had no time for their bread to rise, thus the tradition. Jews are able to eat leavened bread other times of the year. It is only during Passover that they must abstain.

Sprouted Grain Bread, Anti-nutrients and Wheatgrass

The most nutritious form of bread is sprouted grain bread. Grain becomes sprouted by soaking it in water. Like any seed, grain is dormant until the seed senses that conditions are correct for it to begin germination. The germination process awakens the genes of the seed to start directing the growth of the seed that eventually will become a plant. The genes direct a complex symphony of proteins and enzymes that determine its growth. A sprouted seed is one that has just begun this complex process and is half-way between a seed and a plant. The process of germination begins when the seed is soaked in water and the enzyme inhibitors it contains are dissolved and removed, thus allowing the enzymes to awaken and start the seed's growth .Seeds that are dormant (not germinating) in the soil, need to protect themselves.

As you can imagine, they do not have many options; how they do this is quite interesting. Seeds protect themselves by containing what is known as anti-nutrients. Anti-nutrients are chemicals within the seed that make the seeds less attractive to predators. They do this by causing toxicity in some cases, such as raw soybeans. Anti-nutrients also bind up many nutrients such as proteins and minerals, making them unavailable to animals that consume them. They also can interfere with the digestive enzymes of animals, making it more difficult for animals to process any seeds they have eaten. Cooking does not eliminate many of the anti-nutrients, but sprouting does, in addition to which, sprouting also increases the healthy nutrients such as minerals, trace elements, proteins, and enzymes.

Raw soybeans are toxic because they contain anti-nutrients and also two chemicals known as goitrogens and phytoestrogens. Goitrogens are substances that interfere with normal thyroid function and thus lead to an enlargement of the thyroid, or goiter. Phytoestrogens are plant-made estrogens and ingesting these leads to havoc with your body's own sex hormones, in both men and women. In Asia, soybeans are an integral part of their diets, but like most ancient societies, they developed means to utilize the food they were blessed with. The Chinese and Japanese would soak their soybeans for some time then rinse them off and put them through a process of fermentation, thus allowing the microbes to partially digest them and increase their nutrient content while at the same time removing their harmful anti-nutrients. In this manner soy sauce, natto, miso, and tofu were made not only more nutritious but delicious! Sprouted grain bread is the kind that was eaten in biblical times and as you can see is much more nutritious than modern versions of bread that are made by refined wheat or pulverized wheat that has not undergone the chemical process of germination and as such the anti-nutrients are all present and the enzymes, minerals, and amino acids (proteins) are bound up and not released and thus not available even after digestion. Modern bread is made from non-sprouted grain flour, whereas ancient bread was made from ground up sprouted seeds and thus was much more nutritious. For those of us interested in good health thru good nutrition, this certainly is the way to go. In fact, it is not only much more nutritious but it is easier when starting from scratch.

Seeds also contain carbohydrate in the form of starches that provide the fuel for the germination process; sprouting seeds reduces their carbohydrate content because the sprouting process utilizes this carbohydrate to grow. Sprouting also reduces the amount of gluten in the bread. Sprouted bread also is made without sugar, making it better for you.

The last thing we need is more sugar in our diets. The combination of no sugar and less carbohydrates leads to very little spiking of blood glucose levels and in turn insulin, thus these breads have a low glycemic index.

One of the primary anti-nutrients in grains is phytic acid. Phytic acid binds up minerals in the seeds such as calcium, magnesium, iron, and zinc, making them unavailable even after digestion. Soaking a seed for a few days will release the plant's own enzymes such as phytase, which inactivates phytic acid.

In her excellent book, *Deep Nutrition*, Dr. Catherine Shanahan describes one of the consequences of ingesting phytic acid along with a poor diet. In the 1960s in Turkey there was a sharp spike in the number of children who were dwarves. It was originally thought to be due to a genetic mutation, however upon further investigation, it was found to be due to diet. The dwarfism was striking poor families -- that was the first hint that it was not a genetic mutation -- why should only the poor develop this mutation? It was found that their diets, due to the cost involved, was poor in meat. They also ate unleavened bread which was very high in phytic acids. This produced the "perfect storm"; low zinc and magnesium from their low-meat diet and then whatever zinc, magnesium, and other minerals that remained in their diets were bound up by the phytates or phytic acid. This lack of minerals in their diet prevented the expression of genes that controlled growth and hence their bone structure did not develop to its full potential. Once this was corrected it eliminated the epidemic of dwarfism.

How to Sprout Seeds

Wheatgrass is sprouted wheat seeds, also known as wheat berries. Wheat berries are very hard and need to be softened by soaking to be able to grind them down, unless you have modern equipment available. Wheatgrass contains increased amounts of soluble fiber, beta carotene, folate, and vitamins such as vitamin B complex and vitamin C. Wheatgrass is also high in enzymes and chlorophyll and is highly nutritious and easily digested and assimilated by your body.

For we health conscious individuals, mastering the art of sprouting will prove very beneficial. Sprouting can easily be done indoors for little cost. Sprouting indoors can give you the advantage of having a steady supply of green, nutritious food that is loaded with enzymes, vitamins, minerals, trace elements, amino acids, and chlorophyll.

Chlorophyll is what gives plants their green color; it has an identical structure to hemoglobin, the pigment that gives human blood its red color. The only difference between chlorophyll and hemoglobin is that hemoglobin has iron in its center and chlorophyll has magnesium. Otherwise their structure is identical. Some believe that ingesting chlorophyll allows the body to easily convert it to hemoglobin, however, nobody has been able to explain how that happens, so for now it remains conjecture.

Sprouting of beans, grains, nuts, and seeds is an easy skill and is similar for all four. Many of these four have been pasteurized and irradiated and are not raw; soaking these will not result in sprouting but will still improve their nutritional content and eliminate anti-nutrients.

Step 1: Soak the beans, grains, nuts, or seeds overnight in a bowl of water. Just put enough water to cover the seeds.

Step 2: The next day, drain out the water and rinse the seeds several times with fresh water. This will help eliminate any mold spores.

Step 3: Take the seeds (or whatever you are sprouting) and place them in a clean Mason jar or other glass jar and keep them moist. A wet paper towel will do the trick, just change it daily to prevent any mold from forming. Cover the opening of the jar with some cheesecloth or breathable mesh, if you are using a Mason jar, keep the metal rim to the lid and remove the center metal piece and replace that with the cheesecloth so the jar can "breathe".

Step 4: Twice daily rinse out the jar with fresh, clean water, once again to remove any mold that might be forming.

Step 5: Make sure the sprouts never dry up; this will kill them and prevent proper germination and sprouting.

Step 6: Once you see them sprouting, which will take several days to a week, then rinse them off with fresh water and they are ready to either eat or to make into your bread.

LACTIC ACID BACTERIA/LACTOFERMENTATION

Fermentation is also done by lactic acid bacteria (LAB) which produce lactic acid….this makes the sour taste of some fermented foods like sauerkraut, dry sausages, yogurt, and kimchi.

Kimchi is the national food of Korea and is made by fermenting various vegetables that have been mixed with a variety of spices, placed in underground containers and allowed to ferment for many months.

The vegetables used can be scallions, radishes, scallions, or cucumbers, and depending on the spices can be either sweet- or sour-flavored. LAB are able to tolerate very low pH (acidic) conditions that kill other bacteria. A by-product of fermentation by LAB is lactic acid, which further acidifies the food that is being fermented, but this also kills off all the other competing bacteria, making the food resistant to spoiling. The process of LAB fermentation is also known as lactofermentation.

Lactobacilli are also one of the only bacteria that do not require iron for their growth and reproduction; they use both cobalt and manganese. Cobalt is part of vitamin B12, so adequate B12 levels will help provide lactic acid with its much- needed cobalt. Cobalt is quite common in foods and is contained in green leafy vegetables, especially broccoli and spinach, fish, nuts, and cereals such as oats. Manganese is also found in green leafy vegetables such as peas and runner beans, bread, cereals, and nuts. By far the most common source of manganese in most peoples' diet is from tea. So, try to make an effort to eat those foods listed above to maintain adequate intakes of cobalt and manganese, and for the same reason I cannot emphasize enough the importance of taking a multi-mineral and trace element source every day such as Supreme Fulvic, which will provide you with everything you need. You can always supplement any item you need more of but at least you are guaranteed to be getting them all.

PICKLING

Fermentation is also the process by which foods are pickled. Pickling is usually done using brine or vinegar in a closed container (anaerobically), and leaving it for months to allow for fermentation. The resulting pickle can have either a salty or a sour taste. In parts of Southern Asia they add edible oils to vinegar, giving the pickles a different flavor. Brine is just another word for salty water which ranges from 5 percent to 26 percent in its salt content. Adding salt or brine to foods draws out more of the water from the vegetable by osmosis and adds to the pickling process....this is done by Germans to produce their beloved sauerkraut and by Koreans for their much beloved kimchi.

The pH of pickled foods is quite acidic due to the lactic acid produced by the lactic acid bacteria used. Once the pH falls below 4.6 as it is in pickled foods, you will kill off any bacteria present; that is why pickled foods do not spoil and can be stored for quite some time.

This easy preservation method for vegetables in a healthy medium teeming with enzymes, vitamins, minerals, and probiotics, and without the need for any electricity, makes fermented and pickled foods so ideal for us. You can easily make foods such as whey, kefir, and kombucha and ferment their own organically grown vegetables, and it can be done on the cheap. Fermenting apple cider or perry (pear cider) into hard cider is easily done and will provide you with a ready source of relatively healthy alcohol. Online there are many suppliers of the materials you need and I suggest you familiarize yourself with fermentation since it is so useful and may very well save your life as well as the lives of your family if you were ever find yourselves in a situation where you had to preserve your own foods.

WHY EAT FERMENTED FOODS?

Our diets were previously filled with organically grown fruits and vegetables and game or free-range meats along with plenty of fermented foods and alcohols. The soils were full of microbial life and hence the foods were full of enzymes, mineral, and trace elements, along with fulvic acid. Contrast that with today's foods, full of sugar and salt, processed, lacking minerals, trace elements, and fulvic acid, with little vitamin content, and laden with chemicals and preservatives, grown on dead soils. Is it any wonder that people are tired, obese, and riddled with diseases of modern man such as diabetes, hypertension, arthritis, and cancers of all types. Look around you.

Americans are horribly obese, bloated, and sick-appearing; not just the old, even young children are obese and unhealthy looking. We are being starved of essential life-giving nutrients, while at the same time being poisoned with chemically saturated, toxin-laden foods. Our only recourse to regain our health and vigor is to return to those foods that enhance our health and

provide all the nutrients and minerals and trace elements that we so desperately need.

Let's take a look at some of the benefits of fermented foods for our bodies. Fermented foods are jam-packed with various strains of beneficial probiotics, enzymes, B vitamins, and omega-3 fatty acids. The fermentation process also helps to partially digest the carbohydrates in the food being fermented, which aids in our digestion as well.

The nutrient content in fermented foods is also naturally preserved and thus readily available upon digestion by our bodies.

Scientists are finding ever more benefits to the ingestion of fermented foods, such as:

1. Improved intestinal tract health and prevention of GI infections
2. Enhanced immunity

3. Synthesizing and enhancing the bioavailability of nutrients and vitamins
4. Improving lactose intolerance
5. Helping leaky gut and thereby reducing the symptoms and the severity of allergies, asthma, and autoimmune diseases. Reducing the risks of certain cancers.

HOW TO MAKE FERMENTED FOODS AT HOME

As a natural health enthusiast this information is invaluable to your health and is quite easy to master. The good news is that it is really inexpensive and the cultures can be used indefinitely to make more and more of whatever you are fermenting. Let's look at some relatively simple examples of fermented products you can make at home. The time to master this skill was yesterday! This is not only a lot of fun, but will supply you and your family or friends a load of delicious, healthful foods to supplement their dinner tables.

Kefir

Kefir (pronounced key-fer) is a liquid drink made from fermented milk, similar to the way yogurt is made. Kefir originally comes from the Caucasus Mountains of Eastern Europe. Kefir is made by using kefir grains or a powdered kefir starter packet. The "grains" have nothing at all to do with grain like wheat or corn and are actually bacteria and yeasts wrapped in a jelly-like coating. Kefir is thought to be much healthier for you than yogurt, due to the fact that it is made from over twenty varieties of yeast and bacteria.

In yogurt, the probiotics it contains do help your GI tract by fighting off bad disease-causing bacteria, but do not stay in the intestines and take up residence but just pass through. The probiotics contained in kefir, on the other hand, take up residence in your intestines and reproduce, providing ongoing health benefits. Kefir also provides a large amount of calcium to help build strong bones and teeth.

Kefir also contains tryptophan, which is an amino acid, the same one that is contained in large quantities in turkey, which relaxes you and is the reason your wife is mad at you for falling asleep on the couch watching TV after Thanksgiving Day dinner.

Tryptophan is also contained in milk and is released by heating it; that is the reason warm milk at bedtime helps children sleep. Tryptophan also works in adults, but we tend to have a nightcap that contains alcohol rather than warm milk. I pass no judgment here, just stating the facts. So, what I am saying is that you can use kefir to relax at night as well, and you don't have to heat it up. Kefir also contains lots of protein and B vitamins such as thiamine (B1) and B12 as well as another B vitamin called biotin, which helps absorb the other B vitamins. Thiamine is wonderful for helping treat stress, and let's face it, what could be more stressful than trying to survive in our current world!

Kefir also contains lots of phosphorus, which our bodies need for multiple reasons but primarily for energy production as well as carbohydrate and protein metabolism. Remember the energy molecule made by your cells' powerhouses, the mitochondria, is called ATP or adenosine triphosphate, which means it contains three phosphate or phosphorus molecules, hence our need for phosphorus to produce energy.

How To Make Yogurt And Kefir

Yogurt is made with either of two types of methods, mesophilic or thermophilic. Mesophilic means it is cultured at room temperature, while thermophilic means heat-loving, so it needs to be heated in an incubator-type device such as a yogurt maker at around 110 degrees (Fahrenheit). Kefir is made by the room temperature or mesophilic process and does not require a heating machine of any type. Kefir is basically made by adding kefir grains to milk at room temperature and allowing it to sit for from twelve to forty-eight hours. Since kefir is made with both yeasts and bacteria, it has a slightly different taste than yogurt, which is made only by bacteria. The taste of kefir has been described as a cross between buttermilk and yogurt, and is slightly more sour. The flavor of kefir can be changed by adding blended fruit, honey, or vanilla extract.

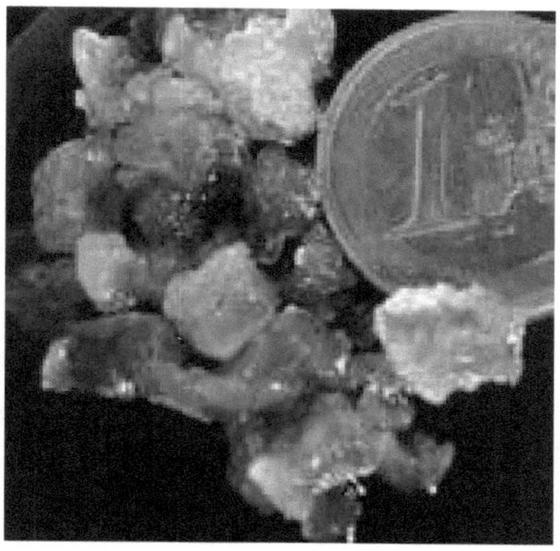

Close-up Photo of Kefir Grains

Both yogurt and kefir can be made thicker by the draining off of whey. The draining of whey from yogurt will produce a Greek style yogurt and if more is drained off, a yogurt cheese, also called labneh, will be produced. By the same token whey can be drained from kefir to produce a pudding-like consistency or a kefir cream cheese or, if more is drained off, a kefir hard cheese can be made. Whey is the liquid remaining after milk has been curdled and strained. Whey is what is used to make Ricotta cheese, one of my favorites. I am slowly facing the fact that I love most cheeses. Do not discard the whey you remove from your kefir or yogurt production; it is full of protein, vitamins, minerals, and traces of fat, and one of the cardinal rules of prepping is to never waste anything, especially foods. Whey can be fed to your pets or utilized for your own nutritional needs.

There is a wonderful website called Cultures for Health that I highly recommend. They have all the cultures you need to make your own fermented foods as well as great background information on each food and free e-books that describe how to make yogurt, kefir, kombucha, and hard cheeses. I recommend downloading those e-books now and printing out hard copies of them for your library. As tempting as it is to leave everything in digital form, there is a very good chance that you will have no electricity at some point and will need a hard copy, so print it out now and save it. I also recommend learning the various techniques now for the production of the different foods; it is fun and is very healthy for you and your family.

Kombucha

Kombucha is a sweetened tea that has been fermented by symbiotic colonies of bacteria and yeast (SCOBY), which are sometimes referred to as "mother" or "mushroom" due to its appearance. It is relatively new in the western world but has been drank in the China for two thousand years and is also known there as "The Immortal Health Elixir". The Chinese feel it helps prevent and treat cancer, arthritis, and other degenerative diseases. The Russians also use it for health and there it is known as "tea kvass".

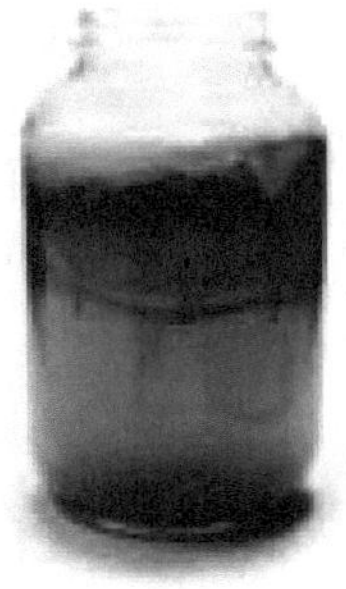

Kombucha with culture floating in it (Photo by Mgarten)

Nutritional studies on the components of kombucha have shown that it contains large quantities of B vitamins, antioxidants, and acetic and glucaric acids. Actual studies on its benefits are lacking and all the benefits reported anywhere, including here, are anecdotal, meaning they are people's personal experiences, not scientifically verified. Kombucha is also full of enzymes and acids produced by bacteria, both of which help detoxify your body and thus at the same time aids your liver. Kombucha supposedly helps prevent cancer as well as delay its spread, and was used for just that purpose by President Reagan starting in 1987, and he died of old age in 2004! Oh, how I wish we currently had a president like Ronald Reagan in the White House, but that is a fantasy for another day. Kombucha also contains significant quantities of glucaric acid, which has been shown to prevent cancers. Glucaric acids are found naturally in many vegetables and fruits; it is also made in small quantities by our bodies. Glucaric acid helps the body remove toxins. It does this by enhancing a process whereby the liver attaches water soluble molecules to toxins called glucuronidation. Once these toxins are made water soluble by that conjugation, they are known as glucuronides; then they can be excreted into the urine by the kidneys. Presumably that is the method whereby Kombucha exerts its anticancer properties. Glucuronidation is one of the primary pathways the body utilizes to rid itself of dangerous toxins. If you think about it, it is quite an ingenious method, attaching a water soluble molecule to something that is not water soluble and thereby allowing the kidneys to dissolve it into urine. The absolute genius of the design of the human body never ceases to amaze me, which is probably a good thing, since I am a physician!

Kombucha also contains a lot of glucosamine, which helps joints by increasing the production of hyaluronic acids which nurture cartilage and lubricate it by vastly increasing the amount of moisture cartilage can hold, thus keeping cartilage supple and flexible, thereby decreasing stiffness and the resulting inflammation of arthritis. Since kombucha is essentially a living colony of bacteria and yeast, it therefore is a strong probiotic, introducing these helpful microorganisms to your intestines, aiding in digestion and boosting your immune system as well as helping diseases like fibromyalgia, anxiety, and depression. Kombucha also is chock-full of antioxidants and thus helps your immune system and also helps disease and cancer prevention.

Kombucha tea can be made at home and is quite simple. There are many websites online with kits containing all the necessary items, and this can be easily done by anyone by following their recipes.

Once again the time to start learning to do this was yesterday!

Kombucha can be made quite easily following these steps for making a quart bottle (change the ratios for making larger quantities):

1. Take a glass bottle and fill it with 3 cups of very hot water, not boiling but just hot enough to steep the tea. The water you use has to have no chlorine or fluoride in it or it will kill the culture.
2. Add half a cup of sugar and stir it in well. I prefer to use raw sugar.
3. Add either two tea bags or a one and a half teaspoons of loose tea: add this to your mixture and allow it to steep.
4. Allow your mixture to cool to about 70-80 degrees F. You can leave the tea in the mix to make it stronger tasting or remove it after a short time for a less robust taste.
5. Remove the tea bags or strain the loose tea out of the mixture.
6. Add a half cup of starter tea (from a previous batch) or use a half cup of distilled white vinegar
7. Add active Kombucha scoby
8. Cover the jar with cheesecloth and put a rubber band around the neck of the jar to secure it in place. A coffee filter can also be used.
9. Place your jar out of direct sunlight and keep it between 70-85 degrees F . Allow it to ferment from one to four weeks. Note: the longer it ferments the less sweet it will be and the closer to vinegar.
10. When it is ready, pour out the Kombucha from the top and use the scoby and the thicker liquid on bottom as your starter for your next batch.

Lacto - Fermentation of Vegetables and Fruits

Unlike the fermentation of beers, ciders, and wine, that is done by yeast, the fermentation method known as Lacto-Fermentation is done by bacteria. The lacto part of the name comes from the specific bacteria used in this process known as the Lactobacillus. The family of Lactobacillus includes many different strains, many of which are found on the surface of plants, especially those grown near the ground. Lactobacilli are also found in our gastrointestinal tracts (our gut), mouths, and vaginas of humans and many other animal species.

In those areas of the body where it naturally resides, it prevents infections by other bacteria by lowering the pH and outcompeting other bacteria for that terrain, and that is why patients frequently develop vaginal yeast infections and oral yeast infections (thrush) after they take antibiotics which kill off the lactobacilli, thus raising the pH and allowing invasion and colonization by fungi and other types of bacteria. That is also the rationale behind doctors recommending that patients eat yogurt while they are on antibiotics, to help recolonize your body with lactobacilli. Lactobacillus gets its name from its ability to convert the milk sugar lactose into lactic acid; however, it is also capable of converting many other sugars into lactic acid by the process of fermentation.

Many of you are aware of one type of lactobacillus known as lactobacillus acidophilus, which is commonly called acidophilus and is responsible for making yogurt from milk. The term acidophilus means acid loving, and is so named because lactobacillus is capable of survival at a much lower pH than most other bacteria. Before the advent of modern refrigeration, foods that were not immediately consumed needed to be fermented to prevent their becoming spoiled by putrefying bacteria and this was one of the primary methods of food preservation besides smoking, drying, and salting foods. Without lacto-fermentation people would not have been able to store and preserve foods they grew during the summer months in order to prevent starvation during the long, lean winters. Besides preservation of foods, lacto-fermentation also increased the nutritional value of foods by providing greater amounts of vitamins, enzymes, and probiotic bacteria and yeasts. Lacto- fermentation also increases the digestibility of foods because the food is already partially digested by the fermentation process and also contains greater amounts of enzymes that aid in digestion.

Remember that cooking foods above 125 degrees F for a half hour will essentially destroy the enzymes that all natural foods contain, and forces our bodies to produce digestive enzymes such as amylases for starches, lipases for fats, and proteases for the digestion of proteins. I earlier touched upon the consequences of eating foods devoid of their natural enzyme content when I told you about Dr. Pottenger and his experiments on cats and the devastating chronic illnesses and infertility they suffered as a result of their enzyme-free diets. Nature does not do anything by mistake; there is a reason the foods we live on contain such enzymes. It is by design, not by accident, and we ignore such designs of nature at our own peril.

How Is Lacto-Fermentation Done At Home?

Home lacto-fermentation is one skill everyone should master. It is not particularly difficult, so let's review how it is done.

The first thing you need is a source of lactobacillus such as fresh whey, kefir grains, freeze-dried powders, or an existing culture containing lactobacilli. This is not essential, but will speed up the process and insure that you will have enough lactobacilli. Remember, the skins of fruits and vegetables are not sterile and are home to large amounts of bacteria including the lactobacillus we need for our lacto-fermentation. Now you need something the lactobacillus can eat or metabolize, so you have to provide sugar (carbohydrate) and these occur naturally in fruit and vegetables. When you finish one batch of vegetables and would like to start fermenting another, you can use a couple of tablespoons of the ferment liquid from your old batch and just spoon it into the new batch and add your salt, etc. Just add a little salt (unrefined sea salt or pickling salts) to make your brine (salt and water mix) and provide a container that is without oxygen (closed container will shortly become anaerobic or without oxygen), and then give it some time to work.

Do not use kosher salt because this contains sodium ferrocyanide to prevent caking of the salt, and is potentially toxic to the culture mix. Do not use iodized salt, which is common table salt that has been fortified with iodine. Iodine inhibits bacterial growth; that is why we use it to clean wounds, etc., and so, it will inhibit the lacto-fermentation process by interfering with the activity of the lactobacillus. Unrefined sea salt is the best option, unrefined means it still has the full complement of minerals from the sea, you can tell it is unrefined by the multiple colored flecks mixed into it. So, the ideal salt for fermenting is whole, unrefined and full of all the natural minerals and trace elements it originally contained

NOTE: The use of greater amounts of salt will slow the fermentation process, so keep that in mind. Salt is added primarily to inhibit the growth of bacteria (and mold) that is not involved in the fermentation process but does not affect the lactobacillus, which is unusually salt tolerant. Salt also, by its osmotic force, will draw water out of the fruit or vegetables you are fermenting. This gives them that wrinkled appearance and also makes it more difficult for bacteria to infect the fruit and destroy it. Salt also hardens the pectins in vegetables and thus makes them crunchy. Think the snap of a pickle when you bite into it!

Pectin is a sugar found in the cell walls of plants that has a jelly-like consistency and is therefore used to thicken up jelly and jams. Not using enough salt will accelerate the fermentation process by allowing the addition of other bacterial species, thus aiding the fermentation. There will be less yeast and mold suppression, and you may find a layer of white, scummy material on the surface of the ferment. This is harmless yeast and does not mean the ferment is spoiled and this can just be scraped off. You can make a ferment without salt and this will naturally leave many strains of bacteria in your ferment, making it more biodiverse, but the vegetables will be a lot more mushy. Alternatively, you can use a 50/50 mix of celery juice and water as your brine or you can use seaweed for its salt content, but neither of these will prevent the vegetables from being soggy.

The container should only be filled about 80 percent of the way, and usually a rock or heavy weight of some kind is place on top of the vegetables to keep them submerged under the brine. There also has to be some opening to allow gases to escape the mixture as carbon dioxide is produced by the fermentation process and must be gassed off. Some glass bottles will come with an airlock system to allow gases to escape but prevent oxygen, which will ruin the fermenting process, from entering. As you remember, this has to be anaerobic, or without oxygen. If oxygen gets into your fermenting vessel it will cause mold and spoil the vegetables or fruit you are fermenting.

You should only use glass or ceramic vessels; most plastic vessels will leach harmful chemicals into your food and metal will react with the fermentation process. The only plastic containers you can use have to be food grade and not used previously. Old slow cookers sometimes utilize ceramic liners and these are wonderful for fermenting. Specialty vessels made specifically for lacto-fermentation will come with the lid and internal stone or weights to keep the vegetables adequately submerged under the brine. The lids for these ceramic vessels have a water-trough-airlock system built into them to allow gases to escape and prevent the entry of oxygen. Once the lid is on, then I recommend wrapping the top of the container with a tight weave towel such as a tea towel or cheesecloth, and applying a rubber band to the neck. This will keep curious insects out of your ferment. This length of time of lacto-fermentation can vary from a few hours to a few months. The usual length of time for the lacto-fermentation of vegetables is from two to twenty-one days. There are other variables which affect fermentation, such as temperature; an ideal temperature for lacto-fermentation is about 72 degrees F.

Any colder will slow it down, warmer will speed it a little. Remember what I said about fever, your body creates a fever to kill off bacteria because most bacteria live within a narrow temperature range. The same holds true for Lactobacilli. A good rule of thumb is if the vegetables taste tart and tangy then they are ready; of course each individual has their own palate of likes and dislikes. Keep in mind, the flavor of vegetables that are lacto-fermented increases over time, so you will have to taste your veggies often to find the optimal flavor for your palate.

You must keep in mind that oxygen will ruin your fermentation, so be careful when opening your batch of veggies, most of which are contained in airtight containers or they use a water seal in a large ceramic crock. You can still buy large ceramic crocks at most flea markets. If they are chipped you can get them quite reasonably. As long as they hold water and have no cracks through and through, then who cares if they are chipped.

You don't have to worry about getting sick from lacto-fermented foods unless they smell putrid; in that case do not hesitate to throw that batch away, it has become contaminated .Lacto- fermented vegetables are alive and continue to develop nutritionally over time. Since the sugars in the fruit or vegetables you are fermenting are used up by the bacteria, this eliminates sweetness and makes all fermented veggies somewhat tart. The lactic acid produced as a by-product of this fermentation also adds to the tartness. Since the sugars have been basically eaten up by the bacteria, fermented foods are excellent low carbohydrate foods, especially good for diabetics and for weight loss. A fermented batch of veggies with between a 1 and 2 percent salt content will keep nicely in a refrigerator for from four to nine months. A 2 percent salt brine will be okay for a root cellar or a cool basement corner and last from three to four months, but keep in mind, the vegetables need to always be submerged in the brine or they will spoil. Any vegetable can be lacto-fermented individually or mixed together, it does not matter. Many people have their own favorite combinations, and the Koreans are masters at fermenting their vegetables into kimchi into a tasty variety of dishes. You can also add dill and garlic to your cucumbers that you are fermenting into tasty pickles. Germans have been known to add juniper berries (the source for gin) and caraway seeds to their sauerkrauts.

The Differences between Lacto-Fermented Fruits and Vegetables

Lacto-fermentation of fruit is more difficult than vegetables, due primarily to the high sugar content of fruit. Fermented fruit will only last about two weeks if you refrigerate it, or it will wind up changing to alcohol. That is the basic problem with fruit fermentation; it can either go the lacto-fermentation route or can go the alcohol fermentation route. Keeping the salt content low will help the lacto-fermentation route. Another method is to mix fruit and vegetables together; since veggies have a lower sugar content, this will allow for longer storage of the mix without spoilage.

Pickles and Pickling

Pickling is the anaerobic fermentation of foods for their preservation by using either brine or vinegar. If brine is used, the resulting pickle will be salty. If vinegar is used, the resulting pickle will be sour in taste.

Using salt will do the same things as with lacto-fermentation. It will prevent many species of bacteria from flourishing and it will also draw water out of the vegetable being pickled and thus shrink it, and also make it crunchy from the effect of the salt on the pectin in the vegetable's skin. Unlike canning, pickling and lacto-fermentation do not require the vegetable to be sterile before being placed in the vessel where it will ferment.

Several important factors are in play here to prevent contamination without sterilization. The main factors involved are the pH and the salinity of the brine. The lactic acid produced naturally lowers the pH, the temperature will kill off many organisms, and finally, the lack of oxygen in this anaerobic medium will prevent most species of bacteria from surviving. Pickling, like most ferments, also improves the nutritional value of foods by adding enzymes and vitamins like the B vitamins. Many people enjoy pickled foods simply for their taste. Pickling has been going on for over 4,000 years and began in northern India, where the pickles they made from cucumbers were called "Achar", and are still popular today.

Some pickles today are done without fermentation and are called fresh pack or quick processed pickles. These are made by submerging the vegetable to be pickled in brine for several hours or overnight and then removing them and covering them with vinegar and seasonings. Vinegar is a strong acid and will prevent most bacterial species from surviving.

NOTE: Pickles are subject to spoiling by yeasts and molds and also from enzymes and may change color and texture as well as flavor.

If you process the pickles in a boiling water home canning system using standard canning jars with self-sealing lids, this will prevent all of the above problems. When using vinegar, use either white vinegar or vinegar with at least 5 percent acidity. Also snip off one-sixteenth of the blossom end of the cucumber to prevent softening of the pickle. Do not use a salt substitute in place of salt, since this is potassium chloride and will give a bitter taste to the pickles.

HOW TO MAKE A ROOT CELLAR

A root cellar is a low tech, simple, effective way to store foods and preserve them without the need for electricity or power of any kind. If you are going to ferment, jar, or pickle some foods then it will be a really useful thing to have.

Many books will describe in detail how to construct a root cellar, but in truth, it is not very difficult.

What a root cellar is, is a storage area that is naturally cool, insulated from the weather (usually by its underground or into-a-hillside location) and humidified.

An ideal temperature involves either being outside or if inside, have a ventilation system where cool, humid outside air can be circulated through. The reason for the humidity, is to prevent dehydration of the stored fruit or vegetables and their subsequent shriveling and getting a dried out, wrinkled, ugly appearance. The ideal humidity level should be quite high, on the order of about 90 percent. The cool air does its part by slowing the release of ethylene gas, which is responsible for ripening. The cool air also slows the decomposition of the stored foods by bacteria and fungi (which live in a narrow temperature range). The ideal temperature range should be just above freezing. You can also build a root cellar in a cool corner of the basement. In most homes the coolest corner is the Northeast. If your home has one end underground that corner will trump the Northeast. Dampness also helps since we are looking to promote humidity. If you can build the two new walls of stone, brick, or cinder blocks then all the better, but normal plasterboard will do, you will just need to insulate it as best as possible. If you can, try to use "green board", which is the waterproof plaster board that is used in showers; rot-resistant wood like cedar would be ideal as well. The upper shelves will be warmer and dryer and the lower will be cooler and wetter. You will need a ventilation system to both bring in cold air and to prevent the entry of any warm air from the house.

You will need to put two ventilation pipes through the wall, one as high as you can closest to the ceiling and the other about a foot off of the floor. Three-inch pipes are the best; PVC will work just fine and is easy to cut and fit elbows and ends. Attach a closed blast gate, which is a valve, to each pipe so that in the event that it gets too cold outside you can close one (and allow partial ventilation) or both if it is really cold out. This ventilation system will allow nice passive, continuous ventilation without the need for any power. Insulate well around the pipes to prevent any other water or air leakage.

Building into a hillside is the easiest and has other advantages such as natural drainage which is very important; you don't want your root cellar to flood. If you build it into the ground, sandy soil is the best because it will drain easier and prevent flooding. In cold areas like where I live in New England and others, you have to keep the frost line in mind. The ground here in Connecticut will not freeze down beyond a foot and a half, so your ceiling will need to be below that point. You will have to dig it away from any significant-sized trees to avoid their roots, which will be tough to dig through and could break through your walls once the root cellar is established.

You can line the hole with straw or pack it with leaves to create a moisture barrier and some insulation, cover the opening with a thick wooden lid and cover that in turn with soil or some straw or just a wooden door , basically anything will do depending on your preferences.

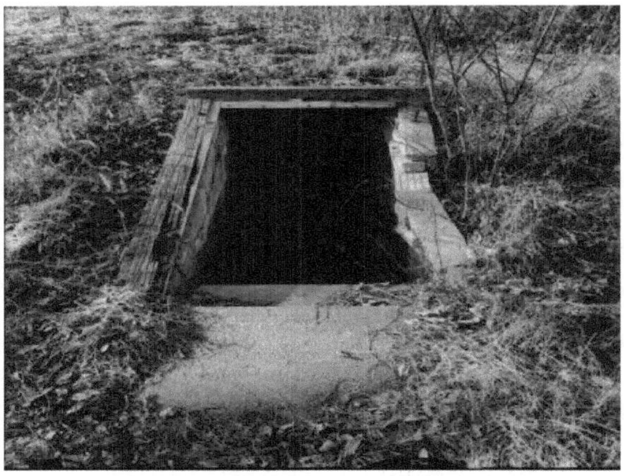

The shelves in a root cellar should be well spaced and a few inches from the walls in order to allow good air circulation, which will prevent mold formation. If you go over ten feet down, you will have persistently cool temperatures without much variation. That being said, if you are doing this by hand, that is one hell of a hole to dig. Burying a garbage can or other barrel in the ground will also work well.

Dig the hole slightly larger than the can and once the can is inside, fill the outside of the can and pack the dirt in well. Put straw on the bottom of the inside of the can and over the lid. Remember to bury the can low enough that the lid is below the frost line. You can cover the lid with lots of straw and a plastic tarp to waterproof it even more. Another idea is for the door; if built into a home or even the side of a hill, if you make it two pieces, opening the top only will prevent loss of a lot of cold, wet air from the bottom. You should have both a thermometer and a hygrometer (to measure humidity) to help keep an eye on the environment inside your root cellar. It also helps to dig a ventilation pipe to the outside and also conceal this to prevent any unwanted discovery of your root cellar. An earth or concrete floor and wooden shelves are ideal.

YEASTS: BREWERS, BAKERS, AND NUTRITIONAL

Yeasts have been used by mankind for thousands of years, to ferment sugars and produce alcohol as well as in baking to make breads rise when cooked (due to the release of carbon dioxide) and also as a whole food nutritional supplement.

The Difference between Yeast and Fungi

Both yeast and fungi belong to the fungal kingdom, as do molds and mushrooms, which are just the above ground "fruit" of a fungus. Yeasts are unicellular (one cell) organisms but sometimes develop into long chains of cells. Fungi also have cell walls that contain chitin, which is also found in the exoskeleton of many insects. The cell wall of fungi (pronounced fun-gee) is stiff and not pliable like the plasma membrane of human cells and is more like a

plant cell wall. Scientists originally thought that fungi were part of the plant kingdom, but now put them into their own kingdom like bacteria, animals, and plants. Fungi reproduce by spores, and yeast by division of their cells either sexually or asexually. People often confuse the two and often describe yeast infections as fungal and vice versa. Yeast infections such as candida, thrush, athlete's foot, jock itch, and ringworm have nothing to do with these types of yeasts and they cannot cause these type of infections.

Yeast for Fermentation

There are two kinds of yeast used for fermentation; baker's yeast, which makes dough rise and also produces sourdough bread, and brewer's yeast, which produces ethanol, the alcohol we drink.

Both brewer's and baker's yeast ferment sugars into alcohol (ethanol) and carbon dioxide, which either makes bubbles in drinks or causes bread to rise.

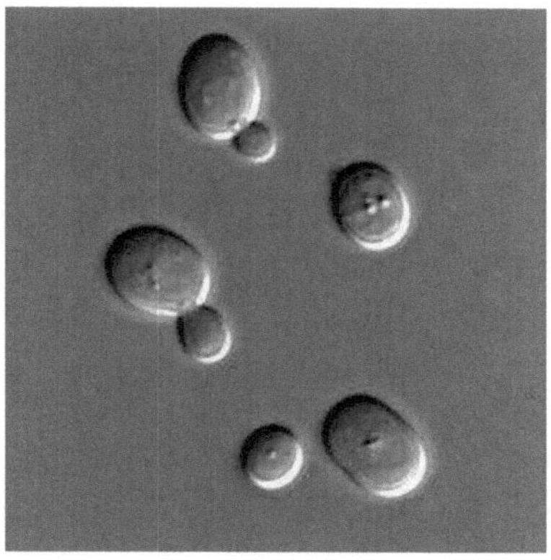

Microscopic photograph of Saccharomyces cerevisiae

Both brewer's and baker's yeasts come from Saccharomycescerevisiae, but from different strains of this fungus. You see, different strains of Saccharomyces c. produce varying amounts of carbon dioxide and alcohol. Baker's yeast is a mix of various strains of Saccharomyces c. that make more carbon dioxide, which is what you want to make your dough rise, and less alcohol. The different strains found in baker's yeast were also chosen for their flavor. The alcohol produced by baker's yeast evaporates during the cooking process. Sourdough bread is actually made by a different strain of yeast known as Lactobacillus Sanfrancisco. On the contrary, brewer's yeast is chosen for the opposite traits; that is, more alcohol and less carbon dioxide production. The flavor of brewer's yeast is also bitter. As you might have already guessed, brewer's yeast is made to brew homemade wine and beer.

You cannot use baker's yeast to produce alcoholic beverages nor can you use brewer yeast to make bread. There is a fungal probiotic made from the yeast Saccharomyces Boulardii which colonizes the intestines and becomes part of the normal probiotic population. The prescription probiotic known as Florastor is made of Saccharomyces Boulardii. Unlike bacterial probiotics, this fungal probiotic has tropical origins; it thus thrives at body temperature but is killed by cold and therefore cannot survive refrigeration and needs to be stored at room temperature.

Brewer's yeast has been pulverized and dried and is dead and considered inactive and therefore does not make carbon dioxide, baker's yeast has been dried (by a much lower temperature) and not pulverized, and is alive. That is why you cannot take it as a nutritional supplement. The process of cooking bread will kill off the baker's yeast; bread will therefore contain no living yeast.

Nutritional Content

Nutritional content is always improved by any type of fermentation. Cheese has more protein than milk, wine has a greater content of antioxidants than grape juice (Now there is a good excuse to drink more wine, not that many people need one.). The reason for the improved nutritional content of fermented foods is the amazing contribution of the bacteria or yeasts involved in the fermentation process. These wonderful microorganisms use their enzymes to convert sugars, starches, and cellulose into an entire array of vitamins, essential amino acids, fatty acids, and nucleic acids (from their RNA and DNA). When we are digesting them we kill off a significant number of these microorganisms and their body parts add to our nutrition, along with their enzymes and their nucleic acids, etc. This is all on top of the enzymatic conversion of the sugars they have already completed, so it is readily evident why the end product, like cheese, has more protein than the starting product, milk.

This once again goes back to the same argument I have been trying to drum into you, my readers, "whole natural foods, unprocessed, grown or raised organically without pesticides, herbicides, and fungicides, and fermented or prepared with as little processing as possible will result in nutritious, life- sustaining foods that are chock-full of vitamins, enzymes, essential amino acids, essential fatty acids, minerals, and trace elements." These types of foods will always trump man-made, inorganic, processed, and synthetic vitamins that your body has great difficulty recognizing as a food, and even more difficulty absorbing and assimilating for its many needs. If you add a natural, multi-mineral supplement either to the soil or take it orally, this will round out your nutrition and provide insurance against any mineral or trace element deficiencies that may exist in your soil.

You cannot use baker's yeast as a nutritional supplement, it can actually cause many deficiencies as it is alive and active and can colonize your intestines and continues to reproduce. Brewer's yeast on the other hand has a long history of medicinal use.

Brewer's yeast contains all the B vitamins (B complex) as well as many minerals including calcium, phosphorus, selenium, potassium, chromium, and iron. No yeast contains vitamin B12, which is made by bacteria, but some nutritional yeast supplements have B12 added to them. Brewer's yeast is a very rich source of chromium, unlike man-made. Chromium picoliniate, the form in this yeast, is very easy for your body to assimilate. Baker's yeast does not contain chromium. Chromium is very useful in helping the body better control its blood glucose levels. Brewer's yeast is also an excellent source of all of the essential amino acids, and is therefore an excellent source of protein.

Neither baker's nor brewer's yeast cause yeast infections such as thrush, candidiasis, and others. There are spreads made from brewer's yeast that are very popular in Australia, England, New Zealand, and other former British colonies. There are two main brands, Vegemite and Marmite. Vegemite was originally used to brew beer. Marmite is supplemented with vitamin B12 and sometimes sweetened. I had an Australian girlfriend in medical school who used to rave about Vegemite, telling me Aussies eat it like Americans eat peanut butter. Trust me; it is no peanut butter and definitely an acquired taste!

Nutritional yeast is different from both bakers and brewer's yeast. Nutritional yeast is yeast that has been grown in a growth medium that is enhanced with various vitamins and/or minerals that the yeast readily absorbs and is therefore available as a nutritional source that your body recognizes as food due to its microRNA content, and readily absorbs into your body at a much greater rate than inorganic minerals or vitamins. Nutritional yeasts contain all the B vitamins except B12, but many times this is added as a supplement to the other B vitamins produced by the yeast. Nutritional yeasts are heat-inactivated or killed in their manufacturing process, and are available either as extracts or flakes.

Nutritional yeast is also grown on molasses or sugar cane, which depending on the variety used, can become either sweet, nutty, or cheesy in flavor. You have to be careful with your intake of nutritional yeasts since greater than three tablespoons daily may cause gout by raising your uric acid levels.

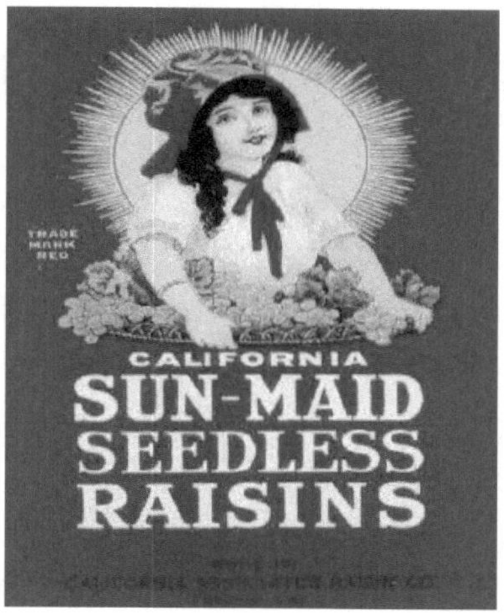

Ways to Make Your Own Yeast

Most fruits, grains, and vegetables have yeast naturally growing on their surfaces or skins. These same yeasts are responsible for the breakdown of the fruits, grains, and vegetables and, their rotting. It seems lately we can never be sure of a supply of any item and need to be ever resourceful and improvise whenever possible. Yeast is no exception, and we can exploit their presence on organically grown foods to find a ready supply for our various needs. Fermentation of foods and drinks will be necessary for you, not only for preservation but also to enhance flavor and nutritional content.

One easy way is to soak any organically grown fruits, grains, or vegetables (potatoes, for example) in the amount of water you will need for your baking. Wild yeasts like these will naturally separate from the surface of the plants when soaked and now are alive and active in the water/yeast mix. The reason I am emphasizing organically grown is because if fungicides are sprayed on these plants, it will kill the natural wild yeasts living on the plants' surfaces. Raisins and other dried fruits have been touted as excellent sources of these wild yeasts; you can also mix different plants together when soaking them to get a broader mix of wild yeasts.

Organic grains can be made into flour and soaked in water, put in a large ceramic crock or a glass container, and covered with a cheesecloth, placed in a cool corner of your basement and allowed to ferment. Depending on the conditions involved, this mix will, over time (sometimes as long as a week), begin to ferment and bubble as the carbon dioxide is produced by the wild yeasts, eventually causing this dough mix to rise.

Many different kinds of fruits can be used to make baker's yeast. These will also change the flavor of the bread somewhat, depending on the type and quantity used. There are three kinds of fruit that cannot be used: pineapples, papaya, and kiwi. The reason these three cannot be used is because they contain actinidain, a protease (protein-devouring) enzyme that will cause the dough to break down.

To use fruit, take a handful of unpeeled fruit and put it in a clean glass container and cover with a cheesecloth. You can add sugar, molasses, or honey if you want to speed up the process. Only fill the jar about three-fourths of the way to allow room for gas production, bubbling, etc. Keep an eye on it, just like with the dough mix. Taste it periodically if you are not sure.

EPIGENETICS

Until the last several years the overwhelming consensus among scientists and physicians had been that our genes determine much of our destiny and many illnesses were inherited from patients with "poor genes".

It was a very discouraging scenario for anyone with a disease that was considered genetic or gene-based and even autoimmune. Over the last several years an entire new paradigm has arisen, known as epigenetic. Epigenetics states that your genes have on and off switches, that are controlled by a combination of factors, mainly your diet and your environment and the toxins you are exposed to. One very important factor is what is known as microRNAs which are microscopic genetic material found in foods of plant and animal origin (not man-made foods) and also of viral origin. Genes are able to exert their influence by direct communication with the cells of your body; this process is known as gene expression. As it turns out, they appear to be in continual contact with an ongoing dialogue. Gene expression in turn is controlled by the microRNAs found in whole, nutritious, natural foods such as raw foods, organs, glands, and other animal and plant material. Supplements such as brewer's yeast and other whole food supplements that are made of organic, chemical-free plant and animal material are chock-full of microRNAs that send the right chemical messengers to your genes telling them to turn on certain genes and inhibit or shut off others. In addition, these are not "generalists" having general effects on the genes and in turn the body, but rather these microRNAs have specific targets such as the thyroid or the liver, etc.

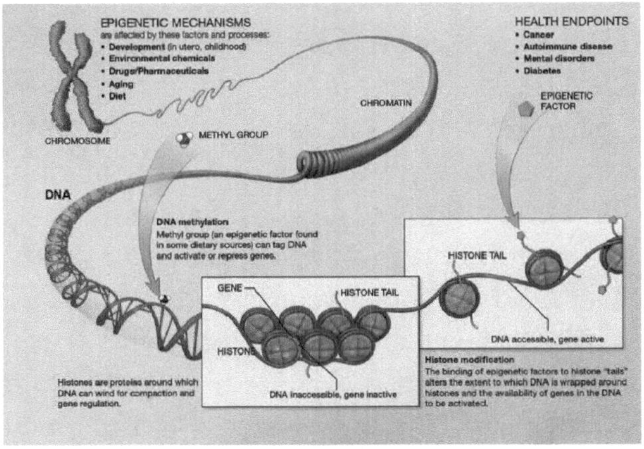

The National Institutes of Health (NIH), starting in 2007 and continuing until present day, has been doing amazing work on this topic and has made an entire host of new discoveries while studying the human microbiome, or the entire complement of probiotic bacteria and yeast that colonize our bodies, especially our intestines, and communicate constantly with our immune system as well as our DNA.

Why Epigenetics Is So Important

Epigenetics and the Human Microbiome Project have made it very clear that we need to eat whole, unprocessed, organic foods to maintain our health. These foods need to have the full complement of minerals and trace elements to do their job. Inorganic, processed, synthetic, and man-made vitamins and supplements can never compete with whole foods and supplements made from them because of their utter lack of microRNAs and therefore their inability to carry on a conversation with your genes and exert positive epigenetic effects upon your DNA. When your DNA is left without this vital communication, it has no choice but to shut down certain processes and turn on others, leading to the chronic disease states that modern man is afflicted with such as obesity, hypertension, autoimmune diseases, and diabetes to name but a few. For this reason, we need to nourish our bodies with raw, fermented, or correctly prepared foods to provide ourselves with the microRNAs our genes need to maintain healthy bodies. This is the only way we will remain vibrant and strong and avoid all the degenerative diseases of previous generations and be able to not only survive but to flourish!

PART TWO

SOME ESSENTIAL TOOLS

CHAPTER SIX

BAKING SODA (SODIUM BICARBONATE)

INTRODUCTION

TABLE OF CONTENTS:

You will discover that baking soda is an essential medicine for your alternative medicine chest for a myriad of reasons that I will go into shortly. What is sodium bicarbonate? It is derived from the mineral natron and is found in nature dissolved in many mineral-rich springs. It has a long history of many medicinal uses as well as household uses.

pH AND YOUR BODY'S HEALTH

It is an alkaline material that helps raise the body's pH. This more alkaline environment is much less receptive to all types of infections including bacterial, fungal, and viral, as well as cancers. The typical American diet results in a chronic low-grade metabolic acidosis. The ideal pH for human blood is 7.4. This is just slightly alkaline. (See the section on Epsom Salt and alkaline minerals for a full explanation on pH and how it works).

The body works to maintain this pH in the proper range and will buffer either a low pH (acid) or a high pH (alkaline) by extracting either acid or alkaline minerals from bone, body fluid, saliva, and soft tissues. Since our bodies have become progressively more acidic over time, sodium bicarbonate has become vital to our bodies' efforts to maintain homeostasis (optimal balance).

If you are going to check your pH with a pH strip, I recommend using saliva. Saliva is more accurate for the measurement of pH than urine. Urine tends to be acidic due to the nature of the waste acids that are excreted in it by the kidney, hence less reliable than saliva. The best way to take salivary pH is either one hour before a meal or two hours after. Take your salivary pH several times a day and average the values.

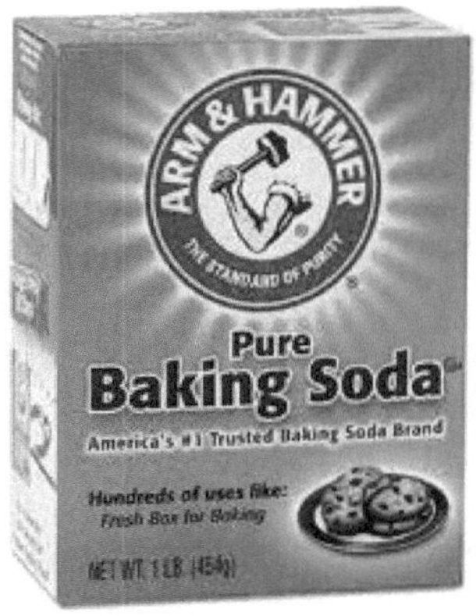

HOW DOES BAKING SODA WORK?

The chemical formula for sodium bicarbonate is NaHCO3. Once it dissolves in water it breaks off the Na ion, which is positively charged, and is the body's major cation (positively charge ion) in the extracellular (outside the cell) fluid. The Hco3 part is bicarbonate, which is a normal part of the body's fluids and is essential to maintaining the correct pH in humans due to its buffering action on acids. The Arm & Hammer baking soda that we all grew up with is a perfect example of sodium bicarbonate.

What you vitally need to understand is that a sick body is almost always acidic. A lowering of pH or metabolic acidosis in the body causes oxygen levels to drop (by moving the oxygen dissociation curve) this drop in oxygen leaves us tired, rundown, and fatigued. It also creates a very receptive environment for molds, fungal infections, parasites, bacterial and viral infections, and cancers.

Magnesium and calcium are leached from your body as it utilizes these two positively charged ions to buffer and neutralize the acid load. This increased acidity will therefore lower both Mg and Ca, which are two of the most vital minerals in your body. As the pH drops and the body becomes more acidic, it will also accelerate its aging.

A major source of acid from by-products of metabolism is from our high consumption of proteins. This acidity, combined with the epidemic lack of minerals and trace elements in our diet from food grown on depleted soils, is a perfect storm for poor health.

Has anyone sat up and looked around at our families? Despite huge increases in household income and wealth over the last three generations and the resulting explosion of food choices, we are becoming a progressively sicker population. Look at the epidemics raging among our offspring (not even touching on the subject of widespread infertility) such as the skyrocketing rates of autism, ADHD, depression, bipolar disorder, anxiety, diabetes, obesity, hypertension, degenerative arthritic conditions, allergies, asthma, and especially cancers.

ENZYMES AND THE WORK OF DR. POTTENGER

All of this was predicted many years ago by the work of a little known dentist in California named Dr. Pottenger. In a nutshell, he studied a large group of cats over many generations. He divided the cats into two groups; one was given cooked, processed foods and pasteurized milk, while the other was given a raw food diet and raw milk.

The cooking and processing of foods destroyed all of the enzyme content and many of the vitamins and minerals, which was not the case with the raw food group. Over the course of several generations the cooked food group became progressively sicker and developed skeletal abnormalities and all of the chronic diseases that Americans currently suffer from such as hypertension, arthritis, and diabetes, to name but a few. By the fourth generation the cooked food group was so sick that they were becoming increasingly infertile with reproduction rates falling through the floor and the experiment had to be discontinued!

Does this sound vaguely familiar? Does anyone know a family that is spared from any of the above ailments? In your own experience, have you seen any families getting collectively healthier over generations with increasing vigor and fertility? I certainly have not, in my over twenty-five years of medical practice I have watched children from each generation with more illnesses, more allergies, more infertility, more obesity, more mental illness -- not less. This is shocking to most folks unless you read the works of nutritional pioneers such as Dr. Pottenger and Dr. Weston Price and their fascinating studies that were done all over the world.

Dr Price studied the facial and dental structure of primitive tribes eating natural foods and followed them as they were exposed to western diets. He documented his work with amazing photos of beautiful natives with perfectly aligned teeth and wide smiles, contrasted with crowded teeth and narrow jaw and facial structure, demonstrating the structural changes a poor diet has on previously healthy villagers.

The use of chemical fertilizers primarily since WWII has resulted in a devastation of our most valuable resource...our soils. They are now seriously depleted of most minerals and most trace elements. From poor soils come poor foods...plain and simple. You cannot grow strong and disease-resistant plants without these essential minerals and trace elements in healthy soil that is teeming with microbes! The result is sickly plants that unfortunately can only be grown in pesticide-soaked soils, with chemical fertilizers. Plants grown in this manner are loaded with these toxins and this contributes significantly to the flood of toxins that our bodies have to handle. Our bodies tend to store these toxins in fat, leading to one of the other contributors of our current obesity epidemic (one of many). The toxin obesity connection would require another book to properly explain.

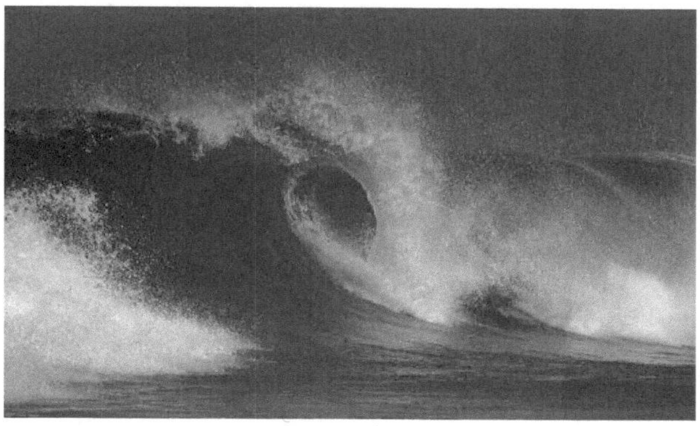

Our human evolution is a story that begins in the world's oceans. These same oceans are alkaline and contain bicarbonate ions, iodine, and high concentrations of calcium and magnesium. These are all things we need to maintain good health. Human blood is alkaline and is quite similar to ocean water in its composition. At no time was that more evident than during WWII when desperate United States Navy doctors used clean seawater as a substitute for blood serum when they ran out of supplies. That does not mean that you can drink seawater in place of fresh water. However, in a survival situation like on a life raft, if your fresh water supplies are dangerously diminished you can dilute it with one part seawater to four parts fresh in order to make it last longer (in a last ditch effort at survival).

Giving sodium bicarbonate to pregnant women, the elderly, children, or patients with renal disease should be done cautiously, at a maximum of half of the ordinary dose. There are definite dangers of prolonged high alkalinity and this can be just as fatal as severe acidosis and should be carefully avoided. High alkaline levels could result in headaches, muscle twitching, nausea, vomiting, confusion, irritability, and muscle spasms similar to tetany. Tetany is the severe involuntary contraction of muscles.

People with high blood pressure who are on salt-restricted diets should also be careful due to the high sodium content of baking soda. Common table salt is also known as sodium chloride; this is the culprit in many patients with hypertension or high blood pressure, since it draws fluid into the blood vessels and causes an increase in the blood's volume. The heart and blood vessels are essentially a closed system, so any increase in volume will exert increased pressure on the blood vessel wall.

MEDICAL USES OF SODIUM BICARBONATE

Gastrointestinal (GI) Problems

Sodium bicarbonate is very useful in treating stomach acid problems such as gastritis and peptic ulcer disease.

Gastritis means inflammation of your stomach lining. Think about it, the stomach is a gastric pit with a pH that can fall as low as 2. This gastric acid pit is able to dissolve meats, yet it does not dissolve itself...why? The reason is the lining of the stomach secretes a mucous film filled with sodium bicarbonate that helps protect its own cells from the acid produced by other cells in the stomach. Sodium bicarbonate is a very strong base or alkaline solution...the opposite of an acid. It effectively neutralizes the stomach acid before it reaches the wall of the stomach. When this does not happen, the acid eats away and irritates the stomach lining and leads to gastritis. When this is long lasting and severe it will erode a hole in the lining, which is an ulcer.

There are many opportunities for treating various conditions with a simple, inexpensive substance such as sodium bicarbonate. It can effectively replace many of the medications you currently use, such as the H2 blockers and the Proton Pump Inhibitors that many people currently take such as Pepcid, Zantac, Prilosec, Protonix, Prevacid, etc. This is a safe and effective way to raise the pH of your stomach and your entire body.

Remember, pH is the way an acid/base balance is measured in your body. A pH of 7 is neutral (water), anything lower than 7 is acidic; anything higher is alkaline or basic. Since the stomach pH is very low because of the acid it is secreting...and if there is a problem such as gastritis or even ulcers...then we need to raise that pH in order to allow healing.

NOTE: Do not take sodium bicarbonate if the powder is not fully dissolved, and never take it when your stomach is full of food and you are bloated. It has the potential to release gases and rupture your intestines.

How To Take Sodium Bicarbonate Orally

When taking sodium bicarbonate for an upset stomach, it should be spaced out approximately every six hours, and only taken as needed. To make your treatment solution, take one teaspoon of baking soda and mix it in a full glass of water. Maximum dose would be around four teaspoons in twenty-four hours. Do not take it for more than two weeks at this maximum dose; at half that dose or less you can take it indefinitely. That being said, if you are taking it long-term I would monitor your urine pH at least once a week.

You need to be careful because too much of a change in pH in either direction is dangerous. Over alkalinizing by raising pH with baking soda is very dangerous and should be avoided. Low dose sodium bicarbonate intake is very well tolerated and is not only non-toxic, but very beneficial to your body.

Your body's most healthy state is an alkaline one, rather than acidic. Our modern diets are very acidic, as is our environment which is burdened by the addition of acidic, man-made toxins being dumped continuously into our air and water supply.

When your body is acidic it makes toxin removal much more difficult. This all works to compound the problems with which your body must cope. If you are able to alkalinize your body it will greatly facilitate its detoxification.

Another useful tip is if you are taking your sodium bicarbonate once daily, the ideal time is right before bed. Your body is most acidic at night as it processes your daily production of waste products, and choosing that time to alkalinize will reap the most benefit.

Toothpaste

Let me stress one thing to you, there is no good health when you have bad teeth. Rotten teeth and sick gums are never found in a healthy person. Cavities and gum disease lead to colonization of your mouth by pathogenic (disease-causing) bacteria that spread throughout your body and act as a source for further infections that can enter your GI tract, other tissues, and even directly into your blood, causing blood poisoning, or sepsis.

Always take the time to maintain your oral health; even if you have to use a piece of rag in place of a toothbrush, it is better than nothing. In a pinch you can even take a small branch with a quarter of an inch diameter and chew one end, making it frayed, then use the frayed end as a toothbrush.

You can make an effective toothpaste by just mixing baking soda with water until you have a paste-like consistency, and then apply it directly to your teeth and gums and rub it in thoroughly and rinse it out with fresh water. Another variation is to mix six parts baking soda to one part sea salt and add some water until you have the paste and then rub it in as directed. Baking soda will also help whiten your teeth.

Another variation is to make an oral rinse using baking soda. It is currently used in many mouthwashes. It will deodorize your mouth (and also your breath), and neutralize acids that damage your teeth's enamel. It will also act as an antiseptic, preventing bacterial, fungal, and viral infections in your mouth and upper throat.

Treatment of Sunburn and Other Burns

Add some baking soda to water and then soak a piece of cloth with it and make a cool compress that you can apply directly to any burned area.

An alternative method is to soak in a bathtub with baking soda dissolved into it. Mix a half cup of baking soda into lukewarm water. When you emerge from the tub, air dry, do not towel dry. The friction of the towel on your burnt skin will not help.

Treatment of Various Skin Conditions

Sodium bicarbonate is very useful for us, especially when it comes to the treatment of almost every type of skin ailment, skin conditions as diverse as psoriasis, eczema, skin irritation, chafing, insect bites, poison oak, poison sumac, and poison ivy. You can treat skin conditions in various ways. You can soak in a bath similar to the burn treatment described above. Or you can make a cold compress just like for a burn. A paste can be made by mixing three parts baking soda to one part water. If the poison ivy is severe (trust me, I know all too well about severe poison ivy) then I suggest making a paste and covering it with a cold compress and leaving it overnight. Urushiol is the oil that is found in the leaves, stems, and roots of all poison ivy, poison oak, and poison sumacs; it is what causes the allergic reaction to these plants. This oil needs to be removed from the skin in order to stop the irritation. These plants have three leaves and hence the very useful saying…"Leaves of three let it be". Touching any part of the plant can lead to a skin irritation.

In Connecticut where I live, patients frequently come into my office with poison ivy in the middle of winter. Usually it is from touching firewood that has remnants of poison ivy stems connected to the bark; the dead giveaway that it is poison ivy is hairy roots. Poison ivy roots are covered with thousands of small root suckers that help anchor it to trees. If you see a hairy- looking root on a tree, let it be. I highly recommend a cleansing solution for your medicine chest called Technu. It can be bought in many garden centers and pharmacies. As soon as you feel any irritation developing, or if you think you might have been exposed, use this to remove the urushiol oil and prevent the poison ivy from developing. I would keep several bottles of it handy if you or your family has a problem with poison ivy and sumac in the east and poison oak in the west. Another useful trick for treating insect bites that my late father in law, Charlie Insalaco, taught me is to put some lemon juice on them, which quickly takes the sting and the pain out. I keep one of those plastic lemons in the refrigerator for just such emergencies. As fate would have it, as I was writing this section I took a break and took a nice long swim in my pool. As I was emerging from the pool I noticed a large white-faced hornet drowning. Like a total idiot I felt compassion for this little bastard and tried to scoop him out of the pool to save him, needless to say I was rewarded with a vicious sting to the palm of my hand.

The pain was immediate and severe. I ran in the house and put some cold lemon juice on it and within seconds it was as if I was never stung; it is simply amazing how well this trick works. Alternatively you can soak in a bath with several cups of sodium bicarbonate dissolved in it.

Deodorant

To make your own deodorant, mix a small amount of baking soda and water together and apply it to your armpits daily. This will help kill many of the bacteria that lead to underarm odor, and is not irritating to your skin.

Armpits and skin folds are also frequent sites of fungal infections, especially in the summer months. Since baking soda is strongly alkaline it will kill most fungal infections on contact. An even stronger antifungal can be made by taking some Borax and mixing it with water and rubbing it into any topical fungal infection. Sprinkled in shoes or boots, baking soda is a wonderful natural deodorizer.

Splinter Removal

Splinters are a common problem that you will encounter, they occur not only in fingers but also commonly in your toes. I know this from personal experience due to my love of walking barefoot. Here is how to get rid of them. Take a tablespoon of baking soda and mix it in water. Soak the area with the splinter in this mixture twice daily. After a few days even deep splinters will work their way to the surface, where you can get them easily.

Diarrhea, Vomiting, And Fluid Loss

In these situations not only is rehydration (getting your fluid levels up to normal in your body) very important, there is also your mineral and salt losses to consider. To replace those lost minerals you can use a good colloidal mineral mix, which you can make yourself with Azomite. Azomite stands for A to Z minerals and trace elements. It is mined from an ancient sea bed in Utah that had dried up long ago. Azomite will replenish all those minerals lost as well as all your trace elements. It is also great to mix into your vegetable garden soil to remineralize and replace any mineral and trace element deficiencies.

You will also need some sodium bicarbonate. The best mixture for replenishing gastrointestinal (GI) fluid and mineral losses is to make a mixture of the following: To each quart of boiled water you must add the following:

1. One level teaspoon of table salt
2. One rounded teaspoon of baking soda
3. Four rounded teaspoons of sugar.

Stir this mix until clear and then flavor with whatever you have available: Kool Aid, Gatorade powder, molasses, agave syrup, etc. (Taken from *Baking Soda: Over 500 Uses,* Vicki Lansky, 2004)

Potassium is also a primary electrolyte lost with diarrhea. Bananas are a wonderful source of potassium as are beans, potatoes, squash, yogurt, avocadoes, citrus fruits, dark green leafy vegetables, tomatoes, coconut water, all dried fruits such as prunes, dates, raisins, dried cherries, and dried cranberries, as well as others, are excellent sources of potassium.

Remember, potassium, magnesium, and calcium are all alkaline minerals and as such will help to raise the pH of the body, or alkalinize it. Refer to the sections on diarrhea and dehydration for full details on how to treat both of these common conditions.

Sore Throat

Melt one aspirin (325 mg) in two teaspoons of hot water, add a level teaspoon of baking soda and an additional half cup of hot water, and mix it gently. Gargle with this mixture; the aspirin will act as a painkiller and soak into the tissues of the throat giving you pain relief, the sodium bicarbonate has antifungal, antibacterial, and antiviral properties and will also soothe the throat.

Alternately, you can use the following mix: mix equal parts of baking soda, brown sugar, and salt in a glass, add water, and gargle. My personal favorite that I have used for over twenty-five years in my practice without problems is the following: Mix half a glass of hydrogen peroxide (3 percent commonly found in your bathroom cabinet) with half a glass of water and gargle it deeply and spit it out four times or more a day; if you swallow a little it is not the end of the world. (See chapter on uses of hydrogen peroxide.)

As a little side note: Alka-Seltzer can be used to make a nice effervescent drink which can also be used as an antacid; Alka-Seltzer is sodium bicarbonate and aspirin.

Another alternative treatment for sore throat is the following mix:

Mix in one glass: one tablespoon of vinegar
half teaspoon of sugar
half teaspoon of baking soda:
all this mixed in a half cup of water.

Vaginal and Anal Infections and Irritations

Prepare a douche with a mixture of two tablespoons of baking soda to one quart of warm water and douche two or more times a day for relief. It will also work for anal itching; lie on your stomach and reach back and spread the cheeks of your buttocks and gently pour a small quantity of this solution onto your anus; this can be done as often as you need it.

For rectal irritation and burning I have found nothing to work better than a barrier cream...whether that is Bag Balm, any diaper creams or my personal favorite Calmoseptine (which is a mix of zinc oxide and menthol). It is amazingly soothing on contact and alleviates burning and itching almost immediately. It will stain your clothes white, but it is worth it for the relief. Another good cream to help deep clean as well as soothe a rectal or perianal (around the anus) itch is Noxzema. It works very well to deep clean the anus even if you have a problem with hemorrhoids and the area is very sore.

Bladder and Urinary Tract Infections

These are very common, especially in sexually active females. That is why nature usually makes women want to urinate after sex; this allows them to flush out their urinary system and prevent UTIs (urinary tract infections) by literally washing the bacteria out. However, things happen and frequently women do have infections and need treatment. Hydration is key and should be part of any treatment of the urinary tract.

That being said, there are other modalities you can employ to also make the urinary tract less attractive to those hungry bugs. One way is to change the pH. All bacteria, fungi, and viruses live within a narrow pH and temperature range. Changing the pH either up to make it more alkaline or down to make it more acidic will frequently make life inhospitable for the various pathogens (bacteria, viruses, and fungi that attack the body) to survive, thus wiping out the infection.

For many years high dose ascorbic acid (vitamin C) was utilized to help acidify the urine, along with cranberry juice which actually contains a substance that prevents bacteria from sticking to the bladder and urinary tract walls. Another modality is to raise the pH; this can be done with baking soda. Mix baking soda (one or two teaspoons) in a tall glass of water and hydrate yourself with that mix until the symptoms subside.

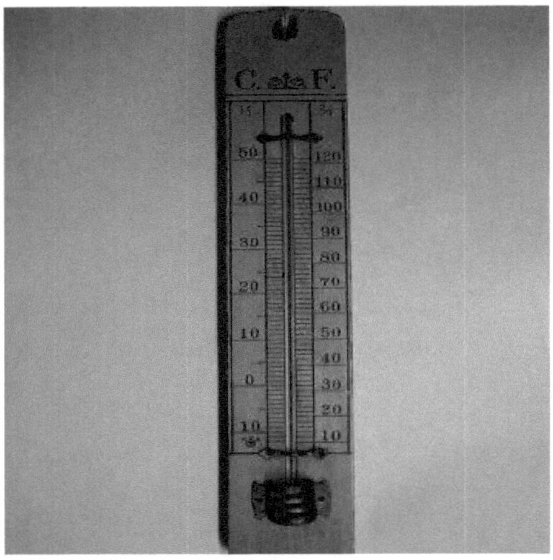

Fever is Your Friend

Fever is one of the body's primary tools for killing off an infection. Your body basically raises its core temperature and cooks these germs. Remember, your body is exquisitely designed and does nothing by accident; it is defending itself with a fever. Unless a fever is above 103 F try never to give anything that will lower it; in effect by lowering it you are prolonging your illness, not helping it.

THE WORK OF DR. MARC SIRCIUS

One of the absolute masters of the use of sodium bicarbonate is Dr. Marc Sircius. He is the director of the International Medical Veritas Association. Veritas is Latin for truth. He also wrote a great book on all of the multiple benefits obtained from the daily use of sodium bicarbonate. I highly recommend his books to anyone looking for a much more in-depth analysis on this subject.

He touts the use of iodine, selenium, magnesium, and sodium bicarbonate, among others, as daily requirements to maintain good health, all of which almost every cell of the body requires for optimal performance.

He notes that sodium bicarbonate acts as a powerful, natural, and safe antifungal, but when combined with iodine it enhances its antimicrobial effect enough to cover almost the entire spectrum of microbial organisms. Sodium bicarbonate at concentrations of 5 percent (one part sodium bicarb to nineteen parts water) would be effective in a 99.99% reduction in viral titers on surfaces with a contact time of one minute.

Sodium Bicarbonate and Cancer

He even covers a very controversial topic of cancer being a fungus and the usefulness of sodium bicarbonate to eradicate cancers. Most of this work was done by a very pioneering Italian physician named Dr. Tullio Simoncini.

Dr. Simoncini has done amazing work with cancer patients and has written a very interesting text on the subject called *Cancer is a Fungus: A Revolution in Tumor Therapy*. I highly recommend it as further reading to anyone interested in this fascinating cancer treatment. Dr. Sircius does not believe that sodium bicarbonate is a cure for cancer, but he does feel that every cancer patient should be taking it. His reasoning for the use of the combination of baking soda with magnesium is fascinating. Magnesium and sodium bicarbonate work together by their complementary actions in the cell. Magnesium acts as a cotransporter of sodium bicarbonate into the cell (they combine and carry each other into the cell) and the bicarbonate then returns the favor and acts as a cotransporter of magnesium into the mitochondria. Mitochondria are the power-producing organelles within human cells, inherited from your mother. The mitochondria then do their job and produce the ATP molecule that our bodies utilize as an energy source.

OTHER BENEFICIAL EFFECTS OF SODIUM BICARBONATE

1. Increasing pH (making you more alkaline) will help the body's immune system kill off bacteria.
2. PH controls the speed of our body's biochemical reactions. pH is responsible for rate control in enzyme reactions in our body as well as the speed of electrical conduction of nerve impulses. Even our mitochondria (the cell powerhouses) suffer under acidic conditions. Enzymes work ideally in a narrow pH range; this is because changes in pH change the way chemical bonds function.
3. Sodium bicarbonate is effective in treating poisonings, chemical exposures, and even overdoses of pharmaceuticals,by canceling out the cardiotoxic (heart-damaging) and neurotoxin damaging nerves) effect. Most of the body's waste and toxins are acids, thus your body needs to combine them with alkaline buffers like sodium bicarbonate in order to neutralize them and excrete them. An increasing acid load lowers the pH and leads to many of the degenerative diseases that Americans currently suffer with such as reflux, kidney stones, diabetes, hypertension, cancer, gout, and heart disease, to name a few. Sodium bicarbonate is capable of absorbing heavy metals and toxins such as dioxins and PCBs (polychlorinated biphenyls). Most patients have dioxins in their body's tissues. These accumulate over a lifetime and persist in people even without continued exposure. Dioxins are known carcinogens, or cancer-causing agents, and greater exposure translates to greater risk of developing cancer and other health problems. Sick patients often have elevated levels of these and other toxins in their tissues since we are constantly exposed to toxins that have entered our waters and our food chain.
4. Sodium bicarbonate is also effective in radiation damage. It will help prevent radiation damage to the kidneys. Currently the United States Army is using it for this to protect its troops.
5. Sodium bicarbonate also helps treat radiation-exposed soils to neutralize the damage, where it can be mixed with the top two or three inches of soil where it has been found to bind up radioactive particles for removal and remediation of the soil. At Los Alamos National laboratory in New Mexico, researcher Don York has used baking soda to clean soil contaminated

with radioactive uranium. He has shown that sodium bicarbonate binds with this uranium, enabling him to separate it from the soil. Using this method he was able to remove approximately 92 percent of the uranium from contaminated soils.

6. Hay fever and chemical and food allergies are also improved with alkalinization of your body with sodium bicarbonate.
7. Headaches and pain relief: Sodium bicarbonate has potent analgesic (pain relieving) properties. Take one teaspoon dissolved in a glass of water. It works very well for migraine headache relief. Migraines are frequently caused by neck pain, sinus and allergy problems, and magnesium deficiency. When taking any medication for a migraine (I highly recommend Excedrin: which is Tylenol, aspirin, and caffeine) Take it immediately, as soon as you feel the headache starting. Most migraineurs learn this eventually; migraines, once they start, cannot be ignored, they always worsen until you are down and vomiting and clutching your throbbing head. Ice packs or anything cold you can apply to your forehead and top of your neck where it meets the base of your skull will help. A dark, quiet area will also help.
8. Earwax: A mixture of sodium bicarbonate and warm water when flushed into the ear gently with a turkey baster or something similar will dissolve and dislodge the wax blocking your ear. Do this several times until it opens up. Some people use some warm mineral oil to get the same result.
9. Constipation and colitis symptoms have been known to improve with the use of sodium bicarbonate enemas. Mix a half a cup of sodium bicarbonate in a quart of warm water and put it in an enema bag and instill it into your colon. This will act as a natural cleanser and help any bowel irritations as well. I also highly recommend Epsom salt orally for constipation, see the section on Epsom salt for complete details.

CHAPTER SEVEN

DMSO: DIMETHYL SULFOXIDE

INTRODUCTION

TABLE OF CONTENTS:

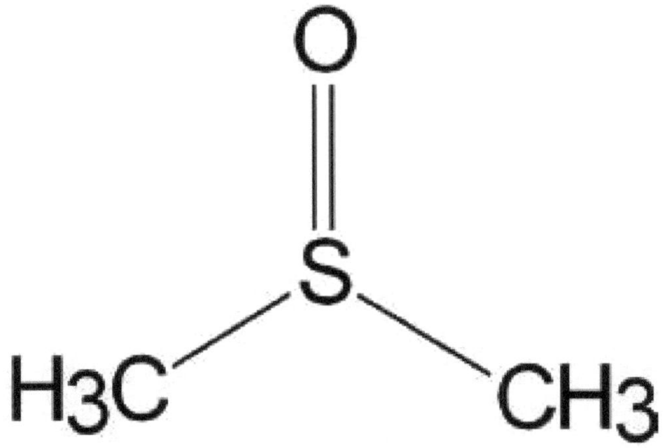

DMSO is a by-product of the wood industry, but its use as a medicine dates back to the early 1960s. At that time it was discovered that it was capable of crossing the skin and other membranes without causing any damage. It was not long before it was noted that it could carry other compounds as well as increasing their absorption through the skin; hence its use in transdermal (crossing the skin) delivery of drugs into the body.

It is essential to our natural medicine chest because of its multiple and varied uses. Even though it is not natural and is a chemical byproduct it still has wonderful use as an alternative to prescription medications.

There is an excellent book covering all its uses by Dr. Morton Walker called *DMSO Natures Healer*. He states that in the pharmaceutical and medical literature DMSO is declared to have the widest range and greatest number of therapeutic actions ever shown for any single chemical.

HOW DMSO WORKS

Here is a partial list of some of its amazing uses: It works to block pain by interrupting its conduction in the small c fibers.

1. It is anti-inflammatory.
2. It is bacteriostatic, fungistatic and virostatic. This means it inhibits the growth of bacteria, fungi, and viruses.
3. It helps carry other pharmaceuticals across membranes and especially the skin.
4. It decreases platelet thrombi (clot formation) in blood vessels.
5. It affects cardiac contractility, hence reducing the workload on the heart.
6. Simply rubbed into the skin it acts as a tranquilizer.
7. When combined with antifungal and antibacterial medicines, it enhances their activity.
8. It stimulates the immune system.
9. It is a potent diuretic, especially when given IV.
10. It helps stimulate interferon formation (helps with immunity).It helps wound healing.
11. Rubbed on painful areas of your head, it will rapidly relieve a headache.

CAUTION WITH FAIR SKIN, BLONDE OR RED HAIR

A Note of Caution: If you have fair skin, especially those with blonde or red hair and blue eyes, you may be more sensitive to DMSO than the general population. In these cases you should cut the concentration of DMSO in half. Also use 50 percent less of DMSO, especially around your face or neck. Also, there are no studies of the use of DMSO in pregnant women or very young children.

WHY THERE ARE NO ALLERGIES TO DMSO

Sulfa allergies: This is absolutely not a problem with DMSO. Believe me, I am very allergic to sulfa-containing antibiotics (Bactrim, for example) and have no problems with DMSO. You cannot be allergic to the mineral sulfur because it has no protein component, unlike the antibiotics or the sulfites used to preserve wines or other foods. Sulfur compounds are found in all body cells and are indispensable for life. They are essential for many chemical reactions and also are critical in the detoxification of harmful toxins.

THE IMPORTANCE OF DMSO

As you can see from the above list, for our purposes it is essential. It is cheap and readily available on the Internet through either eBay or others. You can easily find it in its almost pure state (liquid) as well as gels or creams mixed with aloe vera. It is also used extensively by veterinarians on horses, as my wife can attest to; it works wonderfully (on her horse). The veterinarian preparations are also quite cheap and readily available. It is also available at Tractor Supply.

THE SMELL AND CAUTION OF TRANSPORT OF UNWANTED SUBSTANCES ACROSS THE SKIN

The major downside, in fact the only significant one, is its foul odor. It smells something like a crushed garlic clove, but if you are in pain, that might be a minor nuisance, especially if you are injured or in significant pain. The body odor you may have from it can be weakened by drinking large amounts of water.

Given the large number of people addicted to opiates one can readily see the critical need for replacements for pain treatment and given the multiple other uses of DMSO besides pain, it will indeed be indispensable.

Another important fact is that DMSO will carry any impurities on your skin across it into your blood. So, always clean the area being treated before applying it. After topical application DMSO will almost instantaneously give a warm sensation to your skin.

You may also taste a faintly garlic flavor in your mouth, also attesting to its almost instant absorption. It will not only absorb across your skin into your blood, it is also one of the few substances that will cross the blood-brain barrier. This is how your body keeps substances from entering the brain; it is a very selective barrier that few substances can cross.

This might be how DMSO works for headaches. Applied topically, apparently it works within minutes to alleviate severe headaches. It can be applied to hairy areas like the scalp as well as to around the eyes without any problems. For headaches, whether they are sinus headaches or migraines, you simply rub some of the solution over the painful area. You may repeat this in several hours if it returns.

A good thing to know is that DMSO has an almost indefinite shelf life in the pure form. I would recommend always keeping it in a cool place away from heat and sunlight just as an added precaution. That is a good general rule for many substances.

USES FOR DMSO: SPRAINS, MUSCLE PULLS, BACK AND JOINT DISCOMFORT

For these, naturally a topical preparation is best. When applied directly to the sore muscles and joints you should feel a positive response within five to twenty minutes and will last from four to six hours depending on the severity of the injury.

You can then reapply it. Remember, you might feel a tingling warm sensation at the injury site. Mix a 70 percent solution of DMSO (and distilled water) in a volume of 8 to 12 ml. Applying this to a wide area around the injured area at least three times a day will provide a major reduction in swelling and pain.

Apply it with some cotton balls. When solutions of DMSO are 60 percent or better, then there will probably be some redness and slight irritation to the area of application. There might be some hives for a short time. These go away and are nothing to worry about. Your muscle pain is now gone and you traded it for a little transient skin irritation. Suck it up, don't be a wimp!

How To Make Your Own Distilled Water

Distilled water is simply water you have purified by boiling it and then condensing the steam or water vapor. Any water can be made into distilled water. You can use sea water, well water, stream or lake water, tap water, or any other water (you get the idea). Boil it, cool the vapor and voila, you have purified water.

Rainwater and snow are two natural types of distilled water, since they have already evaporated and then condensed in clouds and have come down as either snow or rain.

The simplest method is to collect either one (won't work if you live in a polluted city environment). In a clean container and let it sit for two days or so. This should allow any impurities to settle, and then pour off your distilled water into a clean or sterile container and it should store indefinitely. **NOTE:** If you are not sure about the quality of the rainwater or snow where you live, then you can take the added steps of either pouring the distilled water through a coffee filter or if you are really unsure you can boil it.

There are various methods of making your own distilled water. One of the simplest is to take a large steel pot and fill it half way with water. Float a glass bowl in this water; it should not touch the bottom of the steel pot. Or you can place it on an oven rack to support it. Take the lid to the steel pot and invert it (turn it upside down) and place it on top of the steel pot. If you have ice, fill this lid with ice. The ice will help keep the lid cool and aid in the condensation from its underside. Now boil the water in the steel pot, if the glass bowl starts to boil, lower the heat, the water in the glass bowl cannot boil or this will not work. The water that is boiled off into steam will condense on the underside of the inverted cool lid and drip into the glass bowl. That water is your distilled water.

Home distillation kits are also available, and these can be easily found on the Internet. If you are so inclined you should purchase one a.s.a.p.

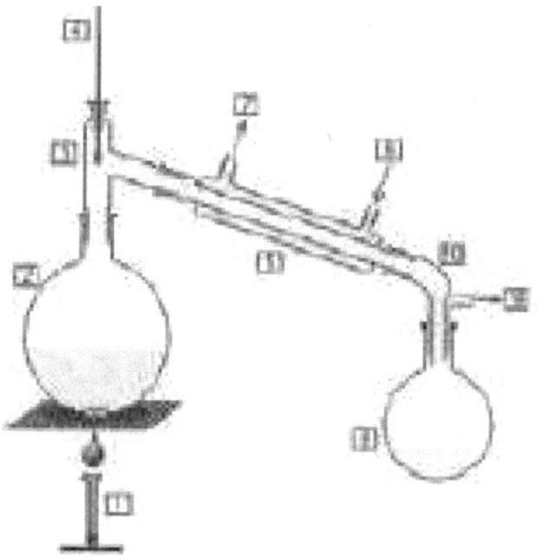

Simple Diagram for Setup to Distill Water

In this illustration, number 4 is a thermometer; 5 is a condenser with cold water going in 6 and out 7; 8 is the distilled water, 9 is a vent, and 2 is your tap water.

Headaches Of All Types

Apply a dose of 20 ml of 50 percent DMSO twice a day to the painful area. **NOTE:** A 50 percent solution is made by taking 100 percent pure DMSO and combining it with distilled water, in this case 10 ml of each. Now you have diluted the 100 percent solution down to 50 percent.

If you wanted to make it 25 percent you would put 5 ml of the 100 percent and mix it with 15 ml of the distilled water. So your resulting mixture would be one part DMSO and 3 parts of distilled water.

Place a few drops directly in the nostrils to open your sinuses. For a headache apply it to the forehead and back of your neck.

Pearl of Wisdom: If you get a migraine or severe sinus headache, if you are able, it is best to lie down and apply something cold (ice pack, cold compresses....anything available) to both your neck and your forehead. Lie down and relax and keep warm. A quiet area is best. If you have any Excedrin take two as soon as you feel the headache come on. Don't be an optimist...learn what every migraine sufferer knows: Once they start they never get better...despite your hopes. Excedrin is a combination of aspirin, Tylenol, and caffeine and works very well for headaches. Either Excedrin or Excedrin Migraine, they are the same. Many headaches are associated with neck problems and the ice to the neck will help those immensely.

Sometimes certain positions will help your neck Strain as well. In my case I found that rolling up a small towel or pillow and hyperextending my neck (bending my head all the way back; bending your head forward is flexing it and backward is extending it) and placing the pillow behind my neck was very helpful. This of course depends on what type of neck injury you have.

You may also discover trigger points. These are very tender areas that will hurt when you touch them. These can be alleviated by applying direct pressure to the area and gently but firmly pressing them. You will feel these trigger points melt away. That is why sometimes holding your neck between your thumb and pointer finger will feel good giving you some momentary relief. This is just an exaggerated version of that squeezing.

CHAPTER EIGHT

EPSOM SALT, MAGNESIUM, ALKALINE MINERALS, ALKALINE WATER, AND THE HEALTH BENEFITS OF AN ALKALINE DIET

INTRODUCTION

TABLE OF CONTENTS:

Epsom salts are different from traditional salts in so far as it is a naturally occurring pure mineral compound of magnesium and sulfate. Epsom salts derive their name from a bitter salt spring located at Epsom in Surrey, England. Epsom salt is an essential tool in your alternative/natural medicine chest due to its multiple medicinal uses as well as its utility in your garden. Epsom salt can be used medicinally both internally and externally. Epsom salt is readily absorbed through the skin and has multiple uses medically. Epsom salt is very cheap and readily available, even at garden centers.

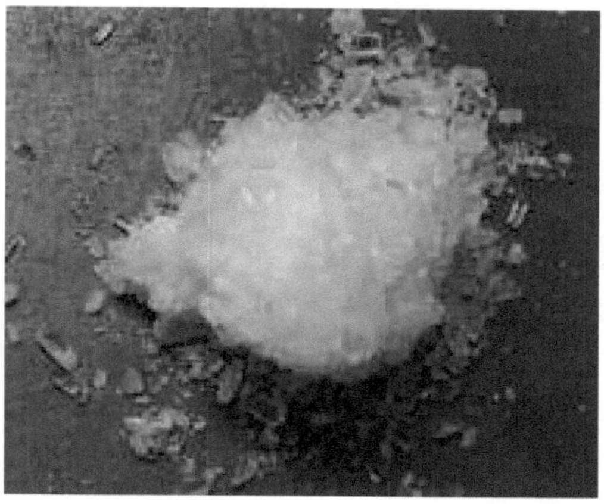

Photo of Magnesium Sulfate

HEALTH BENEFITS OF MAGNESIUM SUPPLEMENTATION

Many health experts say if there is one mineral you absolutely need for good health, it is magnesium. Magnesium is essential for the functioning of over 325 enzyme reactions in the body, helps lower blood pressure, treat and prevent migraine headaches, helps abnormal heart rhythms, helps relax constricted airways in asthma, decrease inflammation, pain, and helps sooth sore muscles an nerves. It also helps healing of cuts, acne, and psoriasis and quickly corrects constipation, and it works equally well for ADHD, insomnia, and restless leg syndrome (a movement disorder where you feel like your legs cannot stay still under your covers when you are in bed). Magnesium has also been shown to benefit pregnant women suffering from morning sickness! Studies have confirmed that most Americans are sadly deficient in magnesium and therefore would benefit from its supplementation.

The widespread deficiencies in the American population is secondary to a variety of factors including magnesium depletion in soils, poor diets, and use of excessive amounts of sugar, which further depletes magnesium levels.

HOW DOES EPSOM SALT WORK?

When applied to the skin via a hot bath or a poultice, the magnesium and sulfates in Epsom salts are readily absorbed through the skin and into the blood and distributed throughout the body. In the brain they will raise the level of serotonin in the same way Prozac and other antidepressants work, but by a different mechanism; this in turn helps elevate moods and leads to calm and relaxation. Magnesium given at bedtime will lead to a nice, deep, restful sleep. In the cells of the body magnesium helps increase ATP, which is the substance via which the cells produce energy. It will therefore increase energy, stamina, and endurance. Magnesium will help patients who are suffering with stress lower their high levels of adrenaline and thereby decrease the irritability induced by stress. In other words, magnesium helps you chill out and be calm.

HOW TO USE EPSOM SALT IN A BATH

Fill a bath tub with the hottest water you can stand without burning yourself and then stir in two or three cups of Epsom salt. You must remain in the water for at least a half hour to get the full effect. That is how long it takes for the magnesium sulfate to penetrate your skin and enter your blood.

NOTE: Be careful on exiting the tub, your legs will be very rubbery due to its relaxing effect. You will feel like you are Gumby! I would also do it right before bed, you will sleep like a baby. Sore feet can be soaked in a bucket with a half cup of Epsom salt, it will soothe aching feet just as it does other muscles. It will also remove foot odors and help athlete's foot. You can eliminate calluses by using a pumice stone after soaking your feet. Daily baths will also help lower blood pressure, help migraine headache and will help relieve the bronchospasm (tight airways) of asthma.

The same baths will also help eliminate harmful toxins from the body. It does this by a process known as reverse osmosis, where it actually draws these toxins out of your body through your skin. Any help we can give our overworked livers in detoxifying all of the dangerous toxins that we are constantly exposed to is a big plus for your health. Your body only has a few options for dealing with toxins. It can excrete them by various means such as urine, feces, sweat, and breathing. It can package them in lipids and store them, or it can detoxify them by various biochemical means in the liver.

The longer these toxins wreak their havoc on your body the more harm they will cause. Your body is also more efficient at functioning at its peak when you are well hydrated and well-nourished with the full spectrum of minerals and trace elements, vitamins, and plants chock-full of a whole array of phytonutrients for your body.

You also need to be alkaline. Acid is not your friend; it has to be excreted by your body just like a toxin, or it has to be neutralized. Either way, it is a problem that your body has to deal with. When your body is alkaline rather than acidic, its full complement of enzymes and chemical reactions will work optimally and your body will not have to lose calcium and other minerals in an attempt to help rectify its acidity.

HOW TO APPLY EPSOM SALT AS A POULTICE

First you need to fill a large container with Epsom salt and add water slowly to it until you have a paste-like consistency. Then soak a small towel or rag in it and wrap it around the muscle or area of the body that is inflamed from an injury. Leave it on overnight and remove it in the morning, or soak it for an hour or two.

HOW TO TAKE EPSOM SALT ORALLY

For Adults: Mix two to four level teaspoons of Epsom salt in 8 ounces of water. For children use half this dose for ages six to twelve. If no satisfactory bowel movements, repeat the dose in four hours. This will generally produce a very good bowel movement in thirty minutes to six hours. Do not take Epsom salt orally if the patient has stomach pain, nausea, or vomiting or if the person is under six years old. Also do not use it in someone with renal (kidney) failure. If several doses of it do not work, or if any rectal bleeding occur, discontinue its use. Do not use Epsom salt as a laxative for more than one week's time.

USING EPSOM SALT IN YOUR GARDEN

Epsom salts will help your garden by providing magnesium to plants. Chlorophyll is the substance that gives plants their green color. An interesting fact is that hemoglobin is the red pigment in blood that carries oxygen. Hemoglobin and chlorophyll are identical molecules, the only difference is that in hemoglobin the central element is iron and in chlorophyll the central element is magnesium. Just like hemoglobin is essential for the life blood of humans, so is chlorophyll for plants.

So, you can see how essential magnesium is for the life blood or chlorophyll of your plants.

If you see your plants' leaves fading yellow, this will help them. Mix two tablespoons of Epsom salt for every gallon of water you use. You can spray it on plants as an insecticide or water plants with it and this will help your plants absorb many of the minerals and fertilizers they need to properly grow. (I also recommend adding liberal amounts of rock dust and/or Azomite to your garden soils.)

Some gardeners recommend adding a half cup of Epsom salt for every 500 square feet of garden (a 25 ft. by 20 ft. garden for example). By mixing it in water and adding it to the soil in early spring, this will keep your soil nice and "sweet" or alkaline.

Some plants require more Epsom salt than others. Nut trees such as walnuts, hazelnuts, butternuts, pecans, and others use a significant amount of magnesium and thrive on its addition to their soil. Simply add two tablespoons at the base of each fruit or nut tree in spring and several times during the growing season. This will help them absorb other vital minerals and nutrients and increase their vigor and fruit set, with no harmful side effects. Some garden plants such as tomatoes and peppers will benefit from two tablespoons of Epsom salt added to each planting hole. You can also add it liberally by adding it to water at two tablespoons per gallon of water and either water the soil or putting it in a tank sprayer and spraying it on the plant leaves themselves through which it will be absorbed readily and utilized by the plants. Later in the growing season you may notice tomato or pepper leaves fading yellow and diminished fruit set; both can be improved by additional feedings.

MAGNESIUM OIL

Magnesium oil is supersaturated magnesium chloride in water. It is a wonderful way to get your magnesium by application to your skin. It is available on the internet in oil form or in flakes that can be reconstituted into oil. It can cause a burning sensation on your skin, and if this occurs simply mix it with a carrier oil to dilute it, or dilute it with more water. The tingling sensation usually only lasts about a half an hour, you could also wash it off after a half hour or so. Magnesium chloride is readily absorbed by the skin and thus is an easy way to raise your magnesium levels.

ALKALINE MINERALS/ALKALINE WATER

Minerals such as potassium, calcium, sodium, and magnesium are alkaline minerals and as such will raise the pH of the body and make it more alkaline or basic. A neutral pH is 7 which is the pH of water, levels below 7 are acids; the lower the number the stronger the acid. Levels greater than 7 are alkaline or bases, and as the numbers go up so does the strength of the base.

pH	Examples of solutions
0	Battery acid, strong hydrofluoric acid
1	Hydrochloric acid secreted by stomach lining
2	Lemon juice, gastric acid, vinegar
3	Grapefruit juice, orange juice, soda
4	Tomato juice, acid rain
5	Soft drinking water, black coffee
6	Urine, saliva
7	"Pure" water
8	Sea water
9	Baking soda
10	Great Salt Late, milk of magnesia
11	Ammonia solution
12	Soapy water
13	Bleach, oven cleaner
14	Liquid drain cleaner

Sometimes foods surprise you and are not what you would think. Lemons are a good example. A lemon is an acidic fruit but surprisingly has an alkalinizing effect in the body due to its high content of the alkaline minerals calcium, potassium, and magnesium. The point I want to drive home to my readers is that to maintain optimal health we need to do everything we can to make our bodies alkaline, taking alkaline mineral supplements or foods with high content is part of that plan. The alkaline minerals also work complementing one another; calcium and magnesium is such a pair. Calcium is required for muscle contraction and magnesium for relaxation; an imbalance between the two will lead to spasms, cramps, weakness, and other problems. The healthiest way to get any nutrient for your body is in foods or drink. It also is a lot more enjoyable than eating a handful of pills. It is no different with your alkalinizing minerals; they are best obtained from foods grown in mineral-rich soils without chemical fertilizers, pesticides, and other toxic exposure. Foods grown in soils enriched with rock dust or Azomite along with manure, compost, biochar, and rich in earthworms (which can by themselves produce tons of their enriched castings annually per acre!) will reward you with not only the full complement of minerals and trace elements, but also with phytonutrients, enzymes, vitamins, and fulvic acid.

Nature is so incredible, these enriched organic soils are teeming with microorganisms which will help turn inorganic minerals into organic minerals that the body can now absorb and utilize. They also produce fulvic acid which, when taken up by the plant, will be delivered to you in these organically grown foods. The wonder of fulvic acid is that it acts like a key, unlocking the portals into cells, facilitating the uptake of all of these minerals, trace elements, etc. Keeping your body fully stocked with all of these minerals and trace elements means it will have all the building blocks it needs when it has to produce the thousands of chemicals that we need synthesized every minute to remain in optimal health. When you are deficient in minerals and trace elements your body does not get hundreds of enzymes activated, thus creating a cascade effect of deficient and abnormal production of protein and other end products by the cells. Ultimately, these deficiencies will lead to both mental and physical diseases. Many mental disorders, including such problems as catatonic states, ADHD, depression, and even schizophrenia, have been cured or at least placed in remission with the use of certain minerals, enzymes, and vitamins. Many of our chronic diseases that we suffer with are also the result of these deficiencies, so the earlier we correct them the greater the benefit. Magnesium helps migraine headaches, cardiac arrhythmias, constipation, insomnia, muscle cramps, and high blood pressure to name a few, so you can imagine the health benefits of just maintaining this one mineral would have on you.

You can also get these alkaline minerals in a readily absorbable form by drinking alkaline water which contains these minerals. The best source of natural alkaline water is from natural springs, not from the numerous ionized alkaline water machines that are being sold on the internet. There is absolutely no evidence that these machines produce healthful water. You may be surprised to learn that some natural spring water is slightly acidic; either acidic or alkaline spring water contains enough dissolved minerals and trace elements to be extremely healthful for your body.

Ionized alkaline water is made by electrolysis, whereby the acidic and alkaline fractions of water are separated. For example, the positive charges on calcium and potassium are all drawn to the negative electrode. There is a danger of excessive pH changes in either direction; either too acidic or too alkaline are both equally dangerous for your body, which has to buffer these solutions in order to eliminate them from your body. The best and often free source of good drinking water can usually be found locally. These waters usually arise from deep underground springs and have been purified by passage through successive layers of soil and subsoils. Spring waters for the most part are not polluted by pharmaceutical drugs, pesticides, and other dangerous chemicals. There is a website that enables you to locate good sources of local springs called FindaSpring.com.

As ridiculous as it sounds, despite the explosion of knowledge and information occurring worldwide, we still do not understand the structure of something so basic as water, which seems to have many properties that just remain elusive to scientific inquiry. That being said, like most things, you will derive the most benefits if you stick to natural, non-man-made sources of water that are as clean as possible.

TYPES OF WATER

Let me clear up some of the confusion surrounding different types of water that are currently available.

Bottled Water: This is the kind you get in every convenience store and gas station. It usually comes from a spring, but not always. Sometimes it is straight from the tap. It is typically made by a process known as reverse osmosis. Reverse osmosis means that pressure is applied to the water and it is forced through a semipermeable membrane where many foreign molecules and ions are removed. Bottled water is the biggest rip- off in history, do you realize that people are bottling tap water in some instances and selling it for more money than gasoline?

Purified Water: Purified means that the water has been put through a process to remove any impurities. These processes can include reverse osmosis, distillation, deionization, and the use of activated charcoal filtration.

Distilled Water: Distilled means it has been brought to a boil which separates the pure water from its dissolved mineral and trace element content. The evaporated water is then put through a condenser and recovered.

Alkaline Water: As I described above, it is water that has been exposed to positive and negative electrodes that separate it into alkaline and acidic fractions.

Hard and Soft Water: Hard water means it just has all of its mineral content. Soft water means it has had all of its minerals removed except sodium.

Demineralized Water (sometimes called deionized water): This is water that has been exposed to electrically charged resins that remove all of the mineral salts from the water by binding them to the resins.

Spring Water: Spring water comes from deep, underground natural springs, the water is pure and usually without chemicals, pharmaceuticals, and other pollutants due to its filtration as it passes through successive layers of soils and subsoils.

HEALTH BENEFITS OF ALKALINIZATION

Let us first take a look at which foods in our diet are alkaline or at least promote alkalinity in the body. Foods such as fruits, vegetables, soybeans, nuts, seeds, tofu, and water all are alkaline or promote raising your body's pH to more alkaline levels. Keep in mind that your blood does not change its pH very much and should remain between 7.35 and 7.45. Your blood is able to stay fairly close to that range due to the numerous systems your body has in place to buffer any changes, which is a good thing since drastic changes in pH to either very acidic or very alkaline are oftentimes fatal! Foods that are acidic include man-made processed foods, alcohol, sugar, meat, dairy, grains, eggs, and canned or packaged foods.

Sometimes determining which foods are acidic and which are alkaline is a bit confusing. Take tea for example. Black tea is acidic but all other teas are alkaline. It is the fermentation process that makes black tea different from the others. Grains are acidic with the exception of quinoa and wild rice. You would think that vegetarians are golden and they are, for the most part, except their major source of protein, beans and legumes, is acidic.

By the way, if you have a pond or lake on your property, planting wild rice as a food source is a wonderful idea. It also attracts large numbers of game birds such as wild ducks which can become another food source for you. One word of caution, I spread wild rice seed in a pond on my property by hand. What a mistake; for some reason, wild rice seed has the most horrific smell to it. There are even warnings on the package (which I unfortunately ignored). My right hand smelled terrible for over a week and nothing I did could neutralize the odor; I even tried using gasoline! So, if you decide you want to plant wild rice, by all means, but remember to wear gloves!

The many health benefits of eating a more alkaline diet include the following:

1. Increased energy levels
2. Increase in mental alertness
3. An alkaline body is a difficult environment for fungi like Candida to survive and thrive.

4. Prevention of osteoporosis, because your body has to leach calcium and magnesium from bones to buffer acids.
5. Prevention of kidney stones for the same reason, as cited under prevention of osteoporosis, above
6. Decrease risk of colon cancer.
7. Decrease risk of diabetes, probably due more to the fruits and vegetables and their phytonutrients along with less exposure to sugar and other processed, artificial foods.
8. Weight loss, for the same reasons as cited above under diabetes
9. Helps alleviate muscle aches and pains.
10. Creates an environment where your body can function at optimal levels including its all-important enzymes.

Bottom line is that adopting an alkaline-dominant diet forces you to eat in a more natural and healthy manner and this in turn provides an entire host of health benefits.

CHAPTER NINE

HONEY

INTRODUCTION

TABLE OF CONTENTS:

First let's define what I mean by honey. Honey is the product of honey bees collecting nectar from various kinds of flowers and transforming it by a process of regurgitation and dehydration and then storing it in their wax honeycombs inside their beehives for their eventual consumption. As it is stored it continues to ferment by the action of enzymes that the bee has added to the honey, in addition to which the bees in the hive will actually flap their wings over freshly produced honey to speed up the evaporation of water in the honey and concentrating its sweetness. That same process of evaporation also eliminates enough water that it stops the fermentation and stabilizes the honey. For this same reason whenever you have honey, you need to keep it covered at all times, otherwise it may draw in enough water vapor from the surrounding air to raise its overall water content and lead to the reactivation of fermentation. Fermentation does not spoil honey; it merely changes its taste and some of its properties. Mead is made from fermented honey and has been a popular drink since the Middle Ages. Honey will also not freeze unless you have it in temperatures of approximately -50 F.

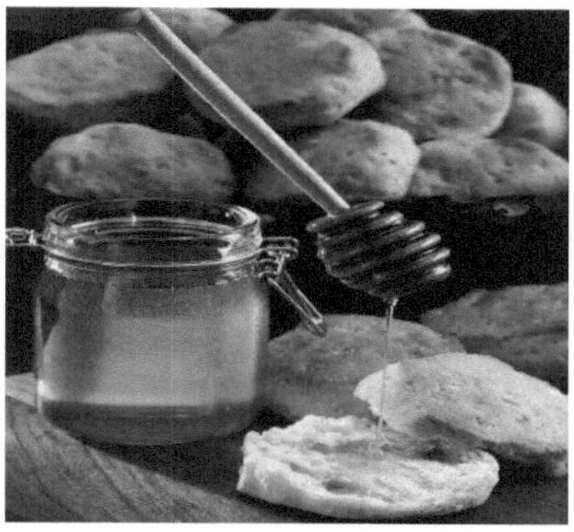

NUTRITIONAL VALUE OF HONEY

Honey is very nutritious for you and contains about 80 percent natural sugars in the form of glucose and fructose and about 18 percent water. The lower the water contents of honey the higher its quality. The remaining 2 percent is vitamins, minerals, pollen, and proteins.

Honey is also jam-packed with digestive enzymes from the bee's saliva as well as minerals and trace elements, depending of course on its floral source. The vitamins in honey are Riboflavin, B6, thiamin, niacin, and pantothenic acid as well as a variety of amino acids, once again depending upon the origin of the floral nectars. The minerals found in honey include calcium, copper, iron, magnesium, manganese, phosphorus, potassium, sodium, and zinc. Honey also has a lower glycemic index than other sugars, meaning that it is more slowly absorbed into your bloodstream, thus preventing spikes in your insulin levels, resulting obesity and other health problems. For this reason if you are diabetic, certainly any type of sugar is problematic, but if you had to choose a sweetener to use, honey would be a better choice than table sugar due to its lower glycemic index.

Honey also has a very low pH of 3 to 4 range, but once acted upon by the digestive system it is said to be an alkalinizing food, which makes it healthier than acid-forming foods. This strong acidic pH also is one of the many reasons for its antimicrobial effect. It has been noted that adding honey to apple cider vinegar enhances the healing properties of the vinegar. Honey is also a very strong antioxidant. Honey contains a unique type of antioxidant called pinocembrin. Pinocembrin has been shown to have many other beneficial properties, including antimicrobial, anticancer, and anti-inflammatory activities. Research has also shown it to have neuroprotective properties in stroke patients, protecting their brains from the effects of decreased blood flow!

Honey is the only sweetener that is not man-made or processed, and has antibacterial properties and a healing effect. Unlike man-made sweeteners like table sugar, honey will not ferment in your digestive tract.

Honey is a monosaccharide and therefore cannot be broken down any further and is readily absorbed by the intestines without any irritation or gastrointestinal upset, unlike other sugars which may cause distress.

THE FRUCTOSE PARADOX

Honey can also be used for weight loss; if taken at bedtime, it will promote your body preferentially utilizing fat instead of protein for its metabolic needs and will promote a deeper more restful sleep. This seems counterintuitive; how can eating something sweet at bedtime promote weight loss? The explanation is a little complicated but involves what is commonly known as the Fructose Paradox, since honey is made up of two simple sugars, fructose and glucose. The fructose is absorbed by the liver and induces the production of an enzyme that helps the absorption of glucose by the liver and the production of glycogen.

Glycogen is a glucose molecule folded like an accordion which prevents the absorption of water and allows an easily stored form of sugar that is readily available by the body. What this honey at bedtime does, in essence, is prevent nocturnal (night time) drops in blood glucose levels with the resulting stress reaction and the release of adrenaline and all the metabolic havoc that involves, which results in weight gain. To do this, take a large teaspoon of raw honey every night at bedtime, I would also take at least 3 mg of melatonin with that to get a real healthy, deep, restful sleep, especially if you are over forty. Melatonin is a natural hormone that helps you sleep, giving you that deep restorative sleep, the kind you had when you were a kid and your melatonin levels were very high. Melatonin levels naturally decline with age, hence the pervasive insomnia among the middle-aged and older. Melatonin also is a very strong antioxidant and is instrumental in the protection of our DNA. When taken along with zinc and selenium at bed time melatonin has wonderful anti-aging properties.

VARIETIES OF HONEY

The type of flower the nectar is collected from will determine the type of honey produced. For example, clover flowers produce clover honey, etc. Many kinds of honey come from a variety of floral nectar sources. There is an entire branch of study of honey that is able to identify its floral source by the pollen and spores which it contains.

Honey bees are all from the genus Apis. Other insects, including other types of bees like bumblebees and even honey wasps make honey, but it is different and does not have the properties we need for our purposes.

THE ANTIMICROBIAL PROPERTIES OF HONEY

Most microorganisms cannot grow in honey due to its osmotic effect, which means that honey draws fluid out of the cells of most germs like bacteria and fungi and therefore they cannot thrive in honey. However, the dormant endospores of the bacterium Clostridium botulinum have been reported to survive in honey. For this reason honey should not be given to children below the age of one; their immune systems have not yet evolved enough to wipe out these spores. In infants this infection will produce endotoxins (bacterial poisons) that unfortunately can be fatal to them. After the age of one there is no contraindication (reasons not to use it) to the use of honey.

Nothing known to man has a longer history of being used as a medicine than honey. As a nutraceutical honey is hard to beat having nutritional, medicinal value as well as being a delicious food, which is why it should have such a prominent place in your medicine chest.

WHY HONEY NEVER SPOILS

Honey never spoils...you could eat thousand-year-old honey if you found it. Why is that, you ask?

The reason is simple ...honey has amazing antibacterial, antifungal, and antiviral properties...so nothing can really grow in it and hence it does not spoil. And that is one of the reasons it is so good to use on wounds.

The Romans were masters of practicality...they did incredibly well with what little they had. Physicians in the Roman army routinely slathered honey on all those nasty wounds their troops had after battles. They did not have the luxury of modern antibiotics and so they used honey and herbal treatments and essential oils.

I have used honey in my practice for over twenty-five years with great success. Wound clinics routinely prescribed ridiculously expensive creams and salves for my patients, and many times with little success. I routinely intervened and told them to buy a jar of raw local honey at the farmer's market or the local grocer. After using my honey treatment they returned to the wound clinics and repeatedly astonished the doctors and nurses there with their speedy recovery and lack of infections.

HONEY AND WOUND HEALING

Here's the science behind honey's amazing properties. Honey is very viscous (thick) and therefore has a very strong osmotic effect (think of osmosis as gravity). Honey is very osmotically active so like gravity, it has a strong pull, so it pulls or draws fluids out of the less osmotically active wound, carrying debris, dirt, and bacteria, etc. away from the wound onto the dressing. That is why it is good to apply the honey directly to a wound dressing and then apply that to the wound. This way you can change the dressing each time it becomes soaked with fluids from the wound. This osmotic effect also helps keep the wound moist, preventing premature scabbing as well as aiding in healing. Honey also has a very strong attractive effect upon water, which it will combine with and make it unavailable to thirsty bacteria, fungi, and viruses. Since all life forms on Earth depend on water you can understand how fatal this can be.

As the bacteria in a wound feed on the glucose in honey they will produce lactic acid, thus preventing the foul smell found in many wounds. As honey gets combined with water it will produce hydrogen peroxide.

This is the same substance that your body's white blood cells produce to destroy foreign invaders. This is why hydrogen peroxide has a strong antiseptic effect. This also promotes wound healing. The hydrogen peroxide in honey is steadily produced and hence has a long-term positive effect on the wound.

Honey also causes the chelation of iron, thus binding it to proteins and rendering it unavailable to bacteria, which need iron to reproduce. Therefore, whenever you bind iron up and make it unavailable to bacteria, you are producing an antimicrobial effect. The lactoferrin in breast milk has a similar function thus rendering it less receptive to a bacterial infection. For similar reasons lactoferrin is also found in other body secretions such as saliva, tears and nasal secretions hence acting to defend the body from infections in your mouth, eyes and nasal passages. Once again the incredible design of the human body is awe inspiring!

Honey also helps promote granulation of wounds. That is the step after the production of a clot to close a wound. Note: Granulation tissue is the yellow tissue in the base of a wound. I have found that even by nurses it is very often mistaken for pus. This is your body's way of filling in a wound gap and allowing normal tissue to grow into that from all sides and heal a wound. You can tell the difference of it from pus because it is nice and uniform, lining a wound with the look of a thin layer of lemon pudding and without any foul smell that pus usually produces.

HONEY FOR BURNS, SKIN ULCERS, AND DRY SKIN

Honey also works very well on burns; use it the same way, covering the burned area with a large gauze soaked with honey. Change it just like the wound dressing, whenever it is soaked with fluids that it has drawn out of the burn. It will prevent the major problem with burns, infection. It will also produce better healing and less scarring, which can be critical in treating burns.

Honey also works very well in skin ulceration. I have treated many patients with large, deep decubitus ulcers (bed sores) and they have healed remarkably well. Honey applied to a dressing along with proper positioning of the patient to alleviate those pressure points will work wonders for patients with bed sores.

Honey has also been used to treat dry, parched, or injured skin of any type. Women as far back as Cleopatra have used raw honey for face masks and to beautify their hair and skin. Ladies, it worked on Mark Anthony and it will work on your husband as well. The great moisturizing effect of honey on dry, aging skin is due to its ability to attract and retain moisture in the skin without making the skin too oily.

For this reason as well as raw honey's antibacterial effects, it works very well in cases of acne. Raw honey has been used for every conceivable kind of skin problem, including athlete's foot.

HONEY FOR AN UPSET STOMACH

Raw honey, when combined with ginger and lemon juice, makes a very potent treatment for nausea and vomiting as well as gastric distress of any type, including ulcers. Raw honey also contains large amounts of amylase which is concentrated in the pollen of flowers. Amylase is a digestive enzyme that digests starches such as bread, pasta, potatoes, and rice, thus it aids in digestion and is an excellent treatment for indigestion.

WHAT TYPE OF HONEY SHOULD YOU BUY?

Raw Honey

There are various types of honey. The best for overall use that is, for eating and for medicinal purposes, is raw honey. Raw honey is honey that has not been processed by man, it is the same honey that is found in the beehive and is not pasteurized with heat; it may however be strained or filtered. Raw honey contains many spores and pieces of wax from the honeycomb as well as bee parts, etc. Raw honey has the benefit of helping people who are suffering with allergies to local plants and many times is used by patients to treat their allergies. If this is done, it has to be raw local honey, which is usually made from either a blend of local hives honey or comes from a single source hive that has collected nectar from local sources and has not been treated with heat to pasteurize it. Raw honey also has the highest antioxidant properties of all honeys. For our purposes raw honey is the type of honey that we should use; it has its enzymes still intact. Heating above 125 degrees F for a half hour usually destroys the enzyme content of most foods. Enzymes are very beneficial to your health and will aid both in digestion and overall health.

Most farm stand and farmer's markets and local beekeepers honeys will be raw and unpasteurized. If you have any doubts, ask the person selling it, but as a general rule they are not pasteurizing their honey.

Pasteurized Honey

Pasteurized honey is like pasteurized milk, it has been heat treated, usually at 161 degrees F or higher. Pasteurization is done to kill the yeast spores that are present in honey and responsible for its fermentation if the water content of the honey reaches 25 percent or higher. That is the reason why you keep your honey covered, to prevent it from drawing in water vapor from the surrounding air and diluting the honey until it reaches that critical 25 percent when the yeast spores will reactivate and begin fermentation. Commercially produced honeys are often pasteurized because this also dissolves any sugar crystals that frequently develop in honey, giving it a granular appearance. People often see crystallized honey and think it has spoiled, but this is not the case, and simply heating it in a pan of water will melt the crystals back into solution. The reheating of crystallized honey is done simply by placing a jar of honey in a small pot filled with water and placing that inside of a larger pot and heating it.

Strained Honey

Strained honey is honey that has been strained through a mesh cloth of some type. This removes many of the particles and contaminants in honey. It does not affect the enzymes and other properties of honey and is merely cosmetic.

Filtered Honey

Filtered honey is heated to about 170 degrees F in order to make it more liquid to pass through the fine filter. The filtering process removes all of the particulate matter, pollen grains, and air bubbles, and it is very clear and more liquid than untreated honey. This is the kind also very often found in supermarkets. It also tends to crystallize much less than raw honey so is felt to be more attractive to shoppers than raw varieties.

Creamed Or Whipped Honey

Creamed or whipped honey is another type of honey that has been processed to remove many of the large sugar crystals and therefore is much less likely to crystallize. The process involves the pasteurization of raw honey and then the blending of it with 10 percent creamed honey to form a honey with very small crystals that usually will not coalesce into larger crystals.

This type of honey is very spreadable and is often used by people for toast and sandwiches.

Honeycomb Or Comb Honey

Comb honey is honey that is still in the wax honeycomb from the honey bee's hive. Chunks of the honeycomb are cut out and packaged raw. It is identical to raw honey with the only difference being that it is still in the honeycomb. It is sometimes known as "cut comb honey".

Manuka Honey

Manuka honey is the most powerful of the various medicinal honeys produced around the world. It originates from New Zealand and is made from the flowers of the tree of the same name. Manuka honey is a monofloral honey, meaning it originates from just one type of flower, as opposed to polyfloral honeys which are the product of many different flower nectars. Another name for the Manuka tree is the Tea Tree and it primarily grows in wild stands in Australia and New Zealand. The name Tea Tree originates from the famous Captain Cook who discovered Australia and upon landfall is said to have made a tea from the leaves of the Manuka tree. It is the same tree from which Tea Tree Oil is made.

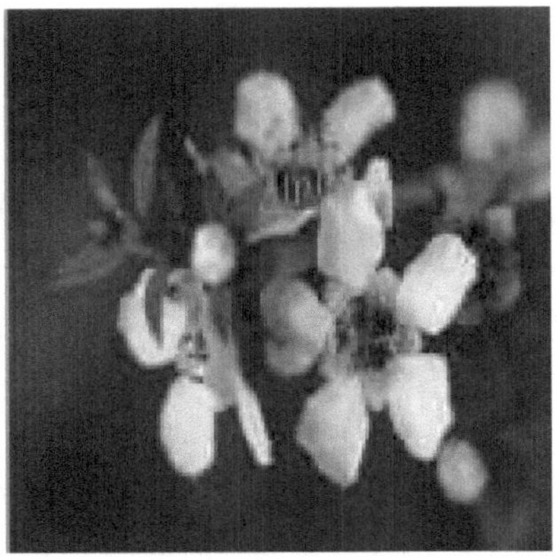

Honeybee on a Manuka Flower

Manuka honey has the highest viscosity (thickness) of any known honey and also therefore has a very strong antibacterial effect, hence its use in the treatment of wounds, where it has been shown to prevent infections as well as promote rapid healing.

I have used it many times and can attest to its superiority over other types of honey. It also has been shown to be quite beneficial for use for skin ulcers as well as for burns, and even has been shown to be effective against MRSA (Methicillin Resistant Staph. Aureus). I highly recommend buying a few jars of this honey and using it exclusively for wounds, burns, and ulcers and use other less expensive honeys for eating and other purposes. It has an "earthy" type of taste to me and I am not particularly fond of it as a food, but that is just my personal preference. Due to the limited number of Manuka trees there is naturally a limited supply of this honey available annually, hence it is much more costly than other honeys. Beware of counterfeit types of this honey and buy it from a reputable dealer preferably from "down under" in New Zealand or Australia. Most of the honey sold worldwide as Manuka is counterfeit and made from floral sources other than the Manuka or Tea Tree.

Manuka honey's strength and healing powers are actually measured by a system known as UMF or Unique Manuka Factor; the higher the value given in UMF labels, the stronger the healing properties. It is usually found in a factor of ten range; for example ten plus, twenty plus, etc.

Pure Honey

Pure honey is honey that has not been adulterated or changed by the addition of glucose, dextrose, molasses, corn syrup, starches, invert sugars, flour, or any other foreign substances. The Chinese have been notorious for adulterating their honey and I would highly recommend not buying any honey from China for that very reason. Unfortunately, there appears to be a lot of tampering with honey, especially from foreign sources. If you can, buy local honey from a reputable beekeeper. There are many around and this should not be a problem. Local honey will also have benefits for anyone who may have allergies. Crystallization of honey is not a sign of adulteration and comes about simply from honey's sugar super saturation. One not very scientific method for determining if honey is pure is to stir it into a glass of water. The adulterated honeys will dissolve much more rapidly than pure raw honey, which tends to coalesce into clumps and take a little time to dissolve properly.

THE GRADING OF HONEY

A word about honey grading: Honey grading is primarily done on the basis of the water content of the honey as well as its particulate content and its color.

There are four grades of honey; A, B, C, and substandard. Grade A honey has the lowest water content, the least particulate matter, and is the clearest in color. Lesser grades have more of all of those factors.

Honey quality can also be easily evaluated by certain characteristics. The honey should flow off of a spoon in a straight stream without breaking up into drops, it should also bead up upon hitting a surface, and when flowing onto a surface should form temporary layers that eventually disappear. This attests to its proper viscosity. If your honey does not do these things then it probably contains too much water and is not suitable for long-term storage.

The color of honey tells you something in general about its flavor.

The lighter honeys have a milder flavor and the darker-shaded honeys have a more robust flavor. The overall color of raw honey is determined by the floral source of the bee's nectar; however, long-term storage may darken a honey, especially if the honey is stored at a high temperature. Honey also lightens in color after it has undergone granulation. This is the reason that most forms of creamed honey are so light in color. Over time many honeys tend to crystallize; this is normal and does not hurt the quality of the honey and can easily be reversed by gentle heating as described above. Depending on the type of honey, some such as Manuka crystallize rapidly compared to tupelo honey, which takes a very long time to crystallize. Crystallization means that the honey forms actual white-colored sugar crystals on the surface, this does not affect the quality or taste of the honey, and you should not discard honey that has done this.

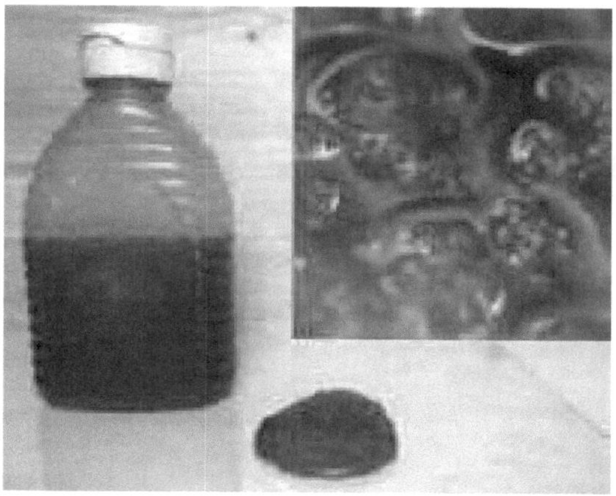

Photo of Crystallized Honey

HOW TO STORE HONEY

Honey should be stored in either glass containers or food grade containers to prevent the leakage of any chemicals from a plastic vessel. You should keep your honey in a cool, dark place out of direct sunlight and away from any heat source like a furnace or space heater. Honey should always be in a closed container with a tight lid to prevent absorption of any humidity which will change the honey and promote its fermentation. You should always use a dry spoon when scooping any honey from its container in order to prevent the introduction of any water into the honey. Some honey purists feel that stainless steel spoons and other implements should not be used with honey, due to some subtle changes in the taste of the honey. Honestly, I have tried tasting honey with a wooden ladle and with a stainless steel spoon and I cannot tell any difference, so in my humble opinion, it doesn't matter at all.

CHAPTER TEN
IODINE

INTRODUCTION

TABLE OF CONTENTS:

Iodine is a trace mineral/medicine that has many uses and should definitely be a well-stocked item in your natural medicine chest. Once you learn about its numerous health benefits, and get some experience with it, you will find yourself turning to it time and time again. Let's see what this wonder halogen can do for us.

WHAT IS IODINE?

Iodine is a chemical element in the class known as halogens. Halogens mean salt producing, and its sister elements such as fluorine, bromine, chlorine and astatine all do just that with great ease. Iodine is essential for human health and the World Health Organization (WHO) has estimated that over two billion people are iodine deficient and this is the leading cause of mental retardation worldwide.

WHY ARE WE DEFICIENT IN IODINE?

Rain leaches iodine from soils depleting them and making the foods they produce iodine deficient. The oceans of the world produce significant amounts of iodine in the form of Iodomethane, therefore it is abundant in seafood. The further a land mass is from the ocean and the greater its rainfall the more iodine deficiency occurs in those soils. The United States government decided to iodize salt in the 1920's to insure that its population would get sufficient iodine in their diets, many governments around the world followed suit. A study of salt samples from 88 different U.S. companies done in 2008 showed that less than half had sufficiently iodized their salt.

The iodine deficiency problem today has been exacerbated by the great increase in chemical farming since WWII causing an exponential loss of iodine and other minerals and trace elements from our soils. Iodine deficiency is further exacerbated by low salt diets, thereby removing the major source of iodine in most American's diets. Many American's cook with salt out of necessity but refuse to add it to their foods because of health concerns. Recent scientific studies have shown that salt used in cooking loses about 62% of its iodine content. Kosher and sea salts have little or no iodine. Eating vegetarian diet is also much lower in iodine than eating meat and fish. How bad is it? A study recently done by the U.S. government showed that iodine levels (measured by urinary iodine excretion) have gone down over fifty percent in the last twenty years.

WHY IS IODINE SO IMPORTANT?

Iodine is used by every cell in our body. Iodine is critical for brain development, an absence of iodine during pregnancy leads to mental retardation and what is known as cretinism. Cretins are short and mentally retarded with numerous other physical impairments. The vast majority of the US population is deficient in iodine and the problem is worsening yearly. Guess what happens when you supplement iodine during pregnancy? Well, I think you are going to find this just as amazing as I did when I first discovered this.......there is on average a twenty point increase in the child's IQ! This was reported by a brilliant physician iodine researcher named Dr. Jorge Flechas, who has done incredible work furthering our understanding of iodine and the disastrous effects of its deficiency. He has a website that documents his important work at www.helpmythyroid.com.

Iodine deficiency is worse in women because estrogen is known to inhibit the absorption of iodine. Iodine deficiency leads to hypothyroidism and not surprisingly women have nine times more hypothyroidism than men. Iodine deficiency is one of the major causes of cysts of all types to develop but especially fibrocystic breast disease. Human breast tissue and breast milk contain higher concentrations of iodine than the thyroid gland. This once again illustrates the importance of iodine; the body concentrates iodine in breast tissue to make it available to the infant in mother's milk, thereby making iodine readily available to the infants growing brain. As I have always said, the human body is such an incredible design, nothing is done by chance. Iodine is supplied to the growing infant's brain because it is critical to its proper development.

Iodine deficiency is a known risk factor for the development of fibrocystic breasts as well as breast cancer. What happens when you supplement iodine in a given population? Let's take a look at Japan where culturally they have a very high iodine intake, twenty five times the intake of the average American; their rates of breast cancer are one third the rate of American women. A healthy breast needs iodine to function properly, one of the reasons low iodine levels predispose to breast cancer is that it causes increased estrogen levels which is a known risk factor for breast cancer. When those same Japanese women immigrate to the U.S. and adopt an American diet their breast cancer rates match those of their American counterparts. If there is any family history of breast cancer and if you suffer with fibrocystic breasts then you should start iodine supplementation immediately.

Iodine deficiency is also one of the major causes of cancers of many types including breast, ovarian, endometrial, thyroid, stomach and esophageal. Supplementation with iodine leads to decreased rates of all of these cancers, this is due to its potent antioxidant activity.

In my opinion it is madness for us not to be supplementing iodine and all the other minerals and trace elements that are essential for normal human growth and development during a woman's pregnancy. Done correctly these are harmless and the upside is incredible. In Japan the average Japanese woman has a daily intake of 13.8 mg of iodine from their diets which contain large amounts of kelp and other seaweed and seafood. They have none of the problems that American physicians are constantly worried about, iodine supplementation is not only safe, but critical to your health in so many ways.

The salivary glands and lacrimal glands also utilize iodine to produce saliva and tears, a deficiency of iodine will lead to dry mouth and dry eyes as well. The skin also uses a lot of iodine and a deficiency will also lead to dry skin and lack of sweat production. The brain also needs iodine as I said for proper development, it also helps with alertness to the brain, for this reason you should not take iodine at bedtime.

Iodine is also critical for cardiovascular health via its effect on the thyroid gland. An underactive thyroid gland leads to a weak heart, elevates blood pressure and causes an increase in bad LDL cholesterol and atherosclerosis (hardening of the arteries), as well as increasing rates of heart disease and stroke. Iodine has also been linked to fatigue, muscle and joint pain and fibromyalgia. White blood cells also utilize iodine and it is thus crucial for proper immune function.

IODINE AND THE THYROID

The most crucial role for iodine in adults is proper thyroid gland function. The thyroid gland needs adequate iodine to produce thyroid hormone. The thyroid gland releases a hormone known as thyroxine, also known as T4. The 4 signifies the number of iodine atoms attached to the parent molecule. T4 is not active, when it goes out to the body it has to be converted to T3 which is the active thyroid hormone. You guessed it; T3 has only three iodine atoms. The enzyme that cleaves one of those atoms off of T4 thereby converting it to T3 is called a deiodinase enzyme and to do its job it needs the mineral selenium. That is why it is so important to supplement all your minerals and especially selenium, even if you are normal, but especially if you suffer with hypothyroidism (a slow thyroid).

THE TOXICITY OF HALOGENS LIKE BROMINE

Other halogens in the same family as iodine also cause problems, especially bromine. In the United States we are exposed to very high levels of bromine. Bread manufacturers are using bromine instead of iodine; it is used in many soft drinks including Mountain Dew where they use brominated vegetable oil. Bromine is also contained in many fabrics where it is used as a fire retardant.

When our bodies lack iodine they will turn to other halogens like bromine. Thyroid hormone containing bromine is not active; it is useless to our bodies. Worse yet, current lab tests of thyroid function will appear normal because they cannot differentiate between thyroid hormone made with bromine or iodine. This unprecedented increase in bromine is causing a condition known as bromism. Bromism results in neurotoxicity (nerve damage) to the brain leading to fatigue, psychotic behavior , seizures, headache, restlessness, ADD ,irritability and memory loss. Look around, our children especially the boys are being ravaged by these type of problems which could easily be reversed by administration of adequate iodine. Iodine can also prevent bromism.

TYPES OF IODINE

Potassium Iodide , Lugol's Solution , Iodoral and SSKI

What is Potassium Iodide?

Potassium Iodide (chemical symbol KI) is a form of iodine that is called reduced because it has an extra electron. Iodide is much more soluble in water than iodine. A French physician named Dr. Jean Lugol was looking for different substances to treat infections. He found that if he added potassium iodide to water and iodine it increased the solubility of the iodine. He made a mix of 5 percent iodine and 10 percent potassium iodide in 85 percent distilled water. This mix over the years has come to be known as Lugol's Solution. Two drops of Lugol's Solution (or 0.1 ml) contains 5 mg of iodine and 7.5 mg of iodide. He treated many infections with this with great success. His standard dosing was two drops per day. This provided approximately 12.5 mg of iodine, which according to Dr. Brownstein in his excellent book, closely approximates the daily human requirement. The combination of iodine and potassium iodide is also available in a pill called Iodoral. It is readily available online. Different organs in the body require different forms of iodine. Supplementation with both iodine and iodide satisfies all your body's needs better than either form alone.

The primary uses of KI include its use as a nutritional supplement, both for humans and animals. Governments long ago began to utilize KI to ionize salt. This was found to be the best method for reaching the iodine needs of the majority of the populace. There is another form of liquid KI known as SSKI or supersaturated potassium iodide. SSKI is made by simply dissolving KI crystals in water until no more of them will dissolve. This process is temperature- dependent and hence the amount of KI in SSKI varies. It usually averages out to approximately 50 mg per drop (assuming there to be approximately 15 drops per ml in this case). Note: Due to its high potassium content, you will find SSKI to be very bitter. It is therefore frequently administered onto a sugar cube or a piece of bread. You can also mix it in a glass of juice.

IMPORTANT POINT TO NOTE: Neither SSKI or KI tablets should be used as a nutritional supplement. They are much too potent. The RDA for iodide is 0.15 mg per day. A single drop of SSKI provides 333x that RDA and a single tablet of KI provides 666x the RDA.

Using Potassium Iodide for Radiation Exposure

In 1982, the FDA approved the use of KI to protect thyroid glands in the event of a nuclear accident or attack. In a nuclear explosion or the result of a bombing of a nuclear power plant, there would be extensive release of volatile radionuclides. One of the most common is Iodine 131. Left unopposed, it will lead to thyroid cancer in many of the exposed victims. The strategy behind the use of potassium iodide is to soak your thyroid with stable, benign (non- harmful) forms of iodine. This prevents the uptake of the radioactive form of iodine by the thyroid gland and actually helps its excretion by the kidneys. The dose recommended is 130 mg of potassium iodide daily. The actual tablet is 160 mg but the remaining 30 mg is composed of fillers and binders. This provides 100 mg of iodide and about 30 of potassium. If you were using SSKI for this protective effect, the dose would be 2 drops per day. Note: You cannot use iodized salt to get your protective iodide dose. The reason is the small quantity of KI in iodized salt would require a lethal dose of the salt to get a protective effect. Potassium iodide should be taken immediately upon exposure, but will still work to protect the thyroid for three or four hours post exposure. Each dose lasts for one day. KI only protects the thyroid; it does nothing for other organs or tissues. In addition, if a bomb like a dirty bomb is exploded it will not produce radioiodine (radioactive iodine 131) and hence KI will not be helpful. Taking a higher dose than recommended also will do nothing but waste your supply.

World Health Organizations Dosing Recommendations:

Over 12 years of age:	130 mg of KI per day
3 to 12 years of age:	65 mg of KI per day
1 month to 3 years of age:	32 mg of KI per day
Less than 1 month of age:	16 mg of KI per day

Note: The WHO does not recommend treatment for adults older than 40 unless they are very close to the detonation site. Also note: Dirty bombs release a different type of radionuclide that does not contain radioactive I 131.

Historical Perspective

Potassium iodide tablets were given out by Soviet officials following the Chernobyl nuclear reactor disaster of 1986 in the USSR. This was done in an approximately 18-mile zone (30 km) around the plant. This worked, and was credited with having permissible levels of iodine in 97 percent of the evacuees. Poland, which is 300 miles from Chernobyl, also gave out KI to its population and had no thyroid cancer among its recipients. In areas not treated the populations developed epidemic levels of thyroid cancer. These increased levels were as far as 300 miles from Chernobyl. The FDA studied various forms of iodine and found potassium iodide to be by far the safest, most effective form. These tablets were also given to US Navy aircrews that were flying within one hundred miles of the March 2011 Fukushima nuclear accident in Japan. Fortunately, no detectable signs of radiation poisoning were detected in US forces.

Helpful Fact: The iodine tablets used to make water potable (safe to drink) can also be utilized for thyroid protection before or following a nuclear accident. This form of iodine is known as Tetraglycine hydroperiodide (TGHP), and usually comes in 20 mg tablets. Each tablet contains approximately 8 mg of free iodine. The dose is four tablets daily for protection of your thyroid.

Adverse Reactions to Potassium Iodide

KI cannot be administered for too long without causing some havoc to the thyroid gland. Ironically it can lead to either overactive (hyperthyroidism) or underactive (hypothyroidism) thyroid gland activity. It is not recommended in those people who have had an allergic reaction to iodine or sensitivity to it. KI also stimulates the salivary glands, and can cause swelling of the parotid gland. This would make you look like when you were a child and had the mumps. The parotids are located in front of your ears below your sideburns. KI use at high doses like this can also cause GI upset, acne, loss of appetite, numbness and tingling in the hands and feet, vomiting, rash, headaches, stomach pain, irregular pulse, and a metallic taste in your mouth. These are all signs that suggest it should be stopped.

How Long Should I Take Potassium Iodide?

After exposure to a single radioactive plume, the recommended dosing time is approximately ten days. You probably will only need it for a few days, but erring on the side of caution in this case is preferable especially since your exposure is based on distance from the initial blast or release and the quantity of mass between yourself and the radioactivity. That single plume of radioactivity will be quickly dispersed by the wind. However, the problem that most people will have is radioactive fallout. This particulate fallout coats everything and is inhaled or ingested from contaminated food-stuffs or water supplies. Radioactive iodine has a half-life of eight days. However, officials fear that it is still significantly radioactive and hence dangerous to you for up to eighty days. You will have to determine, depending on your proximity to the release or explosion, how long you need to take it. Remember, you will need a supply of KI for each of your family members. A bare minimum that I would recommend is a two week supply for each person. The optimal would be a ninety-day or better supply If you find yourself trapped in an area with significant fallout the ideal course of action is to immediately leave the area (if possible) to create the greatest distance between yourself and the detonation/fallout. I would continue to take the KI until you are a safe distance away and probably for a few days after just to make sure. The reason for this is you will still be carrying some radioiodine in your blood until it is fully excreted by your kidneys, which might take a day or two. Also, if you have any renal failure you might want to double the time you take your KI after leaving a contaminated area to four days instead of two.

Can I Take Potassium Iodide Tablets Before A Nuclear Event?

KI can be taken up to forty-eight hours before an exposure and still protect your thyroid effectively. However, if greater than ninety-six hours or three days before exposure, it will have no protective effect. In addition, if you take KI more than sixteen hours after exposure it will not be helpful.

BETADINE / POVIDONE-IODINE

This is a liquid form of iodine complexed with another molecule. It is the predominant type of disinfectant used in medical settings. It works exceedingly well to kill bacteria, viruses, mold, yeasts and even potozoans. It is also used to clean and disinfect wounds. It is great stuff and has a million uses. I have used it on patients with acne and it has worked very well, by both disinfecting the skin and nurturing it when it absorbs the iodine.

NASCENT IODINE

Nascent iodine is iodine in atomic form; it has an incomplete number of electrons and thus has an electronegative charge. It is in liquid form. This strong electronegative charge results in easy absorption of this form of iodine; it has been used since the 1920's. It has been used for everything from skin infections, urinary tract infections, respiratory infections, dental infections, and to lower blood pressure.

It can also be used to displace the toxic halogens such as chlorine, bromine and fluoride thereby preventing their absorption. As I mentioned above it can therefore be used for the treatment of bromism.

DIETARY SOURCES OF IODINE

As I have previously stated, a food source is very often preferable to a supplement. Excellent food sources of iodine are the seaweeds kelp, dulse and bladderwrack. Many types of seafood including shellfish and deep water white fish are known to have high levels of iodine, presumably from its absorption from the surrounding ocean water.

Other foods that are high in iodine are garlic, lima and soybeans, spinach, swiss chard, mozzarella , feta cheese and especially sesame seeds. Haddock is also a good source of iodine, having high levels in its tissues. You can also use dried organic dulse granules as a salt/seasoning on your food to provide iodine.

IODINE AS A TREATMENT

Iodine is here in the essential tools section due to its multiple uses. For our purposes it is a go to treatment for many problems. Let's take a look at some of its myriad uses:

1. Skin Infections: Iodine topically is very useful for any type of skin infection. It will clean and sterilize a wound, abrasion, sting or burn. For these purposes you should use betadine. It is inexpensive and readily available. I would keep several bottles of it in your alternative medicine chest. Simply soak a cotton ball or similar item and generously apply it to the problem area. You can repeat this three or four times daily until it resolves/heals.
2. Mouth Infections: Take your nascent iodine and place ten drops in an 8 oz glass of water and rinse it around your mouth four times a day and spit it out.
3. Vaginal Infections: Use nascent iodine and place ten drops in an 8 ounce glass of water and douche with it, three times a day until resolved.
4. Treatment of Goiter: If you are developing a goiter or enlargement of your thyroid, this is a sign of iodine deficiency and can easily be corrected by oral administration of iodine . I would recommend using Iodoral 12.5 mg a day.
5. Fibrocystic Breasts: All cyst development in the body is a consequence of iodine deficiency. The breasts are exquisitely sensitive to iodine deficiency. To treat this take iodoral 12.5 mg once a day.

6. Radiation exposure: Refer to the preceding section in this chapter on the use of potassium iodide.
7. Internal Infections: using iodine supplements will also boost your immune system, since your white blood cells need iodine to properly function. Iodine is also deadly to all microorganisms , including bacteria, viruses, and fungal infections. Take one 12.5 mg Iodoral tablet daily until resolved. (I would also add Vitamin C 1,000 mg twice daily to start and increase until you get diarrhea then you know your body is saturated. Remember to go up in steps and down in steps, once the infection is over your body will require much less vitamin C and you will get diarrhea from a much smaller dose. Every two days decrease your dose to you are back at your baseline 1,000 mg twice a day.)

CHAPTER ELEVEN

VINEGAR AND ITS MANY MEDICINAL USES

INTRODUCTION

TABLE OF CONTENTS:

In this book you will find certain things will have multiple uses both medicinally and for various other tasks; vinegar of all types certainly fits this description. Vinegar is becoming increasingly popular as a medicinal nutraceutical agent and that is because it is well tolerated, inexpensive, readily available, and guess what folks? It works. Vinegar has endless medicinal applications for everything from colds to heartburn; it also has many uses in the home from pickling to cleaning your stove to removing hard water buildup off of faucets. There are many sources on the internet that describe many of the uses of vinegar in your home; here I will deal primarily with the uses of vinegar as a medicine/nutraceutical.

FERMENTATION AND THE PRODUCTION OF VINEGAR

When speaking about the many medicinal uses of vinegar it is usually apple cider vinegar which people are referring to. Vinegar is a product of fermentation. The fermentation process is carried out by microorganisms such as yeasts or bacteria which metabolize the sugars in the plant being fermented. The first stage of the fermentation of grapes by yeasts will produce alcohol and thus in this case wine, a second stage of fermentation by bacteria, in this case acetobacter, will change the wine into vinegar.

Acetobacters are able to do this chemical conversion by combining the alcohol present in the wine with oxygen thus forming the acetic acid solution giving vinegar its characteristic taste. This second stage of the conversion of wine to vinegar will occur on its own if the wine is exposed to oxygen for any length of time. Anyone who has ever opened a bottle of wine and not drank it all and left it standing for several days will attest to this! Since I have a sulfite allergy and do not drink wine (due to the sulfites put in wines to preserve them), my wife enjoys a glass or two with dinner but frequently the wine changes to vinegar before she can finish the bottle.

Vinegar in French means sour wine. Vinegar can be made from a variety of sources including fruit, vegetables, and grains, but apple cider vinegar is made from smashed up apples. The main ingredient in all vinegars is acetic acid This gives vinegar its characteristic sour taste.

Once the sugars are removed from grapes by fermentation then the remaining liquid has had the sweetness removed and is sour. Vinegars also contain significant quantities of other acids, minerals, salts, and amino acids (which are the building blocks to proteins).

The History Of Vinegar

The use of vinegar as a medicinal agent dates back as far as the ancient Babylonians. The ancient Greeks also used vinegar, and Hippocrates used it both as an antibiotic on wounds, pouring it directly onto wounds and as a disinfectant by soaking bandages in vinegar. He also used it to cure pleurisy, fevers, constipation, and ulcers. The ancient Greeks also combined honey with vinegar and used it on patients who were suffering with various illnesses. As recently as World War I medics in the United States Army used vinegar on wound dressings.

As far back as the ancient Egyptians wine was a popular drink. We know this from the residue of 6,000 year-old jars that contained wine. In the heat of Egypt, grapes must have fermented quickly to produce wine, but how on earth did the ancient Egyptians prevent the second step of the conversion of wine to vinegar?

The answer seems to be by using the resin and berries of the terebinth tree, which grew naturally in the same areas of Egypt as their grapes. The berries and resin of the terebinth tree were harvested at the same time as the grapes and when this resin and berries are added to wine it slows down the second step in the fermentation process. The ingenuity of the ancient peoples of Egypt, Greece, and Rome never cease to amaze me!

The modern use of vinegar as a health-enhancing substance in the United States dates back to the 1950s; at that time a country doctor named D. C. Jarvis wrote a best seller called *Folk Medicine, a Vermont Doctor's Guide to Good Health*. He popularized the use of vinegar for many health problems, and also combined it with honey in what he called "honegar". I personally think Viney would have been a better name. Dr. Jarvis felt that mixing apple cider vinegar with honey enhanced both and was a very healthy tonic. Dr. Jarvis also felt that ingesting vinegar with meals would destroy harmful bacteria in the GI tract; he recommended drinking it with every meal. The book is a classic and easy to find online.

The health benefits of vinegar touted over the centuries are as numerous as those of garlic, but like most natural substances there are few scientific studies supporting the various claims. However, from our perspective, we want to know what will work for us when our usual medicines fail, or instead of them.

Please also keep in mind, whenever I am referring to vinegar it is apple cider vinegar. Apple cider vinegar has been the one most used in folk remedies, although most other vinegars will probably have similar health benefits. So, after that rather roundabout disclaimer, let's take a look at the touted health benefits of apple cider vinegar.

WHY VINEGAR IS GOOD FOR YOU

Nutrient Content

Vinegar has been shown to contain many vitamins, minerals, enzymes, fiber, and pectin and its fans attribute many of its health-enhancing benefits to these ingredients. One of its benefits is its positive effect upon heart disease as well as its lowering of cholesterol levels and blood pressure. The mechanism by which this is done is by pectin binding to cholesterol, which allows it to be eliminated by the body. Vinegar also contains high levels of potassium and calcium, both of which lower blood pressure and thus help heart disease.

Increases Calcium Absorption

Vinegar also helps the body absorb calcium from other food sources. Some reports say that vinegar helps increase the absorption of calcium from green vegetables by over a third. In addition to providing significant amounts of calcium, vinegar also helps the body absorb it better leading to stronger bones and teeth, as well as lowering blood pressure.

Better Blood Sugar Control

Vinegar also helps control blood sugar levels and therefore diabetic control is improved. The means by which vinegar lowers blood glucose level is that it interferes with the digestive enzyme amylase that breaks down carbohydrates into glucose or blood sugar. This slowing of the release of glucose into the blood gives the body more time to handle the glucose load it has and also lowers insulin levels which spike along with any spike in blood glucose levels. Vinegar also has positive effects on the hormone insulin, lowering insulin resistance by increasing the body's sensitivity to insulin. Along with this better control of blood sugar levels and insulin comes a reduced risk of developing all the horrific complications of diabetes including diabetic peripheral neuropathy (nerve damage caused by poorly controlled diabetes) and diabetic retinopathy (diabetic damage to the retina that eventually leads to blindness) and diabetic nephropathy (diabetic kidney disease which eventually leads to kidney failure).

High Fiber Content

The high fiber content (especially the soluble fiber pectin) of vinegar leads to a sensation of fullness and thus causes less hunger, and weight loss. This too helps control diabetes better and leads to improved overall health.

High Beta Carotene Content

Vinegar also contains high levels of beta-carotene (which is a form of vitamin A) which is a potent antioxidant. Antioxidants help combat the damage done by free radicals and therefore help fight cancer, aging, and heart disease.

Aids Digestion and Absorption

The acetic acid in vinegar, like all acids, helps break down foods and thereby helps our bodies absorb minerals and trace elements from our foods. This is the primary mechanism for the increase in calcium absorption with the use of vinegar.

Many of the folk remedies recommended for vinegar involve mixing a tablespoon of vinegar in a glass of water and drinking this mixture before meals to help increase the absorption of minerals from the foods we eat. Dark green, leafy vegetables are good sources of calcium but ironically contain a substance that interferes with calcium absorption, so using vinegar dressing on your salad will help unlock the calcium in these veggies and make them more available to your body. Dairy products are still by far the best source of calcium in foods, but due to lactose intolerance many people cannot eat dairy products without suffering with diarrhea and abdominal cramping.

Cleans Raw Foods

Washing your food with a 10 percent vinegar, 90 percent water mix will help remove the harmful pesticide residue on the fruit and vegetables we eat, and will also decrease the bacteria on the surface of foods, helping to prevent food borne illnesses.

To make a mix of this strength, mix one part of vinegar to nine parts of water. The part is whatever you need it to be, 10 cc, a cup, a quart, whatever you desire, as long as it is a nine to one ratio. Do not wash berries with this mix since they have very porous surfaces and will soak up too much of the vinegar and ruin their flavor.

Weight Loss

Vinegar is very low in calories, only twenty-five to a half cup, and this is why it helps with weight loss when you substitute vinegar for high calorie salad dressings, etc. The pectin and other fiber also increase the sensation of fullness and decrease one's appetite and make you feel full quicker.

APPLE CIDER VINEGAR'S MULTIPLE USES:

Wounds

Vinegar can be used to clean out a wound and also on wound bandages to help wipe out bacterial contamination and promote healing. It worked for the ancients, it will work for us.

Scalp Problems and Bad Breath

Vinegar can be used to alleviate bad breath and also be used as a shampoo to treat both oily and dry hair and keep your hair clean and shiny and your scalp healthy. It will work for cradle cap, seborrhea of the scalp, and bad dandruff. Vinegar will help disinfect your mouth and improve your breath; mix a tablespoon of vinegar with water and swish it around your mouth and spit it out.

Vinegar can also be used to treat dandruff. Dandruff is frequently caused by a yeast-like fungus named Malassezia furfur. Vinegar is thought to change the pH of the scalp and make it less receptive to M. furfur, thus helping your dandruff. Mix a quarter cup of vinegar in a quarter cup of water and put it in a spray bottle and spritz it onto your hair and scalp, thoroughly soaking it, then wrap a towel around your head for approximately one half to one hour and then wash it off; this needs to be done twice a week until healed.

Gastrointestinal (GI) Problems

Vinegar can be used for acid reflux and GI disturbances including "GI Bugs" like gastroenteritis (the proverbial stomach flu). One teaspoon of vinegar in water several times a day will help both reflux and help eliminate harmful bacteria in the gastrointestinal tract (your stomach and intestines, including your small intestine and colon). If you have bad diarrhea you can raise the dose to one or two tablespoons mixed with water or apple juice taken several times a day, this will also help intestinal spasms.

If you suffer with chronic indigestion problems this can be treated by making a mixture of one teaspoon of vinegar and one teaspoon of honey mixed together in a small glass of warm water and taken about a half hour before your meal. This mix will calm down your stomach and soothe it, while at the same time helping any indigestion.

Sore Throat

Vinegar can also be used to treat a sore throat. You need to gargle with a mix of a quarter cup of vinegar with warm water and gargle with this mix as often as you need to. An alternative treatment is to mix a tablespoon of vinegar and a tablespoon of honey and warm water and slowly sip this concoction to soothe your throat.

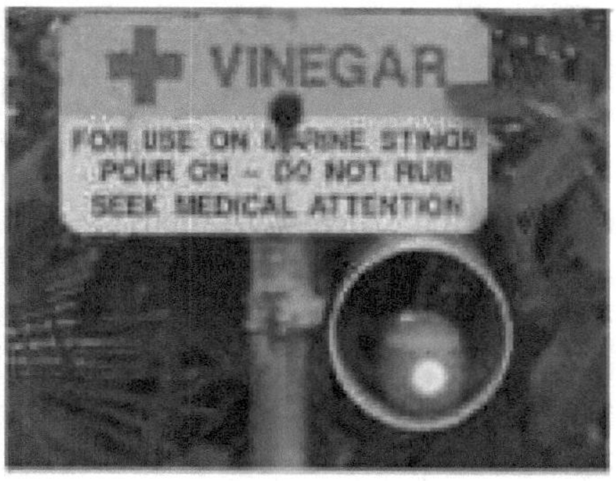

(Photo by Michael Coghlan)

Skin Conditions/Sunburn

Vinegar can also be used for skin problems. It seems to work well when applied with a cotton ball directly to eczema and psoriasis, as well as acne. Sometimes vinegar will cause some burning when applied to acne, so in those cases mix one part of vinegar to three parts of water and apply that with a cotton ball to your acne. Vinegar will also take the sting out of insect stings, as will lemon juice. Lemon juice contains citric acid which probably is the reason it takes the sting out, as opposed to the acetic acid in vinegar. Who cares, both work just fine. Vinegar can also be used to treat sunburn. Just add a cup of vinegar to your bath and soak in it for about fifteen minutes. This will eliminate all the stinging.

Alkalinize Your Body

A very popular but as of yet unproven use of vinegar is to restore an alkaline pH to the body. This sounds odd since vinegar is an acid, but according to its proponents it has an alkalizing effect upon the body. A healthy body is slightly alkaline with a pH in the blood of approximately 7.35 to 7.45 being ideal. How vinegar is used by these patients is to take one or two teaspoons of vinegar in water once or twice a day, depending on how acidic your body is.

Some signs of an overly acidic body are multiple allergies, fatigue, brain fog, arthritis complaints, anxiety and irritability, sinus and nasal congestion, gout, sore throat, and headaches. Most people are acidic because of all the processed foods in their diets, and most have these symptoms. The only way to know for sure is to check a urinary or salivary pH, using pH strips that you can buy in a pharmacy. There will be instructions on how to measure your pH right on the test strip bottle.

Precautions To Take With Vinegar Use

Vinegar is not a benign substance and may cause problems with erosion of dental enamel when taken full strength, as well as burning of the mouth, throat, and esophagus.

No one with an allergy to apples should use apple cider vinegar. You would think I wouldn't have to say that; if you are surprised that you shouldn't take apple cider vinegar with an apple allergy then you are probably the same guy they have warnings on ladders for that say "if you go above the top step you may fall and get injured.

Patients with low potassium and osteoporosis should avoid apple cider vinegar, since it may worsen both conditions.

Apple Cider Vinegar

Unlike white vinegar, apple cider vinegar is a light yellowish brown color and has lots of sediment and is cloudy. Apple cider vinegar is often sold unfiltered as well as being unpasteurized, and is known as "mother" or "mother of vinegar". The dark sediment at the bottom is the acetobacter bacteria that has settled to the bottom, and is not harmful. This is the best form of apple cider vinegar to drink. One of the oldest and best brands out there is Bragg Apple Cider Vinegar and can easily be found in most food stores or online.

Avoid vinegar in tablet form. It is frequently just acetic acid tablets and does not have many of the healthy benefits found in the liquid form, and if these tablets get lodged in your throat they could burn the mucosal lining.

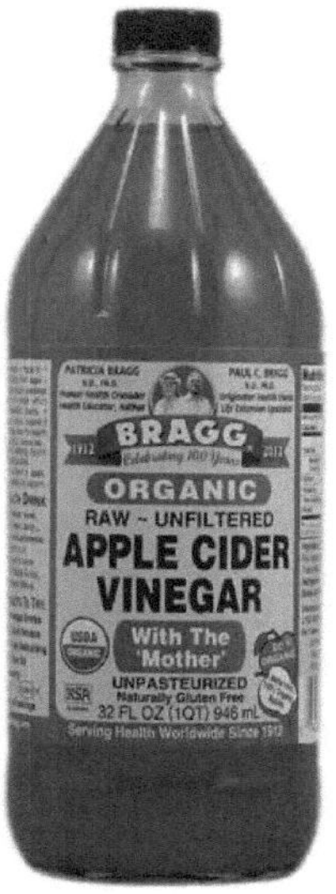

How To Make Your Own Apple Cider Vinegar At Home

In order to practice natural healing and alternative medicine we need to be ever resourceful, and growing our own food and making our own medicines certainly is part of that mindset. Here are some simple instructions in making two things – first, hard apple cider (cider with alcohol) and secondly, further fermenting the hard cider to make apple cider vinegar.

Making Hard Apple Cider

The first thing you need, naturally, are apples. Not just any apple will do, you will need apples that ripen in the fall or winter. These apples contain more sugar than summer and green apples, which don't make good cider. In a pinch you can use any apples; you might just have to increase the sugar content of your ferment, more on this later. Gather up the fruit you need and wash it to remove any dirt and debris from the skins of the apples.

Now, take the fruit and crush it into pulp, if you have an apple press it will be much easier. Drain off the juice from the pulp. If you don't have an apple press, use cheesecloth to strain the juice and separate it from the pulp. You can also make your hard cider from apple cider that you have bought. It can be from commercial ciders because they are usually pasteurized and this will ultimately affect the flavor.

There are two kinds of pasteurization, cold and hot. Cold pasteurization is done with ultraviolet light to kill off the microorganisms and this is the preferable method because it impacts the flavor less than heat pasteurization. At this point you have two choices. You can put the juice in a large glass bottle and cover the top with a double layer of cheesecloth and secure it with a rubber band and place it in a dark, cool place for several months, the ideal temperature being around 60 degrees F. Natural wild yeasts in the air will enter the juice and start the fermentation process. This is slower than the second method of adding active yeast cultures to your juice.

NOTE: Bread yeasts are not good for this. You can use dry wine yeasts which work fine; these can be found online or from any homebrew store. Dry wine yeast packs are very inexpensive and work just as well as cider yeasts.

You can also make your own starter. This is your own active culture which you can add to lots of batches of cider. The formula for your own starter is: First pour out about one-fifth of your cider out of its bottle; you will need this room for fermentation. Crumble one cake of cultivated yeast into the remaining one quart of cider. Reseal the bottle and shake it vigorously for a few seconds and then reseal the bottle. Within five or six hours you should start to see bubbling in the bottle; now fermentation has begun.

Once you see this, lift a corner of the bottle's lid to release the pent up gases within the bottle and then reseal it and put it in the refrigerator. To use it as a starter you will need to take it out of the refrigerator again and let it sit at room temperature for a few hours before you add it to your next batch of cider. This will make enough starters for approximately five gallons of cider. Doing this step is optional, but I recommend doing it because if you have a bad batch of yeast then you have not ruined a large bottle of cider. You will know if it is a bad or dead batch of yeast because it will not begin the bubbling signifying that fermentation has begun.

Only use glass, ceramic, or stainless steel to make cider, do not use other metals or plastic which will react with the ferment and leach out toxins into the cider. The acid in the cider will also corrode most metals except stainless steel.

It is best to sanitize your container or vessel. This step is not critical but highly recommended or you could possible spoil your cider. Sanitizing your container is relatively easy; here is how I recommend it: Pour a cup of bleach into your vessel or container and fill it with cold water and swish it around and then let it sit for about a half an hour and then pour it out and rinse thoroughly with cold, clean water. Repeat this process one or two more times to get any smell of bleach out of the container. Now take your cider and add either your starter or directly add your yeast. Stir the mix with either a plastic or stainless steel spoon for several minutes to mix it well and then seal the lid and affix the airlock. Place your container in a room, closet, or basement.

The ideal temperature for fermentation of cider is about 60 F, but anywhere from 60-75 degrees F will work. If the room is too cold it will stop the fermentation and if it is too warm it will speed it up too much and will change the flavor. The temperature is very important for proper fermentation and you should make every effort to keep it as close to 60 degrees F as you can; doing this correctly now will really pay off in the end. Within a few days you will see gas bubbling from the airlock. This is great news; that is carbon dioxide, a by-product of the fermentation process. We are now on our way to making some great cider. This bubbling will subside after about two weeks, signaling the end of the first step or primary fermentation. Now let the cider sit for a few more weeks to allow the yeast in it to settle out. At this point you can pour the cider off into smaller bottles or jugs that have been sanitized and reseal them and allow them to sit for a week or two and then they will be ready to drink. When performing this step be careful not to slosh around the large container as this will raise the yeast sludge from its bottom and cloud up your cider. This is only cosmetic and does not affect the cider in any other way.

Keep in mind that your cider will most likely be "still", meaning it is not fizzy. However, if you let it sit for several months the fermentation will produce some fizz. Cider is like wine, it does improve with age. The alcohol content of your cider can be raised by raising the amount of sugar that is in your cider for the yeast to ferment and change to alcohol. To sweeten the cider, add either honey or brown sugar before you add the yeast or starter to it. This will raise the sugar content of the cider and once fermented will raise its alcohol content as well. Now you have completed the first step in making hard cider. This step is also known as yeast fermentation for obvious reasons, and is done anaerobically or without oxygen. If you want to drink some of your cider, now is the time. Usually the alcohol content of most ciders is about twice that of beer, so enjoy yourself.

Making Apple Cider Vinegar

Now if you want to go on to make apple cider vinegar, this involves changing the alcohol of the cider to acetic acid of vinegar. This step is known as "acetic acid fermentation" and is carried out by the acetobacter bacteria and unlike step one, this is done aerobically or in the presence of oxygen. The production of apple cider vinegar from apple cider involves two critical factors; temperature and oxygen content. The temperature has to be as close to 60 F as you can get it and you have to stir your brew daily to introduce oxygen into the mix. Also covering the brew with cheesecloth will allow oxygen to enter.

The first step in the conversion of hard apple cider to apple cider vinegar is to pour off the cider into the containers you want to use to ferment your cider. These have to be sanitized as explained above. Only fill the containers about three quarters of the way, and cover it with cheesecloth and keep it out of direct sunlight and as mentioned at as close to 60 F, but no warmer than 80 F. Take a large, stainless steel or plastic spoon and stir the contents daily to introduce oxygen into your mix.

Each time you are finished stirring, replace your cheesecloth cover; this will allow oxygen to continue to enter your mix and will allow the bubbling off of carbon dioxide from the fermentation. A mat of what is known as mother will develop at the bottom of your mix. This is harmless and is a natural part of the fermentation by the acetobacter bacteria. Full fermentation will take about three to four weeks. As the vinegar is maturing, the mix will get a vinegar smell; this is from the acetic acid formed by its conversion from alcohol. The taste will mature over time. You should taste your mix periodically to see how far along you have reached.

When your vinegar is fully fermented you can filter it through either several layers of cheesecloth, or a plain coffee filter will work just fine. The filtering will remove the "mother of vinegar" or the cloudy sediment that has accumulated from the fermentation process. This does not have to be done and is only a matter of preference; personally, I prefer the mother in my vinegar. However, if you choose to remove the mother this will prevent further fermentation and will prevent the vinegar from ultimately spoiling.

Another method to prevent spoilage and insure indefinite storage of your vinegar is to pasteurize it. Pasteurization is done with heat and you have to do it at just the right temperature. This requires a minimum of 140 degrees F and a maximum of 160 degrees F. This will kill off the acetobacter bacteria and allow the vinegar to be stored indefinitely. You do this by placing the bottle of vinegar in a large pan of water and bringing the water to the 140 to 160 F range as stated above. You should use a cooking thermometer to insure the proper temperatures.

As soon as this level is reached, remove your vinegar bottle from the pan of water and allow it to cool and store it out of sunlight in a cool area at as close to 60 degrees F as you can. Remember, the vinegar reacts with its container and can only be stored in glass, ceramic, or stainless steel bottles.

Flavoring Your Vinegar

You can also flavor your vinegars if you like. This can be done with a variety of items including garlic, green onions, ginger, and various herbs.

This will also boost the nutritional content and allow you to make some delicious vinegar that is also very nutritious. Flavoring your vinegars with plant parts whose molecular size are too large to normally use in essential oils is not a problem, and they can easily be introduced into vinegar. The reason this can be done is because vinegar is being ingested, broken down and absorbed by your intestinal tract. This will also allow you a method to introduce larger plant molecules that can be ingested and absorbed in the intestines that otherwise would be too large to cross the skin in an essential oil. To flavor vinegar, suspend the vegetable or herb that you want in a small cheesecloth bag and leave it in the vinegar, usually for four days with the exception of garlic, which is only one day. Make every effort not to overload the vinegar, too much vegetable matter will ruin the acid and ruin the preservation of the vinegar and ultimately cause it to spoil.

A good rule of thumb is to mix as follows:

For every two cups of vinegar add the following for each flavor:

Fresh Herbs, use half a cup

Dried herbs, use one tablespoon

Garlic, use two large cloves

Green onions, use eight small

Four Thieves Vinegar / Master Tonic

Four thieves vinegar has many names; Marseilles vinegar, master tonic, prophylactic vinegar and many others. As the legend goes, depending on which country you are in, this wonderful natural broad spectrum antibiotic, antifungal and antiviral remedy either originated in London during an outbreak of the bubonic plague in 1066 or in Marseilles (or Toulouse) sometime during the centuries of the bubonic plague outbreaks.

As the story goes, here too there are two versions; one where a gang of four thieves were breaking into plague victims homes and robbing the sick and the dying.

Eventually they were apprehended and during their trial they were questioned as to how they never caught the bubonic plague like all the others that is when they disclosed the formula in exchange for their freedom. Another version says that four thieves were already in prison and given the fatal task of burying dead plague victims and came up with this concoction to protect them. Either way, at this point we will never know the true origin of the name.

One thing is true is that the aromatic nature of the tonic probably repelled the fleas that were responsible for spreading the plague and the antimicrobial properties helped treat just about any other infection that they might encounter.

For our purposes, this is a very easy to make tonic that we can do at home and keep on hand either as a daily drink to maintain health and assist our immune system in its fight against any and all types of invaders or as a super-antibiotic/antiviral/antifungal/anti-parasitic drink to be used as needed. With the current widespread over prescribing of antibiotics by physicians as well as the much greater indiscriminate use of antibiotics on factory farms; we have created a perfect storm where multidrug resistant pathogens (germs that cause disease) of all types are winning this arms race and are rendering our antibiotics useless. That is why we need new novel methods of treating diseases of all types, and here is the mother of all natural antibiotics. In addition to being fatal to all types of pathogens it is also purported to increase blood and lymphatic flow as well as being an anti-inflammatory agent.

I would like all of my readers to prepare themselves at least one or two mason jars full of this master tonic to have on hand if they become sick. Face it, you will not feel like making this once you are sick, so the time to do it is now.

Let's take a look at what goes into this master tonic: The original recipe hung in the Museum of Paris in 1937, supposedly it was an original copy of one that hung on the walls of Marseilles during the plague.

There are several minor variations of this formula; here is the most powerful combination of natural ingredients that in my humble opinion would make you the best, most potent four thieves or master tonic brew:

1. Garlic: Garlic by itself is well known for its antibacterial properties from its active compound allicin which has a broad range of antimicrobial activity. Allicin is produced by garlic when the bulb is damaged, either by crushing, biting or cutting. Allicin is what the garlic plant produces to protect itself from predators; it also gives garlic its pungent odor. The good news for us is that it kills many types of bacteria, but does not kill the good probiotic bacteria that live in our intestines. Garlic even has activity against multi-drug resistant strains of E.coli and intestinal parasites.
2. Ginger: Ginger has been used for centuries to treat illnesses, and also has the benefit of helping nausea and vomiting. Ginger is in the same family as turmeric. The root of the plant is what is used medicinally. The active ingredient in ginger is known as gingerol. Gingerol has antibacterial, as well as antiviral activity and has been used as such for centuries as a treatment for colds and flu.
3. Horseradish: Horseradish is a perennial herb that is easily grown in any garden, for our purposes we use the root. For our purposes horseradish adds a powerful immune stimulation to the tonic as well as delivering vitamin C, enzymes and minerals.
4. Onions: Onions possess antibacterial, antifungal and antiparasitic properties that help all of those type of infections. In addition, onions are strong antioxidants as well as being anti-inflammatory.
5. Red chilies: Here you can use red chilies or any other hot peppers such as cayenne, jalapeno, serrano's and habanero's. All of these hot peppers contain the active ingredient capsaicin, which is a natural pain killer as well as being anti-inflammatory. Capsaicin also is known to support your immune system, thus aiding your body in ridding itself of an infection. **NOTE:** You should wear gloves when preparing your tonic because of the capsaicin content of any of these peppers, which will cause severe burning if there is any scratches or open wounds. The only way to neutralize the burning is with milk.
6. Turmeric: Turmeric is the main spice in curry, giving its characteristic flavor. In India, turmeric has been used for many centuries as a topical antiseptic due to its strong antimicrobial properties (it kills germs). Turmeric also boosts your immune system and is a potent anti-inflammatory agent.
7. Raw Honey: Raw honey means honey that has not been pasteurized, filtered or treated in any way. Honey never spoils; you can eat thousand year old honey. The reason for this is that honey has antibacterial, antifungal and antiviral properties that prevent anything from growing in it causing it to spoil. When honey interacts with the water in your body it produces hydrogen peroxide which kills many types of microbes (germs).
8. Apple Cider Vinegar: Apple cider vinegar helps preserve foods by preventing the growth of germs like E.coli. There are many health enhancing benefits of vinegar that I described earlier in this chapter.

The Recipe for Making Your Own Four Thieves/ Master Tonic

Ingredients: This will make one large Mason jar of your tonic, scale it up for larger batches. Try to use only organic ingredients to prevent any toxins from contaminating your brew.

1/4 cup of freshly chopped garlic (wait to chop it until you are ready to use it)

1/4 cup of chopped white onion

2 fresh hot peppers (red chilie, habanero's, serrano's, jalapeno or cayenne peppers)

1/4 cup of freshly grated ginger

2 teaspoons of freshly grated horseradish

1/4 cup of freshly grated turmeric (or two teaspoons of turmeric powder)

3 tablespoons of raw honey

3 cups of Bragg's apple cider vinegar or any unfiltered and unpasteurized organic apple cider vinegar

1 large Mason jar with lid

Cheesecloth to use as a strainer

Preparation:

Mix all the ingredients in a large bowl, without the apple cider vinegar.

Transfer your mix to a large Mason jar, filling it about 2/3 of the way.

Fill the rest of the jar with your Apple Cider Vinegar, leaving a small open area at the top so you can shake it to mix it.

Keep the Mason jar in a cool, dry place mixing it several times a day (this step is critical, if you don't do this it will not work) for about two weeks time. Do not dilute it with water. It will probably reach its maximum potency in about six week's time.

After at least two weeks (any time after which is fine) you should strain your mix through a cheesecloth and pour the liquid tonic into another clean mason jar.

Place your mix in a cool, dark place and it will keep indefinitely. You do not need to refrigerate it, unless you prefer your tonic cold to drink.

Directions in its Use:

You can take your four thieves/master tonic several different ways. You could use it as a daily health tonic to boost your immunity and prevent any infections. It also will provide an incredible array of vitamins, plant nutrients, minerals, enzymes and trace elements. Any of the doses are pretty arbitrary, but use half of what you normally would in a child or a pregnant woman.

For a sore throat you could gargle a tablespoon of it several times a day.

You could make a poultice and apply it as a topical antiseptic to any external wounds.

If you have a severe infection like a cold or the flu you could take a tablespoon (1 or 2 ounces) every four to six hours, depending on how sick you are.

For its immune support and general health benefits you can take one tablespoon a day. If you feel as if you are coming down with an illness, then double or triple your dose.

CHAPTER TWELVE

WOOD ASH, LYE, SOAP AND ACTIVATED CHARCOAL

INTRODUCTION

TABLE OF CONTENTS:

As a physician in private practice for over twenty-five years I have come across a handful of treatments that I have found to be outstanding; it is not a very large group, but activated charcoal is definitely one of them. It has proved itself time and time again to be incredibly useful and quick acting and has helped countless numbers of my patients recover amazingly fast from nausea and vomiting and GI upset. There is no medication comparable in that regard, but the good news does not end there, activated charcoal has many other clinical uses and this is an item that I would rank up there in my top ten as the most useful, versatile, and indispensable. The World Health Organization has even listed it on their list of essential medicines. Activated charcoal is still used extensively in emergency rooms around the country and is also used in filter systems of every conceivable type from fish tanks to sewage treatment plants and is indispensable in our modern world.

Let's take a look at what activated charcoal actually is, and let's examine its structure and why that structure contributes so much to its unique and varied applications. To understand the process of activated charcoal production we first have to see how charcoal is produced and for this we need to examine the structure of wood.

WOOD

Wood is made of four essential ingredients:

Water
Volatile Organic Compounds
Carbon
Ash

All wood contains water. Freshly cut wood's volume is almost half water, dried or seasoned wood is much less. If you ever made a fire you will remember the sizzling sound made by water boiling off of freshly cut wood that had not been adequately dried. Green or unseasoned (not dried) wood will also be much heavier than dried wood because of all the water it contains.

The volatile organic compounds are the sap and the cellulose and other organic chemicals that the tree produces and are found in its wood. Volatile means that the substance evaporates when heated. Carbon is self-explanatory as its own element. Ash is what is left over when wood is burnt and it is composed primarily of non- burnable minerals such as potassium, calcium, and magnesium, among others, as well as many trace elements. The minerals and trace elements in ash will vary depending upon the type of soil the tree was grown in as well as the type of tree, because different trees require different minerals and trace elements for their health.

CHARCOAL AND ASH

Charcoal is created by heating wood to very high temperatures in the absence of oxygen, and this is done by heating it within a closed structure such as a clay or stone box, or a steel box in modern times. Once you heat this wood to approximately a thousand degrees F this will evaporate off all of the water and burn off all of the volatile organic compounds, leaving you with carbon and all the other minerals. You have to remember to have a vent hole in the box you are making the charcoal in. This allows for the volatile organic compounds which are now gases to vent off, otherwise you will have a pressure bomb that will explode at a certain point. The vent hole has to be small enough to allow the gases to escape and yet prevent oxygen from being sucked in; if this happens, you will burn the wood and not char it. Now, if you decide to burn your charcoal you are just burning the carbon and allowing it to combine with oxygen and produce C02 or carbon dioxide, and the only thing remaining once all the carbon has burned off will be the mineral- and trace element-containing ash.

By the way, this ash is wonderful for your garden for all the minerals it contains, and should never be discarded. One of the primary tenets I try to follow is to make do with what you have and also to utilize everything available to you; therefore, why discard ash when it can be put to further use to provide minerals to your garden and ultimately to you?

The value of ash was recognized as far back as the Romans, who added it to their soils to improve them. In the eighteenth century the United States was heavily wooded and the clearing of those woods for farms involved the cutting down of millions of very large, old trees. This resulted in a large wood ash, or potash, industry. The very first patent issued by the patent office of the young United States, patent number one, was for a method of making fertilizer from wood ash and was called "an improved method of making pot and pearl ash".

In addition to the minerals and trace elements named above in ash, it also contains oxides and carbonates that are alkaline, making ash a valuable material to "sweeten" soils by raising their pH. Most soils tend to be on the acidic side and increase in acidity over time and therefore benefit from raising their pH to make them more alkaline, hence their usefulness in our medicinal gardens.

There are large differences in the ash produced by hardwood trees such as oak and ash as compared to softwood trees like pine. Hardwood produces three times as much ash and five times as many nutrients as compared to softwood trees. Ash should be gently worked into your soil and well spread out to avoid concentrating any of the mineral salts it contains in any one area that might damage plants, so work it in to your garden with a hoe and a rake.

Wood ash can also be used to neutralize the acidity of your compost pile and will add minerals to your compost. It can also be used sprinkled around the base of plants as an insecticide. Ash works as an insecticide by drawing water from the bodies of insects, snails, and slugs, and will deter surface feeding insects, but will lose its value once it becomes wet.

Ash can also be used to treat your dog or cat after they have been skunked, and can be spread on ice to melt it. So, as you can see, we are using what would normally be considered a waste product for multiple applications, and that is something that is near and dear to my heart.

POTASH AND LYE

Incidentally, potash is different from ash and in earlier times was made from ash. Potash is actually potassium-containing compounds made from wood ash. The potassium in wood ash is water soluble, meaning it dissolves in water, so in the old days they would soak wood ash in water and then take that water (which was basically lye) and heat it in large metal pots. Once all the water was evaporated off you were left with an ash that was basically potassium hydroxide, which was used for fertilizer and other industrial needs.

Note: Do not use ash on acid-loving plants like azaleas, rhododendrons, blueberries and huckleberries. Also avoid using wood ash on potato plants since it encourages potato scab, and do not use it on new seedlings since it is too high in mineral salts and will kill them. Also, do not combine it with nitrogen-based fertilizers such as ammonium sulfate, ammonium nitrate, or urea, since it may produce ammonia gas.

I have digressed a little here; I just wanted to illustrate the various steps involved and the useful by-products produced. Now let's get back to how to make activated charcoal.

ACTIVATED CHARCOAL

Activated charcoal is actually carbon that has been treated with oxygen to open up millions of tiny pores between the carbon atoms. This is done by first crushing the coal or carbon into a very fine powder and then placing it in a tank and highly heating it, then exposing it to argon and nitrogen gases in the absence of oxygen. In the final step it is exposed to steam and oxygen at high temperatures, which again opens up the pores in the carbon, vastly increasing its surface area. The final product is activated charcoal. There is an alternative process for making activated charcoal by exposing the charcoal to various chemicals and heating it and repeating the process. This second method frequently leaves behind residual chemicals from the original chemical exposure step.

HOW ACTIVATED CHARCOAL WORKS

Activated charcoal comes in three different grades, depending on the size of the final particles. The powdered form is more potent than the granular form because of the much larger surface area. Most people think that any chemicals that get neutralized by activated charcoal is done by absorption (with a B). Absorption means just soaking something up into something else, sort of like a sponge. Activated charcoal actually works by adsorption (with a D). Adsorption involves a chemical bonding on the surface of the activated charcoal, not a soaking up or absorption. Adsorption would be like chalk on a blackboard, where the chalk is bound to the surface of the blackboard but does not soak into the blackboard (that is why you are able to erase the blackboard). Sometimes adsorption is the first step before absorption...an example of that would be wood exposed to rain, at first the rainwater is adsorbed or bound to the surface of the wood then eventually it absorbs and enters into the wood itself, swelling the wood. The reason I am going into this lengthy discourse about the differences between absorption and adsorption is so you understand how activated charcoal works in your body. Think about it, if activated charcoal absorbed substances in your body into itself, it would swell to huge proportions and seriously injure your body. Instead it adsorbs and just binds all kinds of chemicals, microorganisms, toxins, etc. to its huge surface area and eliminates them with your stool.

For medical use, it is best to use the finest powdered activated charcoal because it has the greatest surface area and therefore the greatest ability to adsorb toxins, gases, chemicals, and medicines of all types directly onto its surface. I keep a tub of the loose powder in my medicinal/alternative medicine chest due to its multiple medicinal uses and its unsurpassed ability to filter and purify water. I also keep many bottles of the activated charcoal capsules. You should always have a bottle of these capsules readily available for accidental poisoning, but mainly for nausea and vomiting.

Beware: Since activated charcoal has the unrivaled ability to adsorb huge quantities of substances onto its surface, it will also inactivate any medications or vitamins or anything else you take within about two to three hours of taking it. I try to wait three hours just to be on the safe side. Activated charcoal's ability to adsorb such a huge number of substances is also the reason you cannot take it all the time since it might also adsorb and remove too many vitamins and minerals and trace elements from your body, which is why it should be used with particular caution in growing children. However, that being said, you can certainly use it in emergencies internally without any worries, and you can use it topically as often as you like since it has no consequences when used in this manner.

Activated charcoal is odorless, tasteless, and completely inert and indigestible by humans. The surface area of a one-inch cube of activated charcoal is so great that it unfolds to a thousand square yards of surface. Think about that for a minute...a one-inch cube unfolds to an area of ten football fields wide, by ten football fields long! That is simply amazing, and that same surface area gives activated charcoal its unique ability to adsorb gases, foreign proteins, body wastes, free radicals, poison chemicals, and drugs onto its surface, binding them and then eliminating them.

Activated charcoal is not a recent invention, although the modern methods for making it are much different. Activated charcoal was used as far back as the Egyptians in approximately 1550 BC (I still like using BC better than the new BCE). In recent times one of my favorite anecdotes about activated charcoal occurred in 1831 in the French Academy of Medicine where a Professor Touery drank a lethal dose of strychnine mixed with activated charcoal which completely neutralized it, thus causing him absolutely no harm. What better example of the amazing power of activated charcoal to neutralize poisons (toxins).

A very ingenious use of charcoal for purification of water was employed by the manufacturers of wooden water barrels. The inner sides of the barrel staves were charred before the barrels' assembly. This worked to continuously expose the water to the surface of the charcoal, keeping the water purified -- especially for long sea voyages. Activated charcoal has many uses, including in the garden where it can be used to top-dress soils, where it is then mixed in and it neutralizes any toxins in your soil.

Sodium bicarbonate also is very useful in the same way to neutralize radioactivity in your soil. Activated charcoal can be made from animal bones instead of plant matter like wood, coconut husks, nutshells, and peat. There is a significant difference between vegetable charcoal and animal charcoal and that is the carbon content. Vegetable charcoal is about 90 percent carbon whereas animal charcoal is only about 11 percent carbon. Carbon is the key, so for our purposes it is always vegetable charcoal that we will use, even if we are making it ourselves. There are numerous YouTube instructional videos on how to make your own activated charcoal.

Note: Burnt toast is not activated charcoal, not even close; it is just superheated proteins, fats, and carbohydrates that are in toast. Also, charcoal briquettes like we use in barbecues and outdoor grills are soaked in petroleum distillates (to help them ignite) and should never ever be used because of this contamination and has no usefulness either topically or internally.

HOW TO USE ACTIVATED CHARCOAL MEDICALLY

Activated charcoal has many medical uses. The one I find most useful is for any gastrointestinal problems (GI) such as diarrhea, nausea, gas, and vomiting. For this I prefer to use two capsules immediately and then every six hours or so until the symptoms subside. Remember, you cannot take any other medications orally for the next two or three hours. If all you have is activated charcoal in powder form then take one tablespoon of activated charcoal in a large glass of water. You should maintain your hydration by drinking a glass of water after each subsequent bowel movement. This will also work for food poisoning of any kind and should be used the same way.

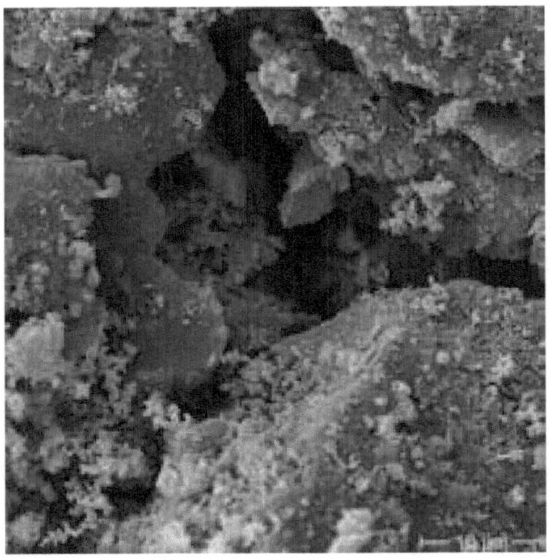

Dark field micrograph of Activated Charcoal showing its huge surface area

Food poisoning is caused by bacterial infection of foods; when you eat food that has been spoiled you are ingesting large amounts of these bacteria. Many of these bacteria release toxins that cause our bodies to try to eliminate them by pouring massive amounts of fluid into our intestines in an attempt to flush them out of our bodies, resulting in diarrhea. Activated charcoal will adsorb these toxins and the bacteria that caused them directly onto its surface, inactivating the toxins and eliminating them from your body.

ACTIVATED CHARCOAL DOSING FOR POISONING OR DRUG OVERDOSES

Infants (under one year old):

The dose is 1 gram for every kilogram or two and a half pounds of body weight.

Children (one to twelve years old):

The dose is 15 to 30 grams if you are not sure of the weight, or 1 or 2 grams for every two and one half pounds with at least 8 ounces of water.

Adults (twelve years old and older):

The dose is 30 to 100 grams or if you know their weight then give between 1 to 2 grams for every two and one half pounds.

BITES AND BURNS

For these, surface application of activated charcoal is ideal and is done by making a poultice. To make an activated charcoal poultice simply mix a paste from several tablespoons of activated charcoal mixed in water. Mix this to a paste consistency, not too dry to crumble and not to wet to be runny. Next, take a piece of gauze or lightly woven cloth or in an emergency whatever kind of material you have available and drench it with your activated charcoal/water mixture. Apply this gauze or cloth over the area that is being treated, completely covering it, and then cover the gauze or cloth with a plastic wrap or other plastic material to keep it from drying out.

Note: Once it dries it will no longer be effective. An alternate method is to mix the activated charcoal and water with flaxseed or corn starch in a ratio of two parts activated charcoal to three parts flaxseed or cornstarch. The benefit of using flaxseed or cornstarch is that it will develop into a jelly-like consistency and be much more resistant to drying out. Keep this mix on overnight or until it dries. Poultices can be placed anywhere on the body including the head, eyelids and face.

LIMITATIONS OF THE USE OF ACTIVATED CHARCOAL

Activated charcoal will not work in poisoning with the following substances: Ethanol (drinking alcohol), methanol, lithium, cyanide, iron, lye, or strong acids; for everything else it will work just fine.

HOW TO MAKE YOUR OWN SOAP

There are several ways to make soap, all of which start with lye. One of the simplest ways to make some soap is, after using a frying pan over a hardwood camp fire, take some of the ashes from the fire and sprinkle them on the fat in the pan, add some water. They will combine and make you a small batch of soap. You cannot use softwoods like pine to make lye because of their high resin content, so stick with hard woods like oak, maple, and ash, for example.

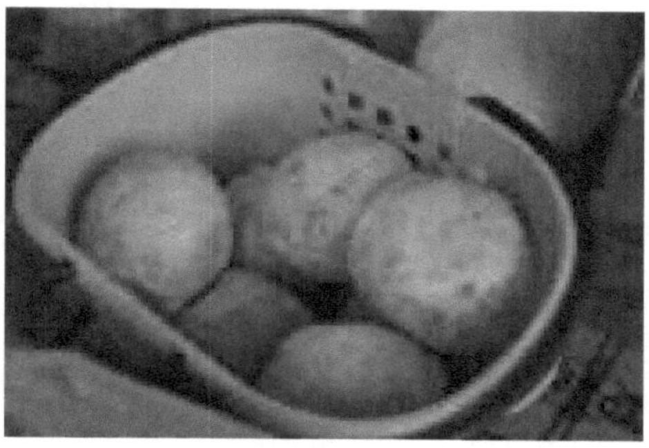

Photo of Handmade Soaps

Larger quantities of soap can easily be made by constructing a lye- leaching container. To make a lye-leaching container you have to use a wooden barrel, or a plastic or a steel container. Lye has a pH of 13 and will eat through aluminum, it is a very dangerous, strongly alkaline solution. Drill or punch holes in the bottom of the container to allow drainage, then fill the bottom of the container with a layer of gravel on top of which will be a two or three inch layer of straw or dried grass, on top of that will go your wood ashes. Tamp down the ashes to compress them and make a depression in the middle of the ashes. Now the top of the container has to be open so you can pour water onto the ashes and allow that water to dissolve the lye from the ash and then pass through the straw and then the gravel for a second filtration. You should fill the depression with water and then wait several hours as the water slowly trickles out of the bottom.

The first batch produced will be the strongest. You can get a second batch of lye by using the same barrel's contents and passing water through it. This second pass lye has to be repassed through the barrel to make it strong enough.

The lye is then combined with animal fat to make soap; you have to keep adding enough fat to consume all the lye. There are actual tables called saponification tables that tell you the required ratio of fat to lye. You can also use any vegetable oil instead of animal fat. Remember, oils are just liquid fat at room temperatures.

Caution: If you get lye in your eyes you have to douse them with milk; if you get lye on your skin douse it with vinegar to neutralize it. Lye is a very caustic substance… meaning it burns like hell! Anything at either end of the pH spectrum will be dangerous…either a strong acid with a very low pH or a strong base or alkali with a very high pH. Lye has a pH of about 13, which is very strong. Lye will easily eat right through things like aluminum.

HOW TO MAKE ACTIVATED CHARCOAL

Activated charcoal can be made from charcoal you have made in your improvised oven and then it needs to be treated with acid and reheated again. From the stage of making charcoal you can also make black powder or wood alcohol or just leave it as charcoal if you want to smelt any metals, since charcoal burns much hotter than wood and thus has been used in forges since ancient times. The best way is to start with the smallest pieces of wood, so cut up your wood as best you can. Eventually, you are going to have to grind these small pieces up into a fine powder, so it is critical to start with very small pieces of wood. A hardwood sawdust would be an ideal place to start.

Whatever you use for making the oven to burn your charcoal, it has to have two common features -- it has to be able to be sealed to prevent oxygen from entering, or you will just completely burn the wood and form ash but no coal. Secondly, you need to have a vent hole, large enough to allow the volatile chemicals in the wood to escape after they have been changed into gases yet small enough to prevent oxygen from being drawn in.

You have to design a setup so your closed oven can be suspended over a fire, allowing it to heat up without the presence of oxygen, to boil off the water and eventually cook off all the volatile chemicals that are in the wood; once these two are gone you will have your carbon and ash left.

Since water boils off at about 212 F at sea level (as you go up in altitude water will boil at a lower temperature), the first thing you will see exiting your vent hole will be steam. Once you see steam coming out you should cook the wood for at least another four hours. This is not written in stone and depends on the amount of wood you have in your oven and the heat production of your fire, etc. After four or five hours have passed and you think you are finished making your charcoal, remove the oven from the fire.

This step is critical. You have to wait until the oven has completely cooled down before you open it, otherwise the char will burst into flame if it is hot and exposed to a sudden rush of oxygen by you opening the oven. At this point you have made charcoal, and if you want to go on to make black powder or use it for smelting an ore, you are ready to do that. For our purposes we need to acid-treat the charcoal and reheat it before we have made activated charcoal. For an acid a good source is battery acid, which you can buy in any auto supply store. Be advised, this acid is very dangerous and has to be handled very carefully to avoid serious acid burns. You should be wearing an apron, goggles, gloves, and a mask over your nose and mouth to keep from inhaling any noxious fumes. Pour the acid into a glass cooking pan, put each piece of coal into the acid bath and allow it to soak for about five minutes, then carefully remove the charcoal and drain off the excess acid and place the charcoal back into the oven. Keep repeating this process until you have soaked all of the charcoal in acid.

As an alternative to battery acid, which is strong sulfuric acid, you can use hydrochloric acid which you can buy in pool supply stores as muriatic acid. It is used to clean the linings of cement swimming pools or you can find it in hardware stores. You can also use nitric acid, but that is harder to find and usually you can only get it from chemical supply stores that probably won't sell it to you.

Now put all the acid-treated charcoal back into your oven, reseal it and reheat it for another four or five hours until it is completely heated. Just like in the earlier step, you need to allow the oven to cool down before you open it and expose it to oxygen or you will have another flash fire as the activated charcoal catches fire. Carefully open up the oven, remove the charcoal and grind it up into as fine a powder as you can, and now you have made activated charcoal.

Note: for the purposes of home water purification, if you are making your own activated charcoal, coconut husks are supposedly the best material to use for this. If you do happen to live in a tropical environment with many coconuts available you should also learn how to make coconut oil which has many medicinal as well as nutritional uses.

An alternative method for making your own activated charcoal involves using two steel barrels, one fifty-five gallon and one thirty-five gallon with its lid, and a few thick, long pieces of rebar. Cut two one foot by one foot holes in the fifty-five gallon drum's sides and then take the thirty-five gallon drum and drill nine or ten holes in its bottom. Now fill the fifty-five gallon drum with your firewood. Fill the thirty-five gallon drum with the wood you want to make into charcoal and seal it up so the only holes are those in its bottom, facing the fifty- five gallon drum fire. Slide the thirty-five gallon drum onto the long rebar rods and place it on top of the fifty-five gallon drum. Now, light the fifty-five gallon drum's wood on fire. Cook it as above for four or five hours and then remove the thirty-five gallon drum from the fire and allow it to properly cool and once it is cooled, open it and there is your charcoal. The difference with this and the previous method is the gas in the thirty-five gallon drum has nowhere to go but out into the fire below, thus stoking that fire and letting it burn even hotter, so in effect you are circulating the wood gases back into the fifty-five gallon drum's fire to make it even hotter.

There are many other methods available to you on YouTube and other websites.

PART THREE

WHATS YOUR PROBLEM?

CHAPTER THIRTEEN

FEVER

INTRODUCTION

TABLE OF CONTENTS:

Fever is technically considered any body temperature greater than the normal 98.6 F (37 C) orally (99 F rectally) and not significant until above 100.4 F (38 C). Any temperature between these two ranges is considered a low-grade fever and not usually considered to be clinically significant. Your medicinal/alternative medicine chest will need to include several mercury thermometers. Digital thermometers are great until you run out of battery power. A mercury thermometer will last a long time and needs no power.

There is one cardinal rule about fever that I want you to remember: You do not usually have to treat a fever unless it is greater than 103 to 104 range or unless the patient is delirious. Fever is your friend. Your body is an amazing machine, fine-tuned and very capable of self-healing. One of its greatest mechanisms for defeating infections of any type is fever. The primary reason for this is that the microbes (bacteria, viruses, or yeast) that cause infections can only survive within a narrow temperature range. Most human pathogens (disease causing microbes) live at approximately 98.6 F. That is the reason they are able to infect us; we are the perfect hosts for them. Your body, being a wizard at curing itself, knows this and utilizes it to defeat these invaders. It jacks up its own temperature oftentimes to levels incompatible with life for those microbes.

FEVER AND YOUR IMMUNE SYSTEM

Fever also has other positive effects on your immune system. It increases the activity and the power of your immune system's foot soldiers. White blood cells like macrophages reside in your tissues and destroy germs by swallowing them whole and then digesting them; hence their Greek-derived name macros, meaning large, and phage, meaning to eat. Macrophages, being the big eaters that they are, will digest cellular debris, microbes, foreign substances, and even cancer cells. This is all done by a process known as phagocytosis. The other kind of white blood cell foot soldiers that next come into play are the lymphocytes. Some are T lymphocytes (or T cells) which directly confront the invaders, and B lymphocytes (or B cells) which stand at a distance and send in their artillery in the form of antibodies that are specific for each and every type of bacteria, virus, or fungus. This is accomplished by an incredible memory for previous invasions by your immune system. When it recognizes an old foe, it immediately starts churning out specific antibodies made just for that microbe. If it encounters a new microbial invader, it notes its characteristics and produces new antibodies specific for it. If the immune system is working properly, this will usually prevent reinfection by the same microbial invader. There are also other added immune benefits of fever such as increasing the pulse or heart rate. This speeds up blood flow by making the heart beat faster. This sends increasing numbers of all of those foot soldiers -- the macrophages, T, and B lymphocytes, into the area of infection, helping to defeat it.

FEVER AND YOUR HEART

You should also note that for each degree F of increased body temperature you will see a corresponding increase of about ten beats per minute in the heart rate. The average pulse rate is about eighty, with a range of sixty-one to ninety-nine being normal. Sixty and below is considered bradycardia, or a slow heart rate, and one hundred and above is considered to be tachycardia, or a fast heart rate. This higher pulse rate produces more heat. After all, the heart is a muscle and increasing muscular contractions generates more heat. Also the movement of the blood cells through the circulatory system also increases body heat and contributes to heat production and therefore fever.

FEVER AND A PATIENTS UNDERLYING HEALTH

Certain facts to keep in mind with Fevers: Fever production is usually tied somewhat to vitality. If you are weak and debilitated, then most likely your fever will be the same way. Strong, robustly healthy patients will spike high, sudden fevers. This is nothing to be concerned about.

TERTIAN AND QUARTAN FEVERS

Some infections (frequently parasitic infections such as malaria) will cause an intermittent fever that will spike every third or fourth day. This is due to the lifecycle of the malarial parasite. It reproduces within the red blood cells where it is inaccessible to the body's immune defenses. After several days of rapid reproduction within the red blood cells the malarial parasites will explode the red blood cells and enter the circulatory system (blood stream) in large numbers. This will trigger a severe immune response in an effort to bring the infection under control; this in turn causes a fever. This cycle takes three to four days to complete. If a fever occurs every third day it is known as a tertian fever, if every fourth day it is called a quartan fever.

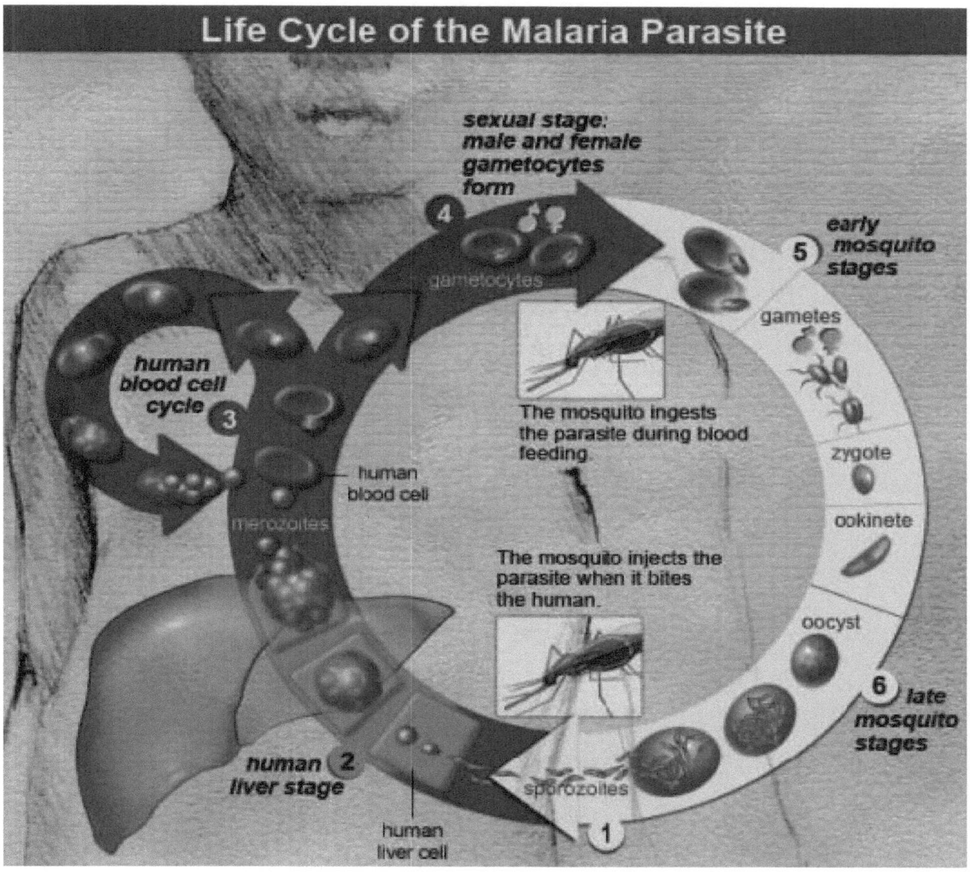

CAUSES OF FEVER

During a bacterial or other invasion of the body there are often toxins produced by the invaders that act as pyrogens (fever-causing substances) and cause fever. As the invaders are killed by our immune systems they also release proteins and other body parts that are foreign to the body and also contribute to fever. These all have to be eliminated by the primary organs responsible for detoxification, the liver and kidneys.

The skin also has a role through its sweat and sebaceous glands, but to a lesser degree. This increased activity of detoxification also produces heat and adds to body temperature. The enzyme systems in the body are also activated and release enzymes that are responsible for the further degradation of these toxins, and their activity also contributes to fever. These pyrogens travel in the blood to the brain and affect the body's thermostat, the hypothalamus. The hypothalamus is the part of the brain that is responsible for temperature regulation. Hypothalamus means below the thalamus, thus denoting its anatomical position within the brain. Once affected by the presence of these pyrogens, the hypothalamus will reset the body's temperature to a newer, higher setting. This new fever puts all the above processes into play; the entire body acts in concert to defeat the invaders. As a medical student, I remember being in awe of this incredibly complex process. It is a beautiful symphony and the hypothalamus acts as the conductor. I want you to appreciate the absolute beauty of this system and remember not to interfere with your body's efforts to heal by mistakenly treating a fever.

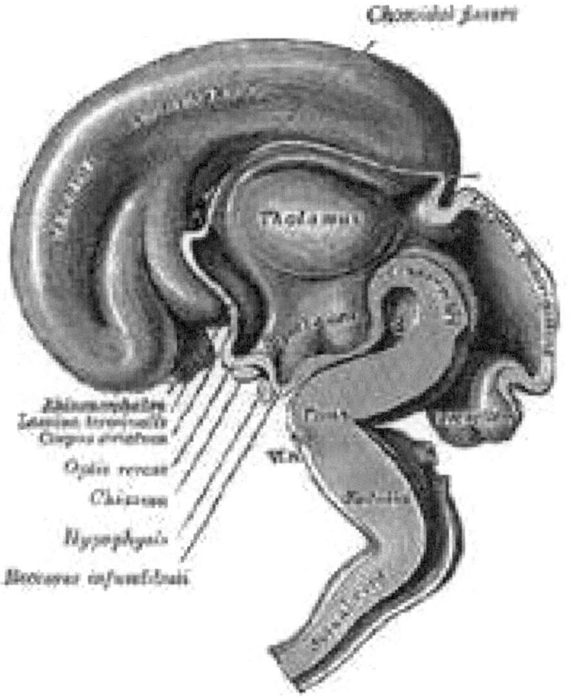

Diagram showing the Hypothalamus within the Brain

Other causes of Fever:

Severe Sunburn
Cancer
Heat exhaustion
Medications
Vaccination

CHILDREN AND FEVER

Children frequently run high fevers without any residual problems. They rise and fall faster than adults. Aspirin should never be used to treat fever in children due to it causing Reye's syndrome. Reye's syndrome is a potentially fatal syndrome caused by giving aspirin to a child with a viral infection. It causes severe hypoglycemia and organ damage, including the brain and liver. The liver becomes damaged and the brain swells, eventually killing the child. These children will develop rashes on their palms and feet, nausea and vomiting and lethargy (they seem sleepy). They may ironically spike a high fever; complain of headaches, and eventually the lethargy progresses to a coma and death. I hope at this point that I have convinced you that you should never ever use aspirin in children.

FEVER AND SEIZURES IN CHILDREN

Children also get febrile seizures (caused by a fever). These are usually benign and not a problem. If one occurs the child should be held by a parent and you should keep their mouths free of any food or drink to prevent them from choking. Any tight clothes should be loosened and the child held on their side or stomach. The child will lose consciousness and will have uncontrolled movement of their arms and legs. These seizures usually are self-limited and will not last very long and usually have no residual effects on the child. When I say not lasting very long, I mean usually for less than thirty seconds. It has been my experience that patients wildly overestimate the length of seizures, usually describing them as lasting five or ten minutes. This is due to their traumatic nature; seeing someone seize scares the hell out of people. Febrile seizures are fairly common in children from six months up to five years of age and are nothing to be overly concerned about, but I would certainly inform your pediatrician.

TREATMENT OF FEVER

Remember that fever should only be treated in rare cases. Examples of this include patients who are delirious, temperatures greater than 103 F to 104 F range, patients who are hallucinating from a fever, are in intense muscle pain or headache, or severe muscle spasms. Sometimes a fever will just be going on too long and has exhausted and weakened the patient. This usually depends on the individual's tolerance, but several days in a row of high fevers will debilitate (weaken) most patients. Treating a fever will most likely prolong the infection by slowing the body's main line of defense, but sometimes you will have no other recourse. Your treatment goal in lowering a fever is not to eliminate it entirely, but rather to lower it to tolerable levels; this way you are limiting the impairment of your body's defenses as much as possible.

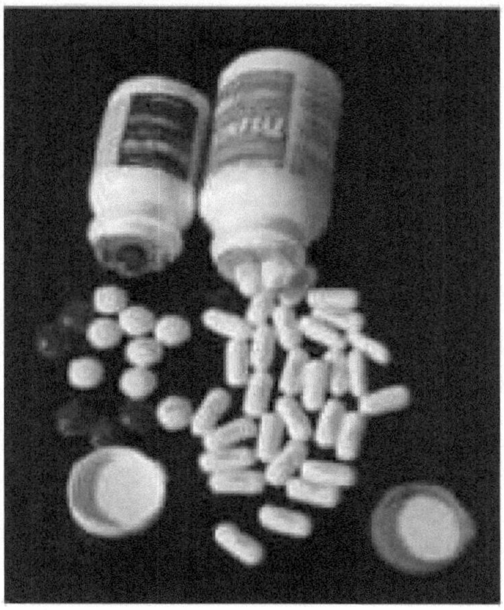

Tylenol (Acetaminophen) and Other Nonsteroidal Medications

Tylenol is the main line of defense. Tylenol works very well to bring down a fever and unlike Motrin, Aleve, and other nonsteroidal anti-

Inflammatory drugs, it will not cause GI upset. Tylenol is toxic to the liver, but the threshold for severe liver damage is approximately 4 grams a day. Remember, a gram is a thousand milligrams. So a dose of less than eight 500 mg Tylenols a day will be below the toxic threshold. Alcoholic drinks will also combine with Tylenol and increase its toxicity. In those cases the 4-gram threshold is off. I would never try to give Tylenol if there is alcohol in someone's system due to this potential liver toxicity (damage).

Any of the other nonsteroidals such as Motrin, Ibuprofen, Aleve (naprosyn) etc will also lower temperatures. I would make sure your medicine chest includes large bottles of these drugs. They are very useful for pain control and cheap to buy in bulk especially at a wholesale club. The government as of this writing just recently mandated lower Tylenol levels in drugs that are combined with Tylenol, the reason being the growing awareness of liver toxicity from Tylenol. For that reason, I would buy several large bottles of the 500 mg Tylenol strength before it is taken off the market. The government has a never-ending zeal for regulating American citizens, and Tylenol seems to be one of the most recent targets in its regulatory crosshairs.

Ice Water Baths, Cold Compresses, and Alcohol Rubdowns

Other methods of lowering temperatures are cold baths, or in extreme cases, immersing patients in ice water baths. This is only employed in extreme cases of hyperthermia (high body temperature). Rubbing a patient down with cool compresses (face cloths) or using rubbing alcohol will also suffice to lower their temperature. It is the same principle as sweating. Sweating releases water onto the skin's surface that evaporates, carrying heat away from your skin and cooling it. Shivering and goose bumps have the opposite effect, increasing your body temperature. As you can see, your skin has temperature-regulatory roles in both lowering and raising body temperature.

Aspirin also works very well to lower temperatures, but as I mentioned it should not be used in children because of potentially triggering a fatal Reye's syndrome. Fever also causes significant fluid loss and eventually will cause dehydration. For that reason maintaining adequate fluid intake during fever is very important. See the section on dehydration for a more in depth discussion on rehydration.

Rest and Hydration

Rest is very important in treating fever. Having a patient lie still and rest (not sleeping necessarily) will decrease the heat produced by muscles involved in movement. The rest should preferably be in the shade if outside. If inside, choose a cool, well-ventilated room with a light sheet on the patient. Keep the patient well hydrated and replace any fluid and electrolyte losses. The hydration will also help the body's efforts at waste removal. Fevers produce large quantities of waste products. If the fever is caused directly by a toxin (or indirectly from a microbial infection that is producing toxins such as Clostridia difficile or C. diff as it is frequently referred to) the hydration will assist the body's removal of these toxins.

HERBAL TREATMENTS

There are some herbal preparations that will lower a fever. Here are a few of the more potent ones.

White Willow

White Willow (Salix alba) is readily available in the United States. It is a widely planted landscape tree and usually lives near a water source. White willow is so named because of the white color on the underside of its leaves. It is originally from Europe and western Asia. The active ingredient in its bark is salicin. White willow can also be made into a tincture by crushing its bark in some ethanol (the kind of alcohol used to make alcoholic beverages). White willow has been used for thousands of years in Europe and Asia including as far back as ancient Egypt. It was used for both pain control and to treat fevers.

To use it, scrape off three-quarters of an ounce of dried bark and add it to a quart of boiling water. Boil for five minutes and then let it steep for ten minutes. Drink two or three cups a day to control a fever and to treat pain. It is also available as a powder, extract, tincture, and in capsules. The capsules are usually standardized to a set percentage of salicin such as 15 percent, take as directed.

NOTE: Aspirin is made from willow bark. Be careful with this drink or any use of aspirin if there is a wound or a bleeding problem of any kind.

Aspirin will make bleeding much worse due to its effect on platelets. Platelets are blood cells that, along with clotting factors in your blood, help control bleeding. They are short-lived blood cells and taking aspirin will affect platelet function (and cause bleeding) for up to a week after a single dose. You can tell the difference between a platelet problem causing bleeding and a coagulation problem by the nature of the bleeding. Platelet problems cause brisk bleeding that can be brought under control by applying pressure to the wound because the coagulation factors are still present and will form a clot. If it is due to a lack of coagulation factors, pressure will not help.

Meadowsweet

Meadowsweet (Spiraea ulmaria) is a perennial herb in the rose family, it grows in damp meadows and has been used medicinally for thousands of years. We use the parts that grow above ground to make it into a medicine. It contains salicin, which is similar to aspirin, in addition to which it contains many tannins that have anti-inflammatory properties and decreases phlegm (mucous) production so it is helpful in colds and respiratory tract infections.

To prepare an infusion use one teaspoon of dried flowers or leaves per cup of boiling water. Let this steep for ten minutes. Drink three to five cups a day to control a fever. This will induce perspiration and reduce a fever. You can buy one-pound packets of this herb quite inexpensively on line. It is also available as an extract. The seeds are very inexpensive; a packet of 6,000 seeds for about three dollars, great to grow yourself in your medicinal garden.

Echinacea

Echinacea is known botanically as Echinacea purpurea and commonly as coneflower, and is widely planted in American gardens, with many new varieties in stunning colors being bred in recent years.

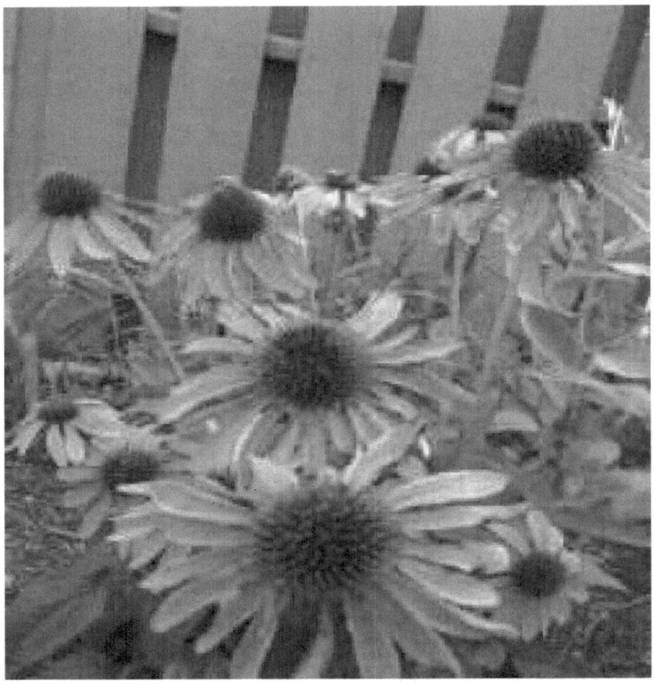

Echinacea was used widely by Native Americans for a variety of problems including fever, colds, flu, and to fight infections by boosting the immune system. It was used topically (on the surface as opposed to being ingested) to treat wounds, burns, and bites. The roots of the plant were even chewed for sore throat and to help alleviate the pain and inflammation of toothaches.

For fever reduction and boosting of immunity use 500 mg of the capsules up to four times daily and as a tincture, 3 ml four times daily.

Garlic

Garlic is also known botanically as (Allium sativum), and it is known to help boost the immune system and help fight off infections as well as scare off vampires. (Hey, you never know what you might need.)

Garlic is a member of the onion family, it is easy to grow, healthy to eat, and wonderful for your health. Garlic is stored warm (greater than 64 degrees) and dry, to keep it from prematurely sprouting. The top stem is kept on to preserve the garlic for a longer period. Garlic is often braided and hung to keep dry. Garlic can be made into oil but if not stored properly or used within one week's time, it could develop Clostridium botulinum, the organism that causes the deadly botulism.

The dose is 300 to 500 mg of the capsules or the liquid equivalent three times daily.

Ginger

Ginger is a spice that is known botanically as Zingiber officinale and commonly as ginger root. It is in the same plant family as turmeric and has many medicinal qualities. Ginger originated in southern China and was spread via trade routes to the Spice Islands (also known as the Moluccas, a group of islands that are part of the Indonesian archipelago), and beyond to Africa and South America. The lucrative spice trade from the Far East through Venice brought ginger to Europe via India.

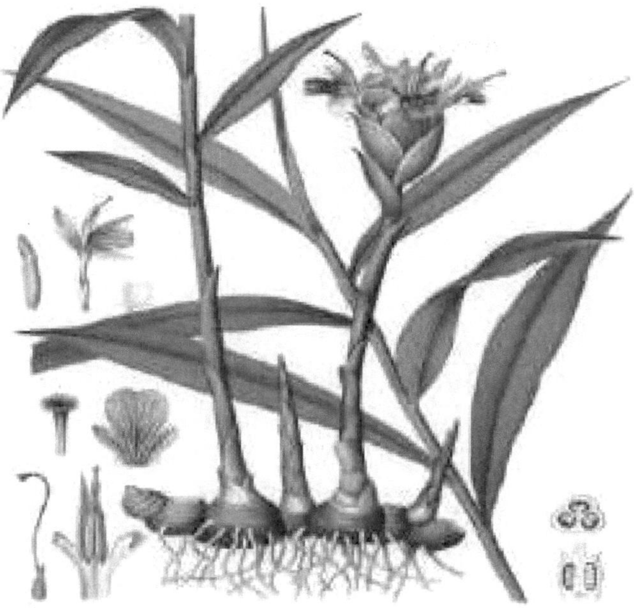

Ginger has many qualities including acting as a potent food preserver. Ginger is also made into a type of candy by cooking the root in sugar until it softens. Ginger root is used traditionally to treat nausea, sea sickness, and the morning sickness that accompanies pregnancy (although the jury is not back on whether ginger is safe in pregnancy, so I would recommend avoiding it if you can). Ginger has also been shown to have analgesic, sedative properties as well as controlling fever.

The dose of ginger for fever control is four times a day of either 500 mg capsules, 2 ml of the tincture or a cup of tea four times daily. It is also available as an essential oil.

Black Elderberry

Black Elderberry (Sambucus nigra): This small tree produces clusters of purple berries. However, it is the flowers that are used to treat fever. Remember that all fruit-bearing plants have to flower first. Then the flower has to get pollinated for fruit production to take place. In a greenhouse, this lack of pollinators can be overcome by the use of electric toothbrushes to vibrate the pollen from the male to the female parts of the flower to induce fruiting. My father-in-law, Charlie Insalaco, pioneered this technique in Connecticut in his greenhouses to produce hydroponic tomatoes as far back as the 1970s.

Elderberries are native to Europe and North America and are easily grown and are quite prolific, bearing large clusters of elderberries that are edible and were used by Native Americans to make healthy tonics to treat fevers, seasonal allergies, and also to boost the immune system. Elderberries are also rich in flavonoids and as such are potent antioxidants. This also helps your immunity by boosting your ability to stave off infections.

In order to prepare an infusion, take a handful (about one and a half ounces) of dried flowers and add them to a quart of boiling water. Let this steep for ten minutes and then drink three to six cups a day to lower a fever. Elderberry also comes in capsules, extract, and as a syrup.

Yarrow

Yarrow is also known botanically as Achillea millefolium and is also called common yarrow. The botanical name Achillea is named after Achilles, the hero of the Trojan war of Greek mythology;

apparently he used it to stop the bleeding and to heal the wounds of his soldiers. For that same reason it is also commonly known as staunch weed and soldier's woundwort (wort means plant in Old English). The leaves of yarrow induce clotting and as such were used not only for soldiers' wounds but to control the bleeding of nosebleeds.

Millefolium means a thousand leaves. Yarrow is very easy to grow and forms dense mats, it is invasive and is considered a weed by many people. It is very easy to grow in your medicinal garden.

Yarrow works by inducing perspiration which cools the skin and breaks a fever. Yarrow comes in 300 mg capsules; take these four times a day to control a fever. As a tincture take 2 ml four times a day, and as a tea take one cup up to four times daily as well.

Linden Tree

Linden tree (Tilia europaea) is also called a Lime tree. These trees produce copious amounts of aromatic flowers much loved by bees. I've loved linden trees since my medical school days in Italy. I lived in a small town outside of Padua on a street named after the large linden trees on either side…via dei Tigli (Linden Street). In the United States these are fast-growing trees as long as you provide them with full sun. Linden trees are inexpensive, so tuck one in a sunny field to give you a steady supply.

Linden flowers have the effect of inducing perspiration. To make a preparation add 1 ounce of flowers to a quart of boiling water, let it steep for ten minutes. Drink three to six cups a day.

Many other parts of the linden tree are used medicinally including the leaves, flowers, wood, and charcoal. The other parts include tannins, flavonoids, and mucilaginous parts that are both soothing and inflammation reducers. It is used as a diuretic, an antispasmodic, and a sweat inducer to reduce fevers.

Roman Chamomile

Roman chamomile (Anthemis nobilis) is also known as English chamomile and common chamomile. It is an herb native to Europe and it has the same medicinal effects as its cousin German chamomile. Chamomile has many healthful benefits including fever reduction, anti-inflammatory, calming of frayed nerves (frazzled nerves or anxiety); it calms an upset stomach and helps diarrhea, nausea, and vomiting, reduces cough, and helps colds and flu.

To prepare an infusion, add three-fourths cup of dried flowers to a quart of boiling water and let steep for ten minutes. Drink two to three cups a day to reduce a fever. You can purchase it loose in a bag to make a tea, or in 350 mg capsules as an essential oil, and also as an extract.

Eucalyptus or Tasmanian Blue Gum

Eucalyptus or Tasmanian blue gum (eucalyptus globulus) is a tall evergreen tree native of Tasmania but now planted widely all over the world. The name blue gum is from a gum-like resin secreted by the tree that has antibacterial properties and also protects the tree from insect pests. This tree is also known as the fever tree for its fever-lowering capabilities.

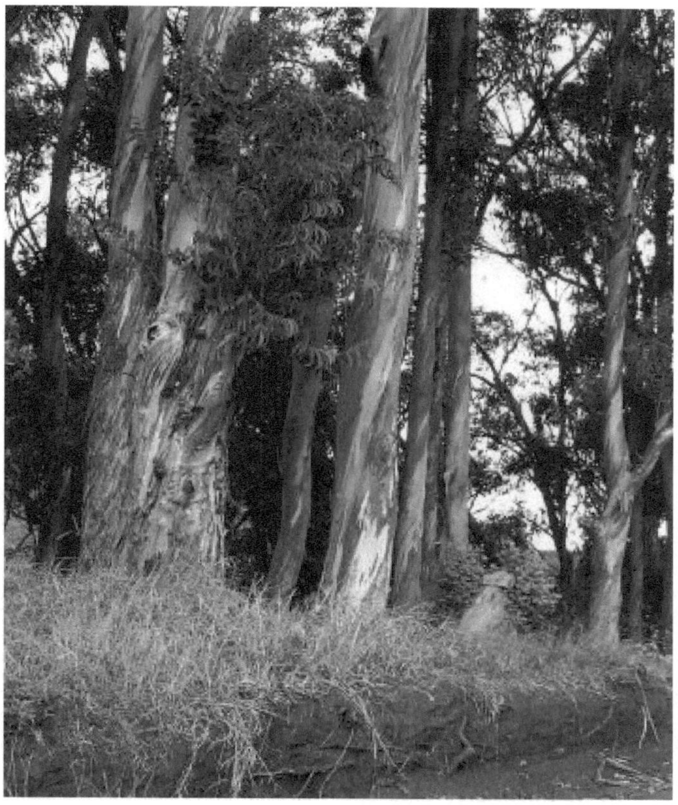

Add 1 ounce of dried leaves to one quart of boiling water. Let it steep for fifteen minutes. Drink three to five cups a day. It will induce perspiration as well as being an antimicrobial.

BOOSTING YOUR IMMUNITY

Another way to lessen a fever or any infection for that matter is by boosting the body's defenses. One surefire way to do that is to take antioxidants such as Vitamins A, C, and E as well as selenium. Also using Alpha lipoid acid, astaxanthin, and COQ10 will also boost your immune system. See my section on vitamins for complete details. Most of these are involved in the antioxidant cascade, which helps boost your immune system as well as regenerating themselves.

CHAPTER FOURTEEN

CONCUSSIONS, HEAD TRAUMA, STROKES AND SEIZURES

INTRODUCTION

TABLE OF CONTENTS:

In our lives unfortunately we will need to know how to treat head injuries of many types and from many causes. In order to better treat them we will need to understand the underlying pathology, once you understand what is going on than the treatments will make more sense to you. These problems almost always require the immediate attention of a physician; I can't stress enough the need for that asap. This information is provided to you for educational reasons and also in the event that a physician was not readily available.

CONCUSSION

What is a concussion? A concussion is a traumatic injury to the brain caused by either a blow to the head, a severe fall, or jarring or shaking of the brain within the skull. Many people have the mistaken impression that you need to have loss of consciousness and that simply is not the case. However, keep in mind that a patient unconscious for more than ten minutes is a very bad sign.

How does a concussion happen? The brain and spinal cord are immersed in a pool of fluid known as cerebrospinal fluid. It is a liquid cushion of sorts that protects the brain from most minor injuries to the head. However, when there is a violent injury to the head, this results in the brain slamming into the inside of the skull. This is what causes the dysfunction (lack of normal functioning) of the brain.

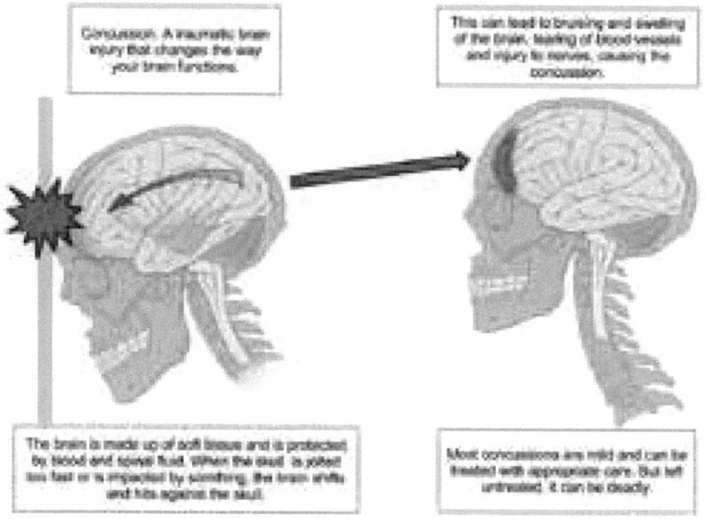

Symptoms of Concussion

It is a commonly held belief that with concussion you will have loss of consciousness but that is not always the case. You may also have a headache and some memory loss. The patient will complain of some mental fogginess with difficulty concentrating and learning new information. Other symptoms are blurry vision, dizziness, perhaps with some difficulty walking...as in a hallway, walking and feeling unsteady and reaching out for the walls to steady oneself. There may be nausea and some vomiting and neck pain. Symptoms of anger and or depression with sadness and increasing emotions may occur. There can also be sleep disturbances and fatigue, with or without insomnia.

In young children they may "act out", be angry or show a change from their normal behavior. Children may act lethargic (sleepy and uninterested in anything around them) and change the way they play. These symptoms may last anywhere from several hours to several months, there is no way to determine how a concussion will play out. The good news is about 80 to 90 percent of concussions will resolve in seven to ten days.

Cerebral Hemorrhage/Subdural Hematoma

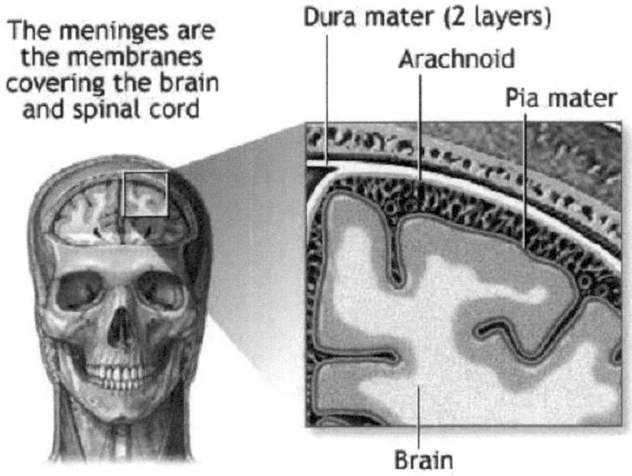

Cerebral hemorrhage means a bleed into the brain. It can come about either from burst blood vessel within the brain tissue or a clot to a blood vessel and resulting necrosis (death) of the brain downstream from that clot (a stroke) and then an oozing of blood into the adjacent brain tissue.

Another even more common bleed within the skull is from the meninges, the triple layer that surrounds the brain (see the accompanying diagram). Bleeds into the meninges are epidural, subdural, or subarachnoid. These technically are outside of the brain, but still within the skull and do exert direct pressure on the brain as they increase in volume. Causes of these bleeds could be trauma such as concussion, skull fracture, or blunt trauma to the head. Elevated blood pressure could lead to a stroke and a bleed from a burst blood vessel within the brain tissue. This is an absolute medical emergency and the patient must be evaluated immediately in a hospital setting with a neurosurgical team ready to intervene if needed.

You do need to remain alert to symptoms that appear to be worsening. For example, if their headache never clears and appears to be worsening, increased nausea and vomiting, severe neck pain, worsening vision, and increasing confusion, along with one pupil (the black part in the center of your eye) being larger than the other, signs of increasing clumsiness or incoordination as well as slurred speech, and difficulty awakening a sleeping patient. These are all signs that there may be a bleed into the brain.

Once a bleed into the brain occurs it usually results in increasing pressure within the skull resulting in herniation of the brainstem and death of the patient. The skull is a closed system, so a bleed of any type into the brain tissue will result in compression of the remaining brain as it increases in volume, at first increasing symptoms of headache, nausea, and vomiting, and ultimately death of the patient.

This type of problem is obviously a medical emergency and will require the unmatched skills of a physician with the full support of a hospital and its resources.

Treatment of Concussion

The most important factor in treatment of concussions is to rest the patient for as many days as it takes until they feel strong, symptom free, and mentally clear. Avoid any alcohol or other medications that would cause sedation. If the patient is asleep, they should be checked about every two hours for the first forty-eight hours. Upon awakening them they should be asked questions about person (point to yourself and ask what your name is (only if the patient knows you), ask what month it is and where they are, to see if they are oriented (aware), and look for signs of worsening outlined above.

Ice packs to any painful areas on the head and neck will help. Always remember not to put ice packs directly on the skin but rather put a thin layer of cloth between the ice and the skin. This will avoid direct cold injury such as frostbite to the skin. Usually about ten minutes at a time will suffice and as often as necessary.

The headache should be treated with just enough painkillers to reduce the pain but not over sedate the patient. Ice packs will also help the headache.

Rest also helps headaches. If you have the opportunity, try to keep the patient in a dark, quiet place to recover. Treat the headache with Tylenol, Aleve, or ibuprofen. Remember to always take naproxen (Aleve) or ibuprofen (Motrin) with food to avoid upsetting your stomach. Tylenol is okay without food and does not cause GI upset.

Sleep is important and will aid recovery. Also make sure the patient avoids any heavy exercise or exertion, which will only worsen the symptoms.

TRAUMATIC BRAIN INJURIES

These types of injuries to the brain are much more severe than a concussion and many times have permanent, irreversible effects on the patient.

Traumatic Brain Injuries are abbreviated TBI. TBIs can occur from a variety of powerful blows to the head. These can be from open injuries that penetrate the skull and enter the brain like shrapnel, bomb fragments, and bullets. These can also result from closed injuries such as violent blows to the head from weapons of various types, severe falls, and motor vehicle accidents.

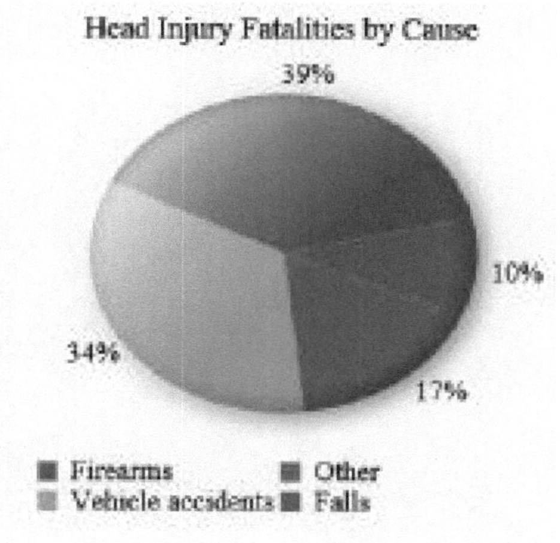

What Happens To The Brain From A Tbi?

The brain is either bruised or bleeding, torn by shearing (tearing) forces, or crushed. As you might imagine, this initial trauma causes significant damage to very delicate brain tissue. Another problem is the second wave of symptoms that may develop.

These include seizures (the patient either stares off into space and is frozen or flaps parts of their body and wets themselves and is confused for a while even after the seizure ends), fever, swelling of the brain tissue, and nausea and vomiting. These patients may bleed from their ears and or nose without trauma to these areas. Sometimes clear fluid may leak from the ears or nose and this is CSF (cerebrospinal fluid, or the fluid that the brain and spinal cord are awash in). Bruising around the ears and eyes without trauma to those areas is known as the raccoon sign and signifies severe trauma to the head. It is so named due to the visual effect of blackening of the eyes, leaving the patient looking like a raccoon. This could indicate a skull fracture with internal bleeding.

Treatment of a Tbi

Treatment of TBI is unfortunately very difficult. These patients sometimes recover but if the TBI is severe may result in permanent neurological (brain and nervous system) damage. Treat TBI the same as a concussion except for the open injuries, which will need to be treated like any wound. The head requires a significant amount of blood flow since it houses the brain and sensory organs such as the eyes, ears, nose, and taste buds, therefore any laceration (cut) of the face or head will bleed profusely. As with any injury, once you have established that the patient is breathing and they have a pulse, then the first order of business is to stop the bleeding ASAP.

Stroke or Cerebrovascular Accident (Cva) And Seizures

Strokes are caused by an interruption of the normal blood flow to areas of the brain from a blood clot or embolism, hence this is known as an embolic stroke, or from the rupturing of a blood vessel and the resulting bleeding into a portion of the brain, which is known as a hemorrhagic stroke. You won't be able to tell which one you have in the beginning. If there is bleeding it will invariably kill the patient. Strokes caused by a blood clot may partially clear on their own from the body's own clot clearing or not.

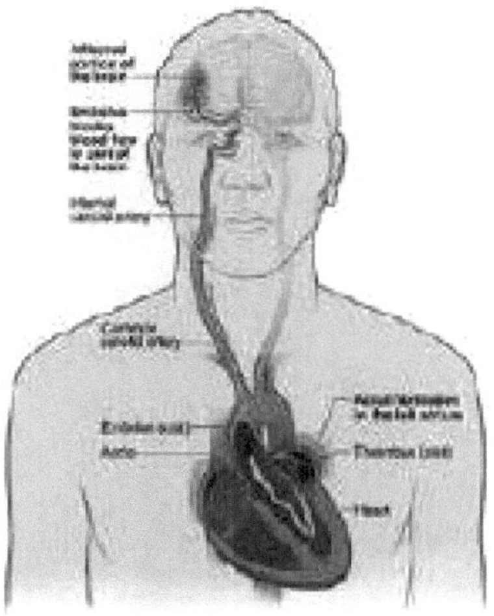

Diagram of an Embolic Stroke Caused by Atrial Fibrillation

What Are Seizures And How Do They Manifest?

Seizures are due to abnormal electrical activity in the brain. Many times a second electrical waves spread out over the brain; this is a continuous series of smooth ripples similar to what you would see if you dropped a stone in a pond. Seizures occur when there is an abnormal area of the brain firing, causing a disruption of the normal electrical activity. Seizures manifest in many different ways. They are also known as convulsions and the disorder is known as epilepsy. Some patients' seizures are simply staring off into space in a trance like state, and like all seizures, one is followed by a period of confusion due to the abnormal electrical activity. Other seizures, depending on the area of the brain involved, will involve involuntary movement of one or more body parts in what is known as a tonic/clonic fashion. Patients often drool or are incontinent of urine and sometimes stool, they may fall to the floor and foam at the mouth, they may all of a sudden suffer an extreme mood change, grunting or snorting, and they may even blackout.

Symptoms of A Stroke And Seizure

Many patients get a headache that many times is described as "the worst headache of their life", it may be accompanied by slurred speech, confusion, inability to speak, vision disturbances, seizure activity, and nausea and vomiting. Depending on the area of the brain which is "downstream" from the clot, the patient may have problems with the function of that area. For example, they may have slurred speech, paralysis, or weakness on one side of the body. The seizure activity may manifest in many ways as described in the above section, anything from staring off, to rhythmic contractions and relaxations of muscle groups causing their limbs to flail about.

NOTE: As large trunks of nerves leave the brain, they cross over in the neck to the opposite side of the body.

That is why a stroke involving the right side of the brain will affect the right side of the face (the nerves cross in the neck below the face) and the left side of the body. You may find a dilated (enlarged) pupil in the eye on the affected side. You may also have what is known as a Babinski sign. This occurs when you run something hard against the sole of the foot. The toes normally curve down towards the sole, but in a patient with a stroke these toes will instead go upward.

TREATMENT OF STROKE AND SEIZURES (EPILEPSY)

Unfortunately many of these patients will become partially or totally incapacitated and for them there are few treatment options. During an actual seizure a patient can be loosely restrained to prevent injury and/or remove any objects around them that may cause trauma. You may have to insert a tongue depressor or any flat object in their mouth if they appear to be obstructed from their tongues (I have treated many seizure patients but have yet to see this); they many times are incontinent (losing control of either their bladder/urine or their bowels/feces) and confused during and after a seizure. Most seizures will incapacitate a patient but not severely injure them. During a grand mal seizure a patient will lose consciousness.

All seizures are followed by a period of confusion. Avoid giving any food or drink to these patients until they are clearheaded; giving it earlier may result in aspiration (choking).

There are not many treatment options for seizure beyond using anticonvulsant medications (seizure-treating drugs), however there are still a few tricks left in my bag of tricks (Felix the cat would be very proud of me).

Avoidance of Hypoglycemia

Avoid hypoglycemia or low blood sugar, as this has been well documented as a cause of some seizures. In patients who are known epileptics (suffering with seizures) they should avoid concentrated sweets that will spike their blood glucose levels and result in an overproduction of insulin and resulting low blood sugar that may trigger a seizure. A concentrated sweet means candy, cakes, desserts of all types, sugar-laden drinks like Coca-Cola, etc. Rapid declines in blood glucose levels have been documented on EEGs (electroencephalograms or electrical tracings of brain waves) to cause seizure activity.

Ketogenic Diet and Medium Chain Triglycerides

Some patients have also benefited from a ketogenic diet, which is a diet that is very high in fat and low in both proteins and carbohydrates. Ketogenic diets have up to 87 percent fat content, and as such causes the formation of ketones which are the partial breakdown products of fatty acid metabolism. It is not clear why, but ketones have been shown to prevent seizure activity in the brain. This type of diet has been used for a hundred years and predates the availability of anticonvulsant medications and in many patients has been proven to achieve complete seizure control. The ketogenic diet is difficult to follow due to its high fat content. Some clinicians have incorporated coconut oil in this diet due to its high content of medium chain triglycerides that are readily metabolized by the brain. Horse milk also is a good source of medium chain triglycerides, so that horse you have been using for your pleasure riding could also supply some nice medicine for your seizure patients, as well as good nutrition. Since they are absorbed readily by the body, medium chain triglycerides are also useful in malabsorption. Palm kernel oil is another source of medium chain triglycerides with a content almost as high as coconut oil.

Herbs for the Treatment of Seizures

Some herbal preparations have been used to prevent seizures in patients:

Valerian Root
Kava Kava
Chamomile
Lemon Balm
Passion Flower
Mugwort
Tree of Heaven
Lily of the Valley
Burning Bush
Marijuana Bacopa

B Complex Vitamins, Omega-3 Fatty Acids, and Magnesium

I have found that B complex (all the B vitamins together), omega-3 fatty acids such as fish oil, krill oil, walnut and flaxseed oils, and magnesium are all helpful for any brain problem, even ADD, depression, etc.

These all have a calming effect on the nerves with little to no side effects. B complex (like vitamin C) is water soluble and you will urinate out any excess; it is not stored in the body. In fact vitamin C is the most nontoxic substance known to man, and there has never been a lethal overdose of vitamin C. The worst side effect of vitamin C over administration is diarrhea.

Patients with neurological problems such as stroke, TBI, concussion and seizures are very difficult to care for and caregivers frequently get burned out. I started to say that our love and empathy are what separates us from the animals, but a recent YouTube video came to mind. The video, I believe, was taken in a large city with a multilane highway in either direction. Two dogs tried to cross and one was run down by a car. The other dog went back for his buddy and repeatedly risked his own life in a vain effort to pull his friend out of harm's way. I can only hope that we can show half as much love and empathy for one another, for that is what makes Man so special and why we were made in God's image.

Aspirin

In regard to treatment of strokes, it normally is determined by the type of stroke a patient has incurred. The vast majorities are embolic strokes (from a clot or embolism) and these can be treated with anticoagulants with aspirin being the king. However, this is absolutely one of those cases where you need a CT scan or a MRI before you know how to treat a patient. If anyone is exhibiting any symptoms at all of neurological problems such as confusion, severe headache, slurred speech, seizure activity, incoordination and verbalizing things that do not make sense then this has to be treated as a medical emergency ...call 911 asap and get them to a hospital for a full evaluation.

The only other treatment you can safely do is to follow the same treatment protocols as concussion. Keep the patient comfortable and resting for as long as possible or your circumstances allow. Many stroke patients will recover partial function after a period of time. How long the period of time is before they begin to recover is anyone's guess, and many times it does not occur.

CHAPTER FIFTEEN

FAINTING, PASSING OUT AND LOSS OF CONSCIOUSNESS, OR SYNCOPE

INTRODUCTION

TABLE OF CONTENTS:

NOTE: ANYTIME A PATIENT FAINTS FROM ANY CAUSE IS A REASON FOR IMMEDIATE MEDICAL EVALUATION TO DETERMINE THE UNDERLYING PROBLEM WHICH COULD VERY WELL BE LIFE THREATENING!

Let's take a look at fainting and all of its causes and see what you can do while awaiting medical attention.

Fainting is the temporary loss of consciousness or loss of awareness of your surroundings or a mental state with complete or nearly complete lack of responsiveness. Fainting is commonly known as blacking out. This is a temporary condition and should not be confused with a coma, which is a complete lack of responsiveness lasting more than six hours and may last any length of time including indefinitely. Coma means deep sleep that someone cannot be aroused or awoken from. Painful stimuli like rubbing their chest or causing pain for the patient in any way will not illicit a response from someone in a coma; that is not the case with someone who has passed out. This is a temporary condition and in most cases lasts only a few seconds. The vast majority of patients will awaken without any other symptoms. If, however, a patient awakens and still complains of chest pain or other symptoms, this may lead you to the cause of his problem, a heart attack for example.

CAUSES OF FAINTING

Blood Pressure

In most cases it is secondary to a brief, sudden drop in blood pressure and with it, the oxygen supply to the brain. The brain is supplied by four main arteries (Remember, arteries carry blood away from the heart and are full of oxygen, veins and lymphatics carry blood back to the heart and are low in oxygen.) The arteries that supply the brain are the carotids on either side of your neck and the vertebral arteries that go up the back of your neck along your vertebral column (spine).

Both the carotid and vertebral arteries come in pairs (right and left side) and join the Circle of Willis in the brain. Picture this as an actual large, circular artery like a stool with the circle being the seat and the four legs being the two vertebral arteries in the back and the two carotids in the front of the neck. It is an ingenious system. Since all the arteries feed the Circle of Willis, if you block any one of them, the blood will circulate around the circle and reach the obstructed area and thus supply the brain with its much-needed supply of glucose (sugar) and oxygen. The brain requires large, constant amounts of both oxygen and glucose for its energy and function; any even temporary drop in the blood flow that carries these two will result in loss of consciousness or fainting.

Vasovagal Response

The vasovagal response is also known as neurocardiogenic syncope (meaning it is mediated by the nervous and cardiac systems). It is the most common cause of syncope, especially in young people. The Vagus nerve is the largest nerve in the body and supplies the digestive system or gut. Any stimulation of this nerve may result in a "vasovagal reflex or response" that will cause a sudden drop in the patient's heart rate and blood pressure and will cause syncope or fainting. This stimulation can be from sudden severe abdominal pain, straining to pass a hard stool, or severe abdominal cramping. Other times it is due to direct stimulation of the brainstem from such things as a needle stick, or can even be from stimuli such as medical students seeing blood for the first time or someone finding out their child or spouse has died. Oftentimes the stimulus is triggered by seemingly harmless things such as hypoglycemia or low blood sugar, severe pain, dehydration, and even menstrual cramps, to name but a few.

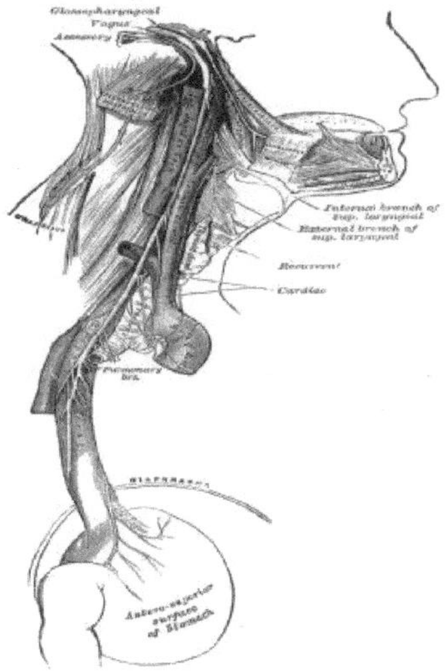

Anatomical Drawing of the Course of the Vagus Nerve

Right before the syncope occurs, the patient will usually have various symptoms such as feeling hot or, less often, cold, sweating, dizziness, slurred speech, confusion, palpitations, or a fluttering in their heart, blurry vision and/ or spots before their eyes, and possibly feelings of anxiety and apprehension. If you see a patient having these symptoms you need to get their heads down and their feet up to quickly restore blood flow and its life-giving oxygen to their brains, it you don't do this they oftentimes will have a short seizure; do not worry, this is not epilepsy and does not mean they have a seizure disorder, it is only a consequence of decreased blood flow to their brains.

Usually these patients quickly regain consciousness, especially when they are lying flat, which once again restores blood pressure to the brain, since the blood flow does not have to fight gravity to reach the brain. There usually are no consequences from these episodes other than injuring themselves if they happen to fall. There are ways to prevent it if you know the triggers from past experience. For example, if a patient recurrently faints from needle sticks, then make him lie down with his legs higher than his heart and his head at the lowest point. A position like that will increase the blood flow to his head and hopefully prevent the vasovagal response from starting.

Postural Hypotension

Hypotension means low blood pressure, the opposite of hypertension or high blood pressure. Postural means your position -- usually this occurs when someone gets up suddenly from a sitting position. This drops the blood pressure to the brain and hence the syncope or passing out. This can also be a cause of vasovagal syncope as described above.

Heart Rhythm Disturbances

Sometimes a change in the heart rate or rhythm will cause a person to faint. When the heart rhythm is very irregular, even very fast, this causes a drop in the actual output of blood from the heart to the brain and can cause syncope. An irregular heart beat is medically known as a cardiac arrhythmia. Arrhythmia means abnormal rhythm to the heart, whether it is irregular or too fast or too slow. You can determine this by checking the pulse. The radial pulse can be taken by turning your hand over so the palm is up and along the thumb side place two of your fingers about an inch from your wrist on your forearm. If you press down you will feel the pulse. You can also listen to the heart by putting your ear to someone's chest or you can feel their carotid artery in their neck on either side. The wrist is the easiest spot. A normal heart rate is between sixty and one hundred.

You can get the rate quickly by counting the number of beats in fifteen seconds and multiply it by four. The time between each beat should be consistent; if this is not, then it is a sign of an arrhythmia.

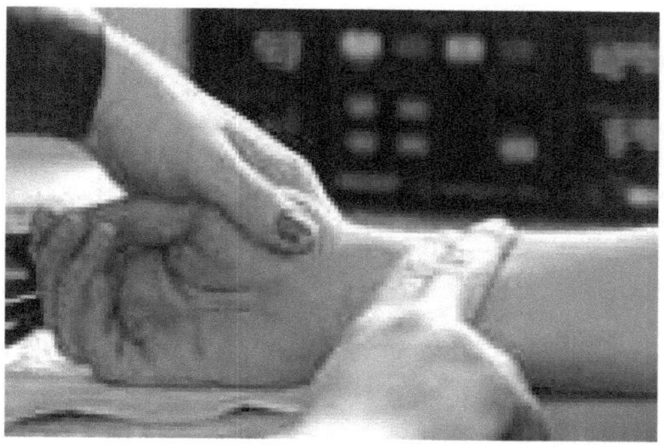

Army Training Photo of How to Check a Radial Pulse

Sometimes a change in the heart rate or rhythm will cause a person to faint. When the heart rhythm is very irregular, even very fast, this causes a drop in the actual output of blood from the heart to the brain and can cause syncope.

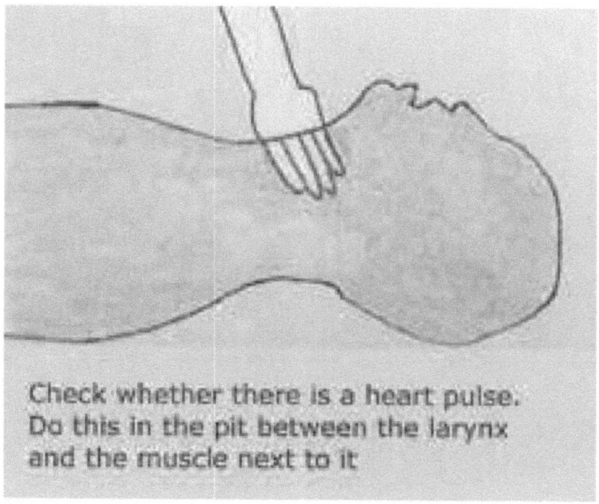

Drawing of How to Check a Carotid Pulse

Myocardial Infarction (Heart Attack)

A myocardial infarction, or heart attack, is another cause of syncope and is a very ominous sign. This almost always will be preceded by chest pain, though not always. It might also present as jaw pain, pain between the scapulae (shoulder blades), pain in the left arm, neck pain, and the most common (other than chest pain over the heart) is epigastric pain (which is pain in the uppermost part of your abdomen directly below your sternum, or breast bone). Upon regaining consciousness the patient will most likely still be exhibiting signs of heart problems such as chest pain or palpitations (pounding heart sensation) or will be sweating, nauseous, and/or weak.

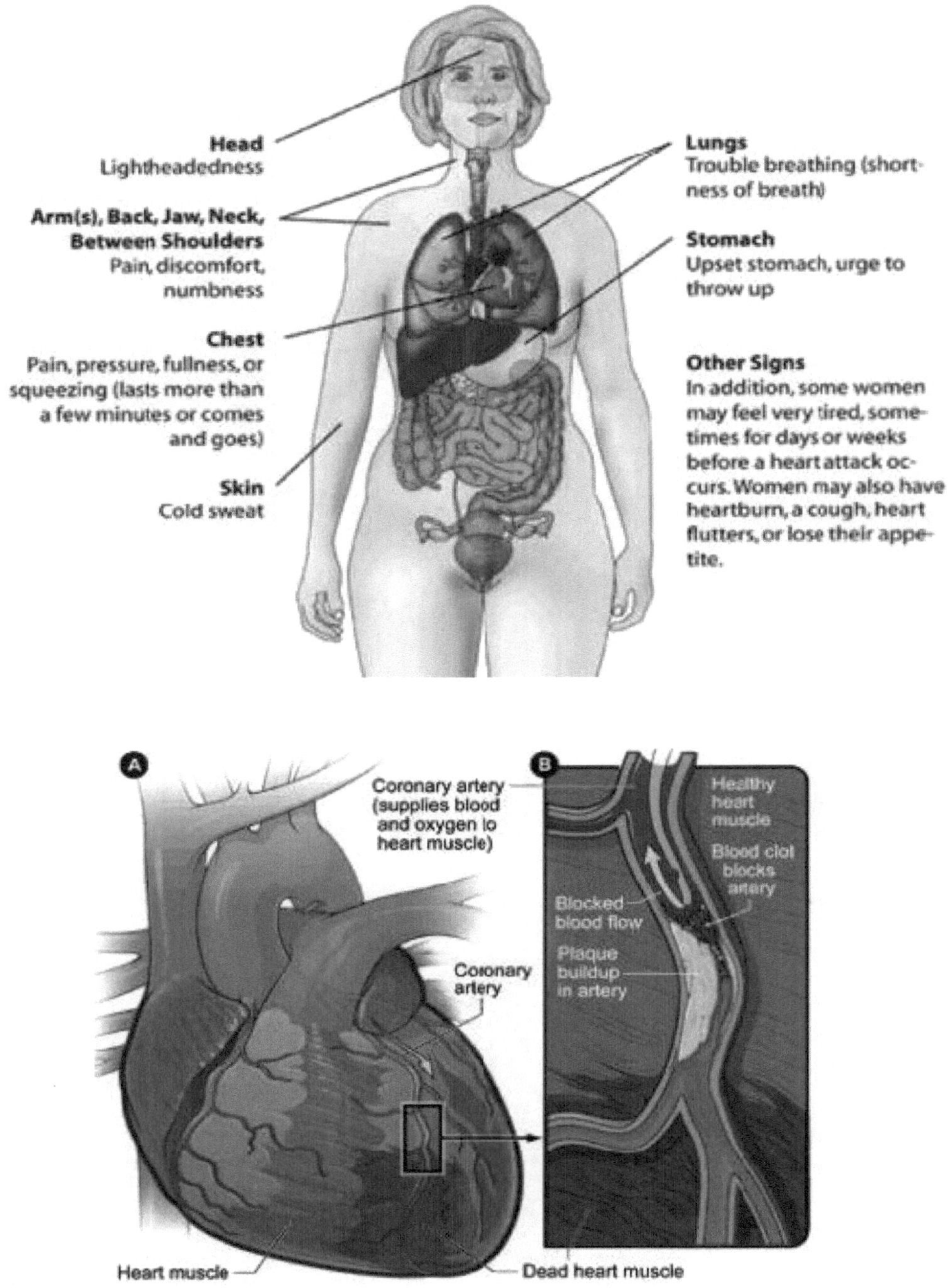

Signs and Symptoms of a Heart Attack

Dehydration

Once dehydration is severe and the body can no longer compensate for the decrease in actual blood volume, then it begins to affect the blood pressure and hence the syncope. A patient with severe dehydration will have sunken eyes and a very dry-appearing tongue. If you pinch a section of their skin on their forearm it will stay up like a small tent; this is another sign of dehydration and is known as "tenting". Unless they are disoriented they will complain of incredible thirst. Be aware that elderly patients do not feel thirst as much as younger patients and oftentimes are chronically dehydrated, remember to check their tongues, they should be wet, that is normal.

Severe Anemia

Anemia means a low red blood cell count. The red blood cells are responsible for carrying oxygen to the cells of the body and especially the brain, which is a voracious consumer of both oxygen and glucose. A person who has lost a lot of blood from a wound, for example, may pass out.

In an emergency situation this will most likely be a fatal situation unless you can stop the blood loss. If it is external (on the outside of the body) it is possible (see the section on wounds and wound care), but if it is an internal injury that is bleeding, you will need a surgeon and an entire surgical suite to back him up. Any internal bleeding is a medical emergency and you need to get that patient to a hospital immediately.

Intoxication from Alcohol Or Drugs

Excessive alcohol intake leads to severe intoxication, and as everyone knows can cause someone to pass out. The same holds true for drug use. A drug overdose needs the administration of Narcan immediately if available, this is life threatening and a medical emergency that requires the patient to be evaluated in the local emergency room asap. In the case of an overdose respiratory suppression (the patients breathing will slow down and eventually stop) will occur, which could be fatal.

Pregnancy

Pregnancy can also cause fainting. The reason is that the developing fetus can compress the mother's inferior vena cava (the large vein that returns blood to the heart from the lower parts of the body) and lead to syncope.

TREATMENT OF SYNCOPE OR FAINTING

The ABCs

The first rule is to follow your ABCs: Airway, Breathing, and Circulation. If someone passes out the first thing you should do is evaluate their airways and then their breathing. If they are not breathing you must first check their airways (mouth and throat) and make sure they have not choked on something and it is obstructing them. The patient should be stretched out lying down on their back. Turn their head to the side and reach carefully into their mouth and make a sweep of it with your fingers to feel for any foreign objects. Examine their chest to see if it is moving up and down as it does with breathing. Sometimes if it is very faint you can put a mirror up to their mouth and see if it gets fogged by their breath. If they are not breathing in an emergency situation you must initiate CPR immediately.

If they are breathing, immediately check for a pulse as I taught you above. If there is no pulse either, then do the chest thump and you should immediately initiate CPR, while having someone else call 911.

Bleeding

If bleeding is evident, naturally that should take priority and be treated ASAP. Apply direct pressure to any wound and, if need be, tourniquets for a brief time. See the section on wounds for complete details. Stemming the loss of blood from one or more wounds has to take priority over any other treatment at this point and should be done as quickly as possible.

Hypoglycemia (Lowblood Sugar) and Other Problems

Once you have checked their breathing and pulse and established there is no bleeding, then we need to do some sleuthing and figure out what the problem might be. For example, if the patient is a known diabetic you could try to administer some sugar, liquid form being the easiest. Even something sweet squeezed into their mouth will get absorbed and could bring them back to consciousness. I once was in a grocery store when my son called me to help a shopper who had passed out in the checkout line. He was unconscious but did have a bracelet indicating he was a diabetic. He was seizing and I sat behind him and cradled him in my arms to protect him. I then instructed the checkout girl to go and get me some sugar ASAP. She incredibly returned with a few packets of Sweet'n Low, which I promptly told her was worthless.

Someone else handed me some sugar and I emptied the packet into the side of his open mouth and within a few minutes he returned to normal and actually refused to go to the hospital and went home.

Elevate Their Legs About A Foot Higher Than Their Body

With the patient lying on their back you should raise their legs about a foot above their body. This will increase the blood flow back to the heart and the brain and help raise their blood pressure. This will be especially helpful in the most common causes of syncope such as vasovagal syncope described above. In many cases this alone will be enough to bring a patient around to consciousness.

Slapping Their Face Or Rubbing Their Sternum

Slapping their face and trying to arouse them oftentimes works, rubbing their sternum or breast bone with the knuckles of your hand also works.

Testing a Patient's Orientation

When they awaken, ask them if they have any medical conditions like diabetes, seizure disorder, or a heart condition. Ask them if they feel okay, see how oriented they are to person, place, and time, with questions like who am I? (only if they know you, or who is the president if they don't know you). Where are you right now? What year is this? If they answer all three correctly then that is the best, they are considered alert and well oriented times three, two questions correct is alert and well oriented times two, and one right is times one. This gives you a quick scale to measure their orientation and the state of their thinking.

Loosen Any Belts, Scarves, or Tight Clothing

Loosen any tight clothing or belts from the patient that may be restricting blood flow. Remove any scarves or ties as well as anything else that might look constricting.

If Conscious Give Fluids/Keep in Shade

If the patient is severely dehydrated then give clear fluids ASAP and keep them in a cool place out of any direct sunlight and away from any heat- generating source that will only exacerbate (worsen) their situation by causing more water loss. Gently give them sips of fluid continuously for several hours. See the dehydration section for complete details.

Smelling Salts/Ammonia

Smelling salts are usually made of ammonium carbonate. Ammonium carbonate is a salt of ammonia made by mixing carbon dioxide with ammonia. Smelling salts in various forms have been used as far back as Roman times, and are very effective in arousing someone who has passed out or in the case of boxers, someone who was knocked out. It is still used on boxers; many other athletes use smelling salts to improve their alertness and performance.

Smelling salts release ammonia gas, which triggers the patient to deeply inhale by stimulating the muscles involved with inhalation (breathing in). Smelling salts cause irritation of the lining of the nose and lungs thus triggering this inhalation reflex. Smelling salts also work by activation of the sympathetic nervous system, which is your fight or flight response. This in turn causes an elevation of your pulse and blood pressure and makes you more alert (since your body perceives this as danger it needs you stronger and more alert). Sympathetic activation works because it counteracts the parasympathetic system activation that does the exact opposite; it lowers blood pressure, your pulse, and makes you at the very least drowsy and at worst you faint.

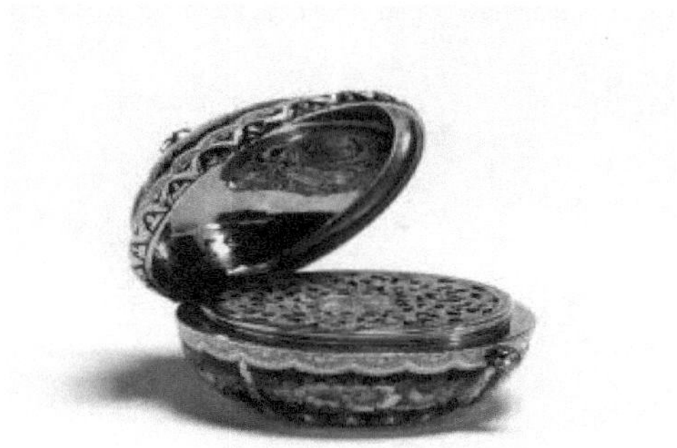

HOW TO MAKE YOUR OWN SMELLING SALTS

The more multiple uses we can find for things the better off we will be. I have always taught my son, Marcus, to improvise and I have to say he has become a master at it, it doesn't always work out but I think it is a valuable lesson for children and many adults. Here is a formula to make your own smelling salts:

Mix one cup of Epsom salt with a quarter cup of sea salt.

Add six to eight drops of an essential oil such as eucalyptus oil, the more drops the stronger the smell and the greater the effect. You can use eucalyptus oil by itself or you can mix it with other aromatic essential oils such as peppermint oil, rosemary oil, and lemongrass oil (two drops of each).Stir the two salts and the oils together thoroughly. Store the mix in a small glass jar, small tin, plastic sandwich bag or a small Tupperware container. You have to keep the container closed to prevent evaporation and weakening of the smelling salts.

You can just hold a small rag soaked in ammonia under a person's nose for a second or two. Do not do it too long; it is irritating to the nasal passages and lungs, and it only takes a few inhalations to do the trick.

Alternatively, you could just open a bottle of the following essential oils and place it under the patient's nose for a few seconds to revive them: Eucalyptus, peppermint, neroli, basil, lavender, black pepper, or rosemary.

CHAPTER SIXTEEN

HEADACHE

INTRODUCTION

TABLE OF CONTENTS:

One of the most common medical complaints that will need to be evaluated and treated is headache. As with all things I teach you to treat, I want you to understand the underlying mechanisms that lead to headaches. I also want you to understand proper nutrition and other medical basics that will prevent your headaches, then finally learn how to treat headaches.

Most headache sufferers are women, especially migraine headaches and in both women and men they tend to decrease with advancing age.

CAUSES OF HEADACHES

In your everyday life there are multiple things that act as triggers causing your headaches, of course your spouse is one of them but let's take a look at some others.

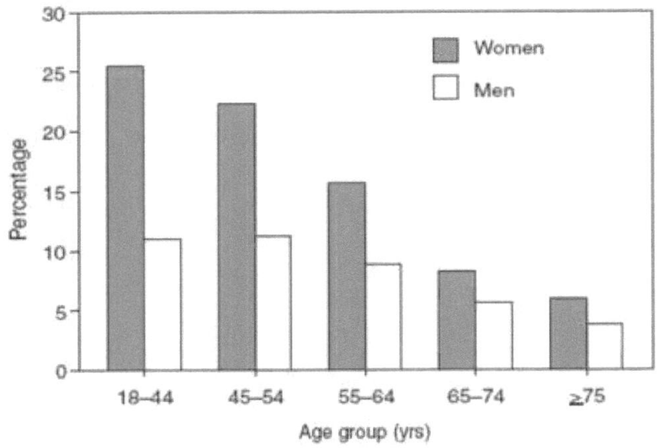

Percentage of persons over 18-years-old reporting severe headache or migraine in the prior 3 months grouped by age and sex. 2004-US

Dehydration

Dehydration will be a very common trigger and you should always be monitoring your body's water content. The easiest way is to look at your tongue, it should be wet. If it is like sandpaper or dry and furrowed (grooved) then you are dehydrated.

NOTE: As you age your awareness of thirst declines and you will not feel thirsty as you did in your younger days. Dehydration can also be caused by diuretic (water pills) use, alcohol, and caffeine. Interestingly, over 60 percent of headache sufferers got relief within a half an hour of drinking a few cups of water. There is no downside to drinking a glass or two of clean water, for that reason I would advise you to have all headache sufferers do this,. Hydration is almost always a good thing and we get the win –win of helping headache sufferers.

Hunger/Hypoglycemia

Sometimes hunger will lead to a headache; eating even a small amount of food should give you some relief. This is due to hypoglycemia, or low blood sugar. The simpler the sugar the better, so sugary drinks will enter your bloodstream quickly. Anything with a high glycemic index -- a packet of sugar under your tongue, hard candy or honey will work.

Smoke and Fumes

Many types of chemicals and smoke can irritate your sinuses and lead to a severe headache. There is not much you can do other than avoidance. Covering your mouth and nose with a wet piece of cloth may help filter out some of the offending agents. Naturally, a gas mask or a face mask with a filter would be ideal. In patients with severe allergies, sometimes a perfume may even trigger a headache or migraine.

Infections

In an emergency situation there are significant stresses upon your immune system, from starvation, lack of antioxidants, dehydration, depression, exhaustion, and excessive sun exposure. Any or all of these can lead to infections, especially airborne respiratory infections like sinus infections and bronchitis. Many times both of these infections are accompanied by headaches. The headache of a sinus infection is usually frontal (above your eyes on your forehead), if it is a maxillary sinus infection you will have pain in the middle of one or both cheeks and your upper teeth might feel sore.

Hypertension and Dilated Blood Vessels

Hypertension (high blood pressure) can easily lead to headaches and this often will be the case in primarily middle-aged and elderly people who have a previous history of hypertension and are either poorly controlled or are off of their medications. One in three Americans currently has hypertension and there are also newly diagnosed hypertensive patients who are not aware that they have elevated blood pressure.

Often a headache caused by hypertension will hurt in the temporal area (commonly known as the temples) and back of the neck. I have found that some patients are more sensitive and get headaches with blood pressures only moderately elevated; systolic blood pressures such as the 150-160 mm hg. That being said, there is research that shows only very high blood pressures lead to headaches, but like many things we clinicians in "the trenches" come to conclusions that are quite different than our colleagues in academia.

Elevated blood pressure can also expand or dilate blood vessels and these blood vessels then stretch and trigger the nerves next to them and headaches occur. Many of these blood vessels are in the scalp. As they used to do in the "old days", tying a scarf or belt around your head helps a headache immensely for many people. If you have a migraine you will try anything; give it a shot. Remedies like drinking water and tightening a binding around your head are harmless and potentially could be very helpful. I have found that deep massage of the back of the neck and over the entire scalp help headaches immensely, in my opinion that is much more effective than tying a belt of scarf around your head, but it is your headache, you will certainly find the modalities that work best for you, who cares what studies show.

Trauma

Many injuries, especially to the head and neck, nose, and sinus areas will lead to headaches. These types of headaches will be very easy to diagnose by the obvious trauma, sometimes you have to elicit a history from someone to realize the source of the headaches.

Stress

Stress in general is in ample supply in all of our modern lives, and there is no end in sight. Stress can lead to either migraine headaches or tension headaches.

Stroke

A stroke is also known as a cerebrovascular accident (or CVA). Strokes occur in two ways, an embolus, or clot, travels up to the brain and blocks a blood vessel, causing death to the neurons or brain cells downstream from the clot. The other way is by a blood vessel bursting and bleeding into the brain.

Strokes are most often described by patients as the worst headache they ever had. The pain is usually unilateral (one side of the head), but may be generalized, or on both sides. Patients often complain of dizziness and have symptoms of confusion and disorientation. If there is a bleed it is usually accompanied by nausea and vomiting and death if the pressure is not relieved surgically and the bleeding brought under control.

NOTE: Obviously this constitutes a medical emergency that requires immediate evaluation by a physician.

Eye Strain

Eye strain is caused by reading in poor light, staring at a computer screen, or straining your eyes doing any task that requires prolonged staring at something. It is made worse by poor eyesight and not wearing corrective lenses or glasses. Eye strain is a very common cause of headaches and can be helped by reading in good light and wearing glasses if you need them, as well as looking away from something you are staring at intently every few minutes to allow your eyes to relax and refocus.

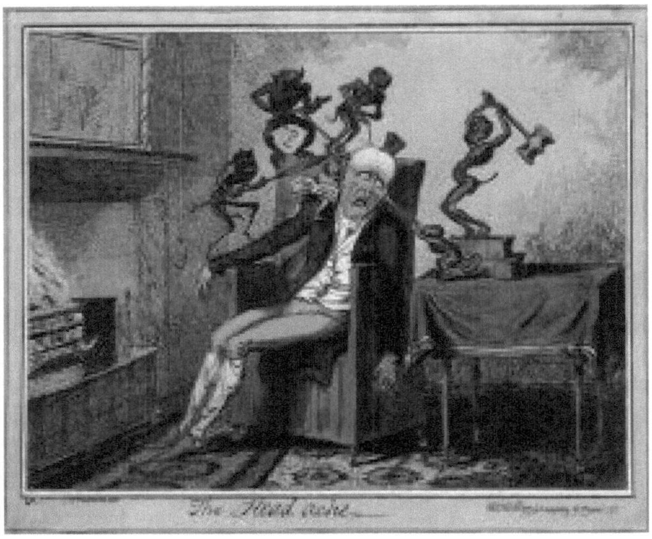

TYPES OF HEADACHES

Sinus Headaches

Sinus headaches are by far the most frequent type of headache suffered by most people. Studies have found that most of these are actually migraine headaches. Migraines affect the trigeminal nerve in the area and leads to nasal congestion and pressure in the area of the sinuses.

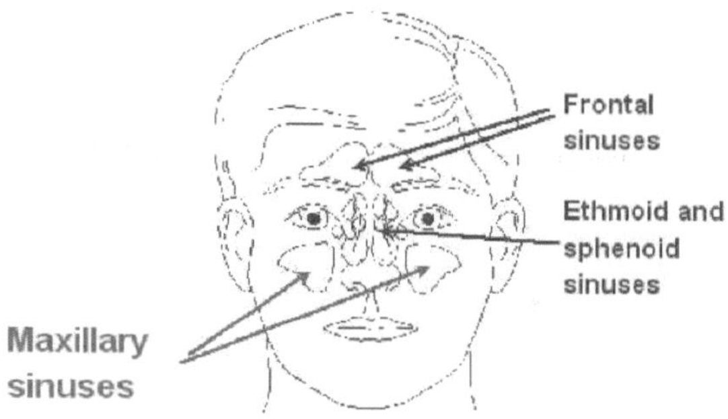

Most people refer to any severe headache as a migraine. The two are often confused. Sinus headaches are often triggered by barometric changes. Patients will frequently comment that they know when a storm is approaching due to the sensation of sinus pressure that frequently leads to a headache. They usually are accompanied by a thick nasal discharge, unlike migraines. They also are located over the sinuses involved.

There are the frontal sinuses located above your eyes in your forehead, your ethmoid and sphenoid sinuses at the top corner where your nose meets your forehead, in your eye socket or orbit, and also behind your eyes. The maxillary sinuses are located in your cheeks above your mouth on both sides. Your upper teeth (first and second molars) roots go through these sinuses, and sinus infections or headaches here can often be mistaken for a toothache, especially when the upper teeth are involved. Sudden turning of your head or bending over may worsen these types of headaches.

Prevention of Sinus Headaches

If you suffer with sinus-type migraine headaches, they will almost always be triggered by barometric changes, such as an approaching rain or snowstorm or a thunderstorm. These will get your head pounding, and your neck will start to stiffen up as well.

Treatment of Sinus Headaches

When you feel a sinus headache starting it is best to be proactive (get off your butt and take something). I suggest either using a nasal spray such as Afrin or a saline spray, or take an antihistamine and a couple of Tylenol or Excedrin. Do not wait, these headaches never get better, act immediately when they begin.

You need to take a combination of an antihistamine such as Benadryl, Allegra, Clarinex, or Claritin, along with a painkiller or analgesic such as Aleve (naproxen), Tylenol, Excedrin, Motrin (ibuprofen). Or you can take something like Tylenol Sinus, Advil Sinus, etc., which is a combination of an antihistamine and an analgesic. You need the combination to eradicate these headaches.

Ice packs on the forehead and also the back of your neck will help. Blowing your nose and keeping your nasal passages open is key to this type of headache. I like using saline sprays; they work nicely. If you have Afrin, all the better. Remember, Afrin only works for a week, after that it causes rebound which means it will shrink your nasal passages like before, but then quickly the swelling will return, worse than it was originally.

Nasal decongestants like pseudoephedrine (Sudafed) will also help clear your nasal passages and relieve some of the pressure-like sensation that accompanies these types of headaches.

Use of a neti pot to clean out your sinus passages is also very helpful. The practice of Neti or nasal/sinus irrigation began quite long ago in India, where it is a daily routine for the prevention of allergies, sinus infections and to clean the nasal and sinus passages of all mucous and other debris. It has been used by practitioners of Ayurveda and Yoga for thousands of years. Neti is one of the six purification rituals performed prior to the practicing of yoga. It is usually done with warm water, sometimes with salt added to make a saline solution, other times with herbs and various essential oils. I advise using a neti pot which is a small pot that looks like a magic lantern, it is filled with neti solution (saline for our purposes), one end is inserted in one of your nostrils and with your head tilted the sinus is irrigated and the solution runs out of the other nostril. There are films on YouTube showing how to properly use a neti pot. What did we ever do before YouTube?

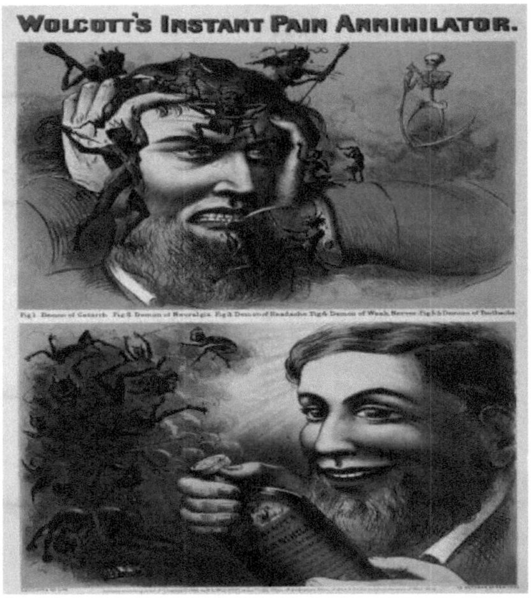

Migraine Headaches

Migraines are usually unilateral (one sided, either right or left) and are frequently preceded by an aura of some type. This aura may involve twinkling light, a smell, or something else. The pain of a migraine lasts between two and seventy-two hours. Migraines also feel like a pulsating pain, with associated photophobia (fear of light, i.e. Light -- especially bright light -- makes a migraine feel worse.), nausea and vomiting. Physical activity makes it worse as do loud sounds.

Causes and Prevention of Migraine Headaches

Migraines in certain patients are triggered by certain foods such as red wine, aged cheese, chocolate, MSG (monosodium glutamate, found in many processed foods and often in Chinese food), dried fruits, which frequently contain sulfites, processed meats (cold cuts, jerky, etc.) which often contain nitrates, any kind of alcoholic beverage and caffeine.

Caffeine is a little controversial since it also helps a headache. I personally do think it is a trigger in those who have developed food allergies to caffeine. Caffeine withdrawal is another cause of migraine headaches. Oftentimes I will see a patient who complains of a headache every weekend and when I ask them they oftentimes only drink coffee at work. When they don't take it over the weekends, it triggers migraines.

If you suffer with migraines, any or all of these foods can be a trigger: cheeses, wine, avacadoes, chocolate, soy foods, msg containing foods, nuts, processed meats, bacon , hot dogs, citrus, olives and vinegars. The primary reason that these foods are the culprits is that they all contain two amino acids which trigger migraines; tyramine and phenylethylamine. Beans sometimes are sited as triggers for migraines, pickled foods along with chili peppers. Artificial sweeteners which contain chemicals that are known as excitotoxins which adversely affect the brain and trigger migraines (they might also be the cause of the explosion of MS).

Avoiding the above named foods will go a long way towards prevention of your migraines.

The changing of the diameter of the blood vessels in your brain has oftentimes been cited as a cause of migraine headaches. Most of the time this is referring to vasoconstriction (tightening of the blood vessel size); some medical researcher's feel it is the opposite or vasodilatation (enlarging of the blood vessels). I personally disagree with them both of them; I think it is a changing of the blood vessel size in either direction that alters blood flow to the brain and/or stretches the nerves associated with the blood vessels.

Eye strain may lead to migraines; reading in good light or wearing glasses will help One of the first things you should do if you are suffering with a sudden increase in the frequency of your migraines is to have a good eye exam by an ophthalmologist..

Treatment of Migraine Headaches

Headaches, Rest, Quiet and Ice Packs

The symptoms of an ailment will often lead you directly to effective treatments. If light and noise are making your headache worse than reverse the symptoms by placing people in dark, quiet rooms and at the same time treat the pain. I also use ice and cold packs quite effectively in treating my own migraines as well as those of my patients. An ice pack strategically placed on the forehead and the back of the neck at the base of the skull will work wonders. Always prevent the ice pack from direct contact with a patient's skin, which can cause frostbite. Just wrap a piece of cloth around it, or even double up a paper towel.

Painkillers

There are various treatments of migraines, everything from nonsteroidal anti-inflammatory drugs like Motrin, to triptans like Imitrex, Relpax, Maxalt, and Frova as well as narcotic painkillers.

I have used them all in every conceivable combination and they all work for certain patients.

There is one other principle that all migraine sufferers quickly learn: ONCE A MIGRAINE STARTS IT ALWAYS GETS WORSE, TREAT IT IMMEDIATELY IT IS NOT GOING TO GO AWAY ON ITS OWN. We are all optimists about our pain, especially headaches. I used to convince myself to ignore the start of a migraine, hoping beyond hope that it would stop on its own. They never get better.

If you suffer from migraine, sinus, or tension headaches, I tell patients to try Excedrin first line ASAP .Excedrin is a great combination for headaches; it contains aspirin, caffeine, and Tylenol. Naturally if you are allergic to aspirin or have any blood clotting or bleeding problems then you cannot use this treatment. Aleve or Motrin will also work but they lack the caffeine component so you could drink a cup of coffee or black or green tea with them. At the same time, go to a dark, quiet room and put the ice packs on your neck and forehead and sleep for an hour. This will fix the vast majority of headaches.

Keeping your nasal passages clear also seems to help both migraine and sinus headaches. This does not just involve blowing your nose, although that is certainly the first step. You need to shrink those nasal passages. Besides topical steroid nasal sprays, this can be done with saline sprays or even snorting homemade saline preparations up each nostril. This needs to be done several times in a row a few minutes apart.

Snort it as deep as you can up both sides of your nasal passages. This will wash out any discharge (snot) in there and help shrink your nasal passages and moisturize them. Ever notice how swimming in the ocean cleans out your sinuses? The neti pot is also wonderful for flushing your sinuses clean and opening them up nicely. A dab of DMSO to the opening of each nostril will also work well, be careful only use a little bit or you might get a burning sensation in your nasal mucosa.

I also have found that the deep massage of certain areas on the head and neck, as well as applying direct, steady pressure to these trigger points, will help a headache immensely. Others report an acupressure point on the web of your hand between your thumb and your pointer finger, when rubbed, will bring headache relief.

Migraine headaches can also be triggered by a magnesium deficiency. Migraines are caused by a vasoconstriction (or tightening of blood vessels) and magnesium causes blood vessels (and the rest of your body) to relax or dilate.

Taking magnesium daily will help decrease these headaches considerably and also has other beneficial effects on your body since there are approximately 300 enzymatic reactions in your body that require magnesium. In addition to which magnesium helps muscles relax, helps constipation, and helps lower blood pressure. You can even get the magnesium that you need by soaking in a hot bathtub with several cups of Epsom salt (magnesium sulfate) dissolved into it. You need to stay in this hot bath for about a half hour to fully absorb your magnesium; that is how long it takes to cross your skin and enter your bloodstream.

Alternative Migraine Treatments

Vitamin B2 (riboflavin) 400 mg daily in addition to a B complex 50 mg a day. Take this for at least three months to help prevent and treat your migraines. Since all B complex vitamins are water soluble you can take these on an empty stomach. Vitamin B6 (pyridoxine) take 50 mg daily of this to treat and prevent migraine headaches. See 5-HTP below, which explains how B6 helps raise serotonin levels, which helps headaches by increasing cerebral (brain) blood flow and relaxing constricted arteries as well as increasing the body's natural endorphins (painkillers). CoQ10: 200 mg daily or 100 mg twice daily (remember, this is fat soluble and has to be taken with a fatty meal or you will not absorb it). 5-HTP (5-hydroxytryptophan): This is naturally made in your body by the metabolizing of the amino acid L-tryptophan (found in foods like seafood, warm milk, and turkey). It is the reason you fall asleep on the couch every year after Thanksgiving dinner. With the help of vitamin B6 this is changed into serotonin. Low serotonin levels lead to headaches, depression, and many other psychiatric conditions such as OCD (obsessive compulsive disorder), ADD (attention deficit disorder) and ADHD (attention deficit hyperactivity disorder). There have been several recent studies that have observed that treatment with 5-HTP did reduce both the severity and the frequency of all types of headaches. Take 50 to 100 mg three times a day.

Note: Do not take this if you are still on an antianxiety or an antidepressant medication, as many of them already raise serotonin levels.

Herbal Treatments of Migraines

Feverfew: 300 mg bid (twice daily) combined with Butterbur: 100 mg daily and White Willow Bark: 300 mg bid (careful with this herb which is the source for aspirin in nature. Overuse of it may lead to bruising and bleeding. Do not take this if you are already on aspirin, Coumadin , Plavix, Xarelto or other anticoagulants.

Feverfew alone can also be taken on a daily basis to prevent or severely reduce the number of migraines a patient has. Take one capsule a day (300 mg).

Magnesium

Magnesium: Take anywhere from 100 to 600 mg of magnesium a day. The higher dose may lead to some diarrhea, in which case you should back off. Play with the dose until you find the right dose to prevent and or treat your migraines. Other than oral magnesium it can be taken trans dermally (across your skin) by taking a bath with Epsom salt. Epsom salt is magnesium sulfate and is very effective as a migraine treatment. I have used it for years on patients who are almost universally reluctant to try it, thinking it is some old wives tale treatment. Using Epsom salt as a treatment has several caveats. You have to dissolve two or three cups of Epsom salt in a bath that contains the hottest water you can stand, and you have to remain in the bath for a half an hour. The reason for the half hour is that is the length of time it takes for the Epsom salt to cross your skin and enter your body. For my male readers, I cannot stress enough the importance of lowering your testicles very carefully into that hot water! The last thing to mention is that when you get out of the bathtub be very careful since your leg muscles will be relaxed and will be very rubbery and you might very well fall, so hold onto something as a precaution.

Sodium Bicarbonate (baking soda)

One of the reasons believed to be the cause of many headaches is vasospasm or constriction of blood vessels in the brain. This is increased in acidic conditions and improved with raising pH to more alkaline levels. Presumably sodium bicarbonate works by breaking down into water and carbon dioxide once ingested. The higher carbon dioxide levels in the blood make blood vessels dilate (to allow more oxygen into the cells) and thus relieving the headache. Oxygen itself has been used for many years for patients with cluster headaches for the same reason. For any headache you can use sodium bicarbonate, just don't take it on an overly full stomach since the carbon dioxide produced may actually rupture your stomach!

For any headache, mix one teaspoon of sodium bicarbonate in a large glass of water and drink it down. I would also lie down and if possible apply ice packs to your head and neck. The baking soda treatment usually works within a half an hour.

Essential Fatty Acids

Essential fatty acids improve circulation in the brain and reduce inflammatory prostaglandins that have been shown to contribute to migraine headaches. Take either cod liver oil, fish oil capsules, krill oil, walnut or flaxseed oil.

Take one tablespoon of any of the oils or 4,000 mg (4 grams) of fish oil daily. A valuable piece of advice is to take the essential fatty acids first and immediately eat on top of it; this will prevent burping up any unpleasant taste.

Melatonin

Melatonin is a hormone that is involved with the body's sleep and wake cycle and its daily biorhythms or its biological clock. Melatonin is not only a wonderful natural sleep aide, but it is also a powerful antioxidant and helps protect both nuclear and mitochondrial DNA. Melatonin use also helps improve daytime functioning and helps treat and prevent migraine headaches. I recommend taking 3 or 5 mg at bedtime, but you can take up to 10 mg if you have severe migraines or intractable insomnia.

Dr. Walter Pierpaoli from Italy is the foremost expert on melatonin in the world and has written a masterpiece on melatonin called "The Melatonin Miracle". I have personally discussed the benefits of melatonin with him; he is an endless source of new information on melatonin. He feels taking melatonin along with zinc and selenium at bedtime has amazing anti-aging benefits. I highly recommend his fascinating book to anyone interested in this subject.

Menstrual Migraine

Menstrual migraine is a variation of migraine headaches and naturally occurs only in women. (Sometimes you just have to state the obvious, you wouldn't believe some of the questions I get at my lectures.) When women have their menses (or period) it is a consequence of a sudden drop in their estrogen levels. This monthly hormonal variation many times leads to what is known as menstrual migraines.

Seventy (70) percent of migraine sufferers are women and many suffer with monthly menstrual migraines. It is a very common problem. Half of women who suffer with menstrual migraines are magnesium deficient, so just as I described above, taking magnesium will be very helpful in their prevention and treatment.

Birth control pills will prevent this sudden drop off in estrogen and will help menstrual migraines but not those that are accompanied by an aura (lost vision or blurred vision made worse by flickering lights, spots, or zigzag lines). Even though these menstrual migraines are caused primarily by a drop in estrogen, they too may also be triggered by foods (see prevention of migraines) such as alcohol, cheese, chocolate, and others. Limiting your premenstrual salt intake will also help these headaches.

If you are a woman who suffers with regular severe menstrual migraines there is another treatment option, you can start Aleve twice a day for a week before your menses and continue it for a few days after they end. Remember always to take your Aleve, Motrin, Excedrin or any other nonsteroidal painkiller with food to prevent GI upset; taking it after a meal will suffice. This regimen will prevent the headaches totally or may weaken them to a point where they are at least not incapacitating. I have had great success using this strategy on my patients.

Rebound Headaches

Rebound headaches are headaches that start whenever you stop your current pain medication for your migraines. This always results in drug over usage and is a major problem for some migraine patients. The only way to avoid this is to use more than one pain medication and rotate them. Most patients do not recognize this and think that their migraines are just not ever going away. The only other option is to go cold turkey with no migraine treatment for a period of time, the length is anyone's guess but I would try ten to fourteen days and then gingerly reintroduce one of the meds. Look for food triggers to avoid as well; prevention is much better than treatment in these patients.

Tension Headaches

Tension headaches will feel different than any others. They will often start in the neck at the base of your skull and the area above it on the back of your head called the occiput. They seem to cause a tightening of your scalp and it feels like a band is around your head and tightening progressively. These are caused by a spasm or tightening of the muscles of the back of your neck and scalp. These are very common and no doubt like other types of headaches will increase in stressful situations.

Unlike migraines, tension headaches are not associated with auras, photophobia (light making your headache worse, it literally means fear of light), nausea, and vomiting.

Causes of Tension Headaches

These headaches can be caused by many things but the primary cause is stress (there is also an increase in middle-aged patients). Other common causes of tension headaches are keeping your head or neck in an abnormal position for prolonged periods, head or neck trauma, lack of sleep, and bruxism (teeth- grinding).

Treatment of Tension Headaches

Massage and Application of Pressure

These can be treated in the same way as migraines, however with one big difference; neck and head massage. The deep massage of your head and especially your neck muscles is key here. Even if you are alone, reaching back and massaging the base of your skull and the area where your skull meets your neck on both sides will pay off in spades. Once you relax the tension in those neck muscles, then they will release their tightening on your scalp muscles and therefore your headache. Also massaging your temporal areas (temples) on both sides will help immensely. Many times you will find a knot-like area, or just a spot that is exquisitely painful to touch, these are trigger points or pressure points and applying slow steady pressure to these areas with your thumb will go a long way to alleviate your tension headache.

If you suffer with tension headaches you might benefit from massage therapy, craniofacial therapy or physical therapy to your neck and scalp muscles.

Massage of an area will also relax tense muscles, for this reason try holding a pencil in your mouth like it was the stem of a rose. This jaw position helps to relax the facial and jaw muscles and helps alleviate tension headaches.

Calcium and Magnesium

Both of these minerals will help both prevent and treat tension headaches.

They both work to relax the nervous system, the muscles, and the blood vessels, and they work well together since the same pump regulates their entry and exit from the body's cells. The dose of calcium is 500 mg bid, or twice daily. The magnesium dose is 200 mg twice daily. You can double the magnesium if no benefit is achieved after two weeks. As described above you can also take magnesium via Epsom salt which is magnesium sulfate. You can also use magnesium oil topically to help provide your magnesium trans dermally, many patients report its benefits, it sometimes causes burning sensation on the skin. If that happens to you then add it to a carrier oil like coconut oil and this should alleviate that problem.

Essential Oils

Other treatment options involve massaging essential oils into your neck muscles such as lavender, rosemary, or peppermint oils. Use a few drops of each on each temple and also the back of your neck. Ice packs as described above are helpful. If you find they are irritating your skin then try to add a carrier oil like coconut oil, hemp seed oil, jojoba, evening primrose oil, sesame oil, olive oil and many others.

Find a Relaxing Position

You may also need to find a comfortable position for your head and neck and lie down for an hour or so to get relief. I oftentimes have my patients with tension headaches hyperextend their necks (roll your head all the way back with your chin lifted up); this is best done with a small pillow or a rolled up large towel placed in the back of your neck and flip your head back over it, with the ice pack on the towel and another on your forehead. Doing this along with taking your pain medication will go a long way to give you relief. **Note:** Some patients respond better to a hot pack than cold, however, I have found that these patients are in the minority. Also patients with cervical disc problems may find that flexing their head forward might give them more relief than hyperextending their head backward.

Herbal Teas

Sitting in a quiet, dark room and relaxing and also drinking a relaxing tea such as peppermint, chamomile, passionflower, skullcap, lemon balm and especially valerian, will be very helpful. A gentle massage of your scalp and neck muscles from your significant other will also go a long way in relieving your headache.

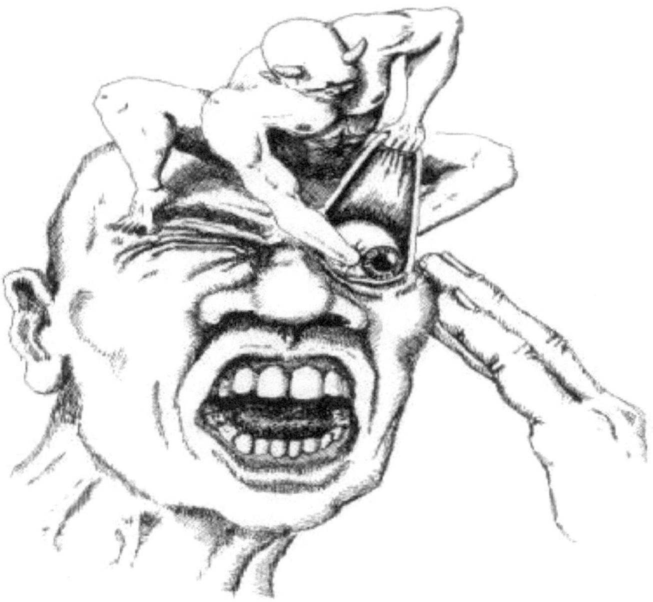

Cluster Headache

Cluster headaches are one of the most difficult to treat due to their sudden onset without any warning, or prodromal symptoms. They usually are over one eye and are piercing and totally debilitating (you cannot do anything when these strike). They occur in clusters that may last from days to weeks or even months.

Treatment of Cluster Headache

These headaches are very difficult to treat; the only treatments that I have found useful are oxygen delivered via a nasal cannula, narcotic analgesics. Certainly I would try many of the above treatments but more than likely you will need the immediate attention of your physician.

CHAPTER SEVENTEEN

THE EYE

INTRODUCTION

TABLE OF CONTENTS:

This chapter covers all the different problems that could happen to your eyes. Most of these should be evaluated by an ophthalmologist as soon as possible and should not be treated at home, due to the risk of permanent damage to the eye and resulting blindness. The presumption in this book as that you do not have access to an ophthalmologist and you are in an emergency situation, or isolated from available medical help.

EYE GLASSES AND CONTACT LENSES

If you currently wear eye glasses or contacts you will need to have an extra pair or set for replacement purposes. There are not many alternatives for eye glasses or contacts. In an extreme situation where you lose your glasses or your lens pops out, you can make pinhole glasses. You can go on YouTube for a full description of this, it is pretty cool. Basically, if you have glasses without a lens, take a piece of duct tape or fit a piece of thin cardboard into the lens frame and secure it with tape. Make a series of small hole punctures. Do this on a piece of paper and determine which size pinhole works best for your vision. What these pinholes do is eliminate scattered light and helps the light that passes through the pinhole better focus on the retina of your eye. Each hole will help, so make a series of them. This will not be as good as your glasses, but certainly will help. Or if you lose your glasses all together you will have to fashion a frame from some wire and use duct tape or cardboard as your lens and punch the holes in that. In a real crunch or a desperate situation you can also improvise this same idea by making a fist and just leaving a small opening to look through and it will surprisingly allow you to read something you wouldn't normally be able to read.

THE BATES METHOD

Another method for improving your vision is the Bates Method. The Bates Method is a series of simple eye exercises developed many years ago by Dr. William Bates that will help your vision naturally and is quite effective. Dr. Bates felt that vision and eye problems were a result of tension unconsciously placed on the eye muscles. He developed a series of eye exercises to reverse this tension and correct the underlying eye condition.

It is beyond the scope of this book and is much easier to watch many of the instructional videos available on YouTube. If you currently do not own a computer, you can either borrow a friend's or go to the local library. I would strongly encourage any of my readers with poor vision to give these exercises a chance. Many people report dramatic improvement to their vision, and it really has no downside. It will not hurt your eyes or further impair your vision, so what do you have to lose?

THE ANATOMY OF THE HUMAN EYE

Here is a quick explanation of the anatomy of the human eye. It is an amazingly complex organ, but learning this anatomy will help you understand problems that arise.

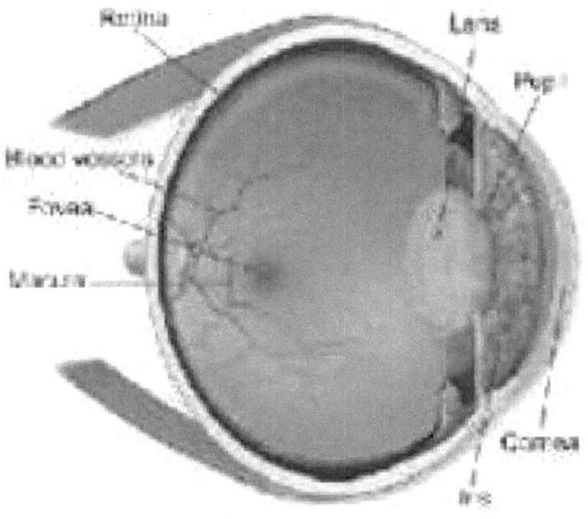

Eye Anatomy

The eye has a clear surface on the front of the eye called the cornea. The cornea is shaped like a dome and lies on top of the iris, or the colored part of your eye. The cornea acts as a camera lens and the cornea helps focus light coming through it (that is why it is clear)…that light passes next through the iris of the eye.

The iris is the colored part of your eye…brown, blue, green, or hazel, or without pigment as it is in an albino, resulting in a pink iris. Sometimes each iris is a different color. No worries, this is genetic and not a problem.

The iris is basically a muscle and some connective tissue that controls the size of the pupil (the black center of your eye). The iris functions just like the diaphragm of a camera, it dilates (expands or enlarges) to allow more light in or constricts (tightens or becomes smaller) to restrict light coming in. By doing so it changes the size of the pupil. You can test this yourself…when you are in a dark room you will have large pupils so there will be more light made available to your eye. When you are outside in bright light, your pupils become tight and small. Doctors test this papillary light reflex by shining light in your eyes during your physical examination.

Once light passes through the pupil it strikes the lens which lies behind it and from there the light is focused onto the retina which lies at the back of the eye. The white part of your eye is the sclera and this is covered by the conjunctiva, which also lines the eyelids.

THE MOST COMMON CAUSES OF EYE PROBLEMS

Conjunctivitis (Pink Eye) and Other Eye Infections

Conjunctivitis (pink eye) and other eye infections are very common problems. The conjunctiva is a membrane that lines your eye lids and also covers the sclera or white part of your eye. Pink eye will be one of the most common eye problems you encounter. It is highly contagious and the only way to effectively prevent its transmission is for the infected person to do frequent hand washing with soap and also to not rub the infected eye thereby transmitting the infection either to the other eye or to another person. Pink eye has two types: viral and bacterial. The two can be identified by the type of discharge the eye produces. A thin watery discharge is from a viral source and cannot be treated with antibiotics (antibiotics only work on bacteria, not viruses or fungi). A thick green, sticky discharge is from a bacterial infection. Both adults and children can get either one, but the bacterial type is more prevalent in children. Viruses have to run their course and will eventually heal, think of the common cold. Both types will remain very contagious until the discharge or tearing stops. Both types will produce symptoms of itchy eyes, some blurring of vision, a gritty feeling in the affected eye, discharge, redness to the eye, pain, and possibly a sensitivity to light.

Treatment of Conjunctivitis

In life your food many times will become your medicine. Here is a perfect example:

Cucumber

Wash your hands first with soap and water and clean under your fingernails as well. Take a raw cucumber, peel it and grate it. Take a large, sterile gauze pad or cheesecloth that has been boiled to sterilize it. Lie down and put your head back and squeeze a few drops of cucumber juice into each affected eye. If it is easier, use an eyecup.

Baking Soda or Honey

You can make a very effective eye wash for conjunctivitis by mixing one teaspoon of baking soda in two cups of cold water. Alternatively you can use honey by dissolving one tablespoon of honey in one cup of hot water, let it cool and use that as an eye wash.

Chamomile Tea or Eyebright

You can also use chamomile tea or eyebright tea (Euphrasia officinalis). Make a double strength version of the tea (use twice as much tea as normal, with the same amount of water). Let it cool and using an eyecup, instill it into each affected eye four times a day until the discharge (water and pus) stops.

Note: You can use the leftover tea bags topically (onto the surface) of your eyelids as cool compresses to soothe the eyes. When you are done, do not waste them, throw them into your compost pile. By the way, any leftover coffee grounds are wonderful to add to your compost as well, they are chock-full of many minerals and nutrients.

Boric Acid

Boric acid is another excellent treatment for any eye problems; it naturally soothes and disinfects the eye. It is inexpensive and readily available.

Here is how to use it: Boil a cup of water with one teaspoon of boric acid which comes as a white or clear powder) let it cool and then use it as an eyewash with an eyecup or soak some cotton balls with it and apply it to both eyes. Rinse after with lukewarm water. Repeat this two or three times a day until the eyes heal.

Calendula

Calendula is an herb that has both very potent antibacterial and antiviral properties. It is also soothing to the eye and hence is wonderful for eye infections.

Take two teaspoons of dried calendula flowers and put them in a cup of water and make a tea of it. Allow it to cool and then strain the tea through cheesecloth or a coffee filter. Use an eyecup and apply this to the eye several times a day until healed.

Saline Solution

You can make your own saline solution; take one teaspoon of table salt or sea salt and mix it in a cup of distilled water. Bring this mix to a boil and then allow it to cool and using an eyecup apply it to your eyes three or four times a day until they heal. Alternatively you can use an eye dropper and place three drops of the saline mixture in the corner of your eye three times a day until healed.

Povidone-Iodine Solution (Betadine)

Povidone-Iodine (Betadine 5%) at this strength is ideal to treat eye infections. Do not use a stronger percentage of this; if it is stronger, dilute it with water down to 5 percent. This is an old remedy that works very well for eye infections. It does sting the eye and also will dye it brown for a short time. This actually helps when using as a guide to see where it has spread after applying it. The best way is to have the patient blink several times and with the eyes closed, look up and down and towards the nose and then towards the ears to properly distribute the Betadine over the entire eyeball.

As I explained in the section covering iodine, it has extensive antimicrobial (germ-killing) properties and works against viruses, fungi, bacteria, even MRSA, and also against tuberculosis. Two or three drops of the Betadine in both eyes one time should suffice to wipe out the infection. It is very potent. Make sure the Betadine you have does not contain any detergents and make sure it is only 5 percent or you will have to dilute it.

Blunt Trauma to the Eye and the Orbit or Eye Socket

Your eyes are partially shielded from blunt trauma by their anatomy. The eyeball is surrounded by a bony wall on all sides (called the orbit) that protrudes slightly beyond the eye itself. This provides protection while at the same time not impairing (blocking) your vision. However, there are still many times when blunt trauma does injure the eye despite the orbits protection.

Trauma to the eye is best evaluated by a physician ASAP, especially if there is visual impairment. However, this book assumes that many of the situations do not involve access to a physician and will have to be treated emergently, be aware that you may permanently damage someone's vision, so really consider it carefully before you treat an eye injury.

Upon evaluating a patient who has sustained trauma to their eye, your job is to first make sure there is nothing in the eye, what we doctors refer to as a "foreign body". You can do this visually and if you see something, you should take a Q-tip and moisten it and try to touch it to the foreign body and gently remove it from the eye. Do not press it down on the foreign body, you might accidentally embed it into the eyeball and or scratch the cornea. If this does not work, then flush out the eye with some sterile water. If you have none, take some water and bring it to a rolling boil for a few minutes and then allow it to cool. Take a small plastic syringe and fill it and use it to flush out the eye. You may have to evert (flip over) the upper and lower lids and flush them out as well. Next you should examine the eye and see if there is any abrasion or scratching of the cornea. You can do this by standing to the side of the patient and shining a light sideways over their cornea (the clear covering of the eye overlaying the iris or colored part of the eye) and see if there are any scratches or rough spots. Patients invariably complain of a feeling of dirt, grit, or sand in their eyes. Next, get an eye patch or make one by folding a four by four piece of gauze and taping it over the eye. If you have any topical antibiotic cream for eyes then you may apply a small string of that over the eye and have the patient blink several times to spread it out . Leave this on for twenty-four hours and then remove it and see how they feel. Their eyes will be a little blurry and light sensitive for a few minutes. After this if they still have the same complaint of sand or gritty sensation, then reapply the eye patch and retape it for two more days. By that time the eye usually heals itself. If you have no ocular (eye) antibiotic cream then use one of the treatments mentioned above for conjunctivitis such as povidone-iodine solution (Betadine).

If there is no obvious rupture of the eyeball you should then apply ice packs or anything cold to the eye to decrease the swelling that usually accompanies trauma to the eye. If you have any pain medications such as Aleve or Tylenol or Motrin you should give them immediately. Other than Tylenol, avoid using these other pain medications and other nonsteroidal anti-inflammatory medications if there is obvious bleeding into the eye because they may worsen the situation. You should also keep the patient sitting up or if they are lying down keep their head elevated; this is especially important in patients who report some loss of visual acuity (loss of vision) because this allows any blood to drain to the lower parts of the eye and very well may preserve some of their vision.

Foreign Bodies in The Eye

See the above section on blunt trauma for a full explanation of how to remove a foreign body from the eye without further traumatizing it.

Corneal Abrasion

A corneal abrasion (scratched eye) is most often due to dust or a foreign body in the eye such as dirt, sand, or others, resulting in an abrasion or scratching of the clear cornea. The most common scenario is a patient who gets something in their eye and repeatedly rubs it, what this does is works to drive the sand or other foreign body into the clear cornea, scoring or scratching its surface. This causes significant pain and irritation to the eye, resulting in constant tearing by the eye in an attempt to wash out the foreign body. See the above explanation under trauma to the eye for details on the treatment of corneal abrasions.

Chemicals and Other Eye Irritants

If a patient presents to you who has had chemicals or some other substances that irritate their eyes you should either take or make a sterile eye solution by boiling water as described above in section 2 on blunt trauma and thoroughly flush out the eye. Do this repeatedly, two or three times or more in a row to ensure you washed out all the irritating chemicals. On a personal note this actually happened to me once when I worked in a gas station in college. A woman came in and she parked too far from the pump. The gas hose from the pump was fully stretched out and I asked the woman to back up a few feet.

Instead she pulled forward, the hose came out of her gas tank still pumping, and as I stooped to retrieve it, it sent a fountain of gas right into both my eyes. It was amazingly painful and felt like my eyes had caught fire, I felt my way inside and found the slop sink and ran cold water into both of my eyes for about five minutes before I had any relief.

Allergic Inflammation of The Eyes, Or Allergic Conjunctivitis

Allergic inflammation of the eyes is also known as allergic conjunctivitis. This is usually seasonal, meaning it is in the spring and fall and not all year round (or perennially). It is caused by an allergic reaction to pollen. In the spring it is usually tree pollen and grasses and in the fall it is goldenrod and other allergens. All allergic reactions are mediated by histamine, meaning the release of histamine causes the symptoms. Hence our use of antihistamines to block this histamine and neutralize it, thus helping however it is manifesting (showing itself), as in itchy, watery eyes, sneezing, coughing or urticaria (hives). Hives are small or large round red areas that come and go and cause intense itching. They typically arise anywhere with no pattern to them.

Note: Year round allergies might be due to animal dander. Most often cats are the biggest offenders, followed by dogs, dust, grasses, and food allergies. That being said, I would rather sneeze and have itchy eyes all year round, than part with my dogs, Amos and Charlie. If you can try to rid yourself of the offending agent, for example…get rid of that cat, dust the house really well, etc.

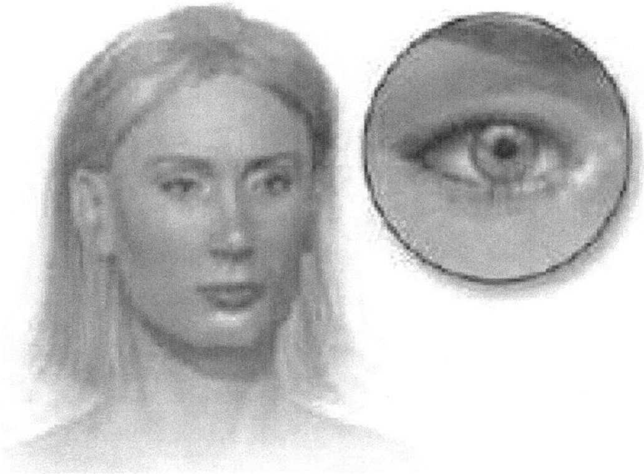

To treat allergic conjunctivitis the first step is to thoroughly rinse both your eyes with a sterile eye solution or sterile saline solution. It will work even better if you can cool those solutions, because a cool solution will help any inflammation caused by the allergens. Wash your face to remove any allergens that may be sticking to your skin and/or eyelids and eyelashes. Apply ice packs or anything cold as a cold compress to both eyes to help decrease the inflammation and provide some relief.

White Pupil

A white pupil is never good; this may indicate a cataract, tumor, inflammation, or a detached retina. You need an ophthalmologist for this and nothing else will be helpful; this is a medical emergency.

Sty

A sty is basically a pimple or white head on the eyelid. The medical term is an external hordoleum. It may also form an internal hordoleum or abscess of the eyelid. A sty usually occurs at the base of eyelashes and is a small "white head".

Stys are self-limited, meaning they usually run their course and go away. You can help them heal by placing warm compresses (a hot face cloth or small towel) directly over them several times a day and then gently squeeze them to drain them. You can also clean your eyelid at the base of your eyelashes with some mild soap and water or if it looks like it is worsening you can use a very small amount of topical antibiotic cream. Usually you do not need to do that.

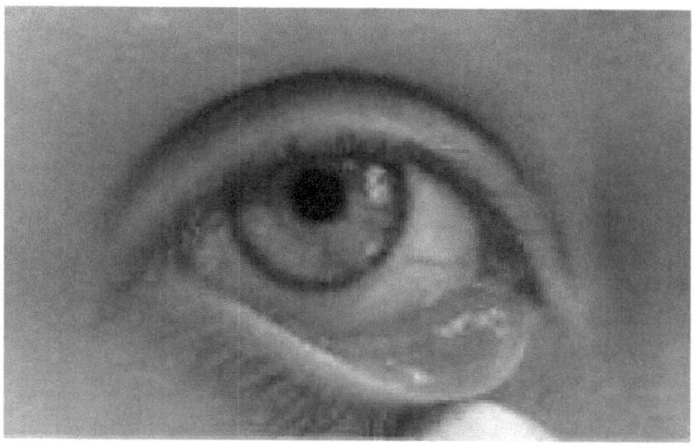

A Hordoleum of the Lower Eyelid

Alternatively you can make a 50/50 solution of baby shampoo and mild soap (Ivory soap for example) and using a hot washcloth wrapped around your index finger, gently clean the affected eyelid margin (where the sty is).

In cases where the sty appears to be enlarging, you may want to surgically drain it. Once again, this is best done by a physician, but if you are in a situation where that is not possible then this can be done with a very small, sterilized needle or a number 11 scalpel.

Carefully and gently hold the lid with your non dominant hand (if you are right-handed this means your left hand) and holding the scalpel or needle in your dominant hand, gently press it against the white head part of the sty and then withdraw it and gently squeeze and try to drain the sty of its pus. Use the same solution mix above and cleanse the sty after you are done.

Eye Strain

Eye strain or pressure sensation in your eyes is a frequent problem and can easily be treated with natural methods. It is caused by prolonged reading, staring at a computer screen, working on small objects in poor light. Eye strain frequently manifests as blurry vision, difficulty properly focusing your eyes, and oftentimes as headaches in the frontal area (your forehead) and behind your eyes.

Here are a few remedies that I like to use that work just fine when your eyes ache or you have a headache from eye strain:

1. Take some raw potatoes (organic, preferably) and grate both the peel and the pulp and take a tablespoon and place it over the eyelid and cover it completely. Take a small clean towel or a piece of gauze and cover it and leave it on for an hour. (a slice of cucumber over each eye also works).
2. Get an old pair of ski or other goggles and clean them well and fill them with any cold fruit, such as watermelon or any type, and strap them to your eyes and lie down for an hour. Make sure the goggles are filled completely so there is no space between your eyelid and the fruit.
3. Take several slices of cold cucumber and apply them to your eyelids, alternatively ice packs or cold compresses applied to the eyelids will also help.
4. Cool compresses of eyebright applied to the eyelids will help.
5. Essential oils such as lemon oil or rose oil: Mix one drop of either of these oils into two tablespoons of a carrier oil and avoiding the eye itself, massage this mix into the bony orbit surrounding the eye and the forehead.

A Bloody Streak on The Conjunctiva

This will no doubt freak out both you or the person who has it. It is due to a broken blood vessel in the conjunctiva or clear surface of your eye and is usually not a major problem. It does not affect a person's vision. The capillary breaks and a small collection of blood pools under the clear surface of the eye where it cannot be absorbed quickly. When you examine the eye you will see a red streak on the white surface of the eye or sclera. It is usually caused by bouts of coughing, vomiting, sneezing, or sometimes blunt trauma to the eye. Even straining to lift a very heavy object can cause these hemorrhages.

It has been my experience in my practice that patients are always freaked out about these bloody streaks and a little reassurance goes a long way. A patient should avoid aspirin or any blood thinners when they have this, otherwise no treatment is necessary. These usually take several weeks to go away; as they age you may even notice a color change from red to orange and yellow (similar to the way a bruise changes with age).

Black Eye

A black eye is a very common occurrence. Basically it is caused by any trauma to the face or head, typically a punch, which causes bleeding below the skin around your eyes. The blackness is caused by the discoloration of the skin from this blood, along with the bruising of the skin and swelling of the soft tissue of the eye socket. The eye itself is not usually damaged and most of these slowly clear over a few days to a week.

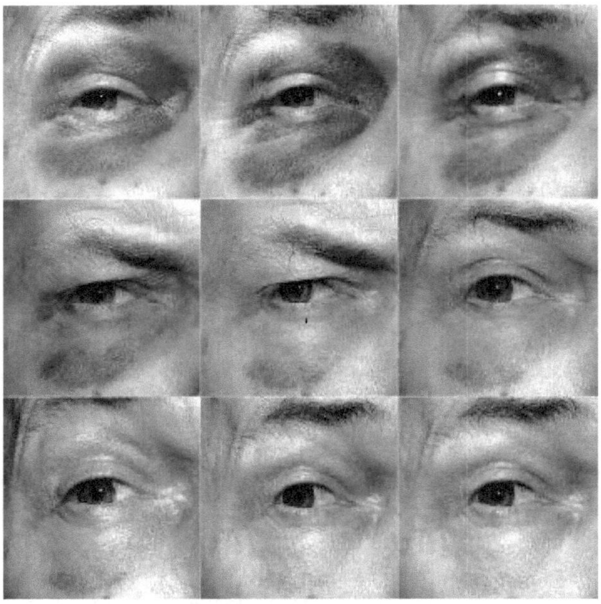

Stages of a Black Eye as It Heals

NOTE: It is of some concern if both eyes are blackened and there has been significant trauma to the head; this may note a skull fracture. Black eyes do not require much treatment and will resolve on their own. Right after it happens the best treatment is ice packs or cold compresses. Do not apply much pressure to the eye itself.

Remember to never put ice in direct contact with the skin, it may cause frostbite. Always use a thin layer of cloth or other material between the ice and the skin. You can take Tylenol, Aleve, or

Motrin for pain, but not aspirin, which affects clotting and might worsen the bleeding. The treatments for eye strain listed above will also work for a black eye.

Swollen Eyelid

The swelling of an eyelid is almost always unilateral (one sided, either right or left) and accompanied by redness, warmth, pain , burning eyes, blurry vision, light sensitivity, crusting of the eyelashes and/or dry eyes. The medical term for this is blepharitis. It is caused by bacteria, blockage of the oil glands of the eyelid, and/or allergies.

This is treated with a clean washcloth soaked in hot water; place this over the affected eye for five minutes at a time. This will help soothe the eye. Then take the same washcloth and soak it in a 50 /50 mix of baby shampoo and mild soap like Ivory Soap for example. Using your index finger inside of the washcloth, wipe away all the debris (pus and oils) on the affected eyelid's margin where the eyelashes attach to your eye.

Any of the cold compresses with cucumbers, potatoes or cold fruit that I described above will help reduce the swelling and soothe any eye inflammation that might be present.

CHAPTER EIGHTEEN

THE EAR

INTRODUCTION

TABLE OF CONTENTS:

In life common problems will remain common, and ear problems, especially among children, will often arise. They are easily treated and you should be knowledgeable about ear anatomy and ear problems and their treatment.

First let's review the anatomy of the human ear: There is the pinna or auricle; this is the medical name for your ear. The pinna helps direct sound waves into the external ear canal (the part that you would slide a Q-tip into, for example)...this leads to the tympanic membrane (eardrum). This eardrum is a thin grayish, slightly shiny membrane on which sound causes vibrations...behind the eardrum lies the middle ear...this has those silly-named three bones called the hammer, anvil, and stirrup, or auditory ossicles. There is a long thin tube that connects the middle ear to the sinuses called the eustachian tube (auditory tube). You can feel this pop when you are on an airplane or change altitude going up a mountain. This is because the pressure is equalizing in your middle ear. Behind the middle ear lies the inner ear...this has two parts, the semicircular canals, which are responsible for balance, and the cochlea, which is filled with little hairs of cilia that vibrate and create the nerve impulse that travels on the auditory nerve which is responsible for hearing.

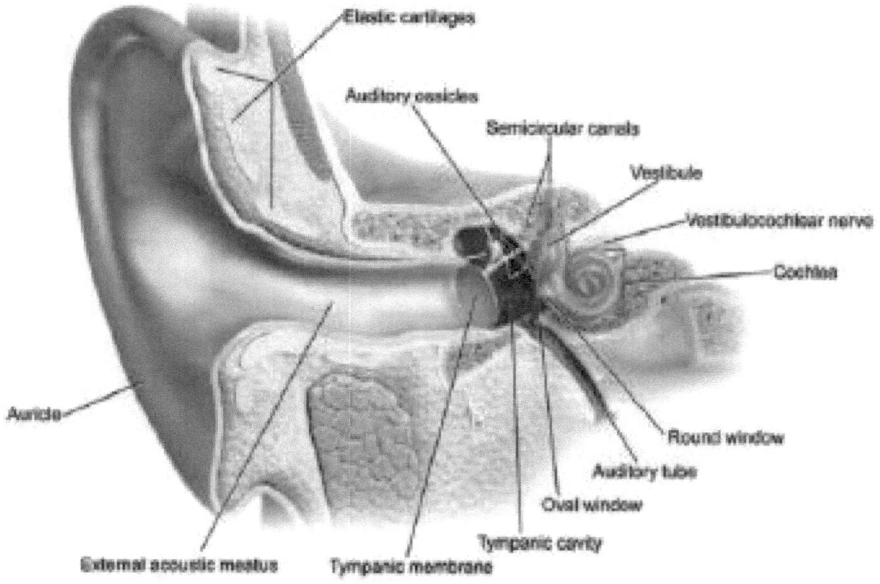

That is ear anatomy in a nutshell.

EAR INFECTIONS

Ear infections are also known as otitis...if it is the outer ear it is otitis externa, the middle ear is otitis media. These are very common problems, especially in children.

Otitis Externa Or Swimmer's Ear

Otitis externa is also known as swimmers ear. This commonly occurs in children, and typically during the summer when they are swimming. It is usually caused by bacteria or fungi in the water they are swimming in, and may also occur from bacteria multiplying in a sweaty ear (although less common).

One of your body's defenses against ear infections is your earwax (or cerumen). Earwax naturally has a waxy consistency and this is your body's ingenious way to repel water. One of the weird facts I recall from medical school, where you are inundated with mountains of information, is that the Japanese have gray earwax.

Classically, when you pull on the affected ear it will be painful. The ear will be painful if you put a Q-tip in the external auditory canal (the canal or passage between your outer ear and your eardrum). The external canal will be reddened as well and also there may or may not be a discharge (pus coming out of the canal). Sometimes there is a feeling of pressure building up in the ear and there may be ringing of the ear also known as tinnitus.

Prevention of Ear Infections

If a child or anyone you know has this as a recurrent problem, then you can consider some preventative steps such as:

Put earplugs in your ear to prevent the contaminated water from reaching your ear. If you don't have earplugs you can improvise with a small ball of silly putty or wax. You can also take a cotton ball and soak it in petroleum jelly and insert this in your external ear canals

Dry your ears well and tilt your head to each side and allow gravity to drain your ears for you. The lesser amount of water you can leave in your ears the better the prevention. You can also dry them with a Q-tip, but you have to be very careful...you know the old saying, "you should put nothing smaller than your elbow in your ear". You can easily perforate (tear a hole) your eardrum. Gently insert the Q-tip and advance it slowly; stopping to gently twirl every so often will pick up a lot of wax and dirt and other debris.

In patients who have a history of recurrent ear infections, you can try mixing one part white vinegar and one part rubbing alcohol. Put about one teaspoon of the solution in each ear both before and after swimming. This mixture will kill most bacteria and fungi that grow in your ear.

Treatment of External Otitis or Swimmer's Ear

Heat Treatment

If you have a heating pad or some way to heat a towel, for example on a stove top or over a wood stove, then apply that to the ear that hurts, several times a day. The towel should be warm but not hot.

Onion Treatment

You can also use an onion as follows: Bake the onion for fifteen or twenty minutes with the skin on it, then cut it in half and allow to cool enough that you won't burn someone, then apply the cut half against the ear. This works very nicely to transmit warmth against the ear. Give the standard Tylenol, Motrin, or Aleve for any pain.

Hydrogen Peroxide

Hydrogen peroxide and water (a 50/50 mix): Have the patient lie on the opposite side from their ear pain, if it is on both sides it doesn't matter, just repeat this on the other side. Using a turkey baster or an infant's ball syringe, gently squirt some of this mixture, about a tablespoon, into each ear. It will foam up as it kills the bacteria. Allow it to remain in the ear for about a minute then have the patient turn their head and drain it out. Repeat this about four times a day until the pain and symptoms subside.

Note: Do not do this if the eardrum is perforated (has a hole in it). Alternatively, you can put a cotton ball in each ear and prevent the hydrogen peroxide/water solution from draining out right away.

White Vinegar

Use a 50/50 mix of white vinegar and sterile water. Mix this together and place a teaspoon of this in a child's ear (a tablespoon for an adult). This can be kept in the ear as well by putting cotton balls in the ear canal to block it running out.

Mullein and Garlic Oil

You can buy this premade or make your own mix. Garlic has wonderful antibacterial and antiviral properties; it also contains natural substances that boost your immune system as well acting as anesthetics to the ear. Garlic is also known to be one hundred times more effective than the two most popular antibiotics for treatment of food poisoning. To mix your own do the following:

Take four or five cloves of garlic and crush and mince them in a pan; allow to sit for fifteen minutes.

Add a quarter cup of mullein (dried).

Add 1 ounce of either olive oil or virgin coconut oil (this, as you recall, has antiviral properties) or you can mix the two.

Mix them all together and put this sauce pan inside of a larger one that is half-filled with water.

Heat it until the oil is warm; do not cook the garlic.

Now strain it through a coffee filter or cheesecloth or some other type of filter. You want to remove all the particles of garlic and mullein.

Use two or three drops of this in each ear two or three times a day until healed. (up to six times a day)

You can also make it more potent by the addition of essential oils which act as carriers and help strengthen the mixture and allow greater penetration. You can use tea tree oil, oregano oil, lavender oil and eucalyptus oil or combine them one drop of each, or use any one of them alone. Store this mix in a glass bottle, dark preferably to cause less breakdown of the ingredients from light. When you need it again, reheat it by placing the entire bottle in a pan of water and heat it to around 100 F (roughly body temperature), check it against your skin. It should not be cold or too hot, both will cause pain. (This recipe was borrowed from a wonderful website: http://creativechristianmama.com.

OTITIS MEDIA (MIDDLE EAR INFECTIONS)

You will discover that this is a very common finding in both children and adults. It most often presents with symptoms of pressure in the ear with or without an earache, fever, dizziness, or cold symptoms. Small children will most likely cry and pull on their ears and may be dizzy with some ataxia (falling over or unsteadiness on their feet). When you look at the eardrum it will appear red and swollen. If you pull the ear and it hurts, this is swimmer's ear, but be aware you could have both an external and middle ear infection. After the common cold this is the most common infection among children, it is also very common with adults.

Treatment Of Otitis Media Or Middle Ear Infections

You can follow all of the above-outlined treatment options for swimmer's ear; all of them will help in cases of middle ear infections as well.

Antibiotics

Antibiotics are overprescribed for ear infections and most except the most severe will resolve on their own in a short time. This book is written under the assumption that you will not have any antibiotics or other prescription medications available, or you are choosing to forego them and treat your infection naturally.

Antioxidants

Some things you can do to help any infection is to boost your defenses by boosting your immune system with antioxidant vitamins such as Vitamins C, D, and E, as well as CoQ10, alpha lipoic acid. Zinc and selenium also help your immune system; both also help your body by the many enzymes that are reliant on each of these to properly function. As I stated earlier in this book, your food is your medicine. Good healthy mineral- and trace element-rich foods will keep you and your children healthy and will enable you to either resist diseases or attenuate (weaken) their effects on your body and therefore shorten both the disease's severity and the length of time you are ill.

Garlic and Raw Honey

First you finely chop a few cloves of raw garlic and mix it with raw honey. Give a tablespoon of these two or three times a day. This supercharges the immune system and helps shorten the length of any infection.

Honey applied to a Q-tip and swabbed around the external auditory canal will also help a swimmer's ear, but you must first flush it out with a fifty/fifty mix of hydrogen peroxide and warm water.

Fermented Cod Liver Oil

Apparently the high vitamin A content of fermented cod liver oil helps ear infections by promoting drainage of the ear. It also contains large quantities of vitamin D and fish oils (omega-3 fatty acids). It is fermented so it is natural and is chock-full of enzymes as well. Take as directed on the bottle. The taste is the problem; cod liver oil, even fermented, has a taste that few people like. You can make it more palatable by adding some raw honey to it.

Eustachian Tube Dysfunction and how to Treat It

Your Eustachian tube originates in the rear of your nose and travels slightly uphill to where it ends in the middle ear. It is named after the 16th century Italian anatomist Eustachius. The purpose of the Eustachian tube is to ventilate the middle ear as well as equalize pressure within it, it also serves as a drain for any debris, bacteria and fluids that may accumulate in the inner ear and have no other way to escape. The

Eustachian tube is lined with the same tissue that lines the nose and thus reacts identically to anything that irritates or infects the nose, by swelling just like nasal mucosa. The Eustachian tube normally is closed, thereby preventing infections going from the nose to the ear, it is designed to open on demand. The Eustachian tube is very thin and any swelling of its lining will invariably close it completely. Many ear infections are accompanied by Eustachian tube dysfunction (meaning it is not working).

When the Eustachian tube is closed completely and not opening as it should, this causes symptoms of a pressure like sensation in the ear, otalgia (ear pain), popping and clicking in the ear. Some patients experience tinnitus (ringing in their ears) and vertigo (a sensation of whirling around when you are not moving). A good example of this is when you are a passenger on an airplane and your ears start building up pressure and your hearing diminishes and you feel a popping, this is all from your Eustachian tube and the resulting pressure changes in your middle ear.

Eustachian tube dysfunction if caused by allergies, and often by infections; both bacterial and viral. In my practice I frequently see smokers with recurrent problems with Eustachian tube dysfunction as well as recurrent ear and sinus infections. Young children and children with Down's syndrome suffer frequently with ear infections and Eustachian tube dysfunction due to the small size of their tubes.

Treatment of Eustachian tube dysfunction in many ways is similar to what you do on an airplane when it occurs. Swallowing, chewing, eating or drinking work to open a closed tube by activating the muscles in the throat which help open the tube. When you drink, if you gulp the liquid down , this helps open a closed tube. Huge yawns also help to open closed tubes. I find swallowing to be the more effective than the other modalities. Another common way to open your Eustachian tubes is to "pop your ears". This is done by pinching both nostrils closed and forcibly blowing out against your closed nose with your mouth closed.

Many times you have to give short toots but forcibly and then a few long toots. Hopefully you will almost immediately feel/hear a popping sensation as the tubes open. In infants the best you can do is to give them a bottle so hopefully their sucking and swallowing will open their Eustachian tubes.

Another method is to use massage to help open your Eustachian tubes. If you are doing it for someone else you should have them lay down on their back and you stay behind them above their head. Gently reach behind both ears and make circular motions with the tips of your fingers, do this from the top of the ear towards the bottom and then a few inches down below the ear. Do this for several minutes and have the patient periodically yawn loudly and or sit up and try to pop their ears by blowing out forcibly against their closed nostrils.

As much as you might dislike it, you might have to take an antihistamine and or a decongestant to help open a closed Eustachian tube. The good news is that this will probably clear up in a few days without any treatment, so don't fret over this too much.

Ear Obstruction with Wax and Foreign Bodies in the Ear

Wax buildup in the external ear canal is a common finding in clinical practice. The wax in your ears can form a plug with hair and other debris and be quite difficult to remove. Foreign objects or bodies in the ear are removed in the same way as the wax, unless you can reach it with the use of an otoscope and a long tweezer, being very careful not to puncture the eardrum. That is not as easy as it sounds, and without a good light source, which you may or may not have, it is very difficult. I find flushing the ear to be the best way to get out wax and/ or a foreign body.

Usually the wax has to be softened to help in its removal. This can be done with a variety of liquids. In my office I typically use a 50/50 mixture of hydrogen peroxide and warm water. Using a 50 cc syringe and a cut down plastic catheter I direct the flow of the warm water (careful not to use water that is either too hot or too cold) gently into the ear, hoping to dislodge the wax plug or foreign body.

Be careful and try not to apply too much pressure when instilling the solution, also try to avoid directing it directly against the eardrum due to the risk of perforation (tearing) it, direct your stream of solution against the edges of the canal. Usually several repeated attempts will suffice to get it clean.

Sometimes you need to use commercial wax softeners if available such as Debrox Otic Solution or similar products.

Other things you can use to soften earwax are:

Mineral Oil
Olive Oil,
Baby Oil
Glycerin.

You basically instill a few drops of these into each ear with a dropper. Do this twice daily for four or five days and this should soften the wax nicely. Now you can get a rubber bulb syringe and squirt the hydrogen peroxide/water mix into the ear to dislodge the softened wax or flush out the foreign body. When squirting this solution in, it will help to pull the ear up and back, this will straighten out the external ear canal and make it a straight shot. After the solution is instilled into the ear, tilt the patient's head to the side to allow it to run out.

You might very well have to repeat this procedure several times to clean out all the wax and debris. Repeat it until there is nothing else coming out of the ear besides the solution.

Note: It is tricky to use a Q-tip to get wax out of an ear. Most times you are just packing the wax deeper into the ear canal and compounding your problems. Softening the wax as described above is infinitely easier and if you have the opportunity you should always soften it first.

Salt

Heat one cup of salt in a pan for five minutes or so. Pour it into a cotton sock and seal the open end with a rubber band or string. Once it cools to the point where it is not burning you...place it against the ear. It will help draw out fluid and open the ear.

Olive Oil and Mustard Oil

Take several ounces of olive oil and heat it in a sauce pan. After it cools to body temperature, place several drops in the affected ear. It will help cut through any wax and debris that have clogged the ear canal. Then clean it out with some Q-tips, taking care not to hit the eardrum or you could easily perforate (puncture) it, especially when it is inflamed as with an ear infection. Mustard oil can also be used in place of olive oil in the same way.

EAR PAIN AND ITS TREATMENT

Heat

The treatment of ear pain can be as simple as lying on a heating pad, which naturally could be substituted with a hot, moist towel or face cloth. An alternative method is to heat up a small ceramic plate and place that cupped over the ear; within a few minutes the heat radiating from the plate will give you some relief. Besides heat, swallowing liquids will help open up your Eustachian tube and relieve some of that ear discomfort, sitting up will also help. Using several pillows at night to keep your head up will allow gravity to work in your favor and assist in drainage of your ear.

Analgesics (Painkillers)

If you have any Tylenol, Aleve, Motrin, or ibuprofen and aspirin, now is the time to take it. Remember, you cannot give aspirin to children under the age of twelve. Also never use aspirin in someone who is bleeding or is on blood thinners of any kind, or is about to have surgery, in which case it should be held for one week prior to the surgery.

Saint-John's-Wort Oil

The botanical name for Saint-John's-wort is Hypericum perforatum. It has been shown that using Saint-John's-wort oil instilled directly into the ear will help treat ear infections as well as alleviate pain. Wort is the old English word for plant, and it is called Saint-John's-wort because it typically flowers on June 24th, which is the birthday of John the Baptist. Gently heat this oil in a small sauce pan or in some other fashion and then instill three drops to the affected ear three times a day.

Pressure

You can apply pressure from the inside out to open up blocked ears. Pinch the end of your nose closed and take a deep breath, filling your mouth and lungs. Blow out through your nose as if trying to blow your fingers off the end of your nose. Using saline spray or a saline solution and instilling that in your nose, with either a neti pot or a bulb syringe (like a turkey baster), will help open up your sinuses and clear your nose and ears.

Do this, wait a minute or two and then blow your nose and then perform the above maneuver; repeat it if necessary. It works well to open your nose, ears, and sinuses.

Ear Candles

An often-touted method of cleaning out ears and blocked ear canals is by use of a lit hollow candle that is inserted in the outer ear canal. The theory is that these candles will heat up as they burn down and create a vacuum that draws wax and other debris out of the ear and kills any microbes with its heat. The only problem is that studies show that this does not work and in fact leaves a waxy debris in the ear canal from the candle. Patients of mine have tried this on their own and most have reported to me that this does not work, a few swear by it, but I have no confidence in recommending this to you. I included it here in order to express my opinion of it and to be comprehensive.

CHAPTER NINETEEN

NOSEBLEEDS (EPISTAXIS)

INTRODUCTION

TABLE OF CONTENTS:

Nosebleeds are a common occurrence and there is a very good chance that you will encounter one personally or from a friend or family member. You will need to know how to treat a nosebleed, it isn't difficult and you will be a hero the next time you use your new skills. The medical term for nosebleed is Epistaxis.

WHY DO WE GET NOSEBLEEDS?

The nose has a lining known as the nasal mucosa. This mucosa is very rich in blood vessels that are close to its surface. The reason for this abundance of blood vessels in the nasal mucosa is to warm and humidify the air that enters the nose before it reaches the lungs. Any rupturing of these blood vessels will cause a nosebleed.

TYPES OF NOSEBLEEDS:

Anterior (front of the nose): This is by far the most common type and the easier of the two to get under control. It involves a network of blood vessels in the fleshy bulb or tip of the nose.

Posterior (back of the nose): This is much less common and much more difficult to get under control, due to its anatomic location and the challenges involved with application of pressure to stop the bleeding way in the back of the nose.

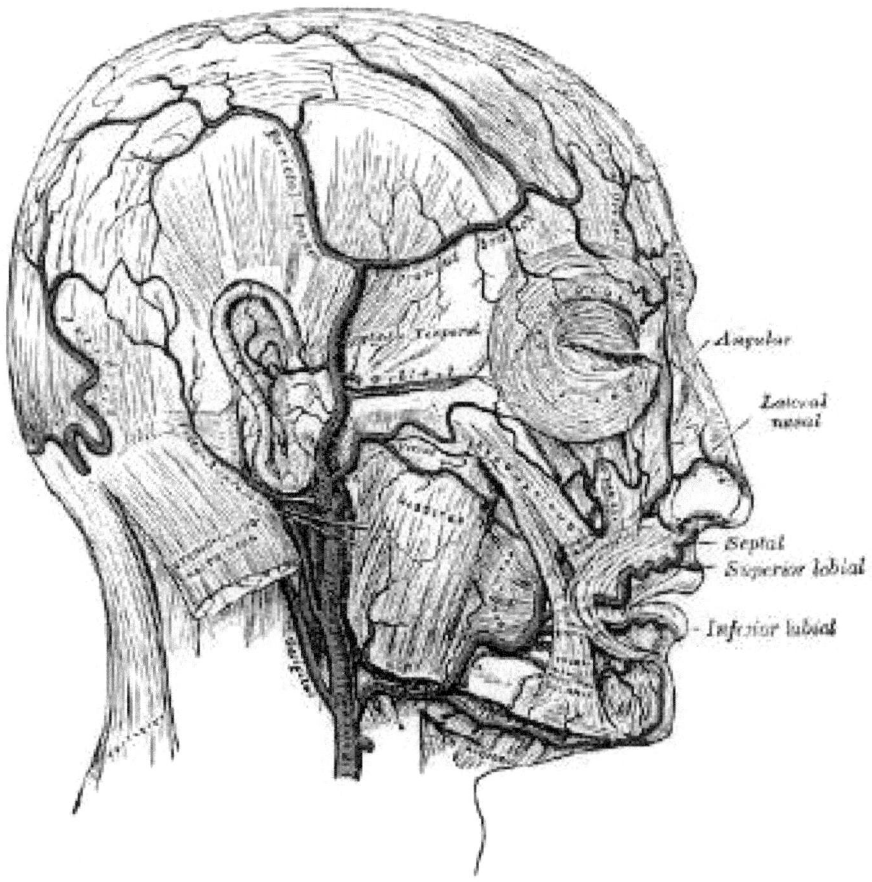

Blood supply to the scalp, Face. Pay special attention to the location of the blood vessels of the tip of the nose. That is where direct pressure is applied to stop a nosebleed.

COMMON CAUSES OF NOSEBLEEDS

Blunt Trauma To The Nose

There are endless ways your nose can be traumatized such as a punch, an elbow during a Basketball game, a kick to the head, striking the nose against something like during a car accident

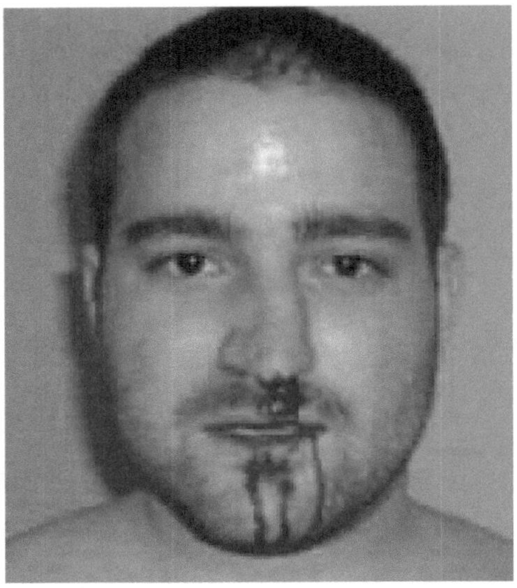

Man with broken nose and nosebleed.

Hot Dry Air

Prolonged exposure to hot dry air can dry out the nasal mucosa and cause it to crack and bleed. For example in homes with forced hot air heat or wood stoves, the air becomes drier than a desert after a short time. The body is not used to this kind of heat without any moisture and it will dry out the noses lining. In these cases even what would normally be insignificant contact with the nose can cause bleeding. Typically these patients will just itch their nose, or rub it and it will start bleeding.

NOTE: Very cold air can also cause nosebleeds. This can be prevented by moisturizing the nasal mucosa several times a day. In my practice I use Ponds Cold Cream and it works better than petroleum jelly which is sometimes too greasy.

Trauma To The Nasal Mucosa (The Lining Of The Nose)

Trauma to the nasal mucosa is most often caused by picking the nose resulting in a nosebleed this is the most common cause, especially in children. Also sticking objects up their noses cause a lot of nosebleeds in kids. Blowing your nose hard can also traumatize it and make it bleed.

Cold and Sinus Infections

Colds and Sinus infections especially with a lot of sneezing and nose blowing can lead to bleeding. The nasal mucosa is already engorged and inflamed and the trauma of repeated coughing or blowing the nose can lead to nosebleeds.

Allergies

Allergies and what is known as Allergic Rhinitis or a runny nose caused by allergies can lead to nosebleeds pretty much by the same mechanism as colds outlined above.

Hypertension

The incidence of hypertension increases with age, this is a frequent cause of Epistaxis or nosebleeds. What happens is the nasal mucosa ages and thins and with increased pressure in the arterioles and capillaries results in them bursting and bleeding.

Medications

Aspirin is the major culprit here as well as Coumadin (Warfarin) and other anticoagulants (Blood thinners) such as Plavix, Xarelto, Eliquis and Pradaxa. Remember Willow Bark is what aspirin is made from and even through many patients consider it "organic and natural" it will lead to nose bleeds just like aspirin. All of these medications decrease the coagulation or clotting of blood via various mechanisms and thus can cause bleeding.

Nasal Decongestant Sprays

Overuse of nasal decongestant sprays can lead to some atrophy of the nasal mucosa and resulting nosebleeds. Some nasal decongestants like Afrin work only for a few days to a week at most, after which point rebound happens and after initially working the nasal congestion returns almost immediately, leading some Afrin users to repeatedly dose their noses all day long in a futile effort to unstuffy their blocked noses, this eventually can cause bleeding.

Intranasal Administration of Drugs

Snorting or intranasal use of drugs such as Cocaine often times causes atrophy of the nasal mucosa and bleeding to occur. The nasal mucosa has an excellent blood supply and as such is a good route for administration of some medications as well as street drugs such as cocaine and heroin. This affords addicts another route of getting drugs into their bloodstream other than intravenous injection.

Nasal Polyps and Tumors of the Nose

Tumors in the nose causing nosebleeds are rather uncommon, but nasal polyps on the other hand are very common. Nasal polyps are benign (not malignant) small fleshy growths inside the nose, sometimes on stalks and other times sessile or broadly attached to the underlying mucosa. Both of these may cause some nosebleeds.

Smoking and Smoke Exposure

Smoking of tobacco or marijuana both can lead to drying out of the nasal mucosa and some atrophy of it resulting in nosebleeds. Also excessive exposure to the smoke of a fireplace or other fire source can severely dry out your nasal lining and cause bleeding. Using a water pipe such as a bong moisturizes the smoke and is less irritating to the nasal and oral mucosas.

BROKEN NASAL BONE

In cases of a newly broken nose, you should attempt to gently put it back in its original position by gently holding the nose between both hands and applying firm steady pressure on one side to push it back. This can be helped by application of ice packs if it doesn't work the first time. The ice will reduce the soft tissue swelling and help reduce (put it back in its original position) the broken nasal bone.

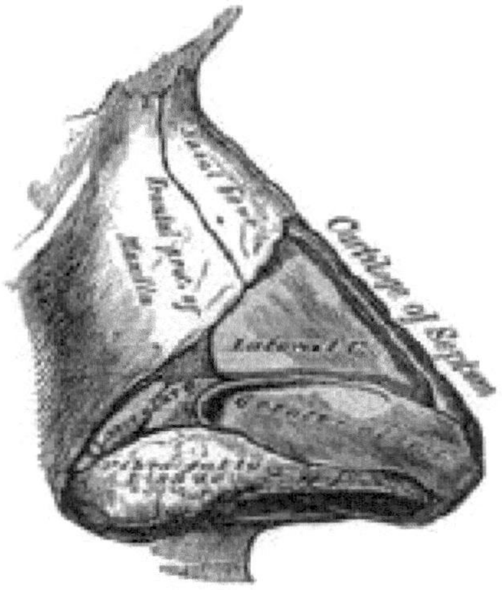

Diagram of the Nasal Bones and the Nasal Cartilage.

HOW TO TREAT A NOSEBLEED

Packing A Nosebleed

The first thing to do with a nosebleed is to take a small piece of toilet paper or paper towel or even a small piece of cloth. Insert it in the side that is bleeding, up on the inside of the bulb or tip of the nose. Do not lean back because blood will flow down the back of your throat and either make you choke and/or make you nauseous and possibly vomit. Leaning too far forward will make you bleed more, so just a little forward. Do not place your head between your legs which is just plain stupid. Breathe through your mouth. If you have any nasal spray such as Afrin, spray this in your nose. The Afrin will constrict (shrink) the blood vessels and slow down the bleeding.

Applying Direct Pressure

Also spit out any blood in your throat, swallowing it may irritate your stomachs lining and lead to nausea and vomiting. Hold the outside of your nose between your thumb and second finger (pointer) and apply gentle steady firm pressure. The direction of the pressure should be towards the center of the nose. Do this for about five minutes, if you have a watch use it. The reason I say this is that it always seems like eternity while you're waiting for a nosebleed to stop and you will think you have held it much longer than you did. After five minutes release the pressure. If it starts to bleed again then repeat the same pressure, but this time for ten minutes. You can do this for as long as twenty minutes.

Ice Packs Or Cold Compresses

An ice pack or anything cold applied to the side of the nose that is bleeding will also help. This constricts (makes them smaller) the blood vessels and slows down the rate of bleeding.

Cotton Balls Soaked In Petroleum Jelly or Neosporin

If the above methods don't work you can take some cotton balls and soak them in petroleum jelly or Neosporin and pack them inside the nostril that is bleeding. Start by packing as far in as you can reach. A forceps will help you do this. Gently push the petroleum soaked gauze to the rear of the nose. Be careful not to traumatize the nose any further.

You can use a few Q tips taped together as your forceps; this will be less traumatic than the metal of a forceps and will bend a little if it strikes an obstruction. I cannot emphasize to do this slowly and methodically and above all gently. You can easily traumatize the nose and cause more bleeding from a new source.

Epinephrine

An alternative method is to use Epinephrine from an Epipen, squirt this onto a thin strip of cotton and pack it into the nose. Epinephrine is a vasoconstrictor (Something that shrinks blood vessels such as arteries) and will slow down the bleeding. Leave this packing in for several hours before removing it.

Catheter Technique For Posterior Nasal Bleeding

The catheter technique outlined below is something that should only be attempted when there is no medical help available and you are desperate to stop a nosebleed. It is difficult to perform and could easily cause more damage if done improperly.

For a nasal bleed that is coming from deep within the nose, what is known as a posterior bleed. This is much more difficult to get under control. If you have a catheter you can try to string it thru the back of the nose into the posterior pharynx (Upper back of your throat). You can attach some petroleum soaked or epinephrine soaked gauze and take the end in the mouth and pull it so the end in the nose enters the nose and is pulled towards the far back of the nose.

NOTE: This is a very difficult and should only be attempted in extreme conditions when a posterior bleed cannot be controlled. In all other cases just try to pack the gauze into the back of the nose until the entire nose is full and see if that works to control the nosebleed.

CHAPTER TWENTY

ORAL HYGIENE, DENTAL CARE, CANKER SORES, THROAT INFECTIONS AND TONSILLITIS

INTRODUCTION

TABLE OF CONTENTS:

If you learn one thing from this book, please learn the importance of proper oral hygiene or dental care.

Many infections enter the body through the mouth and can be prevented with proper care. One thing I have always noticed in my many years of practicing medicine, I have never seen a patient with bad teeth in good health, the two just do not go together.

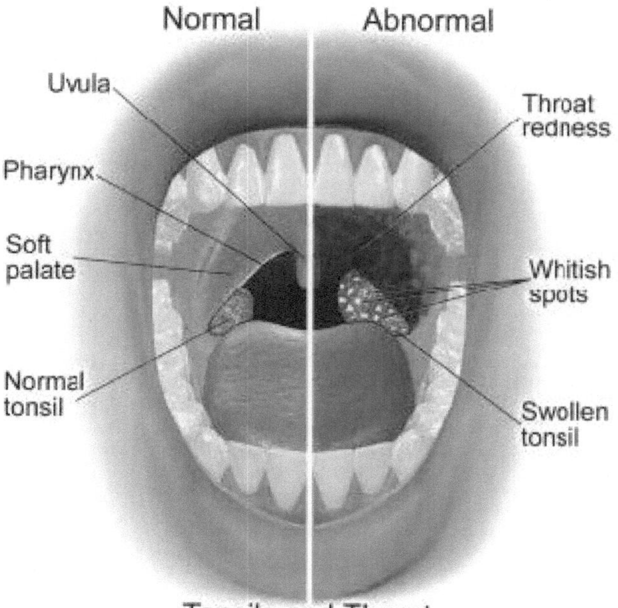

Tonsils and Throat

THE ANATOMY OF THE MOUTH AND TEETH

The human mouth is also known as the oral cavity and the buccal cavity. The mouth is divided into two parts; the vestibule, which is the area between the teeth and your cheeks, and the oral cavity proper. The tongue is attached to the floor of the mouth by the frenulum linguae. Sometimes at birth this frenulum is attached further down the tongue than the base, and the person is "tongue tied". This is usually just partially severed (cut) at that time to prevent further problems.

The roof of the mouth separates it from the nose and is known as the palate. The palate is mostly hard or solid, but in the back of the mouth it has a soft rim with a punching bag-like piece of flesh hanging down known as the uvula. The hard part of the palate is cleverly named the hard palate and the soft part the soft palate. The tonsils lie at either corner where the soft palate meets the sides of the mouth. The oral cavity and the vestibules are lined with a mucous membrane that has three pairs of salivary glands secreting saliva into the mouth to keep it moist and also to fight cavities. On the surface of the tongue lie small raised areas which are the taste buds.

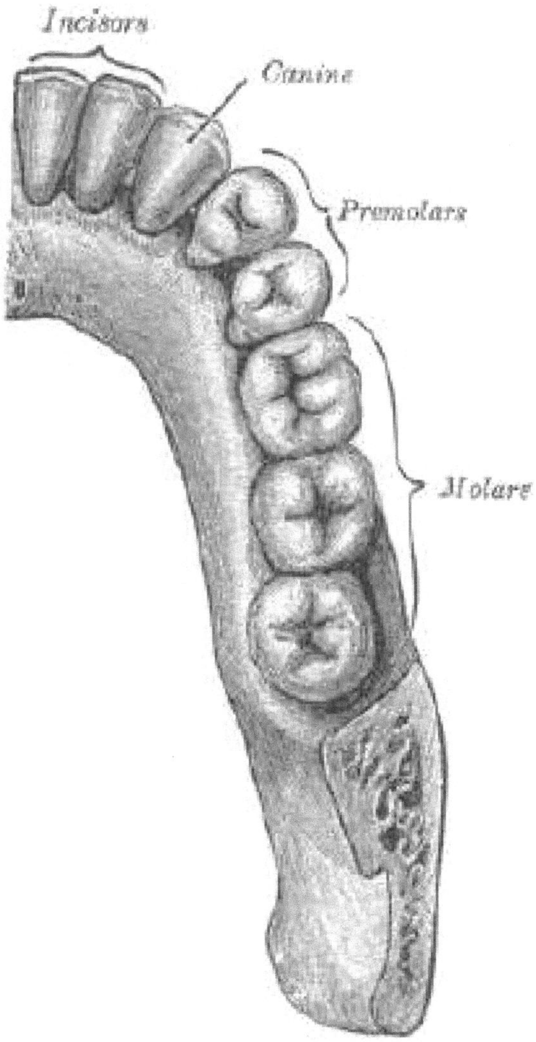

Humans, like many mammals, have two sets of teeth, their baby teeth (also known as milk or primary teeth) and their adult teeth. Baby teeth begin to develop at about six months of age, although some babies are born with a few teeth, known as neonatal teeth. The normal eruption of teeth through the babies' gums at six months is painful and is known as teething.

There are a total of twenty baby teeth and thirty-two adult teeth. The formula for adult teeth is 2, 1, 2, 3. This means two incisors, one canine, two premolars and three molars. Of course this involves only a quarter of the mouth.

The tooth is divided into two parts; the crown, which is the area that you can see above the gum line, and the root, which is below the gum line. The crown is covered with enamel and the root with covered by cementum. The enamel is the hardest substance in the body and it surrounds the dentin, and inside of that lays the pulp. Ninety-six (96) percent of the enamel is made of minerals, thus you can see the importance of having the correct minerals in your diet. Your body has no way to make teeth that have strong enamel without all the right minerals obtained from your food. The enamel is thickest on the cusp or the pointy tops of the teeth, where it comes in contact with food for cutting and grinding.

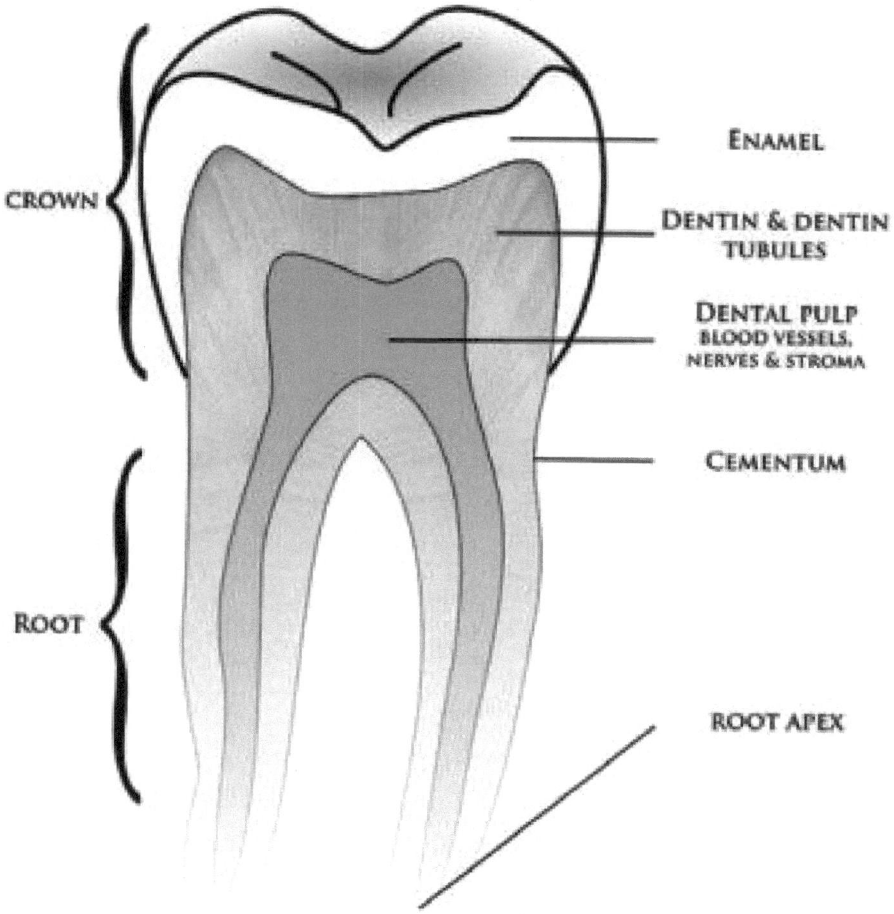

The Anatomy of a Tooth

ORAL HYGIENE

Oral hygiene is the practice of properly cleaning your mouth and teeth; this is necessary to prevent tooth decay, gum infections (gingivitis) and bad breath

Cavities develop when food gets caught in the little nooks and crannies on teeth and the spaces between teeth. Sugars in the food ferment and produce acids that erode the hard outside surface of teeth known as dental enamel by demineralization (dissolving the minerals in the hard enamel's surface). This process is made worse by sticky foods that attach themselves to the teeth and the spaces between them.

Americans currently consume about 150 pounds of sugar in various forms yearly. The only way for your body to process that sugar is by secreting insulin from your pancreas. Insulin has two roles in the body; the first is to help regulate blood sugar levels by driving sugar (blood glucose) into the body's cells. The second role concerns fat. Insulin promotes fat storage by converting those excess calories from carbohydrates such as sweets, bread, pasta, potatoes, and rice into fat for storage in your body. Insulin also protects the fat stores you currently have in your body, forcing your body to metabolize muscle for energy, making you fat and shrinking your muscles. Most people are overly concerned with their fat intake and not their carbohydrate intake and that is just wrong, fat doesn't make you fat (unless you are eating massive amounts of fat) it is your carbohydrate intake that is making you fat due to its effect on your insulin levels.

Alternative Methods of Oral Hygiene

No matter what your living situation I highly recommend good daily oral hygiene. If you have no toothbrush, even a wet piece of cloth worked vigorously over your teeth and gums will help mechanically remove most of the sugars. If you have the luxury of being able to floss, definitely do it at least once a day.

One outstanding way to clean and disinfect your mouth is by a solution of 50 percent hydrogen peroxide (the 3% mixture that is available in pharmacies and is very inexpensive). Simply mix half a glass of warm or cold water, whichever is your preference, and the other half, hydrogen peroxide. Take a mouthful and swish it around your mouth for at least a minute, gargle it, and spit it out. Be careful if you swallow some of the peroxide your hair will turn blonde....only kidding. Brush or clean your teeth after the peroxide rinse. You will see it foaming as it kills off the bacteria in your mouth.

It gives your mouth a wonderfully clean, tingling sensation. This solution works very well for oral hygiene and will prevent most cavities. It also helps to whiten your teeth by reducing dental plaque.

Dental plaque is what causes the yellow/brown discoloration of your teeth. It is actually what is known as a biofilm. A biofilm is a three dimensional dome that is grown by a colony of bacteria to protect themselves from the body's defenses. Eventually as they mature they will cause erosion of the dental enamel and cavities to develop, they also cause gum disease. Incredibly dental plaque has also been associated with cardiovascular disease, diabetes, respiratory diseases and can even lead to problems in pregnancy. Since your teeth only comprise about 20 percent of the surface of the mouth, besides brushing your teeth it is important to use a mouthwash and also to floss between your teeth.

Even rinsing your mouth out with salt water will help keep it clean. Children should be encouraged to brush or clean their teeth and mouth at the very least twice daily from a very young age. Good hygiene habits last a lifetime and will serve them well as they grow older. Don't get me wrong, brushing after every meal and before bed is preferable; when I say twice daily that is the minimum. The reason for the frequent brushing is to remove those sugars and other foods that have stuck between your teeth and in all those nooks and crannies. The longer these foods stay on your teeth the longer time they have to erode your enamel. Making a game out of brushing their teeth will help children. Tell them to tickle each tooth with their toothbrushes, also behind each tooth, try to reach back beyond the last teeth on either side and top and bottom, and brush those areas as well. That is why the hydrogen peroxide rinse is so important, it will kill off the bad bacteria that cause tooth decay and reach those areas that are so hard to reach and easily missed. The hydrogen peroxide rinse is most effective when followed by flossing; the floss will carry the peroxide between each tooth killing the bacteria that will lead to plaque development and all its associated problems.

How To Make A Toothbrush

You can also make your own toothbrush by taking a small stick and chewing one end until it is frayed. Then wet it and use it to scrub your teeth. A small, sharp stick can also be used as a toothpick to clean between your teeth. Make sure it is live green wood, otherwise it will just fall apart in your mouth and be useless. Historically this was a common method used for tooth care and these were referred to as chew sticks.

How To Make Toothpaste

An alternative method is to apply toothpaste to your finger and rub it vigorously around your mouth and over your teeth, reaching the back side of your teeth as well as the front and going to the far molars on either side to remove any food particles.

Another alternative is to use sodium bicarbonate, or baking soda. You can mix some baking soda with a small amount of water and use that to brush your teeth.

I think the most potent toothpaste comes from mixing hydrogen peroxide and baking soda. This combination kills many of the bacteria that cause dental problems as well as alkalinizing your mouth helping to neutralize the acids bacteria use to damage your enamel and start cavities.

In a glass, mix:

2 tablespoons of baking soda

1 tablespoon of hydrogen peroxide

Add some flavoring like one-half teaspoon of mint extract.

(Taken from a wonderful little book called Baking Soda, by Vicki Lansky)

Another alternative method of making your own toothpaste is by using all natural ingredients such as:

Coconut oil, bentonite clay, sea salt, and peppermint oil.

Mix four tablespoons of coconut oil and bentonite clay with half a teaspoon of real sea salt in a small bowl with several tablespoons of filtered water. Use your own personal preference for the thickness of the mix by adjusting the amount of water you add. Mix these briskly with a spoon until they are creamy in consistency. Now add some peppermint oil, about ten or fifteen drops. Store this in an airtight container so it does not dry out.A pea sized amount will work to brush your teeth. The coconut oil has both antibacterial and antifungal properties and the sea salt acts as a natural abrasive.

This formula came from a very insightful website known as "Thank Your Body".

If you absolutely cannot brush your teeth at least vigorously rinse out your mouth with water, gargle, and spit it out. This will remove some of the sugars and food particles and will provide a minimal level of protection.

DENTAL CAVITIES

The medical term for dental cavities is caries. Caries are very common problems and will invariable rear their ugly heads from time to time. Unless you are in a wilderness area far from a dentist there is no substitute for a good dentist. I would urge you to seek dental attention as soon as this develops because it will be a very long time before it goes away on its own, and by the time that happens your tooth down to its roots and nerves have been destroyed. Your teeth should be cared for and preserved intact as much as possible, their replacements are never as good as the originals.

TOOTHACHES

Usually the first indication of a cavity will be a toothache. As most people are well aware, toothaches can be extremely painful. They must be dealt with immediately because they are not going to go away or improve on their own. The origin of the pain felt in the tooth can either be from the decay of the tooth itself or trauma to the mouth, the fracturing (breaking of a tooth) or inflammation and or infection of the gums of the mouth (gingivitis) or the formation of an abscess.

An abscess is a collection of pus and to be treated needs to be drained. This can be done by identifying the area around the tooth that has the abscess and then lancing it with a properly sterilized sharp needle or even a very small knife or scalpel. This will relieve the pressure in the abscess and drain the pus out of it and allow healing to take place. After any dental procedure such as this you should thoroughly rinse out your mouth with a 50 percent solution of hydrogen peroxide and water to help clean the area. For those of you who are math-challenged, a 50 percent solution means half a glass of hydrogen peroxide (3%) and half a glass of water. You can quickly sterilize a needle or small knife by soaking it in hydrogen peroxide for a minute or so.

Treatment of Toothaches

You can take analgesics like Aleve, Tylenol, or ibuprofen for some pain relief. Other than the Tylenol, these medications should be taken with food to avoid any GI upset.

You can also use oil of cloves (also known as eugenol). Make sure not to touch your tongue with the eugenol, it will cause burning. There is also an over-the-counter antiseptic containing benzocaine (which is an anesthetic). You can find it in various products such as Anbesol, Cepacol, Red Cross toothache medicine, Dents toothache drops, Orajel, and Hurricaine.

All of these products should be applied carefully to the tooth involved; you might want to apply it with a Q-tip.

Avoid all hot and cold beverages and food, which will only increase the pain. The best treatment for a toothache is extraction of the tooth. In extreme cases you will need to do this to provide any relief. It has been said that about 90 percent of all dental problems can be treated by extracting the tooth. This is not an easy procedure and a dental extractor is the best instrument to do this, but any pliers that can give you some leverage can be used. Try to give any pain medications that you have to the patient before and after.

NOTE: I would strongly advise you never to attempt to extract a tooth, only do so if you are in a survival situation and dentists are absolutely not available. Only attempt an extraction if all other options have failed. Be aware that teeth are held in place by small ligaments around the tooth that will need to be cut away to free the tooth. This will need to be done on all four sides of the tooth. In a severe situation this can be done with a small flat head screw driver, prying each ligament away from the root of the tooth. This will produce a lot of bleeding.

In children, the tooth can be rocked back and forth and loosened. This is not usually the case in adults. Be aware of not damaging adjacent teeth, so any prying motion should be done towards the front of the mouth or towards the cheeks and not towards the tongue or center of the mouth. The tooth should be grabbed as close to the gum line as possible. Remember, the front teeth have one root and the others have two roots. You will probably need to rock back and forth to loosen the tooth before attempting its extraction. You should try to extract the tooth in one swift motion without breaking it off, if possible. You should be wearing gloves and have the person rinse their mouth out before and after with a 50 percent solution of hydrogen peroxide and water.

Alternative Treatments For Toothaches

Cloves can be used whole to treat a toothache. Cloves are the aromatic flower buds of the clove tree, which is part of the myrtle family. Squeeze the cloves against your good teeth to release the oil and soften them up and then press the whole, softened clove against your bad tooth and keep it there for a half an hour.

Peppermint tea can also be used. Peppermint tea is both numbing and soothing and will ease the pain of a toothache. Make a cup of tea using one teaspoon of dried peppermint leaves. Allow it to steep until cool and then swish it around your mouth to ease your toothache.

Red cayenne pepper and some powdered ginger root. These two can be mixed in equal parts (fifty/fifty) in a small bowl and add water until you get the right paste-like consistency. Once you have it mixed into a paste, place a cotton ball in it and soak it and then apply it directly to the tooth that hurts. Be careful, the cayenne pepper might burn your gums. If this happens the only thing that will neutralize the burning sensation is milk. These two ingredients can also be used separately.

Tincture of myrrh is used to treat toothaches as well as helping with inflammation and also being antibacterial. Simmer one teaspoon of tincture of myrrh in two cups of water for a half an hour, let it cool then strain it. Take one teaspoon of this mix with a half a cup of water and swish it around your mouth, especially on the painful tooth. Repeat as necessary.

CANKER SORES

Sores in the mouth are called apthous ulcers and apthous stomatitis, or are more commonly known as canker sores. These are usually shallow ulcers (erosions of the mucosa or lining of the mouth) with a grey or white/grey base to them. They are very painful and are quite common. They may occur on the mouth, lips, or tongue. They are usually preceded by stinging, burning, or pain in the area before the actual ulcer appears.

Zinc

In my internal medicine practice I have treated these successfully for over twenty-five years without fail with the use of zinc lozenges. Health food stores and pharmacies carry these; they are inexpensive and quite useful. I instruct patients to hold the lozenge in their mouth and let it dissolve directly over the canker sore. You should do this four or five times daily until it heals. Medical books will list the cause of these as various infections, low levels of B12, folic acid, or iron, or simply as unknown, but I beg to differ. I am quite sure these lesions are caused by a zinc deficiency.

Zinc is known to help heal all wounds and is routinely administered in hospitals after surgery for this purpose. I have also noted that high sugar intake in the diet does contribute to the flare-up of these ulcers, possibly due to the zinc content of insulin, further lowering the body's zinc levels. Vitamin B complex (which contains B12 and folic acid as well as all the other B vitamins) will also help the healing of these oral ulcers.

Alternative Treatments For Apthous Ulcers Or Canker Sores

1. DGL: an extract of licorice with the glycyrrhizin removed from it due to its harmful side effects. Take about 200 mg of DGL powder mixed in a glass of water and gargle and rinse the mouth with it four times a day until the mouth heals.
2. Baking soda (sodium bicarbonate) and warm water: dissolve one teaspoon of baking soda in a half cup of warm water and rinse your mouth with it several times a day until healed.

3. Liquid Benadryl (diphenhydramine) and either Maalox, Mylanta, or Pepto Bismol: mix equal amounts of both and rinse your mouth with these and spit out. Do this several times a day until healed.
4. Hydrogen peroxide and water: mix a small glass with half the glass filled with 3% hydrogen peroxide (the usual percentage that is sold in pharmacies) with half a glass of water, rinse out your mouth four times a day until healed.
5. Milk of magnesia: soak a Q-tip in milk of magnesia and apply it directly to the canker sore several times a day until healed.

SORE THROATS, THROAT INFECTIONS AND TONSILLITIS

Sore throats are usually caused by either bacterial or viral infections. They can also be caused by dry air (and mouth breathing) and allergies can cause a scratchy throat. When the tonsils are infected and enlarged, this is tonsillitis. Most sore throats are relatively harmless and are self-limited (they go away by themselves).

Most sore throats are viral infections (colds and flu, for example) and resolve after a week, when the body has time to build up the right antibodies to fight these infections. Antibiotics do not work against viral infections, only bacterial infections. These viral infections may have a fever or not and many times are accompanied by cough, runny nose, headaches, and muscle aches. Bacterial infections are most commonly caused by streptococcal bacteria and are highly contagious and can be very dangerous. If left untreated, these may progress to rheumatic fever and kidney infections known as glomerulonephritis.

The symptoms of bacterial throat infections like strep throat are much more severe than viral throat infections. In cases of strep throat there will be white patches on the throat or tonsils (the tonsils look like pink-/red-colored balls on either side of the back of your throat.

The size varies depending on the enlargement and may even be large enough to obstruct swallowing.). It will be painful to swallow and the lymph nodes (glands) in the patient's neck will be enlarged. You can feel the lymph nodes by running your fingers under their jaw and along both sides of their neck starting at the angle of their jaw and moving downward. They will feel like small balls under the skin, frequently in a chain. With strep throat there is usually fever greater than 101 F and often the patient will have chills. In general they will be very sick and usually incapacitated and usually have severe myalgia's (muscle aches and pains). Frequently patients will describe how they feel with strep throat as, "Doc, I feel like I have been hit by a bus". Strep throat symptoms are not usually mild, although every clinician has been fooled at one time or another by a case of strep throat that has just a few symptoms that is why they call it the "Practice of Medicine".

Once again in the case of a severe sore throat, I would strongly advise you to go to a physician and get it cultured for strep asap. Strep throat is a nasty infection and as I mentioned it can easily spread and damage your heart and kidneys. It will require antibiotics for a ten day course followed by a repeat throat culture to insure its eradication.

Treatment of Throat Infections

With all throat infections, whether viral or bacterial, I like to use a fifty/ fifty mix of hydrogen peroxide and water. Either with cold or hot water (it makes no difference in the treatment, but rather is only a personal preference), mix with half a glass of hydrogen peroxide. Swish this around your mouth and gargle it deeply, leaving it in your throat for as long as you can and then spit it out. It will produce foam as it kills off the germs in your throat. Do this four times a day until the infection subsides. As you will see in this book simple treatments like hydrogen peroxide are very useful and also very effective. For your natural medicine chest you should keep a large supply of this in its concentrated form and learn to dilute it properly to its 3% strength. I describe how to do this later under the section on hydrogen peroxide.

With any throat infection you want to prevent drying of the mucosa lining your mouth and throat. If it dries it will become more sensitive and sore and only worsen your symptoms.

Your saliva also contains enzymes and antibodies that will help the infection. Thus avoid caffeine and alcohol both of which will dehydrate you further. Honey mixed with warm tea and lemon juice also helps soothe a sore throat. Drink this mix up to four times a day to soothe your throat.

Honey is another item that has endless uses medically as well as nutritionally, and should keep a nice supply of it. It should also be one of your primary sources of sugar for sweetening foods and drinks. If you are so inclined I would recommend bee keeping as a hobby. Bees are essential for pollination of any crops you grow and as a bonus give you honey and other products

Gargling with a mix of salt and warm water will also help your sore throat. Mix a half teaspoon of salt in a glass of warm water and gargle this up to four times a day. Avoid smoking and excessive talking. Talking can help avoid any irritation of your larynx or voice box. A throat infection can spread to your larynx and lead to laryngitis; in this case the person will develop hoarseness.

Boosting Your Immunity to Treat a Throat Infection

As with all infections, treatment should be looked at in two ways, offensive and defensive. Most of the above treatments are offensive, that is, attacking the infection. I like to treat infections both offensively and also defensively. Defensive treatment involves supporting the body's immune system to aid it in fighting these microbial invaders. There are several ways to do this. Rest is very helpful in treating any infection, leaving your body's strength to fight the infection. A good night's sleep often is enough to help your body fight off any infection and you awaken feeling rejuvenated and back to your old self. Also, adequate hydration is important, as mentioned above.

A third way is to support your body's immune system by supporting what is known as the antioxidant cascade. Dr. Les Packer discovered this fascinating system that the body utilizes. It essentially has two branches, a fat soluble and a water soluble branch. At the head of these two branches is a unique substance known as alpha lipoic acid (or ALA). ALA is unique due to it being both fat and water soluble. This speaks to its importance in the body. It is able to cross all the internal barriers of the body, from cell walls to the blood-brain barrier.

Here is how it works: ALA helps regenerate on the fat soluble side vitamin E and Coenzyme Q10 (which also help regenerate each other). On the water soluble side ALA helps regenerate vitamin C and glutathione (which also regenerate each other).

That is the antioxidant cascade starting from the top and flowing down both branches and supercharging the body's immune system. What you need to take is ALA, Vitamins E and C, and CoQ10. You cannot take glutathione because it is almost immediately metabolized by the liver and unavailable. However, if you take the other four it will boost your immunity and shorten the length of any infection.

Another substance that greatly enhances your immunity is vitamin D. Vitamin D, as we are learning, is much more than a vitamin, and acts more like a hormone in the human body. Vitamin D works very well to help boost your immune system; in fact, taking vitamin D is eight times more effective in flu prevention than the flu vaccine itself! There is even a theory that flu, which typically strikes in the winter when our vitamin D levels are the lowest due to lack of sunshine, is actually due to this drop in vitamin D making us vulnerable to the flu. There was an interesting study of this done inadvertently in a prison. There were two large buildings in the facility, each of which had its own physician. In the one building the physician was a big believer in the immune-enhancing qualities of vitamin D and gave it to all the inmates; the other did not. When a flu outbreak hit in midwinter, the building where prisoners were given vitamin D had zero cases of the flu (only among the guards who did not get the vitamin D), the other building had an epidemic of flu. Now mind you, there was communication between the two buildings by sick guards, etc., but no transmission of the flu to those prisoners protected by vitamin D. Remember, vitamin D, along with all other vitamins except B and C, is fat soluble and needs to be taken with food to absorb it properly, otherwise it will pass right through your body unabsorbed and wasted.

Another recently discovered potent antioxidant is Astaxanthin. Astaxanthin has been studied and found to be 6,000 times more powerful than vitamin C. This is measured by using an ORAC scale. ORAC stands for Oxygen Radical Absorbance Capacity, which is a method for measuring antioxidant capacities of biological samples. The ORAC scale has been controversial at times since it measures the antioxidant capacity of a substance "in vitro", which in Latin literally means in glass, i.e. a beaker or test tube, as opposed to "in vivo", which means in a live subject. It is exceedingly difficult to measure ORAC in vivo and thus we realistically settle for in vitro results. A dose of 2 or 4 mg of Astaxanthin daily, with a fatty meal since it too is fat soluble, will boost your immunity and help ward off infections.

CHAPTER TWENTY-ONE

SKIN PROBLEMS

INTRODUCTION

TABLE OF CONTENTS:

ABSCESS, BOILS, INFECTED WOUNDS, SKIN INFECTIONS, AND FUNGAL INFECTIONS LIKE JOCK ITCH, ATHLETE'S FOOT, AND RINGWORM

The first thing you must learn is what is causing a skin reaction. Any change in the skin invariably has inflammation involved. When there is inflammation you will find the skin area you are examining to have several features in common. The signs of inflammation are redness, pain, heat, swelling, and loss of function.

ABSCESS

Sometimes you luck out and the skin you are examining has an obvious cause. Things like thorns or splinters of wound with a clear entrance track and a collection of pus swelling the area and a ring of red inflammation around that. Other times you may see what looks like a large "white head" with a bulging around and below it. This is an abscess. What basically has happened is the thorn entered the skin with a nice load of infectious microbes hitchhiking on its surface. These microbes are rejoicing they have landed in the Promised Land. All around them is healthy tissue soaked in blood and they naturally feast. The result is a short time later these germs have launched a major invasion of that area. Your body then rushes in all its troops: tissue macrophages and large numbers of neutrophils and other white cells. The healthy cells on the perimeter pitch in and all produce large shields, that together interlock and form a hopefully impenetrable wall. Now your body is hoping to starve out the invaders. It has successfully, for the moment, sealed off the invaders in a tomb of their own. The area is a wasteland of cellular debris and large numbers of dead white cell defenders and live and dead bacteria...a pus collection. From the outside it appears to be a painful swollen mound or a really large white head, with a volcano of swelling around it. It is walled off from healthy tissues but also from any other defenders the body wanted to throw at it.

How To Drain An Abscess

In my experience the best way to heal these is to drain them. Draining them clears out all the pus and debris and lots of the bacteria from within.

Removing the dome and draining out the pustular material lowers the pressure within the wound and allows your white blood cells (your offensive line) access to the infection. After I clean them out I flush abscesses with hydrogen peroxide. This effectively is a wave of sudden death for the remaining bacterial invaders. It is your best way of cleaning a wound. It doesn't even usually sting. Alcohol stings severely, not peroxide. It is a large quantity of the same stuff the cells of your body release to kill invaders they have ingested. We are just sending in a wave of it.

You can also use Betadine or iodine in its many forms to clean a wound area; just like hydrogen peroxide, iodine solutions do not burn. I clean the surrounding area as well. Now you are doing several things. Many of the germs that have caused the infection are anaerobic (live without oxygen) These do wonderfully in dead and dying tissue that is very low in oxygen. They now find themselves engulfed in an entirely new aerobic (oxygen-containing) world that is toxic to them. You have also ruptured the outer wall that was made by your body to keep the invasion out. This destruction of the abscess capsule during your draining of it, has allowed your body to once again charge in with its various white blood cells and finish off whatever germs have survived.

Now is the time to clean out the entire wound area. If you have ice you can apply a piece of ice directly to the area until it is numb. Take a sterilized instrument (you don't want to introduce a new infection into the wound) and scrape out the area. Your next step is to take a Q-tip and dip it into some honey and apply it into the former abscess. This will seal it off from the outside, and honey is toxic to bacteria, fungi, and viruses. The honey will also provide vital healing enzymes from the bee's digestion. These enzymes will help keep the area clear of infection. Honey also produces hydrogen peroxide when exposed to water. This too will help keep it infection free. Take a small piece of gauze or any thin clean cloth you can find. Soak the underside with a small amount of honey and apply it to the surface of the abscess. It is best to overlap the abscess and cover the rest of the red skin area with the gauze. Now take a clean, dry piece of dressing and cover the outside with that. The honey is very osmotic by nature. It will draw water into the area from the clean tissue surrounding it.

This will also draw in cells from your immune system that will promote healing. Honey also works wonderfully to keep a wound area moist. Periodically you will notice that the dressing is soaked and the dry outer layer is now wet. That is the time to change your wound dressing and reapply it the same way. Eventually the wound will heal in from its edges. The healthy tissue will send in an army of its construction workers to build new healthy tissue identical to previous tissue.

Platelets from the blood will combine with fibrin and seal off any bleeding points. Then fibroblasts go to work. During this process they will produce a scaffolding of collagen and other proteins. Vitamin C is critical for collagen production as well as being a strong antioxidant, thereby helping the infection as well, hence its importance in helping wounds heal properly. This process produces granulation tissue. Over the years I have seen it mistaken by patients and even nurses to be pus of an infection. Granulation tissue looks more like a very thin layer of custard pudding. It is uniform and does not smell foul. Pus appears more cellular…more lumpy so to speak and even runny, more liquidly. The granulation tissue is good; leave it alone. It is the scaffolding your body is going to use to now send in the new cells and form your new tissue. It is the matrix on which the body builds its new tissues. Its technical name is the extracellular matrix.

Your body might develop its own leather-like dome or scab on the wound. Do not pick any scabs off…doing so will only prolong healing and promote scarring. Let a scab fall of naturally. When it is getting ready to fall off the edges will curl up and it will slowly break off any connections it has with the new skin. This is done beautifully from the edges towards its center. Leave it alone.

In addition to honey and iodine products you can use essential oils such as tea tree oil or lavender oil. You can also use a paste made from Epsom salt and a little water. You can pack the wound or abscess base with this paste. It will disinfect the wound and will also draw out fluid necessitating changing the bandage regularly as well. If you have nothing else then use some alcohol on the area. Ethanol (the alcohol that is in drinks, a name I will never forget because of my high school gym teachers favorite phrase…"Ethel is not a lady.") Be advised this will burn like hell, but it will disinfect wounds. The stronger the alcohol content, the more potent. Do not waste that bottle of Grey Goose whatever you do!

If there is a splinter or any other foreign object …bullet, shrapnel, etc.it needs to be removed as soon as possible, if possible. For splinters if you can see them usually you will find the way they entered. That end of the tunnel they have made will usually be open. Take them out the same way they came in. It will be much less traumatic and painful. If there is no opening, make one. Use a sterilized pin or sewing needle or knife. If there is a large abscess, once you take the dome off and have squeezed it out is the time to also scrape any pus and other necrotic (dead) material from the abscess. It is not doing any good and a lot of harm left in there. Now take your finger and try to get it under the far tip of the splinter and gently apply pressure in the direction of the skin's opening.

It may come right out as has happened for me many times. Or if a small piece of it protrudes, try to grab it with a sterile pair of tweezers. You can then pull it out. Frequently the splinters will break off. If that happens just repeat the process until you get it all. After it is out and you should re-cleanse the base of the wound then you can apply your honey, etc. Other times you may have to make a small incision over the length of a splinter and remove it that way.

BOILS AND CARBUNCLES

Boils are infected hair cells. Surrounding the hair cell's base, a large area forms, similar to an abscess. If there is a cluster of infected hair cells together, this is a carbuncle. These need to be treated in the same way as an abscess. Sometimes they have not yet come to a head and you should then cover them with a dressing soaked in warm salt water. The hotter the better, without burning your good skin. This should be changed several times daily. Eventually it will soften up and you can then gently squeeze it and drain out its pustular material. These should be squeezed until the pus is out and you are getting out a runny mixture of blood-tinged fluid. Then cleanse the area and apply a dressing as described in the section on abscesses above.

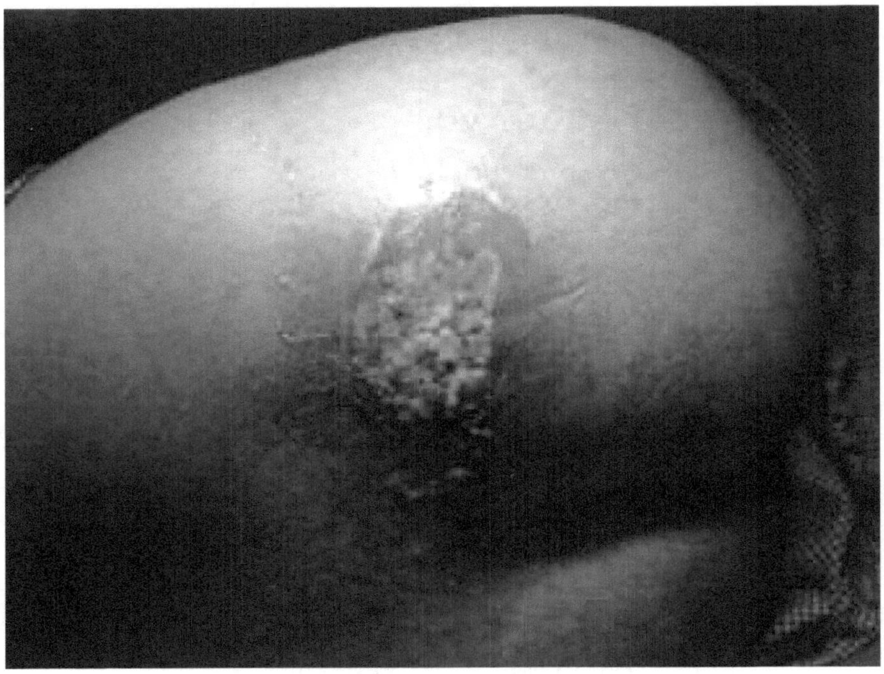

Photo of a patient with a large carbuncle on the buttocks

SKIN INFECTIONS/CELLULITIS

Frequently there will be redness and tenderness to an area around a wound or sometimes an area of skin will be involved by itself. This skin inflammation/infection is called cellulitis. It is an expanding area of warmth, tender and red. Cellulitis is frequently found on the limbs, feet, and spreading from an abscess or boil. Cellulitis starts on the skin's surface and may spread internally to local lymph nodes and eventually may enter the bloodstream at which point infections of this type are known as sepsis (blood poisoning); it can also infect the nearby bones causing what is known as osteomyelitis. This is best treated with antibiotics to prevent its spread to deeper tissues.

Do not get intimidated by these medical terms, they almost all have either Greek or Latin origins. Take osteomyelitis for example, osteon is Greek for bone and myelo means marrow, the suffix -itis means infection or inflammation, so taken all together you have an infection of the bone and its marrow. Once you learn and understand science, it is a beautiful thing!

As you have just read, treating this without antibiotics will be more difficult than draining an abscess. These infections are dangerous and often are overlooked by patients until they are in a critical stage. As with most things, early treatment has much better outcomes. Treating a cellulitis of the leg early may save that leg, letting it fester could cost that person either his limb or his life, especially in patients whose immunity is compromised such as diabetics, HIV positive patients, cancer patients or anyone who is critically ill and thus debilitated (weakened).

The first thing you can do is to clean the surface of the area involved as well as the surrounding area. Many times there is an area of skin breakdown at the point of entry of the bacteria causing the cellulitis. Clean the area with hydrogen peroxide if available, several times a day. If not, then use soap and water, really lathering up the involved area. Also avoid any other abrasions or damage to the skin if possible. See the Essential Oil (Aromatherapy) section for essential oils that can be used. Tincture of iodine works wonderfully for covering any area involved, or Betadine or poviodine would work wonderfully. You can make your own antiseptic mix by mixing some Lugol's solution with water and applying that to the area. Do not use straight potassium iodide (KI); it is too strong. You can mix some KI with a carrier oil and utilize this to attack the infection. This will allow the KI to penetrate the epidermis or outer layer of skin and reach the dermal layers and below, through which the infection is spreading. The KI is frequently irritating to the skin without dissolving it in a carrier oil.

The carrier oil is so named because it "carries" whatever is dissolved in it across the skin, which otherwise is a formidable barrier. This type of therapy is called transdermal, which means across the skin. If you utilize essential oils and your carrier oil, you get the double whammy of the antiseptic effect of the oils themselves coupled with the killing power of iodine, a very potent combination. This illustrates the importance of you building the complete medicine chest of items I have suggested. In this way you will have several treatment options.

FUNGAL SKIN INFECTIONS: JOCK ITCH, ATHLETE'S FOOT, AND RINGWORM

Fungal infections of the skin include many of your old favorites...jock itch, athlete's foot, and ringworm, among others. They are all moderately to severely itchy, and very annoying. Remember, a mushroom is a fruit of a fungus. Where do mushrooms grow? Where it is wet and dark, and the warmer the better. It is the same with these infections. If you are sweating a lot and your feet or groin or skin folds are soaked with perspiration, this is the perfect growth medium for a fungus. Most of the time these areas are "where the sun doesn't shine" Hence, you develop athlete's foot and jock itch and fungal infections in your skin folds. They are also very contagious, as especially evidenced by the spread of athlete's foot from feet exposed in infected locker-room showers.

Athlete's Foot

Fungal infections can frequently be identified by a red spreading edge, where the edge is a deeper red color then the interior areas of the infection, many times it is slightly raised as well. In the case of athlete's foot it is most often found between the toes, but may be anywhere on the foot's surface. The medical name for athlete's foot is Tinea Pedis. When you spread the toes the skin will appear white and/or macerated (chewed up looking), the foot may appear red with cracking and splitting of the skin. The skin oftentimes appears to be dry and is scaling (peeling off in spots) and is oftentimes mild to severely itching. On occasion small blisters will appear, especially on the soles of the feet, but they could be anywhere on the foot; they are filled with fluid and many times are painful.

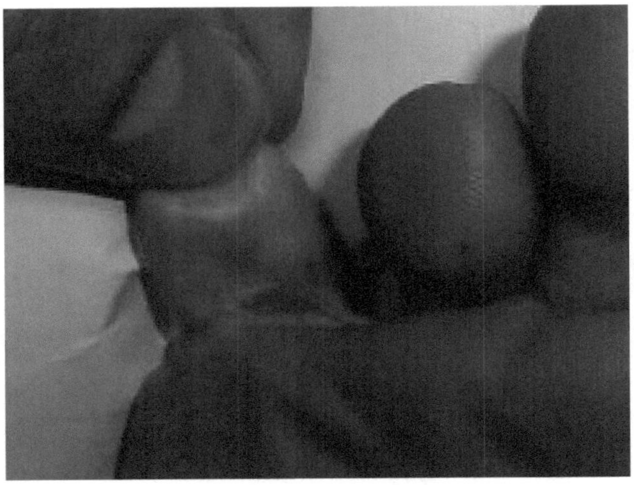

Photo of patient with a severe athlete's foot infection

Tinea Pedis was originally only found in parts of Southeast Asia, Africa, and Australia. After colonization of these areas by humans, the dermatophyte that causes athlete's foot was picked up by colonial troops and brought back between their toes and on their feet to Europe. The first case of athlete's foot was not reported in the United States until the 1920s in Birmingham, Alabama. It was thought to spread rapidly in Europe and the United States from the practice of wearing occlusive footwear (closed shoes), which makes the feet sweat and creates the perfect environment that is warm and wet for the dermatophyte to flourish.

Jock Itch

Jock itch is caused by a fungus called Tinea, hence its other name Tinea Cruris. Like all fungal infections it thrives in a warm, wet environment. Athletes frequently suffer with this due to their profuse sweating, but even nonathletes often get these infections. Jock itch occurs on the inner thighs, the inguinal area (which is the skin folds where your thigh meets your abdomen), scrotum, and buttocks. Jock itch often manifests as chafed, burning, red skin that is also very itchy. You can easily see the skin discoloration and its red spreading, slightly raised edges. Many times it is evident in the perianal area (the area surrounding the anus), causing intense anal itching.

Ringworm

The medical term for ringworm is Tinea Corporis. It has nothing at all to do with any worms, and gets its common name from its circular appearance which resembles a small worm.

Like all fungal infections it is contagious, usually by direct contact.

Ringworm can infect you anywhere on your body, hence the Latin name Corporis, which means body. You can also get ringworm infections from vectors such as clothes, pets, and even exposed furniture besides direct contact with someone's infected skin.

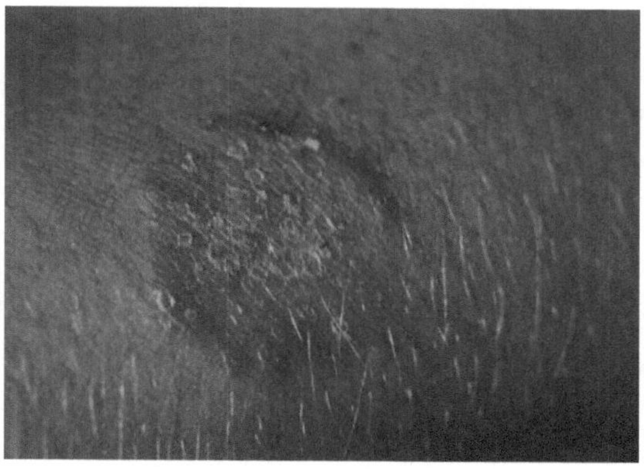

Photo of typical lesion of Ringworm

The skin will have a reddened (not always), flat, circular area of skin. Many times these ringworm lesions are spread out, far apart on different areas of the body, other times they may be in a cluster even with overlapping margins, making a diagnosis more difficult.

Candida Yeast Infections

Candida as a cause of yeast infections most often occur in diabetic, obese patients and patients just recently treated with antibiotics. Antibiotics kill the good bacteria that colonize your body and with their absence there occurs an overgrowth of yeast. The good news is that they are not contagious on contact. They often involve axillary areas (armpits), the groin, and other areas prone to sweating. If serious enough they may cause some moderate blistering of the skin. They oftentimes cause some oozing of clear fluid from the infected areas as well as some burning sensations.

Thrush and Vaginal Yeast Infections

Candida can be both internal and external. Internally it may be systemic (through large areas of your body) or just involve your throat in what is known as thrush, or a vaginal yeast infection. Thrush is easily identified by a careful examination of the tongue, cheeks, mouth, and the back of the throat or oral pharynx area; it will appear as white streaks or patches.

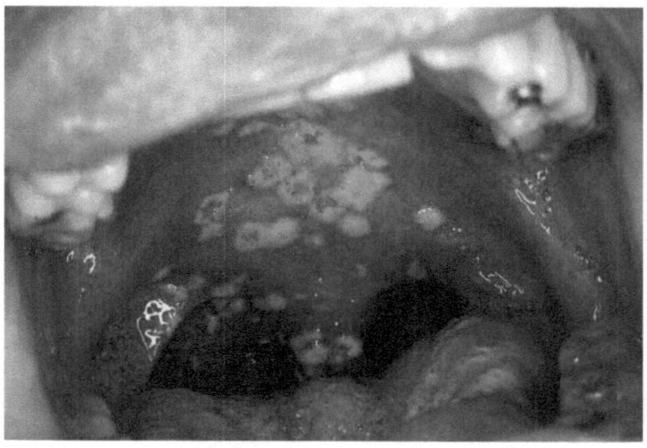

Photo of typical infection with thrush on a patient's palate, tongue, and uvula

Vaginal yeast infections will have a "cheesy" discharge of white or yellow material. Most women who have been on antibiotics for urinary tract infections in the past have experienced vaginal yeast infections. It is often accompanied by a burning sensation and what is often described as a "raw" sensation.

TREATMENT OF ALL TYPES OF FUNGAL AND YEAST INFECTIONS

Topical antifungal creams such as Lamisil, Mycelex, Lotrimin, Lotrisone and Monistat-Derm all work well to eradicate these fungal infections. In this entire book I am working on the assumption that you either do not have any of the above medications or prefer natural/alternative treatments.

The best course of treatment for all fungal infections is to exploit their weak points against them. In the case of fungal infections, their weakness is their pH. Fungal and yeast infections thrive in an acidic environment; they also make their environment more acidic by actually secreting organic acids to dissolve substances around them to eat. This love of acidity makes them extremely susceptible to changes in pH such as applying alkaline or strong bases to them. Utilizing this vulnerability to our advantage works wonderfully to eradicate these infections. The alkaline pH substances I most often use are either baking soda or my personal favorite, Borax laundry detergent.

Borax is used by making a solution of a cup of Borax in a bucket of water and soaking your feet in it to eradicate athlete's foot. An alternative method is to wet the area you want to treat with water and then mix some borax with water, making it into a paste-like consistency and rubbing it into your feet, groin, armpits, or skin. The patient will notice almost immediate relief from any itching or burning or chafed sensations. Keep repeating this until the infection is healed.

For vaginal yeast infections you can make a solution of Borax and water and flush out the patient's vagina with this twice a day until healed.

A teaspoon of Borax mixed into a liter of water will make a good strength douche. An alternative method is to fill some gelatin capsules with Borax and insert them vaginally at bedtime nightly for one to two weeks, you can end it sooner if it heals faster.

To treat systemic candidia infections you can make the following concentrate of Borax and water; you should follow these instructions carefully to insure that you make the proper mix: Mix one and a quarter teaspoons of Borax in a liter of water (unchlorinated) and mix this well and then drink it over the course of an entire day (spacing it out). Drink this mix for five days a week for an entire month and this should eradicate any candida; the boron content will also help any arthritic complaints you might be suffering with.

When treating systemic yeast infections one of the cornerstones of any successful treatments is to use a good, broad-mix probiotic formula. My personal favorite is VSL #3, but any probiotic will help by colonizing the areas where the candida has taken over. Remember to take any probiotic mix with food since they are alive and will need to eat as well.

Topically, baking soda can be used in the same fashion as Borax. Take a couple of tablespoons of baking soda and add water to it until you have the consistency you want and then apply it to the affected area several times a day until healed.

Another topical treatment for fungal infections of the feet and toenails is to make a mix of bleach and hot water. Mix one cup of bleach in ten cups of hot water, immerse your infected feet into this solution for five minutes or so daily. Remove the foot and towel it dry. Repeat this on a daily basis for one to two months and it should eradicate any toenail fungus. Remember, it takes twelve to eighteen months for the infected toenail to grow a new nail, so be patient; you don't have to treat it that long, the initial treatment should last the entire time.

Tea tree oil is also antifungal and applying it undiluted directly to the infected area on the feet daily until the infection clears will work well. Tea tree oil also comes as tea tree oil soap and this can also be used to treat both athlete's foot and fungal toenail infections.

Oregano oil also is antifungal and can be used topically to treat athlete's foot. A foot bath can also be made by adding some of the following oils to some warm water and immersing the patient's foot in this solution.

Any of the following essential oils can be used for this treatment such as tea tree oil, eucalyptus oil, geranium oil, patchouli oil, myrrh oil, and lavender oil, all of which have antifungal properties. Garlic oil is also known to have antifungal properties and will eradicate fungal infections, but you might not smell very good!

Some alternative practitioners have used direct applications of yogurt to athlete's foot and jock itch. Apply this yogurt daily until healed. The yogurt must contain "live cultures", which almost all of them do.

CHAPTER **TWENTY-TWO**

BITES: ANIMAL, HUMAN, INSECT, SNAKE, AND SCORPION

INTRODUCTION

TABLE OF CONTENTS:

Any of us who spend time outdoors either gardening, hunting, fishing, hiking or foraging for plants will expose themselves to bites of many different types. These will primarily be from insects such as ticks, fleas, spiders, mosquitoes, wasps, bees, and others. Animal bites of all types both domestic and wild do happen as well.

All of these bites have the potential to develop into very serious infections and in some cases can be fatal (think rabies). One thing you can do right now is to make sure every one of your family members is properly immunized with a tetanus vaccine. No matter what your thoughts are about vaccines, tetanus is one that is indispensable. A tetanus vaccine is given every ten years with a booster every ten years until you are sixty-five years old. Now is the time to get your tetanus vaccine; do not wait.

Why do you need a tetanus vaccine? The bacteria that causes tetanus is ubiquitous (this means it is everywhere) and comes from the bacteria Clostridium Tetani. Clostridium t. is a normal inhabitant of soil and this explains why it is everywhere. Clostridium tetani enters the body through open wounds, bites, etc. Once in the body it produces a toxin (poison) called Tetanospasmin which is a neurotoxin (a toxin that damages the nervous system). This results in such violent muscle spasms that it can cause your jaw to lock closed in a violent clenching of your facial muscles, hence the common name lockjaw. The spasms are so violent they can break bone, teeth, tear muscle, and before the advent of the tetanus vaccine was frequently fatal.

In an emergency you will not be able to treat this and it will be fatal, and a miserable death at that. That is why I am strongly encouraging you and your family to be proactive and get your tetanus boosters now, not tomorrow. If you are uncertain as to the date of your previous tetanus vaccine then get one now, it will not hurt you if it is too soon.

GENERAL PRINCIPLES FOR ALL BITES AND STINGS

There are certain principles that will help concerning any type of bite you might encounter. All bites should be cleaned thoroughly with soap and water if available or hydrogen peroxide. If no soap is available, flush out any open bite with copious amounts of water. A mix of one part Betadine to nine parts water can also be made and used to flush out any bite or wound.

The application of an activated charcoal poultice to any sting or bite as soon as possible will help immensely. Activated charcoal is always helpful due to its incredible surface area and its ability to adsorb toxins and substances of all types on its surface. These poultices should be changed often, preventing them from drying out. In an open animal bite with a macerated or chewed up surface the activated charcoal should be generously applied to the inside of the wound and a poultice over it. This will insure contact of the charcoal with all areas of the wound in order to better adsorb the various toxins as well as the microorganisms from the animal's mouth. There is no downside to the use of activated charcoal; it is completely inert and cannot harm you in any way. It does make a mess, but under these circumstances who really cares.

When I say make as poultice, all that involves is mixing the activated charcoal with water until it is a thick wet paste, sort of the consistency of mud.

In the case of any allergic reactions, as a first responder you will need to access the patient and determine the severity of the reaction. If a patient develops systemic (whole body) symptoms after a sting or a bite then this should be a clue that you may have to intervene to interrupt this allergic cascade before it becomes potentially life threatening. Systemic symptoms such as lethargy (tired and listless behavior), severe swelling at the site of the bite, near it, or in the face and throat, rapid heartbeat, feeling faint, wheezing and difficulty breathing, generalized itching, etc. should all be treated as a medical emergency. If you have an EpiPen this is the time to immediately give it. Also give the patient an antihistamine such as Benadryl. The dose of Benadryl should be 25 mg every four hours as needed for a mild reaction or 50 mg every four hours for a severe reaction.

Limit the blood flow to the area of any bite. If it is on an arm or leg you should keep the limb elevated and if severe apply intermittent tourniquets, for no more than ten minutes at a time. After ten minutes you should loosen the tourniquet to avoid permanent damage to the areas "downstream" from it. Ice or any cold substance should be applied directly to the site to help decrease blood flow and also to decrease swelling.

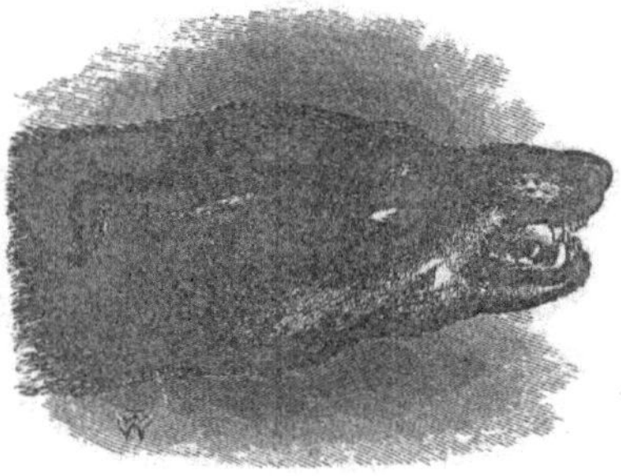

ANIMAL BITES

There are many things in the world that we prepare for that are unlikely to happen; this is NOT one of those occurrences. The odds of you or one of your family members getting bit at some time is very likely.. Either wild dogs or dog hybrids such as coy dogs (a mix of a dog and a coyote) can be very aggressive when they are hungry. There are many other wild animals that have gone feral and produced significant large offspring, such as pigs. Domestic pigs have gone feral and over time developed into very large boars with long, sharp tusks. There are currently four million in the United States and the number rises every day. They are different from their domesticated relatives in so far as they have longer legs, tusks, and dark coats with narrower faces and a dark ridge of hair down their spines… hence the name razorbacks. Some of these have been reported to be several hundred pounds -- up to 500+ pounds. Feral pigs are also the most prolific large mammal on the face of the Earth with some sows having four to six piglets on average 1.5 times per year! Rodents such as mice and rats and bats can often bite humans and bats are known to carry rabies. Rabies can be carried by bats, dogs, cats, bears, wolves, coyotes, groundhogs, weasels, skunks, and raccoons. Rodents and rabbits are not usually infected with rabies. Animals with rabies will look very mangy, with red eyes and foaming at the mouth. They may have self-inflicted bites and generally will not behave in a normal fashion. Normally nocturnal animals like raccoons seen during the day should be considered rabid until proven otherwise. The rabies virus is a slow incubator and may take several months to kill a human. It travels to the central nervous system (brain and spinal cord) and does its damage. Therefore the closer the bite to the head or spine the quicker the manifestation of symptoms will occur.

If a human is infected, he or she will die without treatment. The symptoms usually occur from two to twelve weeks after a bite, but may take longer. It usually begins with a flu-like illness, with fatigue, headache, and myalgia's (muscle aches and pain) and progresses to confusion, anxiety, irritability, and then to paralysis, seizures, and death.

WHAT TO DO FOR AN ANIMAL BITE

The first thing to do with all bites is to clean them as much as possible. Use soap and water and lather it up well. Rinse the wound with large amounts of water. If you have a large (50 cc) syringe, use this to flush the wound under pressure to clean out any saliva, dirt, or dead tissue. Iodine is very useful as well due to its ability to kill viruses, bacteria, etc. Flush out the wound with your iodine solution of choice (see Iodine section). A general principle is to mix one part iodine such as Betadine with nine parts water and use this to flush the wound or bite site. Iodine will kill the rabies virus, so will a chemical called BZK or Benzalkonium chloride. Both are useful in cleaning wounds especially from animal bites. You can buy BZK ready-made wipes on Amazon or eBay. They are cheap and a good thing to have to clean bites, cuts, scrapes, etc., and it does not burn. However, I still prefer iodine for its multiple other uses for health and even for water purification. Any heavy bleeding should be controlled with some direct pressure to the wound. Using whatever cloth or bandages are available, apply continuous direct pressure to the wound until the bleeding is brought under control.

I have been in situations where someone is bleeding and I do not have any cloth or rag or anything to stem the flow of their blood loss and I have taken off my shirt and applied direct pressure to it. Packing a wound or bite with wound packing will also help control bleeding once pressure is applied. Naturally sterile wound packing is preferable, but in a pinch anything will do. If you have time, soak whatever you have with a solution of iodine and water and use that to pack the wound, it won't be as good as sterile material, but it will kill most of the microorganisms.

Never close a bite wound by suturing, stapling, or taping it shut. All bites should be considered to be full of infectious microbes that will fester and breed under the skin of a closed wound and lead to more serious infections, abscesses, etc. A closed infected wound will also eventually cause sepsis (blood poisoning) which, in a situation without antibiotics available, could be fatal.

Any bites on the hands will very likely cause swelling, so ASAP remove any rings or other jewelry. Keep the bite open, and if you have any antibiotic cream/ointments such as Bacitracin triple antibiotic etc., now is the time to apply it to the wound. Clean the bite twice a day with hydrogen peroxide, you will see it foaming as it kills the bacteria. With any bite you should immediately take measures to not only cleanse and treat the wound as outlined above, but also aggressively start to boost your immunity with antioxidants such as vitamins C and D, alpha lipoic acid, astaxanthin, and others. This way you are using both your offense and your defense to attack any infection. This will also promote healing. All of the above measures are naturally assuming that you have no antibiotics available but are all still applicable even if you do have antibiotics.

HUMAN BITES

Human bites should be treated in the same way as animal bites. The human mouth is full of different potentially infectious organisms. Hepatitis, syphilis, HIV, and herpes are just a few of the infections you may get from a human bite. Many human bites occur accidentally during fights, when one person will punch another in the mouth and gash his hand on the person's teeth. This should be considered the same as an intentional bite and treated in the same way. There are no known cases of rabies being transmitted between humans, although it is possible considering their saliva is teeming with the rabies virus.

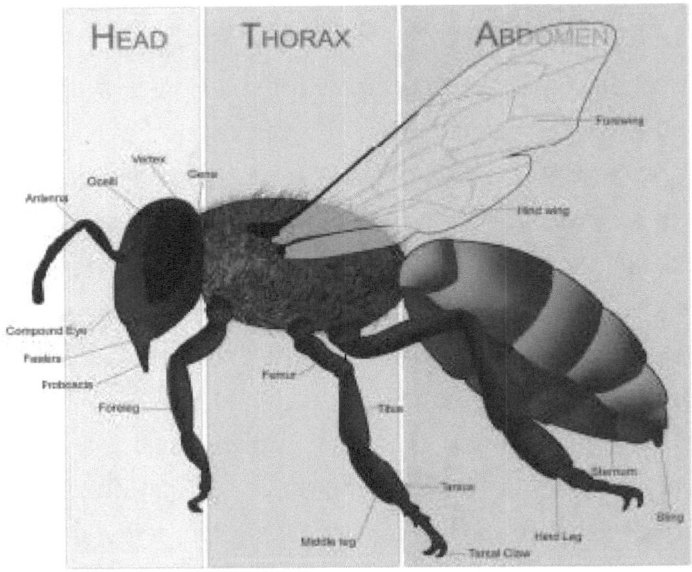

Anatomy of the Honeybee

INSECT BITES

In any outdoor situation you potentially could be exposed to a very large number of insect bites. Most of these fortunately will not be any more than a nuisance. Some of the most benign-appearing bites will potentially develop into some serious illnesses. Avoidance of insect stings and bites is critical for anyone planning to be outdoors for any prolonged period of time.

Several methods will help, such as not wearing any perfumes, hair spray, fragrant soaps, or colognes that might attract insects; since many of these have floral or flower essences that naturally attract pollinators such as bees. For the same reason do not wear bright colors, stick to white, brown, tan, olive drab and khaki as outdoor colors to avoid attracting insects.

Bright shiny jewelry will also attract insects. To avoid tick bites and repel ticks, wear your pants tucked into high socks and also apply DEET. DEET is the primary ingredient in most insect repellents and works very well to deter ticks. Formulations containing DEET currently on the market contain anywhere from 4 to 100 percent. DEET works not by killing insects but rather by blocking any smells that might attract them. DEET was developed by the United States Army in 1946 and has been available for the general public since 1957. Depending on the concentration of DEET in various products, it will protect you from ticks for two to ten hours following each application and for mosquitoes from two to twelve hours. You will not need 100 percent DEET; 30 percent will work to deter most ticks and other insects for about twenty-four hours before you need to reapply it. If you the outdoors type I would recommend having a good supply of DEET on hand, it is inexpensive and readily available. The question of DEET being safe for you is generally, yes, it is relatively safe; studies on rats have shown that it might cause brain cell death in rats, after the Gulf War American troops reported headaches, muscle aches, shortness of breath, memory loss, fatigue, and joint pains.

Just to be safe, I try to avoid applying DEET directly to my skin; instead I spray the clothes I am wearing. Never apply DEET to infants, and as an added precaution I would use it sparingly in children, although that being said, Lyme disease could be devastating for anyone, but especially for children. Other sensible precautions to take when going outdoors: check your clothing for ticks, especially your pants and socks. Using a lint roller will pick up many ticks, wearing light colors will also make spotting those little bastards easier. They are the size of a poppy seed, very small indeed. Washing yourself with soap and hot water will also help flush them away, usually a tick has to "feed on you" for twenty-four to forty-eight hours before transmitting Lyme and other diseases, so checking yourself and your friends and family members will go a long way in prevention. Especially look in moist body creases, hairline, groin, back of your knees, scalp, and body folds will help in catching most ticks. There are several devices on the market, including Tick Twister, which are excellent little devices that slide right under a tick and easily remove them, they are inexpensive and make the job of tick removal quite easy.

HOW TO MAKE NATURAL INSECT REPELLENT

As you have learned I like to use natural products instead of man-made products like DEET. Natural insect repellents are easy to make, keeping a couple of principles in mind.

Essential oils are the primary ingredients; these confuse insects and are repulsive to them. Since the old principle of "oil and water don't mix" these essential oils will need to be either mixed with other oils or with alcohol such as witch hazel. Like humans, insects have different tastes and likes and dislikes, hence if you make an insect repellent that is to be effective it is best to combine different oils to repel a variety of insects. The ratio should be approximately 10 to 20 percent essential oils mixed with alcohol or a carrier oil, for example one part of essential oil to either ten or twenty parts of alcohol or carrier oil.

If you are looking primarily to repel mosquitoes then use the following essential oils: Castor oil, cinnamon oil, citronella oil, or eucalyptus oil. If you are looking to repel ticks, flies, fleas, and lice, then use eucalyptus, rose geranium oil, citronella, and orange oils. For alcohol or carrier oils you can use witch hazel, vodka (please do not waste Grey Goose, use some other brand!), gin, tequila, olive or sunflower oils.

Store the above mix in a dark glass bottle, away from heat and sunlight. You can also thicken this mix into a gel by mixing it with aloe vera gel taken directly from the leaves of your aloe vera plant.

By now I am sure you have realized that I like to find multiple uses for everything. Here is another example, chickens. Keeping chickens in your yard will not only provide you with eggs and meat but also for weed control and tick control. A study done in South Africa showed that chickens ate an average of ten ticks per hour. Using a mobile chicken coop you can move the chickens to different areas of your yard, providing them with food and you with both tick and weed control.

The deer ticks that carry Lyme disease are mostly carried by field mice; these same ticks are also now infected with Babesiosis and Ehrlichiosis.

Bees, unlike wasps, leave their stingers in you after they attack. You should take care to remove the stinger with a tweezers ASAP to lessen the reaction. The stinger will look like a small black dot in the center of the bite. Even scraping it with a fingernail to get it out is better than leaving it. Your body's reaction to insect bites is due to venom that is injected with the bite. Wasps, yellow jackets, and hornets, have stingers without barbs on them that are usually retracted after stinging you. Bees, on the other hand, have barbed stingers that contain a venom sac along their shaft.

Bees leave their stingers in you after stinging you. Approximately 3 percent of people have allergic reactions to bee and other insect stings that range from mild itching and swelling to full-blown anaphylaxis and death.

Africanized honey bees, or killer bees, are a major problem that is growing as they migrate northward from their original release in South America. These Africanized bees are much more aggressive than the Italian honey bee and its European cousin the Iberian bee; they swarm and attack their victims with multiple stings, often killing them. They were originally bred from African honey bees and Italian and/or Iberian (from Iberia, which is the peninsula that primarily includes Spain and Portugal and the British territory of Gibraltar), for increased honey production and better suitability to the hot tropical climate of South and Central America. Unfortunately, they did produce more honey but no one was able to predict that the same behavior that had them more active in honey production also made them more aggressive.

They aggressively defend any perceived threats to their hives and also swarm, which means a young queen bee will leave the colony with a large group of worker bees and form a new colony. They also tend to abscond, which means the entire colony gets up, moves, and form a new hive, in addition to which if food supplies dwindle they will also leave the area. They originally escaped from near Sao Paulo, Brazil, in 1957 and by 1985 they arrived in California on a Venezuelan oil tanker. They have since continued their annual spread and by 2012 have made it as far as Georgia (after crossing the Southern United States).

Bee stings are fatal to fifty or so people in the United States annually. If you know you are already allergic to bees I would once again be proactive and ask your doctor for a couple of EpiPens. If your child has severe allergies, get a few EpiPen Jr.s for them as well. EpiPen Jr. is for children between 33 and 66 pounds. These are syringes prefilled with a standard dose of epinephrine. Epinephrine is what is given to counteract allergic reactions like bee stings. They are pretty idiot proof. You simply uncap the syringe and stick it into your thigh or any other muscle and inject it. You can even inject it through your clothing.

Only use the EpiPen if you are having a severe reaction, such as difficulty breathing or talking, dizziness, faintness, problems swallowing, or facial or neck swelling. Note: There is a delay when you push down the plunger on an EpiPen, so wait a few seconds without moving the needle.

Spider bites such as black widow and brown recluse spiders as well as scorpion bites can also be fatal. It is beyond the scope of this book to identify the different insects and their characteristics, but if you are interested it is easy to find photos of them on the internet.

GENERAL RULES TO FOLLOW FOR INSECT BITES

1. Get away from the area where you were bit. It is very likely whatever bit you is not a loner and has friends around that will do the same. If you are swarmed by a large group of stinging insects like bees, it is sometimes useful to take off your shirt and throw it down and run in the other direction. They often are using the color you are wearing as a target and will go after the shirt (hopefully). If there is a body of water nearby, submerge yourself in it. This will get the insects off of you, and the coolness will help the stings.
2. If it was bees stinging you, take the time to remove the stinger, either with tweezers or scraping it off with a sharp object like the edge of a knife, or even your fingernail.
3. Clean the area with soap and water.
4. If you have ice, apply it to the stings. This will diminish the blood flow by constricting the blood vessels and thereby reduce the allergic reaction and histamine release from the bites. Ice or cold compresses should never be applied directly to the skin due to the possibility of causing frostbite-like damage, instead a thin layer of cloth should be used between the ice pack and your skin.
5. As I said above, I have found lemon juice wonderful for taking the stings out of insect bites. Vinegar will also work to remove the stinging sensation.

Another wonderful method of treating bites and wound infections is using the herb plantain. It is actually more a weed, listed as one of the top three weeds found in lawns in the United States. Plantain is a native of Europe and Asia but has naturalized all over the world. I have it all over my yard;, it grows right out of cracks in the sidewalk and is very common. Look at the photo below and you probably recognize it.

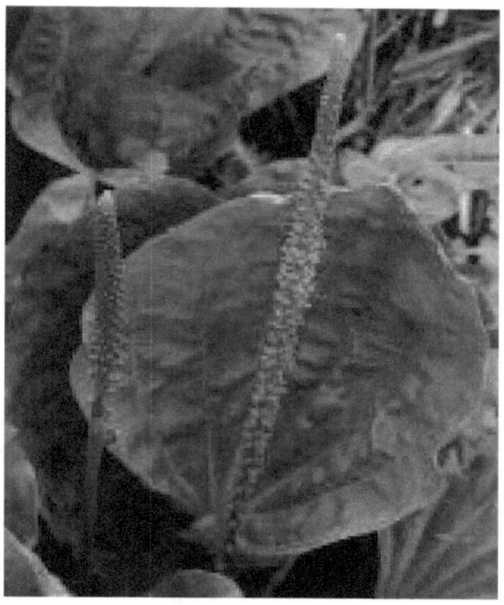

Plantain leaf with flower spike filled with seeds

Plantain's botanical name is Plantago Major, or greater plantain, and Plantago Lanceolata, or lance-shaped plantain. Plantain can be used for any sting, bite, foreign body (thorn, piece of glass, wood sliver, etc.) and the leaves can also be used as a bandage for wounds. For stings and bites of all kinds plantain has several wonderful properties…it is antimicrobial (kills germs), promotes wound healing and will take the stinging sensation out of stings and bites. To use plantain, take a few leaves and chew them in your mouth. This does two things; it breaks up the plant cells releasing its enzymes and phytonutrients and also mixes it with your saliva which activates it and provides its own germ fighting abilities. Some of the many phytonutrients in plantain include aucubin, which is a germ killer or antimicrobial. Plantain also contains allantoin, which promotes healing and regrowth of tissues. Plantain also contains mucilage, which decreases swelling of tissues and decreases pain.

Sometimes plantain leaf is chopped up and mixed with bentonite clay to make a paste for wounds. This works great to take away the pain and stinging of a bite or sting. Chew it up well and then apply the saliva/leaves mixture directly onto the bite or even a wound. It also has styptic properties that will help stem bleeding. For this reason do not take it internally if you are on blood thinners such as Coumadin or others, since it will work against them. Plantain leaves can be used as wound bandages using the entire intact leaf and wrapping it around a wound directly and then securing it with some tape or a string.

Plantain leaf is also used as a poultice to relieve the itch of poison ivy, poison oak, or poison sumac.

6. If you are in significant pain, take a painkiller such as Tylenol, Motrin, or Aleve. Remember the Motrin and Aleve should be taken with food to prevent stomach upset.

7. If you are very itchy, take an antihistamine such as Benadryl. Take 25 mg every four to six hours depending on your symptoms; if it is severe you can use 50 mg. It will make you tired, but it will work very well to eliminate an itch. Benadryl is a very important part of your medicine chest and I recommend several large bottles. It has multiple uses for sedation, allergic reactions, seasonal allergies, itch, and insomnia. It is the active ingredient in many over-the-counter sleep preparations. It even works reasonably well for sedation, if someone is agitated and manic and needs to be calmed down. It is relatively harmless.
8. If you develop a severe allergic reaction (anaphylaxis) with symptoms such as: Facial or lip swelling, hives, difficulty breathing, feeling faint, difficulty swallowing with a sensation of your throat swelling, palpitations (you feel your heart pounding in your chest), rapid heartbeat (pulse) or confusion, then it is time to break out your EpiPen and immediately inject it into your thigh. Do not hesitate. These could be life threatening allergic reactions and hesitation could kill you. Once again this highlights the critical importance of having several EpiPens in your medicine chest. There is nothing else that will work quickly enough to reverse a severe reaction once it gets steamrolling. If you have nothing else then immediately crush two Benadryl tablets and swallow them with a glass of water. It may or may not work in time, but let's face it...you don't have many options right about now. Note: If the person is stung on their hands, remove all rings and jewelry ASAP. Swelling often occurs and the rings might have to be cut off later. If they are tight, apply a little oil or soap to help slide them off. An alternative method can be to use string or dental floss or a folded strip of duct tape. You insert the short end under the ring towards the knuckles about three inches (enough to grab). From the ring outward toward the tips of the finger, you wrap the other end around the finger like a tight bandage. This is done to get the swelling down. At least go to the first knuckle. This should shrink the swelling in the finger that is trapping the ring and enable you to get it off. Married men (and women) seem to be able to get them off easily enough...but that's a whole other book.
9. Most venom from insect stings is acidic, so they can be neutralized by applying a base or alkaline substance. Employing this tactic you can use baking soda (sodium bicarbonate) mixed with water and a few drops of vinegar. Mix this up and apply it directly to the bite, reapply as needed. Using the same reasoning in a pinch you can use toothpaste. This will work on spider bites as well as stinging insects. You can tell if it is a spider bite by the fact that the bite area will swell, become reddened, and will have a small, distinct hole in the center.
10. Meat tenderizer mixed with a little water and made into a paste will also work to neutralize the venom injected by insect or snake bites. Meat tenderizer contains enzymes that break down the proteins in the venom and neutralize it. Take about a tablespoon of meat tenderizer and add just a drop or two of water; remember, you want a paste not a liquid consistency. This also works well for spider bites for the same reason, it is alkaline and will neutralize the acidic venom.
11. Activated charcoal: Any bite, sting, or burn will respond to activated charcoal. The reason activated charcoal works is by adsorption. Adsorption is different from absorption, adsorption involves a chemical reaction on the surface of the activated charcoal where it chemically bonds to toxins, proteins, and other substances but does not involve the absorption of water. Activated charcoal has an amazing surface area and is able to present hundreds of yards of surface from a small amount of powder, thus having incredible adsorption abilities.

If it was absorbing water with this surface area it would swell to an incredible size and burst your abdomen (if ingested) or swell to the size of a watermelon if placed on your skin. It works very well for snake bites and other venomous insect bites by adsorbing the venom and thus neutralizing it upon contact!

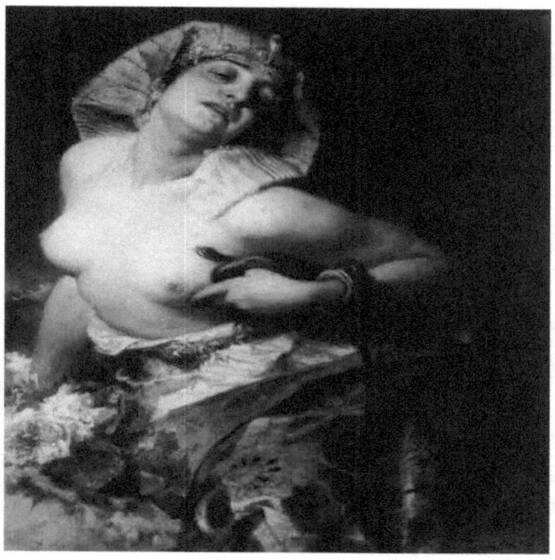

SNAKE BITES

The vast majority of snakes are not venomous and they kill their prey by constriction rather than biting them and injecting venom. For venomous bites please see the section below. The vast majority of snake bites will occur during the summer months and at night when snakes are active.

Most can be prevented by taking certain precautions like wearing appropriate clothing (high top boots and long pants) and also by staying attentive to your surroundings. Naturally, walking in tall grass will make it easy to get bit and difficult to see the snake before it strikes. Snakes do not have ears and cannot hear, so making noise will not help you. What will help is treading heavily on the ground or pounding your feet as you walk. This will create vibrations that the snake is able to detect. Using a flashlight at night will also help. A very important way to prevent snake bites is to also be careful when reaching under rocks or into holes and rotting logs. Also remember that snakes are cold-blooded, so they often have to warm themselves by sunning themselves on a rock ledge or outcropping. Be careful when climbing as you reach up to a rock ledge, especially on a warm day. Dry snake bites and nonvenomous snake bites should still be a major concern for infection.

Note: Even venomous snakes may deliver a dry bite or one without venom. The snake makes the decision as to whether to include venom or not.

If the victim is too large to eat and the snake just wants to scare them off they may not inject venom. This behavior is called venom metering. A snake's mouth is a cesspool of dangerous microbes that can cause severe infections in addition to which most victims are terrified and as a result have a pounding heart (palpitations) and are sweaty and nauseous and short of breath. Most of these symptoms are the result of their anxiety and the resulting autonomic nervous system's activation and not from the venom.

There is no foolproof way to tell the difference between venomous and nonvenomous bites. There are some symptoms that might help. Here are some symptoms that occur primarily with venomous bites:

1. Burning at the site of the bite.
2. A metallic taste in your mouth. Oftentimes patients report it tastes like tin.

3. Numbness at the site of the bite, especially traveling towards the body from the bite itself.
4. Rapid onset of profuse bleeding from the site of the bite and or a nosebleed right after the bite.
5. Generalized bruising and or bleeding from the mouth and recent wounds that appeared to be healing. Tissue necrosis (your flesh turns black and rots).
6. Patient becomes confused, lethargic (sleepy, listless), and develops difficulty breathing.
7. Blistering almost immediately at the site of the bite.
8. Blurry vision and a sensation of numbness throughout the body.

Note: Some snakes fake being dead by lying on their backs with their tongues protruding and will bite after they are handled.

Also, even immediately severing the head of a snake will sometimes not prevent them from reflexively biting. In these cases venomous snakes will not be able to venom meter and can deliver a very large dose of venom.

GENERAL RULES FOR TREATMENT OF BOTH VENOMOUS AND NONVENOMOUS SNAKE BITES:

1. Get the victim away from the snake. This sounds stupid to say, but many snakes stay around and do not flee the area and are able to bite again. Also be aware of where the snake is to prevent getting bit yourself.
2. Clean the wound as thoroughly as possible with soap and water. If you have any iodine solution, such as Betadine, also use this ASAP. Be generous with the iodine solution, pouring it inside the wound.
3. Apply a poultice of activated charcoal as soon as possible Due to its incredibly large surface area, that activated charcoal will adsorb any venom, microorganisms, and other toxins and neutralize them. I cannot stress this step enough! These poultices should be changed every few hours or sooner if they start to dry. Poultices will not work if they dry out.
4. Keep the victim as calm as possible. The vast majority of bites are nonvenomous and the patient should be reassured. If it is venomous, a nervous patient will only hasten the spread of the venom through their body by their rapid pulse.
5. If bitten on an arm or leg, immobilize it (keep it from moving) and keep it below the level of the heart. The idea here is to slow the potential spread of any venom. You can immobilize it with a splint or a sling.
6. Remove jewelry such as rings and bracelets and take off any shoes or boots from the bitten leg. This is because there will most likely be a certain degree of swelling.
7. Apply a pressure dressing to the bite site. This is done with a long bandage or an ace bandage. Start on the proximal side of the bite (the side closest to the heart or body), about three or four inches above the site and wrap it snugly around the limb like a mummy. Wrap around the limb winding it around and up to either the armpit (if doing an arm) or groin (if bitten on the leg) and then back down again over the bite to the hand or foot.

   Make sure you do not wrap it too tight and cut off blood flow.
8. Take a pen or a magic marker and draw a circle around the bite site. This will help later to see if the area gets infected and it is spreading.

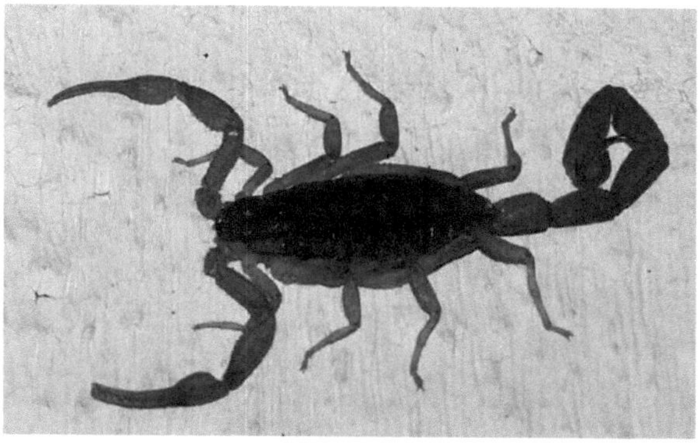

BITES FROM BLACK WIDOW AND BROWN RECLUSE SPIDERS AND SCORPION STINGS

Most of these bites are not fatal in adults but sometimes are in children. The venom of a brown recluse spider is felt by some to be more potent than a rattlesnake's, however they usually inject much less with their bites. Brown recluse spider bites may lead to widespread muscle and organ damage, especially the kidneys, causing death. Once again, this is more likely to occur in children but on occasion will happen to adults. Unfortunately one of my colleagues was on vacation in Florida and was bitten by a brown recluse and ignored the bite. He came home, became very ill, and wound up getting septic. He had an arm amputated from tissue necrosis at the bite site and then his kidneys failed and he died.

Black widow spiders are jet black, one-half inch in length and usually can be identified by the red hourglass marking on their backs. They usually are more active at night. They are not aggressive and typically only bite when sat on or bothered in some way. They get their name from an unusual behavior of sometimes dismembering and eating their male counterparts after mating. Just like brown recluse spiders, the black widow's venom is many times more potent than a rattlesnake's. But just like a brown recluse, the vast majority of bitten victims do not die from these bites. The group most at risk are the very young and the very old (the old bell-shaped curve rears its ugly head again) or the very ill who are already very weakened.

The care of spider bites is the same as other insect bites; however in these cases I would stress the use of activated charcoal poultices as soon as possible to adsorb any venom.

SCORPION STINGS

Of the 1500 species of scorpions worldwide, only thirty are dangerous enough to injure humans, and only one in the United States. The only one in the United States is the bark scorpion that lives in the desert southwest only. Scorpions have no teeth and therefore cannot bite; they do use their stingers to sting. Most scorpion bites are very painful but are relatively harmless. So rest assured the vast majority of spider and scorpion bites will not be fatal and should be treated as any other bite. Just like venomous snakes, scorpions will access a threat and venom meter (determine the dose of their venom delivered). In the case of scorpion stings, Benadryl will help slow the spread of the venom, as well as cold compresses or ice wrapped in a towel or other covering applied directly to the wound. Activated charcoal poultices should be used if available and changed frequently to keep the site wet.

WHEN TO KISS YOUR ASS GOODBYE

There are certain circumstances or conditions that may arise, especially in a survival situation, where the absence of doctors and/or medications as well as a hospital to support their use will make any treatment futile. This is not to say that you don't care or shouldn't continue to give support and try to keep the patient comfortable. It just means that nothing you can do with your limited training and resources will save this patient. Even the most highly trained physician, without IV fluids, medications, oxygen, and a hospital infrastructure to support him, will be helpless. The reality is these patients are most likely going to die despite your most valiant efforts.

RABIES

Any bite from a rabid animal in a scenario where you cannot reach medical help asap will result in the slow agonizing death of the patient. There are no ifs, ands, or buts. After a bite by an infected animal (there are no known cases of rabid humans biting another human and transmitting the virus), depending on its proximity to the brain or spinal cord (the closer the bite to the brain the shorter the incubation period), you can expect to start developing symptoms between two and twelve weeks, the average being about a month.

Once symptoms develop the patient will die usually within a week or so. Even with treatment, once a patient becomes symptomatic (develops symptoms) death is almost universal. So without treatment it is obvious that death will be the outcome. I am assuming that rabies immunoglobulin and rabies vaccines are not available, which I think is a reasonable assumption if you are stranded somewhere and cannot reach anyone for help.

VENOMOUS SNAKE BITES

The vast majority of snakes in the United States are not poisonous (but remember, these still can be serious and can become badly infected.) There are basically three snakes you need to worry about. These are the pit vipers such as rattlesnakes, water moccasins and coral snakes. In Europe the common adder is a venomous snake. According to legend, Ireland has no venomous snakes thanks to the efforts of Saint Patrick. Australia has several kinds of venomous snakes, as does Africa. The only continent without venomous snakes is Antarctica.

There is no easy way to identify a venomous snake from a nonpoisonous snake. Unless you know your snakes and are able to identify it when you are bit, you will not be able to objectively assess your risk. Once again, I am assuming no antivenom will be available, therefore I am placing those victims in this "when to kiss your ass goodbye" category. Venomous snakes deliver different types of venom. Some contain hemotoxins that attack red blood cells and also prevent clotting, resulting in severe hemorrhaging from the nose, mouth, old wounds, and the bite itself. Other snakes' venom contains a neurotoxin that will attack the nervous system. In these cases there will be burning and numbness and blurry vision and confusion, etc. Some venoms contain a mix of various types of toxins. Either way, it is not a pretty picture. Some cause severe necrosis (tissue death) and the bitten limb will turn black and its tissue will essentially rot.

CHAPTER TWENTY-THREE

BURNS

INTRODUCTION

TABLE OF CONTENTS:

Burns are something that we all encounter from time to time. They can be benign like mild sunburn or horrific as in third degree fire burns. No matter the source, my goal is to make you adept at diagnosis and treatment of burns of all types.

There remains the very real possibility of a terrorist attack with a nuclear device of some type that will cause significant burns in the immediate vicinity of its detonation. Other burns will come from cooking fires heating homes with woodstoves, fireplaces, and other improvised heating devices will invariably lead to a number of injuries, especially among children who always mysteriously attracted to fire. Sunburns of varying degrees of severity are a common problem, as are cooking accidents, burns from car engines and motorcycle mufflers and a million other mishaps.

To understand what burns are and how to treat them we must first take a look at ordinary skin anatomy.

SKIN ANATOMY

The skin has essentially two layers, an outer epidermis and an underlying dermis. Below the dermis is the subcutaneous tissue (sub means below, cutaneous means skin) which contains a fatty layer. See the diagram below for full details.

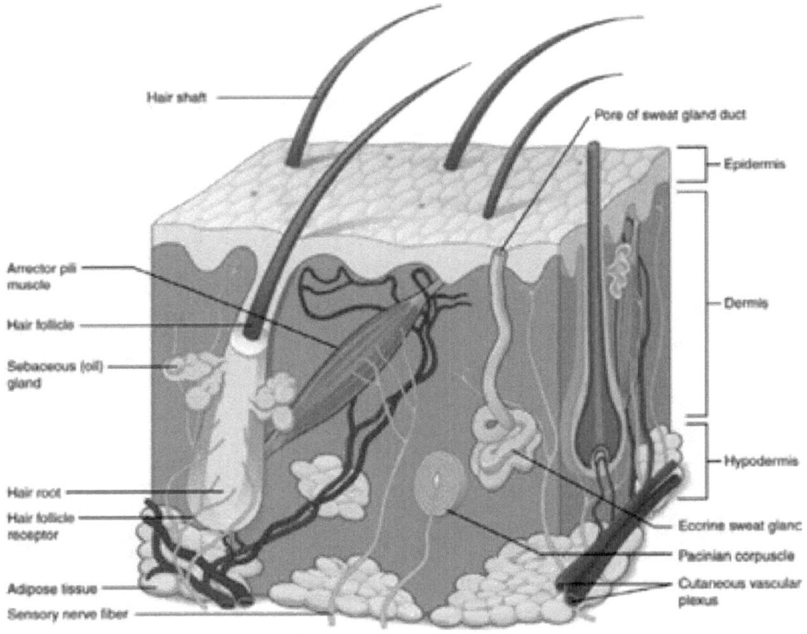

The skin is the body's largest organ. The skin has multiple functions, such as a barrier; the skin acts as a barrier protecting the underlying body structures from dehydration, invasion by germs, chemical exposure, and temperature variations. The skin also produces vitamin D from exposure to the sun and helps control body temperature by controlling sweating and blood flow to the skin.

I am sure you noticed how on warm days or after a heavy workout your skin is red and flushed. It does this by dilating (enlarging) capillary (small blood vessel) networks in the dermis that allow heat to be given off. The enlarged capillaries give the skin a red color. The skin is also a sensory organ and can detect hot and cold as well as touch and pain. The skin also has sebaceous glands that secrete a fatty substance to lubricate and waterproof the skin and hair, known as sebum. Sebum is produced most abundantly on the skin of the face and scalp and is not produced by the palms or soles.

In the epidermis there are cells known as melanocytes that produce skin pigment called melanin, the more it produces the darker your skin. Melanin's primary role is to absorb ultraviolet radiation, especially UVB, or ultraviolet B radiation. The cells produce melanin and put it inside of special vesicles known as melanocytes which accumulate in the cell directly over the cell's nucleus, presumably to protect the nucleus's DNA from ultraviolet radiation damage. The body's incredible complexity and the beauty of its function never cease to amaze me!

Burns are so dangerous because of their potential compromising of the skin and interference with its function. Burns can come from a variety of sources such as the sun, chemicals, steam, fire, hot liquids, electricity, and radiation.

The two most critical factors when evaluating a burn is the percent of the body that it covers and the depth of the burn.

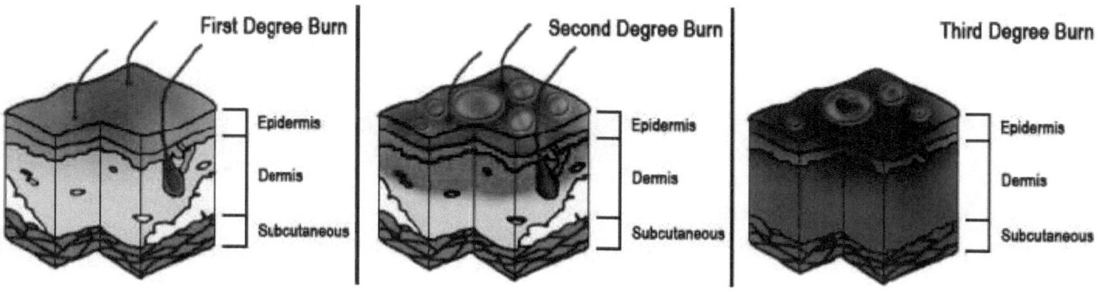

TYPES OF BURNS AND THEIR TREATMENT

As most people are aware, there are three types of burns: the easy way to remember them is by their names. First-degree burns involve only the first layer of skin, or the epidermis. Second-degree involve the first two layers of skin, the epidermis and dermis, and third-degree involve the first two skin layers and the third underlying area and beyond. Here is a more in depth explanation.

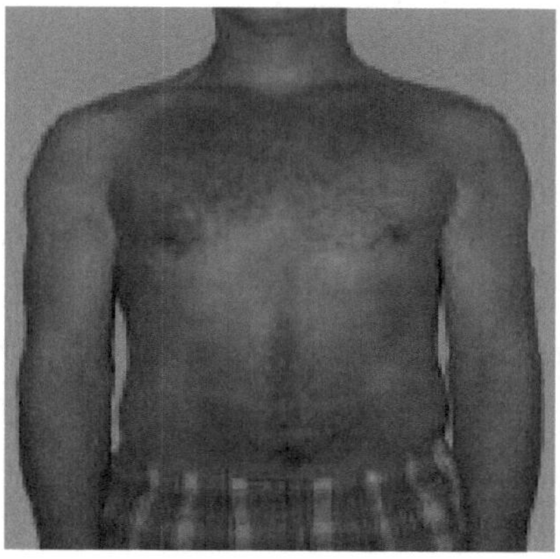

First-Degree Burns

This is the least serious of the three types. These types of burns only involve the outer layer of skin or the epidermis, and have not penetrated through to the underlying dermis. The skin will be reddened and perhaps swollen and painful as well. Usually these types of burns can be treated as minor unless they involve a large percent of the body's surface area. Sunburn is an example of a first- degree burn.

Treatment: Immersion in a cool bath or lake or stream will help, if it is a small area like an arm or leg or both, then running them under cool water will help.Aloe Vera gel is wonderful for these types of burns. I first encountered Aloe Vera during a college spring break trip to Florida. Kevin, a very fair-skinned Irish friend of mine, was as red as a lobster; an old fellow was riding his bicycle past us and noticed his sunburn. He struck up a conversation with us and had us follow him to his home where he split open some Aloe Vera leaves that he grew in his backyard and applied them to Kevin's burns. He also gave us fresh-chilled coconut milk straight from a coconut.

After treating Kevin he bade us farewell and gave Kevin a supply to keep in our hotel room. It saved Kevin from a spring break of sunburn agony and convinced me of the usefulness of Aloe Vera gel. The best source is to grow your own plants. Fifteen years ago I purchased a small Aloe Vera plant for a dollar and still have it, over the years it has grown into a very large plant with practically no care other than leaving it in a sunny window and occasionally watering it.

Like all succulents it loves the sun, the more sun the better. It will reward you with a steady supply of fat, thick, fleshy leaf stalks that can be broken off and used. Take the long sword like leaf and bend it and split it open length wise put a little cold water on your fingers and take the clear gel inside the leaf and mix them together and apply directly to your burns. It is immediately soothing and penetrates the skin nicely. Aloe Vera has been shown to help promote wound healing by promoting production of new skin cells. The leaf can be wrapped in tin foil and kept in the refrigerator or anywhere until you need it again. Nothing feels better on sunburn than pure Aloe Vera gel. You can find it in health food stores as an almost pure 99 percent gel; it comes in glass bottles and should be kept in a cool, dark place. Don't buy most of the commercial preparations that "contain Aloe Vera", they usually contain only a very small percentage of aloe. Aloe Vera juice is also available and this can be drank for GI disturbances and is very helpful in inflammatory bowel diseases such as Crohn's disease and ulcerative colitis as well as irritable bowel syndrome. Aloe Vera juice seems to have a very beneficial effect on the bacteria residing in our guts what is known as our intestinal flora. Aloe Vera juice can also be applied to burns. I personally prefer the gel but if you have a large area the juice can be poured on without incurring as much pain as applying the gel would incur.

Another treatment for burns is zinc oxide cream. Zinc oxide is the white stuff that years ago when I was a kid I remember life guards always had on their noses for sun protection. It is inexpensive and works very well for burns. In addition to which, zinc helps promote healing of burns and wounds.

Silvadene (silver sulfadiazine) cream is also very useful for burns as is its chemical relative colloidal silver. Silver has the unusual property of killing microbes (germs) as well as promoting the healing of burned tissue. The antimicrobial properties of colloidal silver can be utilized to help eradicate bacterial overgrowth or dysbiosis in the gut. If you are suffering with any gastrointestinal infection, ulcerative colitis, clostridium difficile infection (commonly known as C. diff) or Crohn's disease drinking a preparation of colloidal silver will help eradicate the pathogenic or disease causing bacteria in your gut and help heal the infection.

I would take a strong probiotic formula such as VSL #3 to help recolonize your intestines with beneficial probiotic bacteria. However, I digress, let's get back to burn treatments.

Other measures you can take: avoid tight fitting clothing, and wear light material like cotton; in addition, keep the burn moisturized, which will help healing.

Poultices for burns will help, when applying any poultice to the skin, once it has drawn enough fluid through the skin into the wound bandage and has made it wet, then it is time to change the dressing. You can use various herbs to make a poultice for your burns such as chickweed, plantain and slippery elm. The herb calendula can also be made into a poultice either alone or with the addition of Saint-John's wort flowers.

Honey is also useful in the treatment of burns, especially Manuka honey from New Zealand. As stated earlier, honey will not only promote healing, it will prevent infections from bacteria, viruses, and fungi. Honey also acts to hydrate a wound and keep it moist. It draws fluid from the body into the burn or wound site and helps flush out the wound, moisturize it, and along with this bodily fluid comes antibodies and white blood cells that will clean up the wound and prevent secondary infections. Please see the section on honey for complete details.

Vitamin E oil as well as oral antioxidant vitamins such as A, C, and beta- carotene are also helpful, along with the mineral zinc, which helps heal all wounds. If given for a long time, zinc should be supplemented with a small amount of copper, since it will cause its depletion over time. A dose of 30 mg of zinc twice daily along with 2 mg of copper should suffice.

The amino acid L-glutamine at 500 mg three times daily on an empty stomach will help heal burns and prevent infections as well as promote healing.

Activated charcoal can also be made into a very effective burn poultice, it is fully described under activated charcoal and under wound care. It works amazingly well to promote healing as well as adsorb onto its huge surface area many microbes, toxins, and wound contaminants.

Bee propolis can also be applied to burns and is very effective at promoting their healing and preventing secondary infections.

Vinegar is yet another very effective burn treatment. Any type of vinegar will work; it does so by soothing the burn and acting as an antiseptic to prevent infections. Make a fifty-fifty solution of vinegar and cold water, soak a compress (wound dressing) in this solution and apply it to the wound. Leave the compress on the burn until it feels warm and then change it. This can be done as many times as necessary in a given day. If the burn is on the torso you can soak a cotton t-shirt in the same vinegar/water mixture and have the patient wear it and repeat. As I said, any type of vinegar will work but I prefer using apple cider vinegar and my favorite brand is Bragg's, which is readily available in most grocery stores.

Witch hazel is a perennial herb that can be used as a compress for wounds. It is readily available in pharmacies and is inexpensive. Soak some cotton compresses in full strength witch hazel and apply it directly to burns just like the vinegar/water solution. Witch hazel is also a shrub that is both ornamental and easy to grow. I grow it in my Connecticut garden, where it flourishes. I try to grow as many herbs and medicinal plants as edible plants in my gardens; this gives you a nice supply of organically grown herbs and medicinal plants as well as a secret food supply. It is also a blast to walk barefoot in my gardens smelling flowers and eating fruit and berries; for a kid originally from the city, this is truly heaven!

A poultice of comfrey leaves can be made. Comfrey is easy to grow and quite prolific. I have it in my garden and it is very hardy, and its purple-blue flowers are much loved by my bees, as are most blue and purple flowers. Comfrey has multiple medicinal uses especially when made into a tea. It also is wonderful to make compost with comfrey leaves since its roots go very deep and bring up large amounts of different minerals that will make your compost very rich and beneficial for your garden. Borage is another useful herb for your garden and compost heap for similar reasons. Both of them are attractive plants that are loved by bees.A bath can be drawn and a quarter cup of baking soda along with a half cup of cornstarch can be added to tepid water. Soak for fifteen minutes to a half an hour to soothe first and second-degree burns.

Essential oils such as lavender and tea tree oils can also be used. Mix either oil with a small amount of water and apply it directly to the burn (for first- and second-degree burns) and cover with some gauze or a clean cloth. These oils will help the pain and also promote healing of the burn.Full fat yogurt and milk (also whole milk, not 1 or 2 percent or skim) can be used quite effectively to treat a burn, especially if extensive areas are involved. Don't get confused by the percentages on the milk cartons, whole milk is 4 percent milk fat, so 2 percent is 50 percent fat free and 1 percent is 75 percent fat free .They are both used the same way.

You make a compress with cold whole milk or full fat yogurt and soak the clean cloth, cheesecloth, or gauze in either one and apply them to the burn. An alternative method is to spread yogurt or milk (it is easier with yogurt) over the entire burned area, leave on until it turns warm to touch and then soak in a cool tub of clean water. Fermented foods like yogurt are also beneficial to eat due to their high nutritional value as well as their probiotic bacterial content such as acidophilus and others. Probiotics are important to colonize your intestines where they help your immune system as well as help to digest foods and produce vitamins and other nutrients for your body. The amount of good bacteria in and on your skin dwarfs the total number of cells in your entire body. As medicine explores this fascinating relationship, more and more benefits come to light. We even have a large number of bacterial genes inserted in our DNA, demonstrating our symbiotic (mutually beneficial) relationship. It has been estimated that approximately 8 percent of our genome or genes are of viral origin, demonstrating quite conclusively the coevolution of humans along with bacteria, fungi, and viruses In the near future as our knowledge of the human genome and the science of genetics explodes, I am convinced that we will learn more about these microbial interlopers in our genome and their influence upon our evolution.

Lard is made from pork fat whereas tallow is made mostly from beef or sometimes from mutton fat or suet. Both are excellent for your skin and will help healing, tallow being the better of the two, if I had my druthers. Tallow is made from animal fat and therefore is full of the fat soluble vitamins A, D and less so for E and K. Your tallow needs to be from free-range, organic cows otherwise there will be too many industrial toxins, pesticides, and hormones and less omega-3 fatty acids (if any) and less vitamins, minerals, and trace elements. If you apply tallow from cows produced in a nonorganic manner then you will be applying tallow mixed with multiple toxins to your skin, which will absorb them, causing your body to have to rid itself of this toxin load.

Tallow is outstanding for burns and will help rapidly heal them by providing all the nourishment a burn needs (supplemental oral zinc always help heal any burn or wound, along with B complex vitamins which contain both B 12 and folate). Tallow also has antimicrobial properties from its palmitoleic acid content as well as anticancer and anti-inflammatory properties from its Conjugated Linoleic Acid (CLA) content. Tallow is very similar in configuration to sebum, which is the oily substance produced by your oil or sebaceous glands of your skin. Skin produces sebum everywhere except on your palms and soles, and it has a high triglyceride content similar to tallow. In fact, sebum is the Latin word for tallow. Your skin cells and your body cells in general all need a variety of fats to remain healthy. What I mean by variety is the full spectrum of saturated, monounsaturated, and polyunsaturated fats. Saturated fats are mostly solid at room temperature, monounsaturated fats are softer and polyunsaturated are very soft. This combination gives the cell membrane the stiffness it needs for structure and the flexibility it also needs to keep from breaking and is vital to your body's health. Remember all disease begins at the cellular level.

Don't get confused by this terminology. Mono means one, so monounsaturated fats also known as monounsaturated fatty acids (MUFAs) have one double bond in their carbon chain, all the remaining bonds are saturated or single bonds. Poly means many, so polyunsaturated fats (PUFAs) have many double bonds in their carbon chains. Some tallow has olive oil added to it which helps make the tallow softer and more spreadable at room temperature. As always, I highly recommend extra virgin olive oil that is cold-pressed which is olive oil of the highest quality with the greatest nutritional content.

You can also blend essential oils with your tallow to give it even greater medicinal qualities, but this is an individual preference. Mastering the production and the utilization of essential oils is a very important skill to have and if you have an interest in it, I highly recommend that you explore some of the great texts on Essential Oils that are listed in the bibliography.

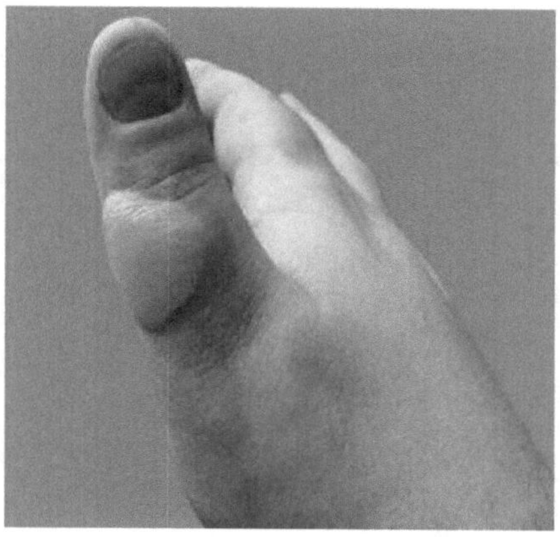

Second-Degree Burns

Second-degree burns go through the epidermis and deeper into the second layer of skin, or the dermis. This type of burn has both blister formation and a blotchy red, raw appearance to the skin. These usually produce some significant swelling and moderate to severe pain.

Treatment of second-degree burns is the same as above only with a few differences. Blisters should be left intact unless they are in an area of the body with frequent contact such as the hands or feet. Then the idea is to drain the blister without removing the overlying skin covering. Take a pin and sterilize it with some alcohol and perforate a small hole on the bottom of the blister and gently press the dome of the blister until it runs out your bottom hole. Drain the blister completely until it collapses like a deflated balloon. Then cover it with some topical antibiotic cream or honey and place a dressing over it to protect it and to keep it moist. If you use honey, apply it to the dressing that is in direct contact with the skin and put a second dry dressing over it.

As the honey pulls moisture out of the skin, it will moisturize the wound, and it will eventually saturate the inner dressing. When the outer dressing is saturated, then it is time to change it.

You can apply anesthetic ointments such as Lidocaine or Benzocaine topically to the burn. For second-degree burns you will need some painkillers if available, such as Motrin or Aleve or Tylenol. I also highly recommend Spenco second skin burn pads; these will not only soothe the burn, but they will protect the skin as well.

Spenco also makes a wonderful line of foot pads for blisters, a definite must for any serious outdoorsman, along with a couple of pairs of good hiking boots or army boots (both of which you should wear now to break them in properly), along with some waterproofing material for your new boots Anyone who has ever owned army boots or hiking boots knows that they need to be broken in before they are fully comfortable, so now is the time to wear them and acclimate your feet to them and them to your feet! Inevitably you will develop some type of blister or raw area on your feet and this is why this Spenco line of pads is so vital to your comfort, have you ever tried to hike with an open sore or blister? It is incredibly painful and before long you will be limping or incapacitated.

An alternative treatment for second-degree wounds is to mix some baking soda in some ice cold water and soak some clean cloths in this and apply it to the burn until it is no longer hot to the touch. This also has been shown to decrease the amount of blistering that second-degree burns produce.

Third-Degree Burns

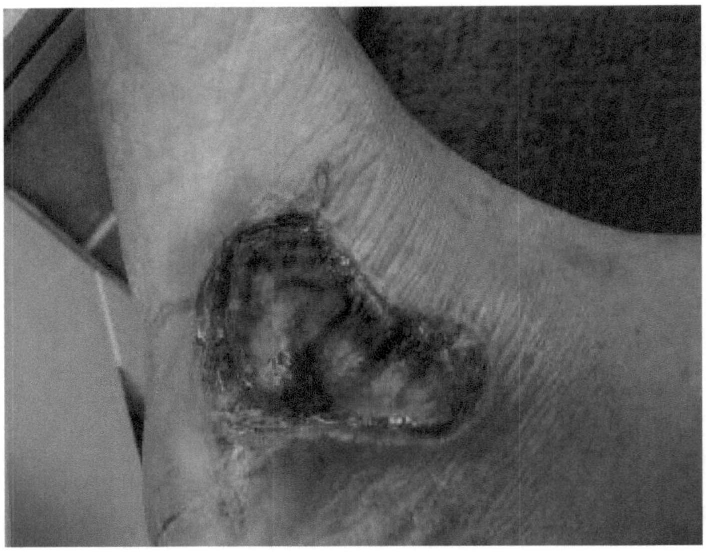

Third-degree burns are the most serious types of burns and involve all layers of the skin. This type of burn has gone right through the first two layers of skin, the epidermis and the dermis, and now involves the underlying subcutaneous tissues and deeper structures. They can either be a charred, black color or a dry, white color. Usually these are very painful, but if significant nerve damage has occurred they may be painless. This is a medical emergency and you should immediately seek professional medical attention. However, as with many treatments in this book I will outline how to treat these burns as if you did not have professional medical care available.

Treatment of third-degree burnsis the same as first and second with a few notable exceptions. Since by nature third-degree burns have fully compromised the skin they will result in severe dehydration, so the treatment involves administering fluids. The hydration will most likely need to be done orally since there will most likely not be any IV fluid and sterile tubing and catheters available where you are (unable to reach medical attention).

Oral fluids with adequate electrolytes, such as Gatorade, should be encouraged as much as possible. Gatorade powder is cheap to buy and easy to store; kept in a cool dark area it will have a very long shelf life and is easier to store and reconstitute than keeping it in liquid form. It has many uses such as this with burns and with dehydration and even for nutrition.

Spenco second skin burn kits are once again very useful for second- and third-degree wounds, first-degree burns don't usually need these unless they are on a very sensitive area, like man's best friend, his penis. They are easy to apply and come in a variety of sizes in the same kit. You can readily find these online at Amazon or other supply houses. I would highly recommend having a few of these kits in your alternative/natural medicine chest.

SPECIAL TYPES OF BURNS

Chemical Burns

Chemical burns are of two varieties, those caused by an acid chemical and those caused by a base or an alkaline chemical. As you will recall, the pH of substances is how the strength of an acid or base is measured. Water is considered to be neutral with a pH of 7. Substances with a pH below 7 are considered acidic, the lower the number the stronger the acid. Those substances with a pH above 7 are considered bases or alkaline, the higher the number the stronger the base or alkalinity. Alkalinity is the measure of the capacity of an aqueous solution to neutralize an acid.

If the burn is caused by an acid then you should use water to wash it off and clean and dilute the acid. Make sure the water does not flow onto other areas of the skin, which could cause other areas to become injured. Also remove any clothing or jewelry that may be contaminated with the chemical. Then take baking soda and sprinkle it on the burn or make a poultice of it with water.

If the burn is from a base or an alkaline substance (such as metallic lithium, sodium, potassium, or magnesium) then do not use water because the alkaline substance will react with the water and cause increased burning of the skin. Brush away any of the dry chemical as best as you can to get as much of it off the burn area as possible. Remove any pieces of those metals with tweezers and cover the area with mineral oil or soak a piece of clean cotton with mineral oil and apply it to the burn.

Note: Be extra careful not to get any of these chemicals on your skin, or you will be in the same situation.

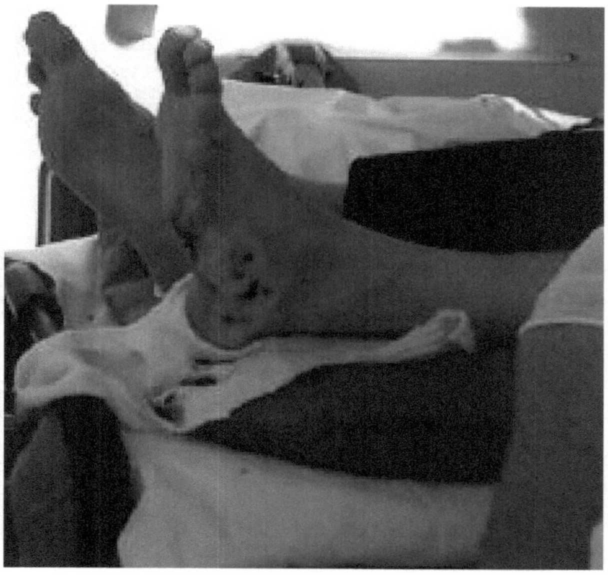

Electrical Burns

Electrical burns are caused by exposure to electricity and the resulting electrical shock. These types of burns are very dangerous because of possible disruption of the body's own electrical impulses, particularly that of the heart, which is controlled by its own pacemaker which sends an electrical impulse for the heart to contract or beat.

Any outside electrical shock has the potential to throw the heart into an abnormal rhythm and could kill the victim; these types of shocks can also cause respiratory failure (you stop breathing).

Electrical burns also have the unique characteristic of not showing much damage on the surface, they seem to damage internal organs more than the surface.

Lightning strikes will have similar characteristics. I have treated a few lightning strike victims in my practice and they are exceedingly difficult to treat due to their multitude of cardiac and nervous system problems.

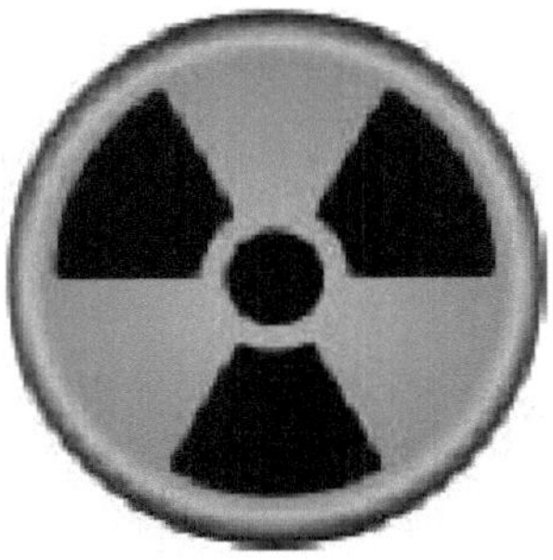

Radiation Burns

A radiation burn is damage to the skin or other biological systems from exposure to radiation. There are four types of radiation that cause most radiation burns:

1. Thermal radiation
2. Radiofrequency energy
3. Ultraviolet light
4. Ionizing radiation

Let's take a look at these different types and their sources.

Thermal Radiation

Thermal radiation is the electromagnetic radiation produced by the thermal motion of charged particles in all matter above absolute zero. Absolute zero, for you nonscience types, is approximately 460 degrees below zero! That's even colder than my ex-wife's heart!

Without getting too technical, thermal radiation is produced by the motion of charged particles such as protons (positive charge) and electrons (negative charge) within the atom; this motion, or kinetic energy, is converted into electromagnetic energy and thermal radiation. Everything we encounter in everyday life (since they are warmer than absolute zero) emits thermal radiation, including humans. As the temperature of an object increases so does its thermal radiation emissions and the frequencies emitted change as well. A good example of this is if you heat an object like a metal rod it will become red-hot, emitting frequencies mainly in the long wavelengths of red and orange in the visible light range (a range our eyes can see). If you heat the same rod further it begins to emit radiation in the green and blue range, which our eyes perceive as white, and we refer to it as white-hot. Sunlight is a good example of thermal radiation.

Sunlight is composed of visible light (light our eyes can see), ultraviolet, and infrared. Both ultraviolet and infrared are invisible to humans; you can feel the infrared light of sunlight by the warmth it creates. Infrared means below the red frequencies and ultraviolet means above the violet frequencies at the other end of the spectrum.

Ultraviolet light comes in various frequencies. There are three different types in sunlight, A, B, and C. Ultraviolet C, unlike Ultraviolet A and B, is absorbed by the ozone and the atmosphere and does not reach the Earth's surface. Ultraviolet B is also absorbed by the ozone but much less than C, and much of it reaches us on the Earth's surface, causing sunburn on our skin. Ultraviolet A is not absorbed by either the ozone layer or the atmosphere. Before you demonize Ultraviolet B remember, it produces vitamin D3 from cholesterol when it strikes the skin. That is the reason that sun exposure does actually lower your cholesterol levels!

Exposure to Ultraviolet A in sunlight dilates surface blood vessels and lowers blood pressure as well. Sunlight also causes an increase in nitric oxide levels, which relaxes blood vessels and also lowers blood pressure. Overall, sunlight is a very good thing for human health, but it must be doled out appropriately to avoid sunburn, which leads to higher rates of skin cancer.

In the past even fair-skinned people in northern Europe were deeply tanned from spring to fall due to this constant exposure. If we listen to dermatologists today we would all be cave dwellers and never venture outside. If long exposure to sunlight caused skin cancer those folks would have died in droves and that was clearly not the case. Skin cancer in my opinion is due to recurrent burns of the skin resulting in damage to the cellular DNA and the subsequent development of cancer.

If you are fair-skinned, start off with one hour or less of early morning and late day sun and slowly increase your exposure. Remember not to wear sunblock or you are defeating the purpose of the limited exposure, which is to slowly acclimate your skin, which will increase its production of the skin pigment melanin and protect your cellular DNA.

Radiofrequency Energy

Radiofrequency energy is the energy produced by radio waves, microwaves, and also alternating current (AC) electricity, which powers all of our homes. Radiofrequency energy is produced in the range of 3 KHz to 300 GHz which corresponds to the frequency of radio waves and alternating current electricity.High power radio transmitters can actually cause burns to the human body. The reason for this is the body absorbs radio frequency energy and converts it to heat. In the United States radio stations that transmit above fifty watts have to evaluate their transmissions for human safety. There are also a group of frequencies that are particularly dangerous for humans because we "resonate" at these frequencies. Resonating means that the body will oscillate or vibrate at much higher amplitudes with certain frequencies of energy, in this case making them more dangerous.

Ultraviolet Light

In the section above on thermal radiation of which sunlight was an example, I described the various components of sunlight of which ultraviolet light is a major component. Ultraviolet light is electromagnetic radiation with a wavelength shorter than that of visible light but longer than X-rays. Ultraviolet light is invisible to the human eye, but many animals are able to detect it. Ultraviolet gets its name because its spectrum consists of electromagnetic waves with both higher frequencies and shorter wavelengths than the color violet on the light spectrum that the human eye can detect.

Ultraviolet light is produced by sunlight, electric arcs, mercury vapor lamps, tanning lamps, and black lights. UV light can cause chemical reactions and result in fluorescence. As I described above there are three essential types of UV light; UVA (ultraviolet A), UVB, and UVC (which does not reach the Earth's surface for the most part). UVC has the most energy and thus is the most dangerous, followed by UVB and UVA in that order. UVA does its damage indirectly by causing the production of free radicals and reactive oxygen species, both of which have to be neutralized by the body to prevent cellular damage.

UVB can damage the cellular DNA and thus potentially produce skin cancer. UVB is also damaging to your eyes and can lead to cataracts and other eye problems. This is how snow blindness occurs in people outside with the UVB light reflecting off of snow and ice, which is even worse at high altitudes due to less filtering of the UVB at high altitudes. If you are in this type of environment you need to wear sunglasses that are full-coverage protective, meaning they have those side pieces as well to prevent UVB from entering your eyes from the side. Wearing sunglasses in this environment is critical or you will really damage your eyes.

Sunscreen is critical to wear if you are not already tan from previous exposure, and even if you are somewhat tanned, you will need some protection if you radically increase your exposure time. Sunscreen works by absorbing the ultraviolet radiation, primarily UVB, which causes sunburn. Remember B for burn. Sunblock, sunscreen, and suntan lotion are other names for sunscreen and have minor differences. Broad spectrum sunscreen blocks both UVA and UVB, other sunscreens absorb only UVB.

Sunscreens are rated by an SPF factor which means how long they are effective on the skin. You can basically measure the length of time any sunscreen will be effective by using the formula of: SPF factor number x the length of time it takes for you to get a sunburn without protection.

Using that formula, if you burn after ten minutes in the sun without sunscreen and you are wearing a sunscreen of SPF 15…it will be 15 x 10 or 150 minutes of protection or two and a half hours. In the United States our beloved FDA limits the claims of sunscreen manufacturers to a SPF of fifty; they say to limit unrealistic claims.

Sunblock is stronger than sunscreen and blocks both UVA and UVB light and also has a carrier oil to prevent it being washed off. Most of these contain titanium oxide and zinc oxide and are white in color. These metal oxides are inorganic as opposed to sunscreen, which is made of organic substances, and thus do not break down in sunlight.

How to Make Sunscreen

Here are the basic ingredients for making homemade sunscreen. Some of the ingredients are optional, and you can also tweak the formula to change the final end product. You could add beeswax to thicken it and you could add more zinc oxide to raise its SPF rating:

One half cup of either almond or olive oil (which can be infused with herbs if you desire)
One quarter cup of coconut oil
One quarter cup of beeswax Two tablespoons of zinc oxide
(thenon nano version that will not be absorbed into your skin)

This will give you a sunscreen with an SPF of 20.

Raise the amount of zinc oxide if you want it stronger. The nano-sized particles are very small and thus penetrate the skin and disappear not leaving a white film. This is the reason for their popularity with sunscreen manufacturers. There are reports of nano particles being able to penetrate deep enough to eventually enter your blood; for that reason alone avoidance of these sunscreens, in my opinion, is very important. The fewer toxic materials our besieged bodies have to deal with the better.

Optional ingredients: One teaspoon of red raspberry seed oil, one teaspoon of carrot oil, and one teaspoon of vitamin E oil, two tablespoons of shea butter, essential oils, vanilla extract, and other natural extracts to match your taste.

Here is how it is made:

Combine all the ingredients except the zinc oxide into a glass jar (Mason jar, for example) and stir them well. Then place this jar in a medium-sized saucepan with several inches of water in it over medium heat. Keep the lid of the jar on loosely. As the water heats up, so will the contents in your jar and they will begin to melt together; open the loose lid of the jar and stir it occasionally to keep the ingredients well-mixed. When all the ingredients are totally melted, add the zinc oxide, stir it in well, remove the jar from the saucepan, and pour the fully mixed ingredients into the jar you are going to store it in. Stir it a few times as it cools to insure that the zinc oxide is well mixed into the lotion. I suggest Mason jars; they are inexpensive, easy to find, come with a nice lid with a rubber seal, and are reusable. Mason jars are very useful items to have; you will also need them for canning foods, making essential oil, and sunscreen mixes as well as things like tallow. I would buy a variety of sizes for your later use.

This mix has an SPF of about 20, will last approximately six months, should be stored in a cool shaded place, and is not totally waterproof, so will need to be reapplied occasionally or after swimming. Coconut, vanilla extract, or lavender essential oil can be added to improve its fragrance, as per your personal taste.

You can make the same mix without the zinc oxide to use as a skin lotion. Personally I like the tallow made from organically raised animals better due to its high vitamin and nutrient content.

There are several oils, butters, and essential oils that provide a very small amount of sun protection and can be used, but keep in mind these are very limited.

Coconut oil (SPF 4-6)

Shea butter (SPF 4-6)

Jojoba, sunflower and sesame oils, vitamin E oil, Eculyptus and lavender essential oils (SPF 5)

Zinc oxide (SPF 20)

If you have skin lotion already that does not contain citrus oil, then you can make a quick sunscreen by mixing in your non nano zinc oxide powder and stirring it well.

Ionizing Radiation

Ionizing radiation is radiation that has enough energy to liberate electrons from atoms or molecules, thus ionizing them. Examples of ionizing radiation are gamma waves, X-rays, and the upper part of the ultraviolet spectrum, along with cosmic waves from deep space.

Ionizing radiation comes from the decay of radioactive materials like uranium, from cosmic rays, which are essentially very high energy waves coming from deep space, they may come from the explosion of distant stars in huge supernovae. A supernova is an exploding star that is so bright that it briefly outshines an entire galaxy, radiating as much energy in a few weeks or months as our Sun has done in its entire life span. As a supernova explodes it sends forth all of the star's contents in one long burst of energy, creating cosmic waves whose energy is ionizing radiation and eventually reaches us here on Earth.

Manmade ionizing radiation is produced by X-ray equipment and gamma ray tubes, etc. Ionizing radiation is invisible and not detectable by human senses. Radiation detection instruments like Geiger counters are needed to detect their presence.

Ionizing radiation does induce cellular damage that eventually causes tissue and organ damage and can be fatal in high enough doses. However, most people are not exposed to a lethal dose and these people have problems due to the long-term effects. If the ionizing radiation damages their somatic cells, then they will have cancers develop in those tissues; if it affects their germ cells (sperm and eggs) then they will have mutated offspring.

Acute Radiation Syndrome Or Radiation Sickness After Ionizing Radiation Exposure

Most of the effects of ionizing radiation are experienced about twenty- four hours after exposure to high amounts of radiation as in after an atomic bomb explosion. The spectrum of problems that appear is known as Acute Radiation Syndrome (ARS) and is also known as radiation sickness, radiation poisoning, and radiation toxicity. This high dose of ionizing radiation causes cellular damage and problems with the cell's reproduction by damaging its DNA. This ongoing disruption of the body's cells' reproduction results in tissue damage.

The damage from ARS starts within one or two days and may last for months. The symptoms you develop are determined by the dose of your exposure. Small dose exposure will result in gastrointestinal problems such as diarrhea, GI bleeding, nausea, vomiting, loss of appetite, and abdominal pain as well as some reddening of the skin. This is usually followed by falling blood cell counts and resulting infections and bleeding problems.

Larger doses will result in nervous system problems and disruption and eventually in the death of the individual exposed, but first they will develop dizziness, headaches, and then lethargy and decreased awareness, and finally, death.Sometimes exposure to low-grade radiation over a long period will result in radiation sickness months or years later, but this is not the ARS.

Treatment of ARS is beyond the scope of this book ; it requires blood transfusions which themselves require a hospital level of care. There is not much to offer you in the way of alternative treatments other than just making the patient as comfortable as possible; death is a blessing to these people.The skin changes from ARS is strange. Initially the victim will have reddened skin and oftentimes itchiness. Over the next few days to weeks there may be blistering and ulceration of the skin. Sometimes, depending upon the exposure, like in Chernobyl, there was delayed damage to the exposed skin that resulted in full thickness loss of the skin. Damaged skin often has hair loss, loss of sweat and sebaceous (oil) glands, thickening of the skin, pigment loss, and scarring.

Since there are not adequate treatment options for us, then our only option is prevention. This in essence means putting as much distance and matter between yourself and a nuclear explosion as possible, keeping your length of exposure and your body surface exposed as small as possible. Reducing exposure by a gas mask, face mask, and covering of exposed areas along with thorough hygiene for removal of contaminated dust/fallout will help. Potassium iodide will protect only the thyroid gland and must be taken for an extended period of time. See the section on potassium iodide for complete details; it will not protect any other organ other than your thyroid and will not prevent Acute Radiation Syndrome.

Alternative Treatments For The Treatment Of Radiation Exposure

Our options here are rather limited since most of the treatment needed is to support damaged bone marrow and the resulting blood cell problems with transfusions, stem cell transplants, IV fluids, and antibiotics, all of which require extensive inpatient medical care.

There are several seed oils that confer some protection to radiation exposure and damage, such as black seed oil, which has been shown to prevent some of the radiation damage to the brain and central nervous system. The active ingredient in black seed oil is known as thymoquinone and has been shown to protect the brain from radiation induced damage.

Squalene; a component in both olive oil and amaranth oil. See the section on seed oils for complete details on how to use these wonderful oils. The use of either oil topically (on your skin) will protect your skin from both ultraviolet and ionizing radiation damage. Squalene is also naturally secreted with the sebum from sebaceous glands in the skin. How squalene functions to protect us from both ultraviolet and ionizing radiation is presumably by its strong antioxidant activity along with its help in the repair of damaged cell membranes and lastly by its stimulation of the body's immune system. In addition to which, squalene also has strong antimicrobial effects killing off bacteria, fungi, and viral infections. This will certainly help during ARS when the immune system is severely diminished. Squalene should also be taken internally to protect the internal organs from radiation damage. See the section on seed oils for full dosing details.

Another treatment option is curcumin, which is the substance in the spice turmeric which gives both curry and yellow mustard their yellow color. In lab studies with mice, if they were given turmeric prior to a radiation dose there were fewer blisters and burns.

Pure Aloe Vera gel applied to areas after radiation exposure has been shown to help heal the burned tissue. The pure gel is easy to find, or you can apply it directly from the plants, which are very easy to grow. In the northern United States they must be brought indoors and put in a sunny window during the winter months. Do not bother using the gels that "contain some Aloe Vera"; make sure it is almost if not totally pure. An alternative to using the gel is to use the juice; cold juice applied to the burns will be very soothing.

A physician named Dr. Akizuki in Nagasaki, Japan, after the second Atomic bomb was dropped was working in a hospital less than a mile from ground zero. He saved all of the patients in his hospital by putting them all on a strict macrobiotic diet and absolutely no sugar of any kind. His diet contained brown rice, miso, tamari soy sauce soup, wakame and other sea vegetables, Hokkaido pumpkin, and sea salt.

This was all documented in the book, *The Macrobiotic Diet* by *Michio and AvelineKushi*. Sea salt is given a lot of the credit for these patients and their miraculous recovery. I have read some reports about the value of sea salt baths in neutralizing radiation from exposure. I am not sure how credible these reports are, but with our limited options we have little to lose.

Baking soda or sodium bicarbonate is also very useful in neutralizing radiation even in contaminated soils. The sodium bicarbonate combines with the uranium and allows it to be separated from the dirt and removed from contaminated soils. This method has been employed at Los Alamos laboratories on their contaminated soil and it was effective in the removal of 92 percent of the uranium. A post radiation exposure bath with combined sea salt and sodium bicarbonate is a good idea; this should be done daily for three weeks post exposure (or every other day for six weeks). The dose is one half cup of sea salt and the same for baking soda. You must remain in the water for at least a half an hour. Presumably the sea salt works its magic by providing all the minerals and trace elements one needs to help rid your body of these radioactive toxins. If that is its mechanism of action, then I would think you could alternatively use Azomite or Supreme Fulvic blend, which both contain the full complement of minerals and trace elements our bodies need.In studies performed on mice exposed to gamma wave radiation it was shown that high doses of ascorbic acid (vitamin C) was both protective of the mouse chromosomes DNA but also helped in its repair.

Calendula oil derived from marigold flowers has been shown to have a protective effect upon skin exposed to radiation in patients with breast cancer. The oil was applied twice a day during the radiation treatments. Calendula has anti-inflammatory properties and also is used to promote wound healing.

Oral administration of omega-3 fatty acids found in fish oil, especially GLA and EPA, have been shown to be protective of radiation-induced damage. Presumably the mechanism of action is by their induction of the production of prostaglandins, which are anti-inflammatory, and also protect the cell membranes. Prostaglandins have been shown to protect normal healthy body tissues from radiation damage.

As with all damage to skin and mucous membranes as well as wounds zinc is the king. Zinc helps repair all of these tissues and it has been shown that high levels of zinc in the body prior to and even afterwards will help skin repair radiation damage.

CHAPTER TWENTY-FOUR

POISON IVY, POISON OAK, AND POISON SUMAC

INTRODUCTION

TABLE OF CONTENTS:

Poison ivy, poison oak, and poison sumac are all classified as contact dermatitis. Contact dermatitis is a medical term for a rash caused by contact with an allergen. An allergen is an antigen or something that provokes your body's immune response and hence the rash. In all three of these conditions the allergen responsible is an oily resin known as Urushiol. Urushiol is also found in mangos and may cause a poison ivy type of contact dermatitis in sensitive individuals. Urushiol is also found in the black lacquer used to manufacture Japanese lacquer furniture which may provoke an allergic reaction in some people upon contact.

In the United States approximately 85 percent of the population is allergic to these three plants and will therefore develop a rash of varying degrees of severity depending upon the strength of their allergic response. It is possible to lose your allergy to these plants after many years but that is not usually the case, in fact in people who are allergic, each time they are exposed the allergic reaction will be worse.

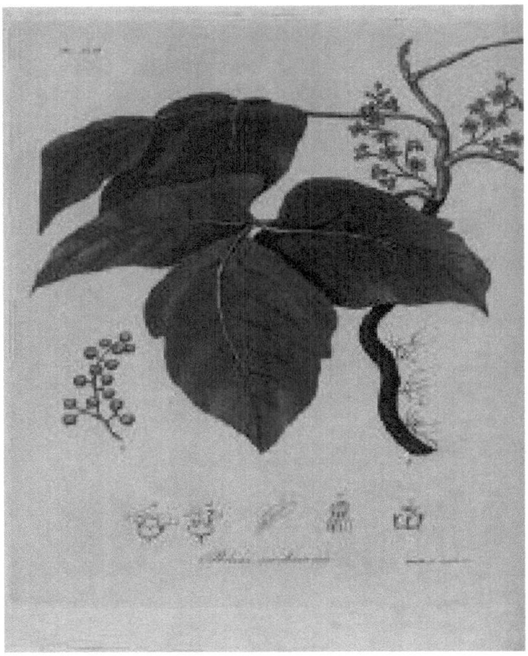

Botanical Drawing of Poison Ivy

These three plants are originally from the western hemisphere and were taken back by explorers to Europe, in fact there is still poison ivy growing in Kew Gardens in London. Other idiots have planted it in England where it has escaped cultivation and is being spread by birds all over England; never underestimate the stupidity of people! The Dutch used the strong roots of poison ivy to stabilize their earthen dikes, which worked very well but also gave it a foothold in continental Europe where it has now spread as far as Germany's Black Forest.

Long ago when the eastern Asian landmass was in contact with what is now the United States, there occurred a migration of these plants to Asia, however due to their overpopulation and resulting intensive land management, these plants have been eradicated. The only allergic reactions to Urushiol are from tree sap that is harvested by workers specifically to make the lacquer used to coat Asian furniture and give it that shiny black look.

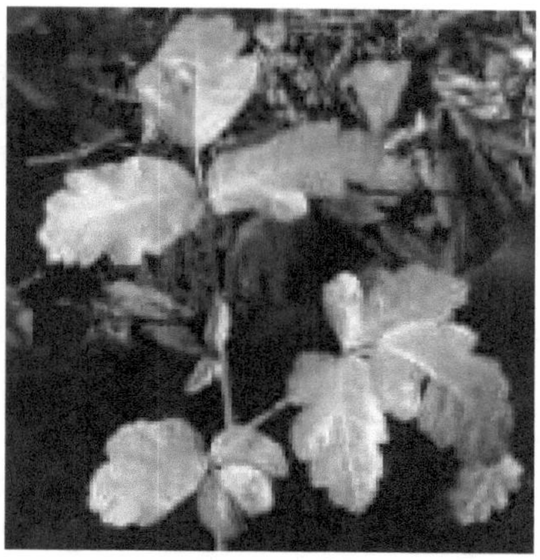

Photo of Young Poison Oak Plant

HOW TO RECOGNIZE POISON IVY, POISON OAK, AND POISON SUMAC

There is a saying that is very important to remember:" Leaves of three let it be". That being said, poison ivy and poison sumac grow all over the country except Alaska, Hawaii, and some parts of the southwest, primarily in desert areas. Poison oak grows as a small shrub in the eastern and southern United States and either as a tall shrub or vine in the western United States. Poison ivy is the most widespread of the three and may grow as a vine, free standing plant, or small shrub; its leaves are in clusters of three but sometimes five and are serrated with a pointy tip. In the spring the new growth leaves are very shiny.

Many people fail to recognize the threat of poison ivy in the winter when the leaves are gone, and get exposed to it from the roots, which are usually very hairy looking with thousands of small aerial rootlets off of the main root stems; those are those hairy looking roots you see on many trees.

Remember, any part of the plant contains the Urushiol resin and thus is able to cause the contact dermatitis. Poison oak also contains leaves of three and as the name might infer, these look like rounded oak leaves (not pin oaks with sharp pointy leaf shapes). Poison sumac is a little trickier to identify and distinguish from nonpoisonous sumacs which are very common. Poison sumac is an exception to my leaves of three warning…it usually has seven to thirteen leaves with one at the point and unlike non- poisonous sumac, the poison variety has red stems. The leaves are always an odd number. The berries of poison sumac are also different from the nonpoisonous varieties. Poison sumac has berries that start green and eventually turn white, nonpoisonous sumacs have green berries that turn red. Poison sumac is less of a problem than the other two because it primarily grows in swampy areas and therefore has less human interaction.

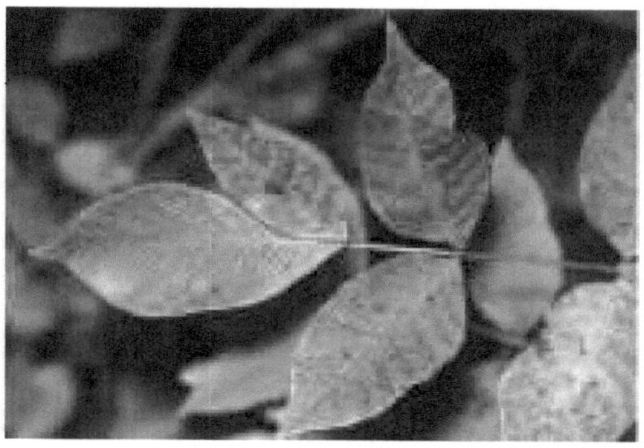

Poison Sumac Plant

HOW DO WE GET EXPOSED TO URUSHIOL?

Urushiol is maintained between the plant cells in all three of these plants under the skin or surface of the plant, it is found in the branches, leaves, and even the roots of the plant. Touching the plant will break up some of these cells and expose the Urushiol and at this point it is transferred to your skin, shoes, tools, or clothing. Urushiol remains toxic on surfaces for almost an entire year and even inside of an old root it will remain contagious for up to five years. Photo below shows the aerial roots of poison ivy.

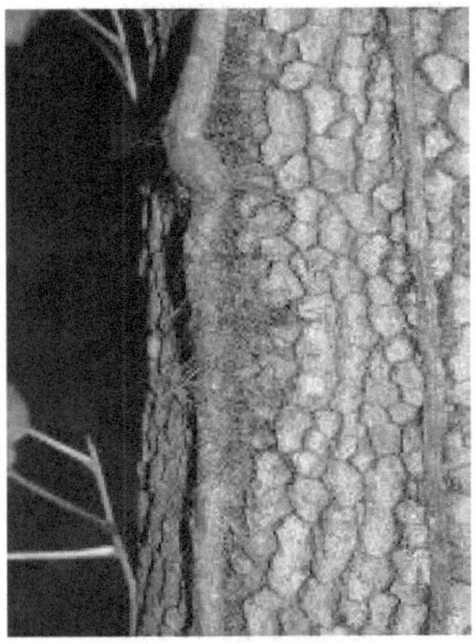

A note of caution, burning any of these three plants is a terrible idea and will result in poison ivy (or oak or sumac) internally in your lungs. Normally this is an occupational hazard for firefighters and requires hospitalization and high dose intravenous steroids. Naturally avoidance is our best deterrent.

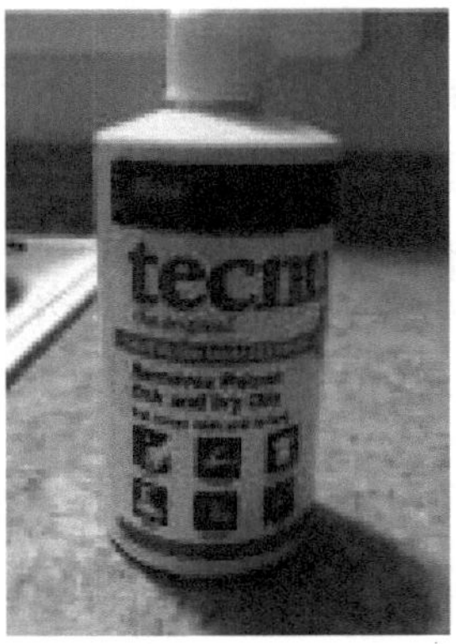

(Photo by Degen Earthfast)

Time is the critical factor here; within ten minutes of contact 50 percent of the Urushiol begins to soak into the skin and penetrate deeper into your skin until it reaches your dermis. Initially you can wash it off with soap and cold water, but once it has penetrated into the skin, soap and water will not work. Dish washing soaps work well because they have grease solvents that allow them to wash off this oil. You can use just soap and water to remove Urushiol from objects, clothes, shoes, bedding, or any nonhuman surface.

The reason for cold water is simply that hot water opens up your skin pores and makes penetration of the Urushiol easier.

You should also note that Urushiol is soluble in alcohol, ether, and benzene, meaning those substances dissolve this oily resin.

A wonderful but expensive topical solution that is alcohol-based is Tecnu, it is used with cold water and works very well to remove the resin. The hand cleaning solution known as Goop also works well and is much cheaper. Since it is soluble in alcohol you can use rubbing alcohol on a cotton ball or other disposable pad and wipe off the resin quite easily. If you use this method then you should be aware that you might transfer or spread the Urushiol by using the same cotton ball, so discard them frequently as you cleanse an area. Since cold solutions and alcohol both work to help remove the Urushiol you could conceivably use beer in a pinch, if you have nothing else, cold, hard liquor would work better due to a higher proof or percentage of alcohol. The alcohol content of beer is quite low, and of course many people would make the argument that it is better to drink the beer and ponder your poison ivy then use it to remove the resin! Personally, I have caught poison ivy since my childhood and would do practically anything to remove the resin.

You cannot get any of these contact dermatitises from another person or from the liquid in your skin blisters, it can only be transferred by the Urushiol resin. Depending upon the thickness of your skin it can take several days for it to appear in other areas, naturally the thicker the skin the slower it will develop.

However, if you fail to clean the Urushiol off of your skin, you may transfer it to other areas of your body, but once it is washed off it cannot be spread any further.

WHAT DOES THE RASH LOOK LIKE?

The rash caused by Urushiol is medically classified as an allergic eczematous contact dermatitis. The rash can be on any area of your body exposed to the Urushiol, and frequently is in streaks where the plant brushed up against your skin (or the roots). The rash is characterized by small bumps, clear, small fluid-filled vesicles (little blister-like bubbles on your skin) and large fluid-filled blisters. Urushiol is so allergy provoking that less than one ten millionth of an ounce will provoke an allergic reaction! Depending upon the degree of a person's sensitivity the reaction might be almost nothing to large areas of their body covered with large weeping blisters. Conversely, some people will show no immune response to their first exposure but will respond to subsequent exposures.

The reason for this is the first time they had no antibodies to the allergen (the Urushiol) and after that the immune memory is there and the body swiftly produces an allergic reaction and attacks the antigen.

All of these three contact dermatitis's will take about two weeks to run their course. Severe cases may result in scarring. Many times the intense itching provoked by the poison ivy will cause a person to scratch themselves raw in areas and secondary bacterial infections may occur. If you see pus coming out of your poison ivy skin patch then you have developed a secondary bacterial infection which will need to be treated.

TREATMENT OF POISON IVY, POISON OAK, AND POISON SUMAC

The first step is very important; you must remove the Urushiol from contact with your skin as soon as possible, as directed above. Initially this is done with soap and water and after that you need a solvent made from alcohol (you can also use ether and benzene but they are hard to find and have side effects).

The second step is to treat the contact dermatitis rash or allergic reaction that has developed which in effect is treating the itching skin condition and the discomfort or pain and also the blisters that frequently develop. You need to soothe your skin and this can be done in a number of ways.

Cold compresses also help reduce the itch and the inflammation. Other products that work to soothe the skin are several of the zinc preparations on the market including zinc acetate, zinc carbonate, and zinc oxide. Zinc helps heal all skin conditions and promote wound healing; it also works wonderfully for oral canker sores which are medically known as aphtous ulcers. Calamine lotion is a combination of zinc oxide and iron oxide, and as the song "Poison Ivy" from the sixties rhymed, "You are going to need an ocean of calamine lotion." Calamine lotion is soothing to the skin and does dry up poison ivy. There are other calamine lotion combinations currently available that include calamine lotion with antihistamines that are very effective.

Soaking compresses (rags or cloth or even paper towels) in a solution of baking soda and water will also help itching and minor skin irritation, as will oatmeal solutions. To make your baking soda cold compresses or poultices you need a mix of 3 parts baking soda to one part water. The oatmeal can be cooked until it is a paste like consistency and then applied as a poultice (with a mud like consistency) to the poison ivy.

Some authors recommend this be done with it warm, I prefer it cool. You can also combine the oatmeal with a few tablespoons of baking soda when making your poultice.

Making your compresses cold has added benefits such as helping to relieve itching by constricting the blood vessels in the skin, thus slowing the blood flow and the resulting immune response.

The coolness also feels good and is soothing to itchy, hot and inflamed skin. That cold soothing feeling can be exploited by drawing a cool (not cold) bath and dissolving a cup of baking soda, soak in that for at least fifteen minutes and you will be amazed at how soothing it is.

Apple Cider Vinegar such as Braggs can also be taken cold from the refrigerator and soaked into a clean cloth and applied to areas of poison ivy, oak or sumac. This provides very quick relief and is very soothing to this inflamed skin.

If you have them on hand, several foods will work very well to soothe hot, itch skin; you can grind up cucumbers in a food processor (first chill them in the refrigerator) and make a poultice that you can apply to your skin. You can also use cold watermelon rinds. I once took the bottom half of a watermelon and ate the watermelon and used the rind on a friend's severe poison ivy, the itch was driving him crazy on his neck and he just wrapped it around it with great success.

Witch hazel from your medicine chest will work fine to sooth the angry skin of poison ivy, just place some on a clean rag and apply it to the various areas for a short time each, it will take away the itch and calm your hot inflamed skin.

Just as I described under sunburns, Aloe Vera can be used quite successfully to sooth your skin. It is a very easy plant to grow in cold climates you can easily grow it as a houseplant. If you place it outside in full sun during the summer, it will rapidly to a large plant. It has sword like leaves that you can break off. Take the leaf at its base and press down towards the bottom of the plant and it will break off easily. Then split the leaf open, you will find a thick clean jelly like material. Mix it with a little water, you don't need much and apply it to your skin. Often times I split the leave length wise and use it directly onto my skin, I cannot tell you how good that feels. Once again, if you put the leaves in some aluminum foil in the refrigerator (not being split yet), they will last a long time and will be nice and cold when you need them.

There are several companies that make the gel, make sure it is 99 percent pure, avoid the others that say, "contains Aloe Vera", the percent they contain is too small and will not work.

The itch is primarily treated with antihistamines, the most popular of which is diphenhydramine or Benadryl; the only drawback is some sedation. Non-sedating antihistamines such as Allegra, Claritin, Clarinex, and Zyrtec work well and are mostly non-sedating. Benadryl by far is the most inexpensive and is available without a prescription, although most of the others are currently available without prescriptions.

Alternative medicine practitioners also use jewelweed to treat exposure to poison ivy and it is touted as a cure by many people, although studies of its efficacy (effectiveness) have been contradictory. The botanical name of the plant is Impatiens Biflora and it is a very common roadside weed. How it is used is to basically make a mash of the plant and apply that to the exposed areas several times until the rash resolves. The famous naturalist Euell Gibbons swore by it and used to keep mash of jewelweed ice cubes in his refrigerator for any contact with the three plants containing Urushiol. That probably was a very good idea considering the cold will also slow down the penetration of the Urushiol from the epidermis to the dermal layers where the immune reaction is initiated.

An interesting fact is that jewelweed contains an anti-inflammatory and fungicide (fungus killer called napthoquinone which is also the active ingredient in Preparation H and also an ingredient in the natural dye henna. That being said I have no personal experience with them and I could not find any references to the use of Preparation H or henna to treat poison ivy.

Other alternative treatments include the use of Bentonite clay. You need to take bentonite clay and mix it with water until you have a mud like consistency or a poultice...apply it to the affected areas of skin and leave it on until it dries and flakes off or becomes itchy and uncomfortable. You can make this poultice more cooling to your skin by adding a few drops of lavender essential oils to the mix. You can make a poultice using activated charcoal with the same directions as above, just without the lavender, which it will just soak up and neutralize.

CHAPTER TWENTY-FIVE
WOUND CARE

INTRODUCTION

TABLE OF CONTENTS:

HOW TO CARE FOR ANY WOUND YOU MAY ENCOUNTER

Wounds are one of those things that you will encounter quite frequently, hence your need to be proficient in their treatment. If deep enough they can be life threatening and even superficial wounds can be incapacitating to you or one of your family members, hence the need to be knowledgeable about all aspects of wound care. The beautiful part is that it is quite easy and you can amaze your family and friends with your adept handling of their wounds.

WOUND CARE BASICS

Understand one thing; your skin is an organ. In fact it is the largest organ in the human body. It is your first line of defense against both the environment and injuries. It serves as a very effective barrier against infections and for prevention of dehydration. It has two basic layers the outer epidermis and the inner dermis, below which there lies the hypodermis.

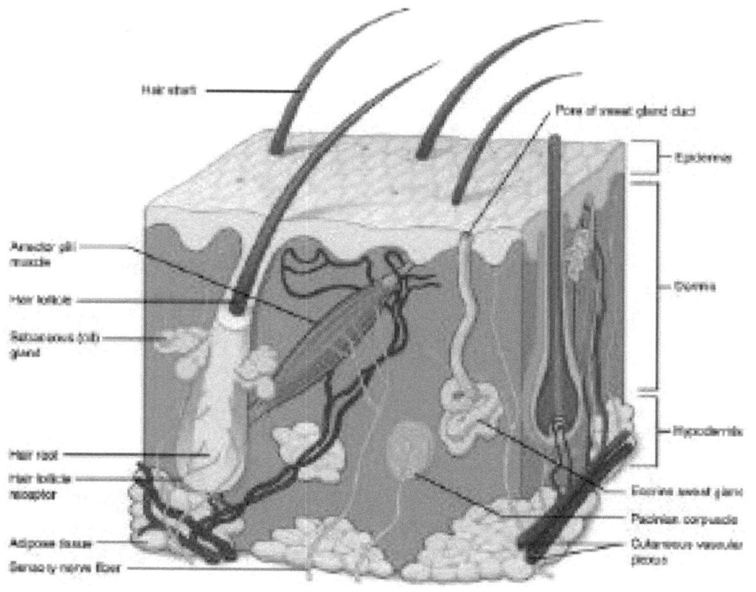

Diagram of a Cross Section of Skin
(taken from Anatomy and Physiology Connextions website)

Step 1: Talk To The Patient

Interview the patient and ask what happened. Every doctor who ever worked in an emergency care setting learns right away that this question is not trivial. It provides you with critical knowledge about the wound and what complicating problems may arise. For example, a simple laceration (cut) on an arm may seem straight forward until you get the history from the patient and he tells you he fell on to some broken glass. Now your focus changes to first stopping the bleeding and then checking for small foreign bodies (in this case glass), before closing the wound. Taking a quick good history will also let you know if the wound was contaminated or exposed to debris or infected by saliva. All of this is important to prevent wound infections down the road. Remember, even the smallest wound left untreated may lead to major problems.

Step 2: Examine The Wound

Do a thorough physical examination of the wound. How deep is it? Are there still active bleeding sites in the wound? Is there involvement of tendons, joints, or nerves? Is there more than one wound? Frequently there are numerous wounds on the same patient and if you are the first one on the scene you need to know this and select the most serious wounds to be treated first. This is known as triage.

Step 3: Clean The Wound

A cardinal rule of wound care is to assume that all wounds have been contaminated and need cleansing. Cleansing a wound has no real down side if done properly; it only takes a few minutes and will pay off down the road with better outcomes of wound healing and infection prevention. Initially this is best done with soap and water with a thorough flushing of the wound area to remove dirt, debris, foreign bodies, and bacteria.

I use hydrogen peroxide for any wound that I think might be contaminated. This is somewhat controversial; some physicians contend that this slows wound healing. I have been doing it for over twenty-five years in my country practice and I have never had any problems. The common name for hydrogen peroxide is simply peroxide. Hydrogen peroxide is outstanding for killing off bacteria and you will see it foaming as it does its work.

Patients have two major misconceptions about hydrogen peroxide; they think it smells terrible and it will burn like hell if placed on a wound. Both are wrong, hydrogen peroxide has no smell hence no taste, and unlike rubbing alcohol does not burn at all. When I advise patients with throat infections to gargle with a fifty-fifty mix of hydrogen peroxide (3% that is found in most pharmacies), I watch in amazement as they crinkle their noses, I then make them smell it to prove it is odorless. This is almost universally met with surprise.

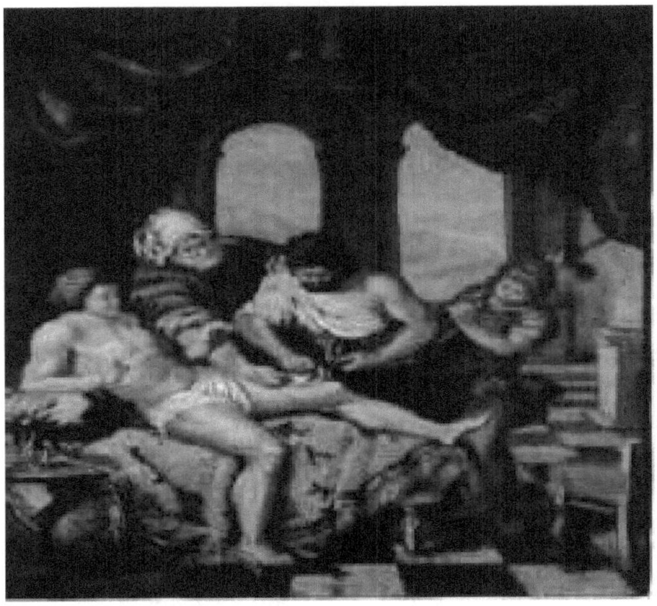

Note: The hydrogen peroxide should be used just for the initial cleansing of a wound and irrigation of a potentially contaminated wound. After that you can use it to clean around the wound area to prevent bacteria from migrating to the wound, but its use in contact with the newly formed cells in a healing wound might prove to be too toxic and therefore slow healing. I would advise if available the use of a bulb syringe (the kind used to clean children's ears or baste a turkey) or a 50 cc syringe. This will allow you to apply a "power washing" or high pressure flow into the wound to dislodge debris and thoroughly cleanse the wound site. Be careful not to blast too hard and tear already injured tissue.

Step 4: Control The Bleeding

Controlling the patient's bleeding is essential to preventing further blood loss and stabilizing the wound. Most superficial (surface) wounds can be controlled by application of direct pressure with your hand to the wound site.

Any bleeding wound on a limb (arm or leg) can be slowed by elevation of the limb above the level of the patient's heart.

The application of direct pressure should ideally be done with sterile gloves; if they are not available then the use of anything else, i.e. handkerchief, bandana.

I have taken off my shirt and applied it directly to heavy bleeding sites and it has worked just fine. In a wide open wound, packing it with some bandages or cloth and applying pressure will help control bleeding without putting your hands directly into the wound Naturally, once again, if you have sterile dressing that is to be your first choice, in order to prevent further contamination. After sterile dressing, the cleanest material you have available should be your next choice.

There are "pressure points" that are areas where a large artery comes close to the surface of the body and therefore can be squeezed to slow bleeding downstream from it by application of pressure. Remember that arterial blood is coming from the heart, so on the proximal side (side closest to the heart) apply a downward pressure to see if this will slow or control the bleeding. Application of manual pressure to these pressure points will slow bleeding dramatically.

Note: The bleeding from a wound will either be from a venous source (a vein) in which case it is a low pressure system filled with deoxygenated (blood that has had its oxygen removed by the cells of the body for their use) and hence dark in color. It will also gurgle out and not squirt out, because the blood pressure in veins is much lower than arteries. Remember, arteries carry blood away from the heart, which in all cases except the pulmonary artery is oxygenated blood and therefore bright red. The Pulmonary artery carries venous blood from the heart to the lungs. Veins carry blood back to the heart that is deoxygenated and therefore dark red; the only exception for veins being the pulmonary vein, which carries oxygenated blood back to the heart from the lungs. A laceration to an artery will spray out blood that is bright red and under pressure. Arterial bleeds will also pulsate as each contraction of the heart will cause a pulsation-eased squirt of blood following the body's pulse rate.

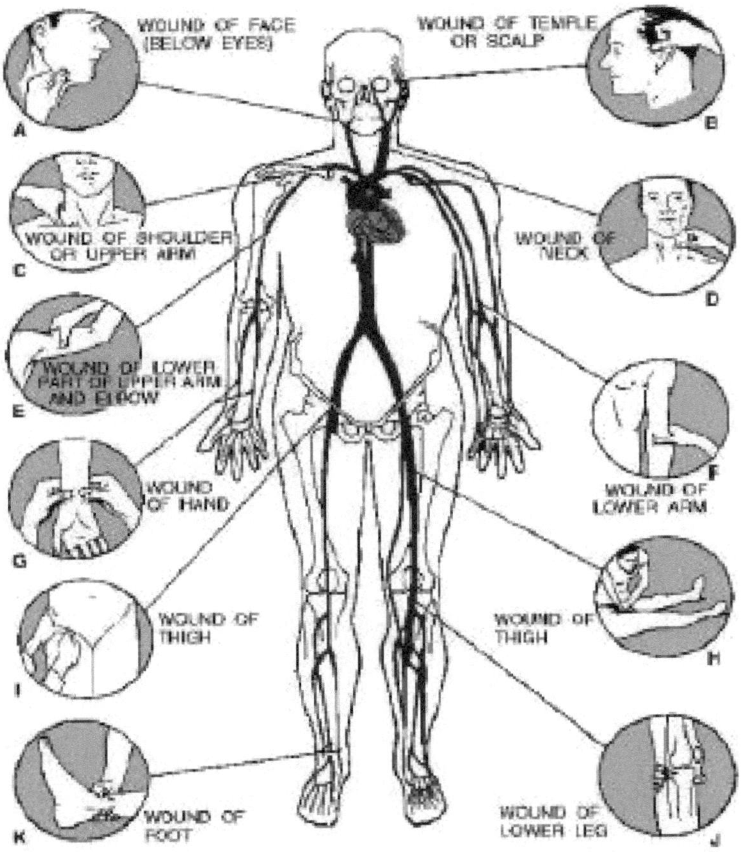

An Anatomical Chart of Pressure Points to Control Bleeding

Tourniquets

If everything else fails to stop the bleeding you will have to learn how to apply a tourniquet. This is not as easy as it sounds. The potential for causing more harm is very easy with a tourniquet. Remember this, when you apply a tourniquet you are shutting off the arterial blood flow to everything downstream from the point of its application. This means that those areas of the patient's body will not have any oxygen from the oxygen-rich arterial blood that you are blocking. This can only be done for maximum ten minutes at a time before serious injury occurs. Hence the ten minute maximum rule for tourniquets; this has two purposes. One, it allows the flow of blood to resume to the tissues to help keep them alive and two, it allows you to assess if you have stopped the bleeding, and clotting has taken effect (in which case you will not need the tourniquet any further). Tourniquets are also painful for the patient and loosening it every ten minutes will give them some much needed relief.

You can make a tourniquet by using a belt or some other strong material about two inches wide, apply just enough pressure to stop the bleeding, in this case less is better. A belt is good because by using the notches you can slowly ratchet up the pressure on the artery.

Any material will work, even a silk tie can be twisted and made very strong and useful for this purpose. Note: To stop a vein from bleeding, you apply pressure directly over it, just like an artery, but if it doesn't control the bleeding then you need to apply pressure distal to the wound (on the far side of the wound, not the side closest to the heart, which is called proximal). The reason for this is simply that veins carry blood back to the heart from the body and arteries carry blood away from the heart towards the body.

If you are serious about being prepared for any wound then I would also recommend getting several C.A.T.s or combat application tourniquets. These are absolutely wonderful battle-tested tourniquets that can be self- applied if you are alone and wounded or easily applied by someone else. You can find them online at Amazon or other sites. The Pentagon tested a variety of different tourniquet systems and this was proven to be 100percent effective.

Another ingenious system was developed by the Israeli military for wound dressing, named the Israeli Battle Dressing…this is an absolutely indispensable addition to your medicine chest and has endless uses as a bandage, and can also be used as a modified tourniquet to achieve hemostasis (stopping bleeding). I would highly recommend buying as many of these as you can afford. They too can be purchased online. There are also some very nice YouTube videos on how to use them. They can be used for head and extremity wounds and are very versatile. Both the CAT and the Israeli Battle Dressings can be self-applied if you are alone and injured.

Alternative Methods to Control Bleeding

Sprinkle cayenne pepper powder or cinnamon powder directly into a wound, this will help clotting for minor bleeding wounds. Remember to apply direct pressure to compress the wound.

Another alternative method to control bleeding is to apply the following essential oils to gauze or if none is available the cleanest piece of cloth you can find:

Cypress oil
Geranium oil
Helichrysum oil
Hyssop oil
Myrrh oil

KEEP THE WOUND MOIST

If possible keep a wound moist and prevent excessive drying out of the wound, which will only delay healing. Also, if a wound dries out the bandage will stick to it and will reopen it when you try to remove it. To keep wounds moist you can use topical antibiotic cream. If you run out of topical antibiotic creams you can always use honey.

Honey is very osmotic (dense and thick and therefore will pull fluids towards it) and will draw fluid from surrounding healthy tissue and keep the wound moist and flushed. Honey is also antibacterial, antifungal, and antiviral and will prevent infections while at the same time nourishing the wound.

Honey can be applied in various ways. If the wound is gaping (wide open) then squeeze some honey directly into the base of the wound and cover with a sterile (if you have one) gauze . The other method is to apply the honey to the underside of a wound dressing and apply this surface directly in contact with the wound. Place another dressing without honey over the honey-soaked one. When the dressing without honey becomes wet then that is time to change the dressing and apply a new one. This combination of wet inner dressing (you can use sterile water, a mix of one part Betadine to ten parts water or Dakin's solution). A dry outer dressing is also known as a "wet to dry dressing". Over the years I have amazed doctors and nurses in wound clinics who have prescribed outrageously expensive wound salves to my patients who asked my advice and I have changed them to honey with excellent results. Honey even works well in diabetic patients.

COVER THE WOUND

Keep the wound covered if possible, Band-Aids for small wounds and dressings for large wounds. This will keep a certain amount of dirt and bacteria from readily reaching the wound and complicating matters. It also mechanically will prevent further injury, especially if the wound is in an area that will receive contact, like a hand or foot. Keeping it covered will also help keep it moist. Change the dressing twice a day if you have the luxury of time, etc. and/or change it whenever the dressing becomes soaked with body fluids or blood.

Note: If possible each time you change a dressing use that opportunity to clean the wound again as described above. Changing dressings or Band-Aids should be done slowly and carefully in order to prevent further trauma to the wound and tearing off any of the granulation tissue (the yellow creamy-appearing substance that your body makes to fill in a wound and allow it to heal from its perimeter) and scabs.

If a dressing is sticking to a wound, moisten it with some water and slowly remove it.

THE MEDIC SHOULD BE CLEAN

A medic should always make sure (once again, if the situation allows) that his or her hands are clean. If you have the opportunity, clean your hands with soap and water and clean under your finger nails. Keep them as short as possible; which will help. This will help prevent further contamination of the wound area and is an essential principle in providing wound care.

Remember: First do no harm. What good are you if your carelessness causes infections in the patients you are treating? Certainly the situation will dictate how sterile the area is in which you are providing your care; a clinic will be a lot different than a hike in the woods. Even a pair of relatively clean gloves will provide a barrier between your contaminated skin and the wound. Sterile gloves naturally would be ideal, but I am realistic enough to know that in certain situations it is unlikely that they will be available.

PAIN CONTROL

Wounds are without a doubt painful, as we all have learned. Burns by far are the worst. If you have an adequate supply of pain medications available, now is the time to use them. Aleve, Tylenol, or Motrin will work just fine for the vast majority of minor wounds. Aspirin should not be used as a painkiller for wound care, since it inhibits the function of platelets (which plug wounds and prevent bleeding) and will cause worse bleeding. Also remember, aspirin should never be used in children under the age of twelve, due to the risk of Reye's Syndrome.

For severe pain, if you have any narcotic analgesics like Percocet, Oxycontin, or morphine type meds, now is a good reason to give them.

Alternative methods for pain control involve the use of essential oils. Make a salve by mixing the following essential oils in a fifty-fifty mix with a carrier oil such as coconut oil or olive oil:

Geranium Oil
Ginger Oil
Helichrysum Oil
Oregano Oil
Rosemary Oil

Remember: The reason for the carrier oil is to allow penetration of the skin. So apply these essential oil/carrier oil mixes around the wound on intact skin to get good pain control. In a winter situation, ice will also help numb the area and achieve pain control (at least temporarily); it will also constrict the small blood vessels and slow bleeding. Never apply it directly to the skin due to the risk of frostbite damage. Always place a piece of thin cloth or other barrier between the ice and the patient's skin.

EVALUATION OF POSSIBLE NERVE DAMAGE

If a nerve is severed (cut) in a deep wound the patient may lose sensation downstream from the wound, the area may feel numb to touch. Involvement of a large nerve may involve loss of movement of the involved extremity (paralysis). In most situations this is permanent and beyond the scope of this book and your capabilities. These patients need to be brought asap to a medical center of some type for immediate care. That naturally also applies to any deep, serious wound that you encounter, especially in those cases where you are unable to control the bleeding.

Once again, it should go without saying, but I am going to mention it again, when I am teaching you how to care for these serious wounds or any serious medical conditions, the presumption is that you have no way to get medical care and are relying on this book. The option with any serious medical problem should always be to seek help from a doctor asap.

PROPER NUTRITION TO HEAL WOUNDS

This is essential and involves adequate protein intake so your body is able to construct new body tissue (which are primarily proteins). In addition to which, your body will need the following vitamins and minerals to promote healing:

Vitamin A: This vitamin is important for wound healing due to its importance in the production of a protein that the body uses for wound repair and healing, called fibronectin. It is also an antioxidant and prevents further tissue damage from free radicals that are produced in abundance with an injury.

Vitamin C: This vitamin is essential for wound healing due to its role in the production of collagen, which is the main structural protein of the human body. Structural proteins are what allow the body to build structures (tissues for healing). Vitamin C is also a strong antioxidant and part of the antioxidant cascade (see Vitamin section).

Vitamin E: Also a strong antioxidant, it accumulates in the cell membranes (the wall of a cell) where it prevents free radicals from oxidizing or damaging the cell wall. It also inhibits prostaglandins and hence has an anti- inflammatory effect. It also is known to prevent or at least decrease scar formation.

Zinc: Zinc is the most essential mineral in wound healing. Remember my use of it in canker sores; it heals them readily and also is essential in the healing of burns. Zinc is essential to the functioning of over 200 enzymes in the body including DNA polymerase which is necessary for cell reproduction.

SIGNS AND SYMPTOMS OF A WOUND INFECTION

One of the easiest ways to determine if a wound is infected is by using your nose. An infected wound will have a foul smell; you can either smell the wound or the dressings you just removed. There may or may not be a pustular (pus-containing) discharge from the wound, with wound tissue that is friable (crumbles). Increased pain and especially fever are all important symptoms of a wound infection. There also may be tissue necrosis (dead tissue) and you may even have gangrene if the blood flow is compromised (cut off). Necrotic tissue will be very dark, even black.

Frequently the wound infection will spread to surrounding previously healthy tissue. You may see a spreading area of redness and especially warmth. It is a good practice to take a pen or magic marker of some type and outline the current edge of infection, that way at a later time you will be able to determine if it is actually spreading. This is a simple thing to do and is incredibly useful when you are watching the recovery of a patient.

Remember the cardinal signs of inflammation: Rubor (redness), Calor (heat), Dolor (pain), and loss of function. A newly infected area will therefore be red, warm and tender, which is very easy even for a person without any medical training to properly evaluate.

You may find enlarged lymph nodes near the wound (lymph nodes will feel like small, round, hard bumps below the surface ranging in size from a pea to a small grape). Just like veins, lymphatic vessels drain tissues and carry fluid back to the heart. They are an essential part of your immune system and when they are fighting an infection they swell in size as your immune system sends in its troops (lymphocytes in this case).

The lymph nodes are small forts along the routes of your lymphatic system that when under attack will swell in size. There are two types of lymphocytes: T cells are responsible for cell-mediated immunity and get right into the fight themselves, attacking the invaders, B cells stand back and produce antibodies and send them in wave after wave, attacking any toxin, infection, and anything it determines is foreign or not self.

An infected wound may also spontaneously start to bleed. The patient may also complain of fever alternating with chills. These are all signs of a serious infection. If the patient becomes septic (blood poisoning), even with the use of antibiotics intravenously there is still a very high mortality rate. Currently about 50 percent of patients die from sepsis, and that is in our modern-day hospitals with the best medical care in the world, so you can imagine why I am pessimistic about the chances of you successfully treating yourself or someone else in this situation.

There is not much you can do for a spreading infected wound other than surgical debridement. This means cleaning out the wound with a sterile scalpel or sterilized sharp knife and cutting away all the dead and dying infected tissue down to clean, uninfected tissue. This should be done only by an experienced medical professional. This is basically a "Hail Mary pass" and should only be done if you see an infection spreading and the patient is becoming septic. This patient might very well be placed in my Kiss-Your-Ass-Goodbye-Category if you aren't able to get them to a hospital.

OTHER SYMPTOMS OF SEPSIS OR BLOOD POISONING

Fever either greater than 101 F or less than 95 F (most often it is fever)

Delirium: the patient becomes delirious and confused, frequently hallucinating and babbling all kinds of nonsense

Pulse greater than 90 and frequently over 100. Note: Pulse will frequently raise about 10 beats per minute for each 1 degree F of fever greater than about 99.

Rigors or severe, shaking chills that wrack the patient's body. Increasing respiratory rate (breathing quickly) usually greater than 20 respirations per minute.

ALTERNATIVE SOLUTIONS EFFECTIVE IN WOUND CLEANSING

Dakin's Solution

During WWI there was an overwhelming demand for methods to clean the horrific number of troops who were being wounded by this newly mechanized warfare. At that time a chemist named Harold Dakin went to England from the United States and volunteered to help the war effort. His contribution stays with us to this day, almost a hundred years later, as Dakin's Solution. It is cheap and effective at wound cleansing and can be made from off-the-shelf materials (the kind of thing we just love).

Formula To Make Dakin's Solution

Take four cups of sterilized water (or 32 ounces). You can easily sterilize water by boiling it for about fifteen minutes with a cover on the pot.

Add one half of a teaspoon of baking soda (sodium bicarbonate).

Bleach (Clorox or regular household bleach): here is the only tricky part.

Depending on the severity of the infection you can make various strengths of Dakin's solution:

For clean wounds, wound dressing changes: Add three teaspoons of bleach.

Mildly infected wounds: Add three tablespoons of bleach.

Severe infections: Add 3 fluid ounces (95 ml).

NOTE: This solution will not last longer than two days. So you will have to mix a new batch when needed. Also remember that bleach rapidly loses its potency over time. If it is old bleach, you may have to double these mixing amounts to get the same strength. Also, remember to wash your hands well with soap and water to prevent accidentally infecting a wound you are trying to clean.

Herbal Wound Cleansers

Another alternative method for keeping a wound clean is the use of herbal preparations as an antiseptic solution.

You can mix a few drops of these oils with some sterile water and wash out the wounds or clean the surface of wounds thoroughly. The following essential oils can be utilized to make this wound cleansing mix:

Eucalyptus oil
Lavender oil
Rosemary Oil
Peppermint oil
Tea tree oil

NOTE: It would be wise to learn how to grow these herbs, some of which like peppermint, lavender, and rosemary, I grow in my garden and are very easy and fun to grow.

I would recommend getting a book on medicinal herbs and keeping a section of your garden open to grow them. Be careful with peppermint, oregano and other mints, they all are very easy to grow and can become invasive. I would suggest using a few old five gallon buckets or large plastic bags that peat moss or manure comes in, and use these as planters to grow these herbs in so they don't take over your entire garden.

Learning how to make essential oils from these is not only fun, but could save your life. Any skills that we can develop will help us be more valuable to you and your inner circle of family and friends, and at the same time it is a blast to learn. These essential oils and tinctures are relatively easy to make for your own natural medicine chest.

One of my favorites is mojito mint, which as you might have guessed is the ingredient in that Cuban summertime drink called mojitos. A curious botanical fact about the mint family, they are the only plants who have square rather than round stems.

When cleansing a wound, take special care to look for foreign material (for example, dirt, glass, bullets, and wood splinters), and remove as much of it as possible, without causing further trauma. Take a tweezer and sterilize it with alcohol (or as directed in the section on sterilization of instruments) and use that to pick out any debris that does not flush out with water.

Note: Burns and bites are treated differently; refer to those sections of this book for complete details.

Betadine And Sterile Water

The formula for this mix is one part Betadine to ten parts of sterile water. Sterilize the water as described above and mix as much as you need. The iodine in the Betadine does a wonderful job of cleaning wounds.

Tetanus Vaccination

No matter how you feel about vaccines and their possible toxicity, the tetanus vaccine is the exception. It is the only way to prevent lockjaw (also known as tetanus) and is essential for everyone since Clostridium Tetani (the bacterium that causes tetanus infections) is ubiquitous (it is everywhere). Clostridium Tetani enters the body through open wounds and multiplies in the wound and releases a toxin known as tetanospasmin, which attacks the nervous system and causes the jaw to spasm and actually lock shut, hence the name lockjaw.

It also leads to severe contraction and spasm of other skeletal muscles, resulting in fractures of bones (breaking) and muscle tearing, incontinence of urine and stool (peeing and defecating on yourself). It has a mortality (death) rate of between 48 and 73 percent and it is a horrible way to die, especially since it can so easily be prevented. Children get their tetanus vaccine as part of a multivalent vaccine called TDAP (Tetanus, Diphtheria and Acellular Pertussis or Whooping Cough). Adults get their tetanus shots every ten years and if you are not sure, now is the time to get a booster. You need the boosters because after time your body's lymphocyte production of antibodies to tetanus falls off with a resulting decline in your immunity. If you get it early it will not hurt you. Therefore I recommend that you get your tetanus booster ASAP.

Activated Charcoal for Wound Healing

Making a poultice (wound salve) of activated charcoal is very effective at promoting wound healing. The surface area of the activated charcoal is so great that it effectively inactivates large amounts of bacteria and toxins on its surface, rendering them inactive. It also promotes healing quite rapidly in many cases. There are two different ways to make a charcoal poultice, either with or without the addition of flaxseed. The flaxseed is used as a thickener and it will keep the poultice moister for a longer time.

Remember: this is critical; poultices only work when they retain their moisture and are in direct contact with the patient's skin.

1. Grind three tablespoons of flaxseed (or alternatively you may use cornstarch).
2. Add to this two or three tablespoons of activated charcoal powder.
3. Add about one cup of water. You can use more or less depending on how thick you want to make your poultice.
4. Let the poultice mix sit for fifteen minutes so the ingredients will thoroughly mix. Or you can put it in a pot and gently heat it up to help the mixing.
5. Spread the poultice mix onto a clean piece of cloth and apply that directly to the wound.
6. Cover the first dressing with a dry clean dressing.
7. Cover the entire dressing with plastic, such as plastic food wrap, overlapping the poultice by about an inch on each side, and bandage or tape it directly in place. You can use duct tape to tape it if you have no surgical tape. The taping is critical, because it prevents air from getting under the plastic wrap and drying out the poultice, rendering it ineffective.
8. Leave the poultice on the wound and change it daily or whenever it dries out.

NOTE: This activated charcoal poultice is also very effective in the treatment of burns; insect bites including brown recluse spiders, scorpions, and black widow spiders; and also works very nicely on contact dermatitis type rashes such as poison ivy, poison oak, and poison sumac. It can also be used for puncture wounds. I would refer you to a wonderful website called *CharcoalRemedies.com*. It is the absolute final word in anything related to activated charcoal.

PUNCTURE WOUNDS AND THEIR TREATMENT

Puncture wounds are treated differently than other wounds. The first thing you should do is remove the source of the puncture. A knife is the only exception; normally these are not removed until in a hospital setting. If you have no choice then and only then would I remove it slowly and steadily, only if you really don't have any other options.

Allow some bleeding so it flushes out the wound by the mechanical motion of the exiting blood, then you should apply direct pressure as described above to stop the bleeding and stabilize the wound. Now clean the wound as above.

Due to the problem of wound contamination with puncture wounds, I would use the hydrogen peroxide initially either full strength (of the 3% hydrogen peroxide) or half-and-half with sterile water if you have it. Alternatively you can use Dakin's solution or a one part to ten parts mix of Betadine and water. If not, use your drinking water as the next best choice.

Do a good job of thoroughly flushing out this wound, taking special care to remove any debris. Look for broken off splinters, glass, and other foreign material. If it is on a limb, I usually squeeze it from both directions a few times to see if anything else comes out. Several times I have been pleasantly surprised by a large sliver of wood coming out with just some pressure.

Now apply some honey directly into the wound, or antibiotic cream if you have any. Cover the wound with a sterile gauze dressing or the cleanest possible material you have. Watch it closely for signs of any infection. I would also apply an activated charcoal poultice to it once the bleeding has been stabilized. See above for complete description of how that is done.

CHAPTER TWENTY-SIX

CONSTIPATION

INTRODUCTION

TABLE OF CONTENTS:

Constipation is the lack of bowel movements or decreased frequency of bowel movements or the passage of hard, dry stool. It is somewhat subjective; men typically have more frequent and larger bowel movements than women. The average adult has one bowel movement daily. It is a commonly faced clinical problem and you will undoubtedly personally encounter it at some time.

You are definitely constipated if you are passing only three stools a week and they are hard and dry. Severe constipation is one bowel movement per week.

CONSTIPATION SYMPTOMS AND COMPLICATIONS

Bloating, Abdominal Cramps, Fecal Impaction, And Vomiting

The usual symptoms are straining to have a bowel movement, feeling of incompletely emptying your bowels and/or feeling of obstruction with abdominal bloating. Some patients experience severe abdominal pain and cramping that is quite incapacitating. Severe constipation can lead to a condition known as fecal impaction, where the feces is actually packed into the rectum and cannot be passed. In these cases many patients have to resort to digging with their fingers into their rectum to remove this stool blockage. Talk about a bad day. Extreme cases of constipation can even lead to vomiting.

When constipation alternates with diarrhea, this is known as Irritable Bowel Syndrome or IBS. This is a very common condition, and you will most likely see many patients complaining of this combination. Most of the time either diarrhea or constipation predominate and this is commonly referred to as IBS-D or IBS-C. IBS is frequently accompanied by abdominal cramping and pain as well as bloating, and the incidence of it increases with age peaking at middle age. Sudden onset of these symptoms after the age of fifty should always be investigated to rule out other diseases.

Rectal Bleeding

The rectal bleeding from constipation is a consequence of passing a hard dry stool which as it passes through the rectum will tear some of the rectal tissue and cause bleeding.

Sometimes patients will notice some rectal bleeding either on the toilet paper or mixed in with their stool. The color of blood in stool tells a lot about its origin. The higher up the GI tract the darker the blood will become. If it originates in the stomach it may exit your anus looking like black tar. This is because it has become digested by the stomach acids and intestinal activity. Bright red blood per rectum is usually from a source very close to the rectum and is most frequently caused by a hemorrhoid; other causes are rectal fissures. A rectal fissure is a small linear tear in your rectum, almost exclusively caused by passing a large hard dry stool. Hemorrhoids are by far the most common cause of rectal bleeding.

There are two types of hemorrhoids, internal (inside your rectum) and external (these you can feel and see on the outside, they look round, red/blue, engorged with blood). There are several other less common causes of rectal bleeding such as a bleeding diverticulum, ulcerative colitis, Crohn's disease, cancer and ulcers.

SIGNS OF CONSTIPATION ON THE PHYSICAL EXAMINATION

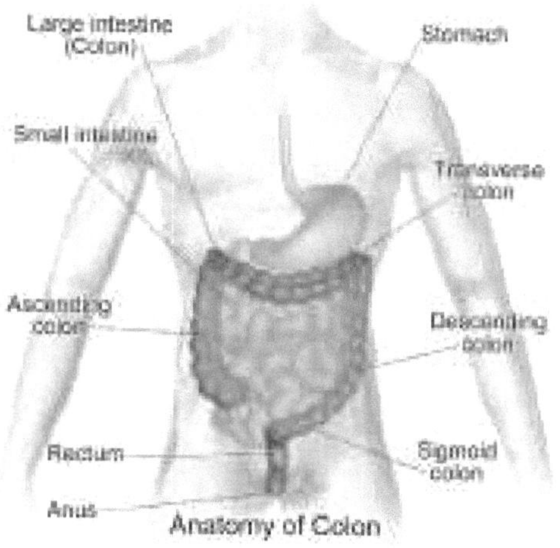

One of the most common signs of constipation on the physical examination is a bloated, distended (it is protruding outward) abdomen. In some patients if they are very thin you may actually be able to palpate (feel) a hard stool in either the ascending, transverse, or descending colon.

Decreased bowel sounds are a frequent sign of constipation. Normally as food is digested and it passes through your intestines, the intestines will make sounds; these sounds are called bowel sounds. Bowel sounds are perfectly normal, however they often are decreased in constipation. If you do not have a stethoscope you can have the patient lie on their backs in what is known as a supine position (lying on your abdomen is a prone position), put your ear to their abdomen and listen to the bowel sounds. Bowel sounds typically sound like water running through pipes, they may also sound like rumbling and even gurgling.

They should be fairly constant, with only a second or so between sounds, when there are more than a few seconds between sounds this is known as hypoactive bowel sounds and is a sign of constipation.

Another sign of constipation that I see quite often is a tongue coated white. The tongue is the barometer of your intestinal tract. A white tongue is a sign of constipation or at the very least very slow intestinal transit time. Nobody is quite sure why this occurs but some say it is due to the lymphatic sluggishness and decreased flow that accompanies constipation. You will notice that once the constipation clears, so slowly will the tongue turn pink once again.

THE CAUSES OF CONSTIPATION

Inadequate Fluid Intake

Lack of adequate fluid intake, especially fresh water, is one of the most common causes of constipation. This often occurs when there is too little water entering the colon. The water in your colon gets absorbed and this can result in a hard, dry stool. A dry stool will also slow the passage of stool through your intestines and will increase the intestinal transit time. Intestinal transit time (also known as bowel transit time) is the time it takes for stool to pass through your GI tract from mouth to anus. Besides the stools water content, the intestinal transit time is also affected by the type of foods we eat; for example it is shorter when the diet is primarily fruits and vegetables and longer when eating a lot of sugar and starches.

Lack Of Fiber In The Diet

Lack of fiber from fruits, vegetables, whole grains and legumes (beans) is another major cause of constipation. Fiber is an indigestible carbohydrate from plants; it is indigestible because our bodies lack the proper enzymes to digest it. It is also known as roughage.

The reason for this is fiber cannot be digested by humans, that is why we cannot graze in a field like a horse and survive. The fiber passes through our bodies but is able to absorb toxins on its surface and absorb water. This keeps your stool soft and also makes it float. Ideally your stools should be a fluffy consistency and be brown in color and float in your toilet and not sink. Okay, this is probably more than you ever wanted to know about stool.

Americans currently eat approximately 10 to 20 grams of fiber daily; we should be eating much more, in the range of 25 to 35 grams daily. Higher intake of dietary fiber has many benefits beyond helping with constipation; it helps lower rates of colon cancer and helps control cholesterol, diabetes, and your weight.

Types of Dietary Fiber

Fiber In Our Diet Comes In Two Types, Soluble And Insoluble.

Soluble fiber dissolves in water, forming into a gel-like consistency, and supports the health of probiotic intestinal bacterial populations by acting as a food for them, or what is known as a prebiotic; they are fermented in the colon to intestinal gases. Soluble fiber helps to control blood glucose levels and also lowers cholesterol levels. Soluble fiber also helps you to lose weight by slowing the release of glucose into the blood, thereby helping to reduce spikes in insulin levels which lead to obesity. Soluble fiber helps constipation by swelling with water and expanding into a gel that exerts pressure on the intestinal wall causing it to contract in response, thus moving along the food/stool.

Insoluble fiber does not dissolve and acts as a bulking agent, drawing water into the colon thus keeping the stools soft and pliable and helps their movement through the intestines, thereby helping constipation. Insoluble fiber also acts as a prebiotic. Insoluble fiber helps weight loss but by a different mechanism than soluble fiber, it acts as a bulking agent promoting satiety (helps you feel full after eating).

Lack Of Exercise

Exercise is essential to maintain proper bowel movements; in fact, lack of exercise is a cause of constipation. The muscles of your abdomen contracting will help pass your stools faster through your intestines; this also decreases the time available for the colon to absorb water from your stools, thus keeping them moist and pliable and preventing constipation.

Even normal walking fifteen minutes daily will help prevent or eliminate constipation problems. Do not exercise for about an hour after eating; if you do it will shunt blood away from your digestive tract towards your skeletal muscles and heart, thus slowing digestion. Any exercising will help, it does not have to be walking, the more aerobic exercise the better.

Narcotic Analgesics

The use of opioids or narcotic analgesics will cause your intestines to slow down and lead to constipation. Narcotic analgesics are painkillers such as Percocet, OxyContin, morphine, and hydrocodone but a few of the commonly prescribed opioids. To make matters worse approximately 10 to 15 percent of patients taking narcotics will have the paradoxical situation where the narcotics actually make the pain worse by sensitizing the nerves in the bowel, this is known as narcotic bowel syndrome. Opioid induced constipation is another term for the syndrome of constipation while using narcotic analgesics or opioid's.

Hormonal Changes And Constipation

Women are twice as likely as men to suffer with constipation problems due to the hormonal changes women undergo around the time of their menses (periods), as well as during menopause where fully a quarter of women have complications of constipation.

Supplements

Supplements like iron and calcium can both lead to constipation. Iron is notorious for causing constipation in patients and often is discontinued for that reason. Many women take iron due to menstrual blood loss and resulting iron deficiency anemia, and women also take calcium to prevent osteoporosis, also causing constipation problems.

Age

As we advance in age due to a decrease in our thirst sensation we take in less water and this oftentimes leads to constipation problems. Many elderly patients are on multiple medications including narcotics and supplements which further worsen their constipation. Children are also more at risk for constipation than adults.

Antacids

Antacids such as Maalox, Mylanta, Tums, and others can cause constipation problems from both their calcium and aluminum content. Alternatively, antacids such as milk of magnesia contain magnesium and may lead to diarrhea.

Hypothyroidism

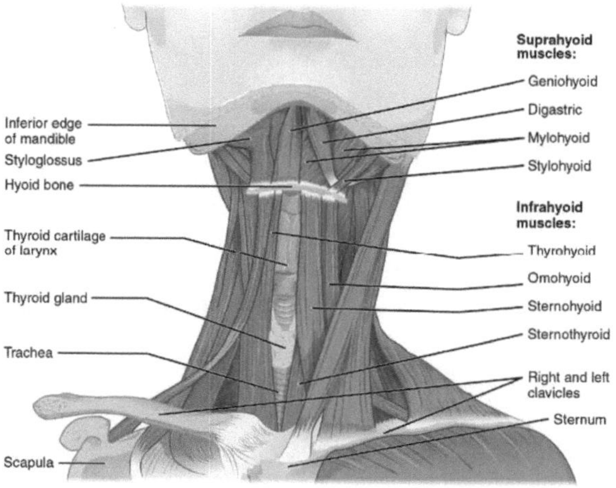

Hypothyroidism (slow or inadequate thyroid function) oftentimes leads to constipation. The thyroid gland controls metabolism and many of the body's functions, when it slows down so do many functions, such as the normal peristalsis or wave-like movement of food from the mouth to the anus. Hypothyroidism can also weaken the normal contractions of the muscles in the bowel wall, also leading to constipation.

How Does the Thyroid Gland Function?

Now for a quick lesson in thyroid physiology (function): The thyroid gland produces T4, which is so named for the four iodine molecules attached to the protein skeleton. When T4 circulates in the body it goes to the body's tissues where a selenium-dependent enzyme cleaves off one of the iodine's and changes it to T3, which is the active form of thyroid hormone. T3 is readily absorbed by all the cells and tissues in our body. Matters get further complicated by free and total hormone levels. Hormones are fat soluble, the blood is primarily composed of water, so most hormones circulate bound to a protein, in order to enter the body's cells these protein-bound hormones have to be cleaved or separated from the protein. Only the free hormone is active, the protein-bound hormone is not.

For example, total T3 measures all the T3 in the blood, free T3 levels measure the free or unbound T3 in the blood, to determine the amount of protein-bound T3 just subtract the free T3 from the total T3.

Sometimes the type of thyroid medications you are taking may contribute to your constipation problems. Synthroid (stands for synthetic thyroid) and Levothyroxine are both standard treatments for hypothyroidism; both are synthetic and both contain only T4. Many patients either are deficient in selenium so the enzyme to change T4 to T3 does not work, or they have genetically low levels of the same enzyme, producing the same end result. In order to avoid this problem I like to prescribe natural forms of thyroid hormone usually made from cows or pigs, such as Armour thyroid, Nature-Throid, and other natural desiccated (dried) forms of thyroid hormone. In this way you don't have to worry if the patient can convert T4 to T3 since you are providing both forms.

Note: The enzymes that are responsible for the conversion of T4 to T3 are known as the deiodinase enzymes and are dependent upon adequate blood levels of the mineral selenium to properly function.

Diuretics

Diuretics or what are commonly referred to as "water pills" are medications that make you urinate. As such they decrease the amount of water in your body and as described above dehydration oftentimes leads to hard, dry stools and constipation.

Dairy Products

A diet that is heavily skewed to dairy products such as milk, cheese, ice cream, and yogurt are without any significant amounts of fiber and as such can cause constipation. They also contain significant amounts of fat which may also delay digestion.

Antihistamines

Antihistamines have several adverse reactions such as blurry vision, sedation, urinary retention, and constipation. The reason for the constipation is the same reason that stops your runny nose and your congestion, it is due to their drying effect.

TREATMENT OF CONSTIPATION

General Considerations

If you can figure out the underlying abnormality then that should be the target of your treatment. For example, if the patient appears dehydrated (the cardinal sign of which will be a dry, furrowed (cracked) tongue, then administer fresh water or other fluids. If the patient's diet is lacking in fiber then give them some fresh fruit, vegetables, or fiber supplements. Note: Fiber administered without water or other fluids will make matters worse. Fiber only works because it absorbs fluids and moistens the stool allowing it to be flexible and pass through the intestines. The ideal daily dose of fiber should be about 25 to 30 grams and contain a mixture of soluble and insoluble fiber. At least one and a half to two quarts of water a day should be given. If you have fiber supplements use them with water, I would also increase the fruit and vegetable content of your diet. There are many sources of fiber that you might not be aware of such as: Bran cereal, psyllium seed (Metamucil), and Citrucel. All of these will work and it comes down to taste and personal preference. In an emergency situation it will come down simply to availability. Remember, take at least a full, large glass of water with each dose of any of these fiber supplements.

Coffee And Tea

Give the patient some warm water in the morning. Most people have a nice bowel movement after they have had their coffee. Coffee and tea, due to their caffeine content, will stimulate your bowels, but it is also a diuretic (makes you urinate). So if you have coffee use it, but just make sure the patient follows it with more water than usual during the day to make up for any diuretic effect of the caffeine. Remember, only black, white, or green tea has caffeine, the herbal teas do not contain caffeine.

Milk Of Magnesia, Magnesium, Potassium, And Epsom Salt

There is a saying that all medical residents learn during the arduous years of their medical training: "If no BM in the PM, then MOM (milk of magnesia) in the AM". It works well because of its magnesium content. Magnesium and potassium both stimulate bowel movements.

A very inexpensive source of magnesium is Epsom salt. I have found very few treatments to be as effective as an 8-ounce glass of water with two to four level teaspoons of Epsom salt (half this dose in children. You can repeat this in four hours. This usually produces a very nice bowel movement from one half hour to six hours. This should be limited to one week's time. Do not give this in patients with renal failure (kidney disease). Another form of magnesium known as magnesium citrate is also frequently used for constipation, it comes in a 10-ounce bottle, they are like depth charges and if you are not obstructed, they will open you right up. If you have magnesium tablets, then 250 mg two or even four times a day will open up most constipations.

Prunes And Other Dried Fruits

Prunes or any dried fruit like raisins or dried figs, cranberries, dates, or cherries will work just fine, but they have to be given with large amounts of water. They have high potassium content and this along with their fiber content causes bowel movements. Prune juice is an excellent choice for treating constipation, and I would keep some readily available as part of your natural medicine chest. A cup of prune juice contains approximately 2.6 grams of soluble and insoluble fiber. Prunes also contain a sugar alcohol called sorbitol which is incompletely digested by the body (it is not an alcohol like ethanol that is in alcoholic beverages and will not give you a buzz), but does contribute to the softness of stools and also helps constipation. Studies show that prune juice is the preferred treatment by patients and even beats out psyllium seed in patient satisfaction surveys.

Psyllium Seed

Psyllium seed works very well for constipation; it acts as a bulk-forming laxative. Metamucil is psyllium seed or husk. Psyllium originated in India and comes from a plant called Plantago ovata, but currently is grown all over the world. Each Plantago ovata plant makes up to 15, 000 small seeds that have a gel-like coating to them. When psyllium seed comes in contact with water it forms a gelatinous (jelly-like) mass that helps keep stools soft and facilitates their movement through the intestines.

Psyllium seed acts like a "normalizer" helping the dry stool of constipation, as well as helping soak up excess water in patients with diarrhea Psyllium husk/seed also helps control blood glucose levels in diabetics by slowing the absorption of sugar and also helps lower cholesterol levels.

Psyllium seed comes in many forms; bulk seed, powder, tablets, and capsules; you will have to follow whatever directions come with each form. If it is the bulk seed then one teaspoon which is about 5 grams taken twice daily should work just fine, as long as it is taken with a large glass of water (about 10 to 12 ounces).

Hyperosmolar Laxatives

Hyperosmolar laxatives such as Miralax and Kristalose are indigestible and non-absorbable compounds that remain in the intestine and osmotically draw water into it, softening the stool and helping bowel movements. If you have chronic constipation currently, you should make a point of stockpiling some of these treatments in your medicine chest because you and I know you will need them. By the way, that is a good idea for any chronic medical problem you have; stockpile more of what you will most likely need. These types of laxatives may lead to lots of intestinal gas (farting). Hopefully you won't find yourself in a crowded elevator, if so your only hope is to get aggressive and blame someone else!

Mineral Oil

Mineral oil can be ingested in small amounts for a short time. They work well to open up constipated bowels. I am not a big fan of them. They also prevent the absorption of fat soluble vitamins by the body like multivitamins, vitamins A, D, E, and K. I would only use mineral oil if no other treatments are available. Mineral oil can also be given by enema but this would require enema bags and tubing and most likely these would not be available.

Probiotics

I would certainly stock my medicine chest with a supply of these valuable bacteria they will certainly help normalize your bowel movements.

A good intestinal flora (living bacteria residents of your gut) is of primary importance and very helpful for both your intestinal as well as your immune system's health.

Fermented foods will provide not only good bacteria but also will provide enzymes that aid in digestion, and fermented foods taste great. The only way we are going to be able to keep probiotics in our diets in the long run will be by continuous fermentation which will also enhance our food supplies. Prior to the modern era the propagation of certain yeasts and other probiotics were passed down within families and communities, in some case such as the yeast responsible for making bread. That yeast was originally wild yeast that was discovered several thousand years ago and was found to cause dough to rise and over generations became domesticated and symbiotic with man.

Yogurt, kefir, and kombucha are good sources of probiotics. Yogurt and kefir can be made from milk as long as you have the proper starting materials and, for kefir, are able to keep a continuous supply of the kefir grains available. Kefir grains are a unique combination of yeasts and bacteria. When added to a milk base the bacteria feast on the lactose in the milk and the yeast help ferment the mix. It is fairly easy to make and a very smart way to turn ordinary milk into a nutrient and probiotic powerhouse. Kombucha is a fermented drink made with tea, sugar, bacteria, and yeast, and as such is chock full of beneficial probiotics.

Bentonite Clay

Bentonite clay is a natural clay found in large deposits in the western United States. It is named for its discovery near Fort Benton, Wyoming. Bentonite is a trade name for Montmorillonite, the active ingredient which is a mineral. It is formed from the weathering of volcanic ash deposits. These types of clays are wonderful for constipation and other bowel problems. Their action is due to their large surface area which is very porous and able to absorb large quantities of toxins. At the same time they provide much-needed minerals to the body.

The mineral content of the clay has a negative charge and many toxins are positively charged, hence their ability to attract toxins and bind them.

Remember, similar charges repel each other (i.e., two negatives or two positives), but opposite charges attract each other. I recommend taking these clays either in powder form or pill form. Take them on an empty stomach at least one hour before or one hour after a meal.

If it is a powder take one tablespoon a day mixed with some juice, this can eventually be increased to four times a day if needed.

Fenugreek

Fenugreek's botanical name is Trigonella foenum-graecum. Fenugreek is an herb that has a long history of medicinal use, used as far back as 1500 BC by the Egyptians. Fenugreek contains high levels of soluble fiber and as such is very helpful in the treatment of constipation. As with all soluble fiber, it absorbs water like a sponge, as it does so it expands and exerts pressure against the intestinal walls, triggering their contraction and thus the movement of food/stool through the intestines, alleviating constipation. The usual dose is 250 mg or 2 ml twice daily with food.

You can also use fenugreek as a poultice, warming it and applying it to painful muscles and joints. The leaves of fenugreek can also be eaten.

Gentian Root

Gentian root is an herb that comes from the yellow gentian plant whose botanical name is Gentiana lutea.

It is a native of Europe, where the root has been used for centuries. Gentian has a very bitter taste. Gentian has long been used to stimulate appetite and to aid in digestion. It has long been used to treat constipation and as such is very effective. Gentian is also used to help alleviate vomiting and heartburn (reflux).

The typical dose of the tincture is 1-3 ml mixed in water and slowly sip this mixture about a half hour before a meal. It also comes in powder form, tea, and extract. As a powder, take 300 mg once again about a half an hour before a meal.

Aloe Vera

Aloe Vera is a very easy plant to grow; in the northern United States it must be taken inside during the winter but it will survive quite nicely if placed in front of a sunny window. Aloe contains two medicinal ingredients, a clear gel from the cells in the center of the leaves and a yellow latex which comes from directly under the thick green skin of the leaves.

Both the gel and the latex help relieve constipation by its laxative effect as well as helping to break down food in the intestines thereby helping with digestion and constipation.

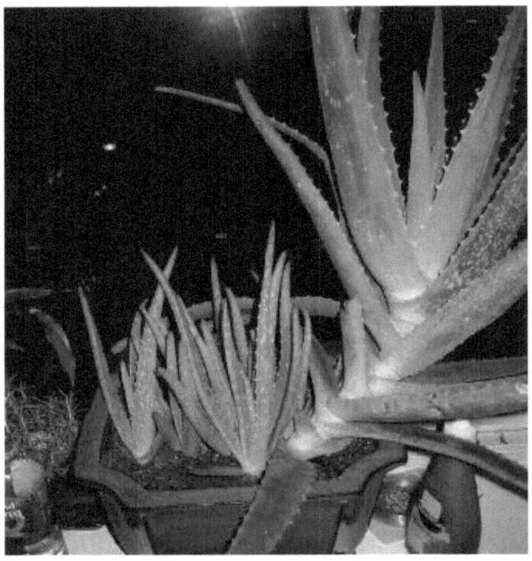

The clear gel in the cells of the leaves also helps soothe any burns or skin ailments. I usually break off a leaf from the plant and split it open lengthwise and scoop out the clear gel and combine it with a little water, making it into a liquid/gel combination.

I apply this to any skin irritations or burns and it rapidly heals them. For constipation many people drink Aloe Vera juice. The usual dose is a quarter cup twice daily. Dried aloe can be taken twice daily as needed, the dose varies and you should play with it to find the right dose that works for you. You can also combine Aloe Vera with Psyllium, the two work very nice together to relieve constipation.

Cascara Sagrada

Cascara Sagrada is the dried bark of the Rhamnus purshianus, this small, woody shrub is native to western and the northwestern United States. Cascara sagrada is Spanish for sacred bark. The bark of this plant is very effective in relieving constipation, in fact the bark is so strong that you have to dry it for a year to weaken it, otherwise the patient's constipation will turn into a very messy diarrhea! Cascara sagrada comes in a tea and in capsules.

For constipation take a 450 mg capsule at bedtime, make sure you drink a very large glass of water to insure it will work properly.

These work well and are inexpensive; for four dollars you can easily find a bottle of 100 of these, for twenty bucks you have a lifetime supply. You can also purchase it in tincture form, as such take

2-3 ml three times a day as needed, once the constipation ends, discontinue its use. All forms have to be taken with a generous amount of water.

Enemas

The use of enemas should be reserved for those cases of constipation where the patient is not getting better with other methods. The danger of enemas is that they will make the bowel wall lazy and eventually unable to evacuate stool. Enemas in various forms have been practiced around the world for centuries.

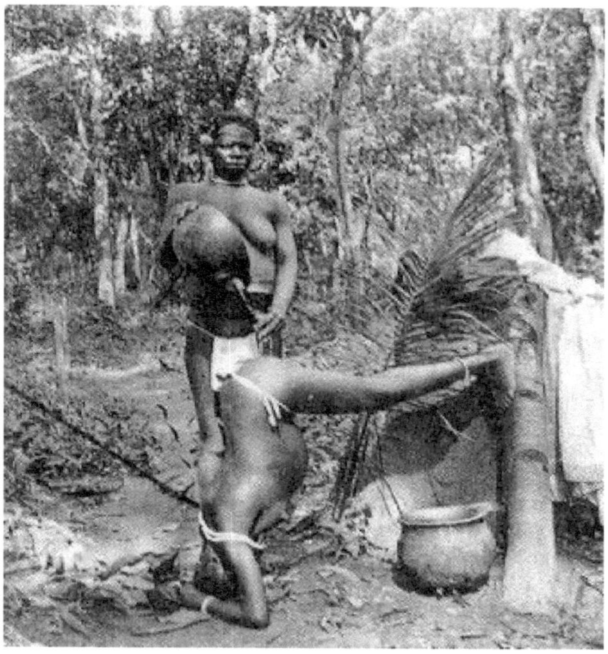

See the photo above of an African native getting an enema.

Enemas work quickly and are safe if done on occasion. The two best solutions to instill are salt water and clear water. Try to avoid the use of soapsuds enemas, the soap may be too harsh for the intestinal mucosa and could irritate it. Done properly, enemas are safe and will help flush stool out of the colon.

If you or one of your family members routinely suffers with constipation then having enema bags and tubing are essential items to have for your alternative/medicine chest. Enemas are composed of a bag to hold the salt water solution (or whatever else you use) connected to clear plastic tubing that gets lubed and slid into the patient's rectum.

Be very careful not to push the lubed tube into the rectum if there is resistance; if so, stop. The patient lies either on their side in a fetal position with their knees bent and brought up to their chest, or on their back with their knees bent. Once the contents of the enema bag are completely emptied into the colon you are done; usually the patient has a bowel movement within an hour.

Try to limit your use of enemas on your patient to no more than once daily, to avoid weakening of the bowels and further exacerbation (worsening) of the constipation. Heating the solution will make it more comfortable for the patient; approximately 100 to 110 F means the water is hot to the touch but will not burn you.

Enema bags are available in reusable and disposable types. In reality both can be reused, especially if you are only instilling salt water or clear water. These bags can also be reused as hot water bottles and the entire setup can be used to douche. Buy a substantial supply of the tubing, if it gets ruined by becoming clogged or some other way then it can be reused as tourniquets. Enema bags come in various sizes ranging from one or two liters up to large four liter bags. Do not instill more than one liter the first time you give an enema to a patient and not more than two liters at any given time. The usefulness of the larger four liter bags is that you only have to fill them once and can use them from two to four times.

In small children even one liter will be too much to instill, do not use more than half a liter and if they are under 80 lbs use a quarter of a liter. What you don't want to ever do is instill too much fluid which could rupture their colon, so it is best to start with very small amounts, less than you think you will need. You could also use a large bulb syringe that holds 500 cc instead of an enema bag. Make sure to lubricate it well.

Be advised that after you empty a bulb syringe into a patient you should keep the bulb squeezed down. Do not allow it to re-inflate, which will suck feces into the syringe. Most enema bags are made of latex but they also can be found made of silicone. Also make sure you have a clamp to put at the top of the tubing near to where the tubing attaches to the enema bag in order to be able to control the flow and shut it if need be.

You can jerry rig an IV pole to hang your enema by attaching an upside down hanger to a broomstick and then attach the enema bag to that and allow gravity to do its work , or it can be held upright until it fully empties.

Salt water enemas are preferable to plain water. Plain water enemas cause electrolytes to be drawn from the colon and can deplete them in the patient's body; salt water does not do that and is considered safer.

Making a solution of salt water for your enema is simple, mix one teaspoon of sea salt into a liter of water, if you are not sure what a liter is use a soda bottle for comparison. Now don't you wish you paid attention in school when they covered the metric system!

Fecal Transplants

If you or if you have someone in your family suffering with Inflammatory Bowel Disease which is Crohn's and Ulcerative Colitis, or are suffering with Clostridium difficile infections or what is commonly referred to as C. diff, then you might want to consider the use of fecal transplants.

Fecal transplants are also known as fecal microbiota transplantation (FMT). A fecal transplant is essentially the restoration of a healthy gut microbial population which has been shown to be very helpful in treating these conditions, so much so that for patients with C. diff there is an over 90 percent cure rate! The Mayo Clinic used these enemas and had 100 percent success, many left the hospital within hours or a day or two after being there for weeks, only two suffered relapses and needed to be retreated.

Fecal transplants can be given from above (through the mouth) via a nasogastric tube or from below via enema infusion. Enemas are the preferred method because they more frequently deliver live healthy bacteria directly to where it is needed; passing through the harsh acidic stomach will kill large numbers of bacteria, as it supposed to. The Mayo Clinic policy was to use healthy family members, and you can either use them or some healthy volunteer from your family or friends. If you have many donors to choose from I would find the healthiest, normal weight, nondiabetic with no autoimmune diseases and use his or her feces to make your solution. National medical societies like the Infectious

Diseases Society of America and the American College of Gastroenterology and others have developed some basic criteria for choosing a fecal donor. They prefer an intimate partner or close family member who has never had any GI illnesses of any type, no cancer, syphilis, HIV, hepatitis, autoimmune diseases like rheumatoid arthritis, lupus, eczema, psoriasis, and has not had any antibiotics within the last three months. The potential donor also must not ever have had intestinal parasites of any type due to the risk of potentially passing parasites to the recipient. The donor should also have normal-appearing stools.

If you are not sure of how stool should look use the Bristol Stool Chart that I have provided below; it is not ideal, but a good way to screen potential donors for ideal-appearing stools. On the chart types 1, 2 signify constipation and 3, 4 are ideal; 5, 6, and 7 represent varying degrees of diarrhea. Type 4 is probably the closest to being ideal. I would add to this that an ideal stool should float in the toilet and be brown in color.

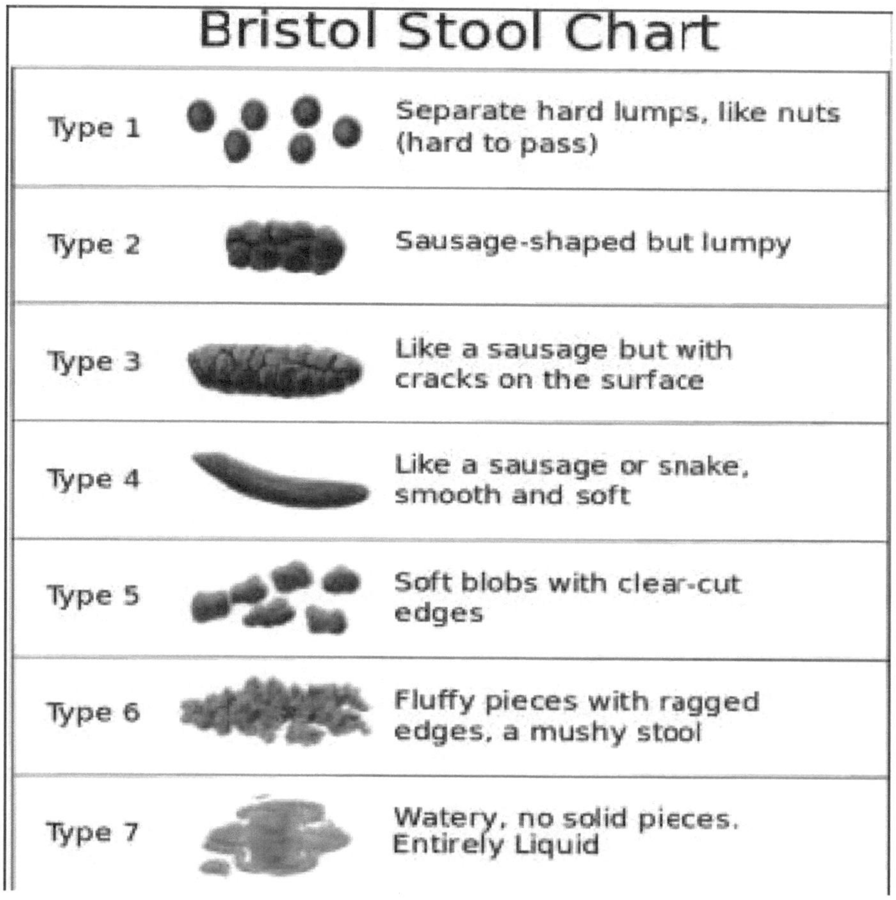

All of this being said, it is still early in everyone's experience with fecal transplants and it appears to be without any significant complications; the biggest risk of a fecal transplant is probably mechanical, perforation of an inflamed colon by inserting the enema tube. Fecal transplants are currently being evaluated for everything from diabetes, and rheumatoid arthritis, IBS (irritable bowel syndrome), multiple sclerosis, chronic fatigue syndrome, Parkinson's disease, constipation, celiac disease, and even obesity!

This will even work for VRE or vancomycin-resistant enterococci, which usually are multi-drug resistant.

How fecal transplants work for autoimmune diseases is not clear, but we do know that fully 70 percent of the body's immune cells lie within the walls of the gut, and there does appear to be some communication between healthy intestinal bacterial colonies (probiotic bacteria) and the immune system. For that reason it appears that a healthy infusion of probiotic bacteria from a healthy donor might just be enough to boost your immunity and quiet down autoimmune diseases, perhaps also by healing the intestinal lining and preventing "leaky gut". The bottom line is that it is just too early and we don't know that much about it other than anecdotal reports from doctors providing this new treatment and patients experimenting with it on their own.

Currently in the United States the FDA prevents doctors from using fecal transplants for any condition other than C. diff, unless they are in a clinical trial of some sort but that is in evolution and by the time you read this it may very well have changed.

I have a patient who had Ulcerative Colitis and became desperate and took some of his girlfriend's feces and mixed it with water and gave himself an enema and had a dramatic improvement, admittedly that is only one case but it has no significant side effects, is readily available from multiple sources, is free and many times has dramatic results.

How To Prepare A Fecal Transplant Enema

First you need to prepare the recipient for the fecal transplant. Make sure the patient is well hydrated and if they have a current infection allow them to take their antibiotics the day of the enema. Ideally a low fiber diet for two weeks before the enema would be helpful. Put the patient on clear liquids including no alcoholic beverages for twenty-four hours before the fecal transplant. The day of the transplant if you have any Imodium give it to the patient to prevent diarrhea and hopefully retain the fecal transplant contents in their bowels for as long as possible.

The day of the fecal transplant find an area that is comfortable for the patient, but at the same time limiting the potential for a spill. Perhaps have the patient lie on some couch cushions that you have covered with a tarp.

The stool of the donor should be similar to types 2, 3, and 4 on the Bristol Stool Chart. Obtain the sample and keep it at room temperature, you must use it within two hours of getting it or you risk significant die off of the good bacteria; if need be you can freeze it. No one knows for sure but it seems that frozen samples will remain viable for at least six months and some reports have used frozen specimens after ten months and they have worked just fine.

Take the donor stool and put it in a large zipper bag or plastic bag and mush it to a soft consistency like mashed potatoes. Avoid using a blender to mix it, this might damage the probiotics and also introduce too much air into the mix. Keep the mix in a sealed plastic bag to avoid too much air exposure which will dry it out and kill off its bacteria.

Take a liter of distilled water and heat it to about 100 F or so, about the same temperature that you would heat a baby's milk bottle. The temperature is important; too hot and you will kill the bacteria. Remember, these bacteria survive at the same temperature as your body, 98.6 F. That is why your body uses fever as a tool to kill bacteria and viruses. If the mix is too cold it will be uncomfortable for the patient and may result in intestinal cramping and pain. I am using a liter here as an example, you need to determine how much water you are going to add to the stool. The ideal consistency of the feces/water/saline mix should be a little more runny than paint, or similar to a thick soup like a bisque. You have to keep in mind that too thick will clog your tubing and too runny will be difficult for the patient to hold in and will just run out his or her butt, defeating the purpose of the fecal transplant.

Add your sea salt to the mix at a ratio of a half teaspoon per cup of distilled water. Do not use table salt unless you are desperate and have no other option, table salt frequently has other additives and does not have the ideal mineral mix that is in sea salt.

Take the mix and using a funnel, pour it into the enema bag. At this point you could use a strainer or some cheesecloth to remove large unwanted material, but this is optional. Be careful that the valve for the tubing is shut so the mix does not spill right out as you instill it.

Take some KY jelly, Vaseline, or other lubricant and lubricate the end of the enema tubing that is to be inserted in the patient's rectum. Have the patient lie on their left side and keep the patient's butt elevated on a cushion so it is higher than the rest of their body. Have the patient raise their right leg up by bending it; insert the enema tube into their rectum. This will be uncomfortable for most patients so be as gentle as you can. If it is painful for them you should put on a glove and lubricate your middle finger and gently insert it in their buttocks and rotate it to stretch it and make it more comfortable and then try again. The discomfort is usually short-lived and will in most cases pass in a minute or two. Encourage the patient to take a deep breath and relax, at this point making sure they are in a comfortable position is very important so they are able to lie still the entire time.

After instilling the contents of the enema have the patient lie still for ten minutes on their left side, while gently massaging their lower abdomen.

Next have them do the same thing for ten minutes while on their back and then lastly on their left side, each time gently massaging their abdomen. The patient should try to retain the enema in as long as possible, hopefully for at least six hours.

Often times some of the contents will ooze out of their anus, do not be overly concerned about this, just wipe them to keep them comfortable.

At this point, if you are using a reusable enema bag it is best to store it in a bucket of water with a pound of sea salt dissolved into it, this will be too saline for bad germs to live and will keep it clean.

You can repeat the fecal transplants as often as needed; each subsequent time should be easier for the patient and as you gain more experience.

CHAPTER TWENTY SEVEN

DIARRHEA AND ITS TREATMENT

INTRODUCTION

TABLE OF CONTENTS:

If there were ever important chapters to earmark, it would be this chapter on diarrhea as well as the previous chapter on constipation. These are two conditions that we everyday American's frequently encounter, and for many is the bane of their existence. Let's take a look at the root of the problem and how to treat it.

Diarrhea is when you are having loose, watery, and poorly formed stool. Diarrhea is always the result of an infection of the GI tract along with toxin production by the infecting organisms or irritation of the GI tract by a chemical or ingested substance. The human body reacts to these attacks on its GI mucosa in various ways; it will induce nausea and vomiting to expel the invaders or irritants as quickly as possible. Another defense mechanism of the GI tract is to pour out fluids into the intestines along with increasing the contractions of the intestines, both of which help expel the offending agent from the anus. The idea in either case is to rid the body of the infection or irritant and decrease the amount of time they remain in contact with the GI mucosa to prevent absorption.

When you are healthy and eating a proper diet, your stools should be well formed and float in the toilet. This means you are eating enough fiber (from fruits and vegetables in your diet). Fiber is not digestible by the human body, it acts like a sponge drawing in water and keeping your stools soft. A hard, dry stool is difficult to pass and unnatural, and many times painful. That is a sure sign that you are not getting enough fiber in your diet. Fiber will act as a normalizer. What that means is it will soak up excess fluid and dry up your stools or it will draw in fluid and keep your stools soft.

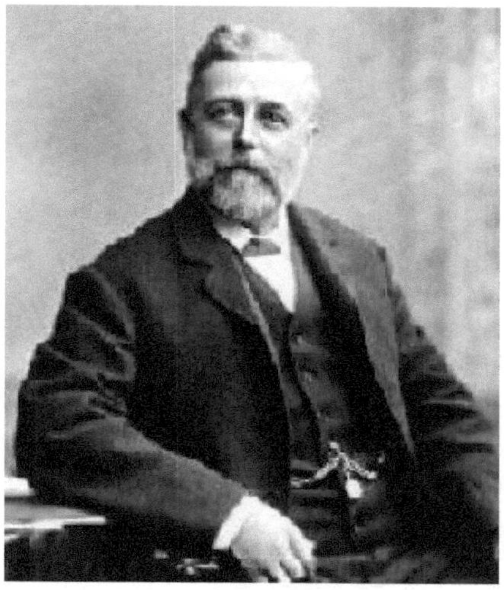

Photo of John Crapper, Popularizer of the Flush Toilet

Diarrhea or loose watery stools is usually self-limited and lasts only two or three days. Diarrhea of this short duration can be caused by many different factors and does not have to be treated, other than by hydration to replace fluid loses. Diarrhea of this short period is usually the result of a viral infection, the proverbial intestinal flu. Prolonged diarrhea is a different story and will need to be addressed.

CAUSES OF DIARRHEA

Viral Infections

Benign (harmless) viral infections: These are self-limited, meaning they only last a short time, viruses such as rotaviruses, noroviruses, hepatitis, herpes, and cytomegalovirus. In children the culprit is most often rotaviruses. The most common way these are contracted is through contact with an infected person (daycare centers are notorious for this) or ingestion of contaminated food or water. In all of these cases the viral infection will run its course over several days with or without treatment. Treatment should be aimed at fluid replacement, and in extreme cases some electrolytes especially potassium and magnesium.

Food Poisoning/Bacterial Infections

In our imperfect world this is a common scenario due to improper preservation of foods and contamination, as well as poor hygienic conditions and food handling. Various bacteria cause food poisoning. The fastest is botulism and this is about six hours. Patients frequently make the mistake of thinking their last meal was the cause of their food poisoning and that is usually not the case. Other frequent causes are campylobacter, shigella, salmonella, E. coli, and listeria.

Botulism comes primarily from canned foods that have spoiled. You should never eat a can of food that appears distended or swollen or rusty, with pinprick holes, or really beat up. The infection can be fatal and it is not worth eating no matter how hungry you may be. Botulism is most frequently found in improperly home-canned foods...especially those of low acidity such as beans, corn, asparagus, and beets. Even garlic packed in oil may get contaminated. You can also catch it from spores contained in an infant's stool. Honey should also not ever be given orally to infants less than one year old because of the possibility of it containing spores of Clostridium botulinum (the bacteria that causes botulism). An infant's undeveloped digestive system cannot destroy those spores and it is possible for them to become infected with botulism.

Since the spores are ubiquitous (all over the place) it is also possible for them to infect an open wound, but that is not very common .Practically speaking you will not have the means to differentiate between the various causes of diarrhea, so a lengthy discussion about the various treatments is pointless. The good news is that most food poisoning lasts only a day or two.

Note: Malaria may present as diarrhea and a fever that occurs every third or fourth day.

Food Intolerances And Alcoholic Beverages

Dairy products are the most common culprits causing diarrhea in many people. Lactose intolerance, which is genetic in most cases, is very prevalent in Sicilian, African, and Asian populations. They lack the enzyme lactase needed to properly digest lactose which is a sugar found in milk and dairy products. Most mammals become lactose intolerant after weaning from their mother's milk; in humans this oftentimes does not happen, however 75 percent of adults do have varying degrees of lactose intolerance, with some being completely intolerant.

In my practice I often see a transient (temporary or short-lived) lactose intolerance after someone has had an intestinal infection, this usually lasts about two weeks after which time they will once again be able to tolerate dairy products.

Excessive alcohol intake may trigger diarrhea in some patients. Food allergies can many times manifest with symptoms of diarrhea after eating the offending food; in these cases the best way to find the offending agent is to make a food diary, tracking what you eat.

Inflammatory Bowel Disease

The two inflammatory bowel diseases are Crohn's disease and Ulcerative Colitis. These frequently are associated with bloody, mucus-laden stools, with bowel movements many times daily, often with abdominal pain and cramping and weight loss. These diseases oftentimes are genetic and run in families, but sometimes they are not.

Malabsorption

Malabsorption is a syndrome where the intestine (primarily the small intestine) is unable to absorb certain nutrients. Malabsorption can be caused by disease, inflammation, injury, and a lack of digestive enzymes. Antibiotic use, diseases such as celiac disease, pancreatitis, gallbladder disease, liver disease, and cystic fibrosis may all cause malabsorption.

Radiation sickness can lead to damage to the intestinal lining resulting in severe malabsorption and diarrhea that is bloody. Your symptoms of malabsorption vary depending upon the substance you are having problems absorbing.

If it is fats you will have greasy, foul smelling stools that are like glue sticking to the sides of your toilet bowl. If it is proteins you will have leg swelling and possibly dry brittle hair and some generalized hair loss. Carbohydrate malabsorption will result in explosive diarrhea, flatulence (farting) and abdominal bloating. If you are not absorbing vitamins you will have many problems such as anemia, malnutrition and cachexia (generalized wasting).

Colon Cancer

The large intestine or colon is responsible primarily for water absorption; when working properly the stool will become progressively more solid (and drier) as it courses the length of the colon, moved along in its passage by the muscles of the colon wall. Basically anything that disturbs this process potentially can lead to diarrhea. In the case of colon cancer the diarrhea is oftentimes bloody, and accompanied by abdominal pain and bloating. It may or may not be associated with night sweats and weight loss. Usually by the time someone has weight loss and severe pain they are "end stage" and in advanced stages of the illness.

Giardia Infections (Giardiasis)

Giardia infections occur worldwide as a consequence of poor hygiene and contaminated water supplies. It is slowly becoming more common as a cause of diarrhea, I am not sure what that says about us as a society.

The infection with this microscopic parasite is known as Giardiasis. Giardiasis is a waterborne infection and as such will be found wherever there are bodies of water such as ponds, lakes, streams, swimming pools, reservoirs, and wells. It can also be spread person to person and through infected foods.

The symptoms of Giardiasis are abdominal cramping and pain, severe diarrhea with large quantities of watery stool, bloating, and nausea with occasional vomiting. The infection itself usually clears after two to three weeks, but many times there are residual gastrointestinal effects. The best method of treatment is prevention and good sanitation.

TREATMENT OF DIARRHEA

Rehydration And Rest

The cardinal rule for the treatment of diarrhea is rehydration. You need to replace the fluid lost; failure to do so will result in severe dehydration and eventually organ damage starting with the kidneys and ultimately death. Death from diarrhea comes quickly in infants and the very young, as well as the very old. In those patients you must be extra vigilant on replacing any lost fluids and electrolytes such as potassium, sodium, and chloride. The patient with diarrhea should also be encouraged to rest, especially if they are in a hot environment where activity will increase their imperceptible fluid losses from their skin and lungs.

Over-The-Counter Treatments

Some items you should include in your medicine chest for treatment of diarrhea are Pepto-Bismol, Imodium, and Kaopectate (made from kaolin clay). All come in both liquid and tablet form. They are inexpensive and available over- the-counter. I would keep a generous supply of these in your medicine chest.

The B.R.A.T. Diet

Diarrhea in young children can especially be fatal, as is often the case in third world countries. In this book's section on dehydration there is information on making rehydration fluids. As you rehydrate an infant or young child you can also start slowly feeding them again. The BRAT diet is a good place to start.

BRAT stands for Bananas, Rice, Applesauce, and Toast. The BRAT diet is easy for an infant or young child to digest and will help them regain their strength, it can also be used in adults. For adults a low fiber diet will also help, along with avoidance of excessively fatty (and greasy) foods as well as spicy foods.

Foods To Avoid

You should refer to the section on dehydration treatment for complete instructions on how to properly rehydrate someone. A few additional details will be useful to note.

Drink your fluids between meals, not with meals. Eliminate caffeine from your diet…that not only includes the obvious like coffee, but also caffeinated teas (herbal teas are not caffeinated), chocolate products, and Mountain Dew. Caffeine will only speed up your digestion, leading to worsening of your diarrhea.

You should eliminate dairy for at least two weeks and then slowly reintroduce it to see your body's reaction. You can drink fruit juice but it should be without any pulp, since pulp will worsen your diarrhea. Soup and broth will help, Gatorade and sports drinks as well, and decaf tea with honey will help as well. Remember, you are not only losing water but potassium, sodium, and chloride as well. All of these will need replacement.

If you develop a rectal or perianal (around your anus) irritation from the frequent stools you may need to use a barrier cream to soothe the area… this can be done with any of the diaper rash creams, white petroleum jelly (which also, like Vaseline, can be used to start fires; since it is a petroleum-based product it is highly flammable) and my personal favorite, Calmoseptine. Calmoseptine is a combination of zinc oxide and menthol which is very soothing and cooling to a burning butt and is very fast acting. Oral zinc administration has been shown to help diarrhea, especially in young children.

Probiotics

Probiotics also help to recolonize your intestines with friendly, health- promoting bacteria. This is especially important after use of antibiotics that are not selective and kill off beneficial as well as harmful bacteria. They should be taken with meals in order to provide prebiotics (food for the probiotics which are alive, good, bacteria, and will need to eat.). Studies have shown that probiotics interact with the intestinal cells and actually help protect them from other bacterial infections. Probiotics are most effective when started as early as possible after the start of diarrhea; they will shorten the length of the illness.

Probiotics can be taken in many forms; they are widely available in both pills and capsular form (capsules). I would not recommend the pills; they are much less viable and frequently the process to produce them destroys most of their probiotic content.

Probiotics also come as either bacteria such as acidophilus, bifidobacteria, or others found in many yogurts and also as yeast such as Saccharomyces boulardii (which is sold under the brand name Florastor). Most bacterial probiotics have to be refrigerated to preserve their potency, but Florastor does not; in fact refrigeration will kill it. It needs to be kept at room temperature to maintain its viability.

Remember, since probiotics are living organisms, they need to eat, so you have to take them with food known as prebiotics. The best prebiotics are made from soluble fiber, which forms a gel-like consistency and feeds the probiotics. Bananas, milk, yogurt, and other foods are excellent prebiotics.

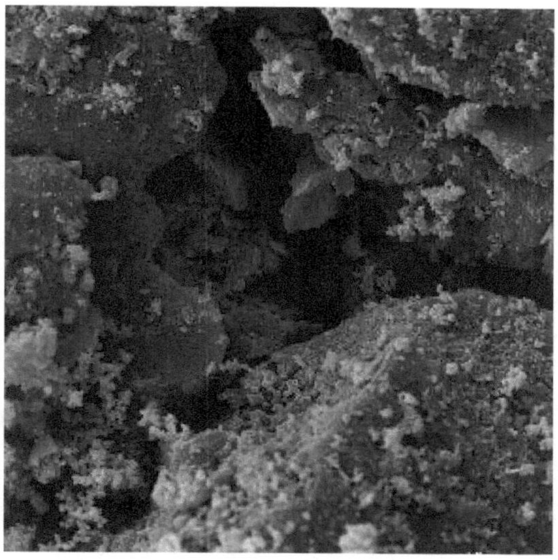

A Scanning Electron Microscope Photo Showing the Incredible Surface Area of Activated Charcoal

Activated Charcoal

My personal favorite treatment of Gastrointestinal (GI) problems such as nausea, vomiting, and diarrhea, is activated charcoal. Take two capsules of activated charcoal immediately upon the start of symptoms and repeat it every eight hours or so until it stops.

Activated charcoal has an amazingly large surface area and will adsorb onto its surface any toxins you might have ingested as well as bacteria or other foreign materials. You cannot take any medications within two hours of using activated charcoal because it will soak up and inactivate the medications. This means two hours before and two hours after you use the activated charcoal. It may cause constipation in some people but that is infrequent and can be treated. See my section on activated charcoal for complete details.

Lemon Juice Or Apple Cider Vinegar

In mild cases of food poisoning you can use several different home remedies. Most of these rely upon the use of acidity either in the form of lemon juice or vinegar to help kill off some of the offending bacteria.

Either squeeze four lemons or use four tablespoons of apple cider vinegar...add either to a large glass of water and add honey, sugar, or any sweetener you have available and drink this twice daily as needed.

I would recommend using Bragg's organic apple cider vinegar; it is the best one out there and has strong antimicrobial effects. It also contains considerable amounts of pectin, which helps heal the GI tract.

Bovine Colostrum

Bovine colostrum is made from cows and is very effective in the treatment of both acute and chronic diarrhea in humans. Colostrum is what both humans and cows produce and is excreted by the breast before normal breast milk or in the case of cows, cow's milk. It is loaded with antibodies to help protect the baby and the calf from infections of various types. Bovine colostrum has been found to contain large numbers of antibodies to bacterial, viral, and protozoal pathogens that cause diarrhea. It has also been found to be effective against a large number of bacterial toxins which many times are the cause of diarrhea. Bovine colostrum will also help leaky gut syndrome and in turn will help those suffering with many food allergies. Bovine colostrum surprisingly contains very little lactose and even those who are lactose intolerant usually tolerate it with no problem.

The good news is that bovine colostrum comes as a powder and does not need to be refrigerated, just keep it in a cool, dry place like a basement or a root cellar and it will be viable for many years! The powder is taken directly into the mouth and then it is washed down with water or it can be added to applesauce, otherwise it should be taken on an empty stomach.

Bovine colostrum is fat soluble so will not dissolve in a glass of water, but it is taken with water to help wash it down. Bovine colostrum can be taken by children and even pets. It should be taken on an empty stomach at bedtime and if a second daily dose is needed it can be taken again upon awakening. The powder is relatively inexpensive; I would look for one from organic sources if possible.

The dose depends on the person; usually if in capsules, 500 mg three per day, usually at bedtime because it does increase serotonin levels and may make you sleepy. If you are taking the bulk powder then it is one teaspoon daily or twice daily depending on the severity of your illness.

L-Glutamine

L-Glutamine is an amino acid that is very effective at healing irritated or infected GI mucosa. It even has been shown to be effective in diarrhea caused by chemotherapy and radiation exposure.

Since L-Glutamine helps heal the intestinal mucosa it helps create a barrier to further infection in addition to which it helps boost intestinal immunity. L-Glutamine also helps the absorption of water and electrolytes by the intestinal mucosa, further helping patients with diarrhea.

Taking adequate supplemental L-Glutamine for your bodily needs is critical, especially after an injury or severe infection.

The dose of L-glutamine in capsules is 1,000 mg tid (three times daily), in powder form take one-quarter teaspoon stirred into a glass of water daily. In severe cases you may double that to a half a teaspoon daily.

L- Glutamine should be avoided in those with kidney or liver disease.

Zinc

Zinc has been shown to be very effective in the treatment of diarrhea, especially in young children. Zinc supplementation works in several different ways to help diarrhea. Zinc reduces the severity and also the frequency of bowel movements, aids in the absorption of water and electrolytes and helps the healing and repair of damaged intestinal mucosa. Zinc supplements come in various forms such as zinc acetate, zinc sulfate, and zinc gluconate; the good news is that all forms seem to work just fine. Zinc is safe and effective for children even under the age of six months where the dose is 10 mg daily, for those over six months it is double that or 20 mg daily and for adults it is 40 mg daily. Any long-term administration of zinc will eventually adversely affect copper levels and copper will have to be supplemented as well. When taking long-term zinc supplementation, I recommend taking 1 mg of copper for every 50 mg of zinc. This will insure that in the long run you do not develop a copper deficiency.

Iodine

Iodine in its many forms is effective in killing many of the microbes that cause infectious diarrhea. Iodine for the treatment of diarrhea can be taken in its various forms, such as Lugol's solution and nascent iodine, which is iodine in its elemental form. As nascent iodine, simply mix five to six drops in a small glass of water and drink this up to four times a day for up to five days; if it stops earlier you can discontinue it earlier. As Lugol's solution, you should mix either six drops of the 5 percent solution or twelve drops of the 2 percent solution into a small glass of water and drink it, repeat this in two hours; you can use this up to four times a day for three days.

For children, use half of that dose. You should swish this mixture around your mouth before you swallow it since it will also help disinfect your mouth; it has a slight medicinal taste but is not too bad. Proper absorption of iodine by the body requires the presence of adequate vitamin C; for that reason I recommend taking approximately 1 to 2 grams (1,000 or 2,000 mg) daily along with your iodine. If you are on a higher dose of iodine, take the 2,000 mg of vitamin C; it is water soluble and has zero toxicity and any excess will just be eliminated in your urine.

Colloidal Silver

What is colloidal silver you ask? Colloidal silver is a mineral drink composed of very small silver particles suspended in a colloid. A colloid is a liquid where all the atoms are spaced due to an electric charge, hence they don't come out of solution and settle, think milk or Jello. The stuff the silver is suspended in is known as the colloid.

Silver has been known for centuries to have antimicrobial properties, meaning it killed bacteria, viruses and fungi well. Up until the advent of the antibiotic age in the 1940's silver preparations were widely used by physicians. Recent studies show it to be effective against MRSA (methicillin resistant staph. aureus) and other bacteria that were multi-antibiotic resistant. It has also been found to be lethal to Avian influenza (bird flu) and pseudomonal infections. We still use them to treat burns and external wound infections with topical preparations of silver sulfadiazine or its brand name Silvadene. Silver preparations are included in a number of wound dressings to exploit their quick killing of many types of microbes.

The big fear often cited by any medical website or authority is Argyria, a condition where the use of silver preparations like colloidal silver or silver dust will permanently dye your skin a blue to blue gray color. Colloidal silver has been often touted in the alternative medicine world to have multiple benefits and people have been using it for decades, without any cases of Argyria that I know of. That being said, I thought I would mention it just to let you know what the supposed risks are.

Colloidal silver has been tested in vitro against all of the typical kinds of bacteria that cause GI problems and found to be effective at eradicating them. The presumption is that it will do this for us.

My experience with colloidal silver for GI infection was personal; I had an abscess develop and was quite ill.

Colloidal silver, L-glutamine, VSL #3, vitamin C along with lots of organic food providing all the prebiotics my gut needed. I did remarkably well and soon fully recovered. Will it work for you? I don't know, or was it just the right combination?

There are many places to buy your own colloidal silver generator, I prefer to buy mine premade. I like a product called Mesosilver made by Purest Colloidals. I have used it for a number of years and have found it to be of outstanding quality and consistency. It is 20 ppm or parts per million of silver. The committee that studies silver is known as the Silver Safety Committee, it is composed of physicians as well as scientists who specialize in silver and its uses. They have an easy formula for determining the maximum silver you can safely ingest in a day. The formula is your weight in pounds multiplied by 12 and then that total is divided by the parts per million of the colloidal silver preparation you are drinking. That answer is the maximum number of drops you can safely take daily. Of course taking way less than that will work just fine. You can either drink it orally or if there is a surface wound or infection it then can be treated topically. I would divide it into three or four times a day if you are treating an infection.

Mucilaginous Herbs

Mucilaginous herbs are herbs that form into slippery, gel-like consistency when they are mixed with water. Three different mucilaginous herbs are used in the treatment of diarrhea, they are psyllium husk or seed (Plantago ovate), slippery elm (Ulmus fulva) and marshmallow root (Althaea officinalis). These three herbs work in similar ways, they contain large amounts of soluble fiber that absorbs water and helps diarrhea, they also coat and soothe the irritated, infected intestinal lining, and they bind up toxins and carry them out of the intestine, decreasing inflammation. They also help to protect the damaged intestinal mucosa and promote its healing. Slippery elm also has excellent nutrient content and will help nourish someone who is malnourished from chronic diarrhea.

Since all three of these mucilaginous herbs have great absorptive capacity you should not take any medications or any supplements for two hours before and after taking any of the three. The dose of these mucilaginous herbs for diarrhea is as follows:

Psyllium husk or seed: One teaspoon mixed into a large glass of water three times daily until healed.

Marshmallow root: Make a tea with one teaspoon of it in powder form in a mug of boiling water, allow it to steep for ten minutes. Drink this tea three times a day as needed for diarrhea.

Slippery Elm: Make a porridge by mixing one tablespoon of powder into a mug of hot water and eat it as a porridge once it cools three times a day until the diarrhea is healed. Slipper elm can also be taken as a tincture 5 mg tid (three times daily), or in capsules at 500 mg tid.

CHAPTER TWENTY EIGHT
NAUSEA AND VOMITING

INTRODUCTION

TABLE OF CONTENTS:

Nausea and vomiting occur quite frequently, so knowing how to treat them is knowledge everyone should have.

We have all eaten foods that are "questionable" in their appearance or smell, sometimes it works out just fine, other times you live to regret that decision. Also, the preparation of your food might be less than optimal, for various reasons. Or perhaps you don't have enough fuel to properly prepare your food or you improperly canned your food from last summer. There are many different scenarios in which you will be confronted with either you or one of your family or friends having a severe case of nausea and vomiting. You will have to learn how to treat it, especially in children, elderly patients, and the severely weakened.

Nausea and vomiting, especially with diarrhea, will lead to severe dehydration and will kill a young child or an old person quickly. It is still a major scourge in third world countries and contributes significantly to their high child mortality. Note: Dehydration will develop into a vicious cycle where it leads to more nausea and vomiting and round and round you go.

CAUSES OF NAUSEA AND VOMITING

The most likely cause is a **viral gastroenteritis**. This is commonly known as "stomach flu". It is contagious (how the hell do you think you got it) and can go through a group living in close proximity to one another like military recruits in a very short time. For this reason the first person to come down with it should be quarantined as much as possible, especially if you and your family are indoors together as during a blizzard for example.

More on this later, along with proper sanitary practices you must employ to prevent and confine such outbreaks.

Food poisoning: I covered a lot of this on the section covering diarrhea.

Alcohol, medications, and toxins: The most likely is alcohol ingestion followed by an infinite variety of other chemicals and prescription and over-the- counter medications that can be toxic or just irritating to your GI tract and will lead to nausea and vomiting. This is your body's primary way of ridding itself of unwanted chemicals or toxins.

Your body will purge the toxin either by making you vomit or will give you diarrhea and get rid of it from your other end.

That is why there is a usefulness to nausea and vomiting and even diarrhea when you are exposed to toxins, but it must be controlled. If left untreated for too long of a time it will result in severe electrolyte losses (primarily potassium, sodium and chloride) and all the resulting problems that go along with that. Taking a good history from a patient will lead you many times to a medication that caused the problem, both prescription and over-the-counter meds.

Migraines: A migraine headache often leads to nausea and vomiting. In these cases you should treat the migraine and that will stop the vomiting. Typically the vomiting associated with migraines is once or twice and not the recurrent vomiting that will lead to major problems. Trust me, I get migraines, it is no fun gagging and vomiting when your head is exploding But once you properly treat the migraine the vomiting will stop.

See the section on headaches for complete treatment details.

Intestinal obstruction: This is fortunately less frequent than the other causes, but especially in the elderly a small bowel obstruction (or less frequently a large bowel obstruction) may occur.

If you suspect this to be the case you must get the patient to a hospital, this is most definitely a medical emergency and should not be something you attempt to treat yourself.

One hint is that they are not having bowel movements due to the obstruction and this will not get better with time. In other words, it will eventually be fatal.

Note: Any intestinal obstruction or stoppage of the usual peristalsis or ileus (the movement of food/feces from your mouth towards your anus in a constant rhythmic fashion) will result in no bowel movements. Sometimes these occur for various reasons that are beyond the scope of this book. The point to remember is that when the bowels are without this peristalsis there will be no bowel sounds (the gurgling sounds you will hear if you put your ear to someone's abdomen or, if you have it, a stethoscope) or they will be very faint. When this stoppage ends, the patient will begin to first pass gas and then within a day or two will have a bowel movement.

Vertigo, motion sickness, and ear infections: These may all lead to dizziness and then nausea and ultimately vomiting. The cause is usually fairly easy to determine. Anyone with dizziness should have their ears checked; look in there with a light. If the eardrum you see is not light pink or white in color and is red and shiny and swollen-looking, that is a sign of a middle ear infection. If you pull the ear and it hurts, that is the sign of a swimmer's ear or external otitis. That comes from swimming in contaminated waters. If there is an earache this is a very good indicator of an ear infection.

Motion sickness is an easy diagnosis, hopefully I don't need to explain that point any further.

Vertigo without an obvious source is called benign positional vertigo, this lasts for weeks. As the name suggests, it is benign, meaning it will not kill you and will cause no significant harm; it is just a very annoying condition. It is made worse by sudden turning of your head to one side or the other, sometimes both.

Radiation exposure: This can lead to severe nausea and vomiting. The source of this will hopefully be obvious.

Head injuries: Concussions or severe blows to the head are unfortunately common occurrences and you should learn their signs and symptoms. The history will be obvious and the head injury may be closed like a blow to the head without a laceration or open with a large cut on the scalp or face, or a combination of the two. If these lead to a bleed within the brain it will cause severe nausea and vomiting that will gradually worsen eventually killing the patient.

This is a medical emergency and the patient must be taken to a hospital asap. One sign that you will see is the patient will develop one pupil larger than the other, this is known as anisocoria. Note: Anisocoria is hereditary in about twenty percent of "normal patients" and thus is not a sign of an intracranial bleed.

Other than drilling a hole in their head at the site of the bleed and relieving the buildup of blood, and opening the skull and stopping the bleeding source, the patient will die. That is the reason you need a neurosurgical team in a hospital setting and nothing short of that .Thus head trauma with bleeds into the brain will have to be placed in the "kiss-your-ass-goodbye-section if you have this and are unable to get to a hospital immediately.

Pregnancy: If it is a female of childbearing age who has been sexually active without protection during or near the time of her ovulation (two weeks after her last menses or period ended) then pregnancy should be considered. There will be other signs as well...breast swelling, hormonal changes, etc.

Note: Nausea occurs in fifty to 90 percent of all pregnancies and vomiting in 25 to 55 percent. It usually occurs in the early stages of pregnancy.

Gastritis and Ulcers: Gastritis is inflammation of the stomach lining; ulcers are erosions of the stomach lining that may or may not lead to perforation (a hole in the stomach or the duodenum or first part of the small intestine that is connected to the stomach). The patient will usually have severe heartburn and a burning sensation in their stomach or esophagus, with bloating after they eat and pain in their abdomen. This can lead to vomiting after eating. Frequently gastritis and ultimately ulcers can be caused by what is otherwise considered harmless medications by the public, such as naproxen, ibuprofen, and aspirin. These should always be taken on a full stomach to prevent this gastric irritation.

Note: Acetaminophen (Tylenol) does not cause GI upset and can be taken on an empty stomach. It does however cause liver damage in doses greater than 4 grams (4,000 mg) daily or with lesser quantities when mixed with alcohol.

TREATMENT OF NAUSEA AND VOMITING

Once again, consider the cause if you know it or can take an educated guess. If they smell like alcohol and are acting drunk it is an easy diagnosis. Ask the patient if they ever had this before and you might get the diagnosis right away.

Food poisoning is a little tricky because of the time frame. It can be anywhere from several hours to a few days after eating something infected. What will be helpful is if several people shared the same food and all became ill…that will make that diagnosis an easy one for you.

If the cause is found treat the underlying condition by eliminating the source of the problem. Alcohol is a ready example. Remove any further alcohol and begin to gently but steadily hydrate the patient. Any questionable sources of food poisoning should be quickly investigated and the source should be destroyed.

If radiation is suspected as the cause the patient may rapidly deteriorate and begin vomiting or passing blood by their rectum and quickly become delirious and die.

Other treatment options, for a patient with a suspected intestinal obstruction, are sometimes effective. If the obstruction is low enough, that is, close to the rectum, you might be able to reach in with a gloved hand and manually disimpact (grab and pull out) the hard stool blocking the colon.

Here we get into some other options that progressively get more difficult, and should only be done if you cannot reach medical attention and are in a desperate situation. One such option is to insert a rectal tube. You can use any wide-mouth tubing that you have. This will only work if the obstruction is a little higher up in the sigmoid colon. Lubricate the tube and gently insert it into the colon; you only have to go in about six inches. The patient should be lying on their side with their legs drawn up to their abdomen, in a sort of fetal position. Your results will improve if you have the patient change from lying on their right side to their left and back again, every few minutes; this increases the effectiveness of these tubes. They often get obstructed and periodically should be removed, cleaned and re-lubed and reinserted. Sometimes, obstructions that are higher will require the insertion of an NG (nasogastric tube) through the nose into the stomach to decompress them just like the rectal tube, but from above. This is a much trickier procedure and has to be done with a well lubricated tube and gently inserted in the nose to prevent bleeding. Before you start the procedure you should measure the distance between the nose and the stomach by laying the tube outside the body and noting the length and marking it. Then when you insert it you will not fall short or go too far into the stomach.

Note: You can use a combination of both NG and rectal tubes to decompress from both above and below. Their success rate is marginal at best, but without the benefits of a surgeon present, this is a viable option, and may very well be your only option. The NG tube should be of a much thinner diameter than the rectal tube, in fact, as small as you can find. This procedure is a little tricky and is best done by a doctor or someone else with experience in insertion of these tubes. The NG tube is usually hooked up to a pump that will help evacuate the stomach contents and therefore decompress from above. Obviously if you are in this emergency situation it is very unlikely you will have a small pump available, thus your only option is to apply suction yourself orally as if you were siphoning gas from a tank. If you have ever siphoned anything, then you already know that quite often the contents come up faster than expected and you get some in your mouth. Obviously, be as careful as you can to avoid this. You could use a small hand pump siphon rather than doing it orally, but once again this depends on what you have available.

The most common types of causes such as gastroenteritis or stomach flu, food poisoning, gastritis and ulcers and toxins will all respond to activated charcoal. I have kept a supply of these in my office for years and give it to patients; I also have used it at home. It works rapidly, in my experience within fifteen minutes to a half hour and gives almost total relief from nausea and vomiting. Activated charcoal is what is used in our nation's emergency rooms, but they pass it through an NG tube and make slurry of it with water. It works very well for overdoses of any medications and helps all toxins. It has such an incredibly large surface area that it adsorbs all toxins, bacteria, alcohol, etc., and inactivates them by irreversibly binding them to the charcoal. I can't stress the usefulness of this activated charcoal to all my readers and highly recommend that you immediately purchase several bottles for your emergency medical chest. It has endless uses that cannot be replaced by other substances. What else can you think of that will work to stop nausea and vomiting, treat burns, and filter water and air as well as detoxify your body?

Once you have controlled the person's nausea and vomiting with the activated charcoal, either by a slurry mixed with water or by two capsules drank with a glass of water, you can then begin to gently but steadily hydrate the patient. Avoid solid food until the vomiting has passed. If the vomiting persists you can try marijuana. Pot has been known for centuries to control nausea and vomiting and is even prescribed for cancer patients to help control their nausea. I am not suggesting you break the law, but pot has multiple uses for our medicinal needs in its various forms, such as marijuana and also hemp oil. Also of note is that hemp oil has been found to have many medicinal uses, beyond the scope of this book.

See the book list at the end for the works of Dr. Marc Sircius. He has written on several subjects including the wonderful medicinal uses of marijuana.

Hydrating a patient can be done with drinks such as Gatorade if you have any available. A cheap way to stock Gatorade and not take up much room is to buy it in powder form and mix it in water. Children sometimes are picky about what they drink and this might make it easier. The same thing can also be done with tea. There are many tea preparations that are relaxing such as chamomile tea and other sleepy time teas. These are inexpensive and can be useful to have to relax someone whose nerves are shot and is nearing exhaustion due to lack of sleep. Marijuana will also be useful for the same purpose.

Pregnant women experiencing morning sickness can find eating a high protein snack at bedtime may be helpful, such as lean meat (venison would work fine) or cheese, and in the morning some crackers before getting out of bed. As a general rule if you find yourself nauseous you should eat several small meals and avoid distending your stomach with a large meal which may not sit well and will result in the recurrence of the vomiting. Avoid rich foods or foods that have a strong smell to them. Keep yourself well hydrated. If lying flat, raise your head a foot or so above your body. This will put gravity on your side and help keep food down.

Avoid caffeine, spicy foods, and fatty foods, all of which may aggravate the problem. It is also very important to eat slowly and chew your food very well. Chewing will break up your food and allow your stomach and digestive enzymes to digest it better and make it easier for your small intestine to absorb. This is a good practice overall that very few of us in our hustle bustle modern world often do not take the time to do properly. The result is an epidemic of indigestion and gastrointestinal problems.

Ginger ale also helps nausea because it contains the spice ginger. Ginger can also be bought in tablet form and works very well for nausea; this should be added to your medicine chest as well. If you grow ginger, then a quarter or a half teaspoon of ground ginger one or several times a day will help. It is easy to grow if you live in a warm climate. If you live in such an area, you might want to make it part of your herb garden as well. Ginger can also be purchased in its raw form (much beloved by my son Marcus) where it is either young (with a soft outer skin, available in many Asian food stores), or in its mature dried form (where you have to peel the outside). It is also available in powder form, candied, pickled, and crystallized. It is very effective in not only treating nausea and vomiting from any source, but especially so in pregnant women, in whom the severe form is known as Hyperemesis Gravidarum. It is safe and effective to use in pregnant women and does not cause any of the potential side effects of traditional anti-nausea medications.

It also helps inflammation, motion sickness, flatulence (farting), and intestinal spasms. All of these benefits and good-tasting as well, can you beat that? For our purposes this is truly a win-win situation and should be exploited by having a good supply of ginger in its many forms in your natural medicine chest.

Antacids such as Maalox, Mylanta, and Tums will help an upset stomach and help soothe it. Pepto-Bismol will also help calm an upset stomach and comes in either pills or liquid. Keep both in your medicine chest. It also helps kill Helicobacter pylori, an infection in your stomach that leads to ulcers. If the cause is gastritis then over-the-counter meds like Prilosec or Prevacid will help, as well as Zantac or Pepcid.

Baking Soda (sodium bicarbonate) can also be used in place of antacids; it is very alkaline and will help neutralize stomach acids and help especially in cases of ulcers and gastritis. The usual dose is half a teaspoon in 8 ounces of water up to six times a day as needed, it should not be used more than that and not for a prolonged period and never use if the stomach is distended, it may lead to violent vomiting.

If you prefer you can also make an effervescent antacid with the following recipe:

Into an 8-ounce glass of water add:

1 tablespoon of vinegar One-half teaspoon of sugar

One-half teaspoon of baking soda

One-half cup of water

Drink this immediately while it is still fizzing.

(Taken from: *Baking Soda: by Victor Lansky*)

Changing position from a lying to a sitting position and giving the person something like ginger ale to drink will also help alleviate some nausea.

If it is winter time or if you have ice available, breaking it into some small chips or crushing it and giving small amounts of this to a person will help with nausea and might be helpful in those situations where the person cannot hold down fluids. If they vomit this, then back off for a few hours allowing their stomach to quiet down and then try again.

Once the vomiting is under control chicken broth, apple juice (do not use grapefruit or orange, they are too acidic), even small amounts of Jell-O will help. You can even dilute the apple juice with half water at first to see how the patient tolerates it, especially in small children.

Milk should be avoided for at least two days after an episode of nausea and vomiting. The enzyme lactase that is responsible for the digestion of milk is produced in the stomach lining and gets depleted by the nausea and vomiting from the wrenching of the stomach. This leads to a temporary lactose intolerance (milk intolerance) and will cause indigestion of milk or any dairy product such as creams, cheeses, or yogurt. I generally advise my patients to avoid these for up to a week or even two weeks to be safe and then slowly reintroduce dairy into their diets

Also many patients benefit from the BRAT diet after a prolonged bout of nausea and vomiting. BRAT stands for bananas, rice, applesauce, and toast. These foods are easy to digest and low in fat, protein, and fiber. The bananas are high in potassium, which is lost in large quantities with nausea, vomiting, and diarrhea and will need to be replaced.

Other foods to be avoided for the first week or so are fatty or greasy foods, dairy, raw fruits and vegetables (due to the high fiber content), spicy foods, and citrus fruits (due to their acidity).

KISS-YOUR-ASS-GOODBYE-SECTION:

Let's be real, you are so screwed if you have any of these, this is why I made this section. Your absolute only hope is immediate massive medical intervention in a hospital setting.

Colon cancer

Intestinal obstruction caused by volvulus (twisting of gut) or a stricture or adhesions.

Brain hemorrhage

Diabetic ketoacidosis

Severe radiation exposure

Renal (kidney) or liver failure

Heart attack

Pancreatic cancer (You are dead with this one even with full medical attention, despite the best attempts of movie stars like Michael Landon, even with endless money and medical attention.)

Perforated ulcer or any severe source of GI bleeding

CHAPTER TWENTY NINE
DEHYDRATION

INTRODUCTION

TABLE OF CONTENTS:

As a health conscious individual one of your cardinal rules must be maintaining adequate water intake at all times. Every cell in your body needs water and is bathed in an aqueous environment. The average adult's body is 60 percent water, and an infant's is 80 percent water! Only oxygen is more critical to your body than water, as evidenced by the Rule of Threes, which is you can live three minutes without air, three days without water and three weeks without food. You must learn to recognize and treat dehydration in you and your family, especially the elderly. This is especially important if you are exerting yourselves in extreme environmental conditions, whether that is a desert, jungle, or frozen tundra.

HOW MUCH WATER DO I NEED?

Your body has water needs that must be maintained and carefully monitored if you are to remain active and effective. The average-sized woman should drink about nine, 8-ounce glasses of water a day and a man about twelve glasses of water daily. This will naturally go up with increased exertion, and in a hot environment water loss via sweating and imperceptible evaporation across your skin could be very significant. An adult male living in a temperate climate (most of the United States and Europe) will have need of approximately three liters (quarts) of fluid a day. For adult women it is 2.2 liters a day...but it goes up to three if she is pregnant or nursing. Others advise to drink half of your body weight a day in ounces of water, so if you are 200 pounds then you will need to drink 100 ounces of water daily or roughly three, 32-ounce bottles of water daily.

Other factors may influence your total daily water needs such as health, environmental factors, exercise, etc. Normally, about 20 percent of your fluid intake needs come from the foods you eat. The more fruit and vegetables you are eating, the greater the percentage of your daily water needs will be met. The water needs of children will need to be ball-parked. This can be fairly accurately done by using their size as a rough gauge. A child of half adult size will need only half of the water and food requirements of a full-size adult. If it is a toddler, then use a quarter of the adult needs, etc. Once again, you can use their tongues and the color of their urine as a rough guide. Your tongue should be wet and your urine should be light yellow in color.

Diarrhea due to illness or infection is a frequent cause of dehydration, especially in infants and young children. Nausea and vomiting will also cause dehydration. Any gastrointestinal loses of fluids either by diarrhea and vomiting will lead to more severe electrolyte losses and result in low levels of potassium, sodium, and chloride. This is why repletion of these electrolytes is of maximum importance and they must be included in your treatment of dehydration. As with most diseases and conditions the very young (infants and small children) and the very old are most at risk.

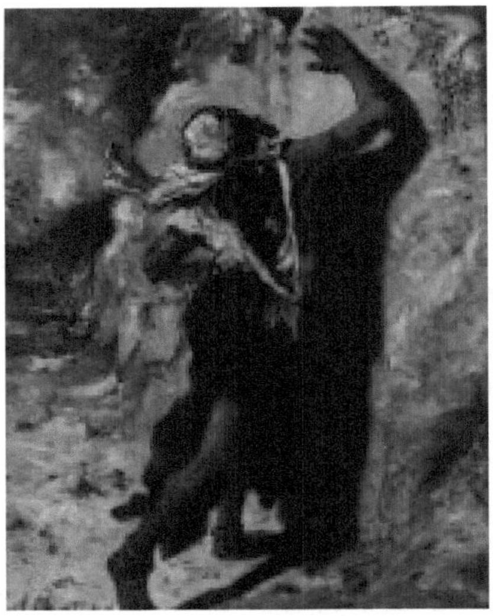

SIGNS AND SYMPTOMS OF DEHYDRATION

The first sign that a person will usually notice is increased thirst. This seems very obvious; however, if you are elderly your perception of thirst declines progressively with age. Many of my elderly patients are very dehydrated and have absolutely no idea since they do not feel thirsty at all. In a normal healthy adult your thirst mechanism will become activated when you have lost only 1 percent of your total body water content. If you are dehydrated, your lips will appear dry and cracked and your tongue will stick to the floor of your mouth and feel thick.

One good way to tell if you or someone in your group is dehydrated is to look at their tongue. A tongue is a very useful barometer of your hydration. If a tongue appears dry and rough looking rather than plump and wet, that is a cardinal sign of dehydration.

Another very reliable method is to examine your urine. You may have noted that your urine is darker yellow in the morning upon your first urination. This is because you have not drunk water for the eight hours or so while you were sleeping and your urine became more concentrated from that lack of availability of water.

You may also have noticed when you are playing sports on a hot day you are not urinating, or barely urinating. This is because you are losing fluids constantly from sweating and panting and rapid respirations as well as imperceptible losses by evaporation across your skin.

Your urine should be almost clear, with just the faintest tinge of golden color. This is normal and is a good way to gauge your hydration. The darker the urine, the more dehydrated you are. If your urine is dark in color, immediately start increasing your water intake until it lightens to an almost clear color. Also if you are urinating only twice a day or less is a strong indicator of severe dehydration.

Note: Frequent clear-appearing urine may be a sign of diabetes. As your blood sugar elevates it draws water into your circulation and also causes more urine to be produced and hence you urinate more often and many times in larger quantities. You should watch your urine color; it will help you determine other possible problems. Urine discolored with a red tinge may be a sign of a kidney stone with resulting hematuria (blood in your urine). The passage of kidney stones is usually accompanied by severe pain (but not always). This pain typically starts in the lumbosacral area (the small of your back) and travels or radiates around your flank and down to your groin. The pain is caused by the movement or migration of the kidney stone. Sometimes the pain localizes in a certain area, frequently just above the bladder on either side; that area is known as the ureterovesical junction or UVJ. The UVJ is where the tubes that carry urine from your kidneys to your bladder (the ureters) enter the back of the bladder on either side. The problem with this area is that it has a dip in its course before it rises up to enter the bladder; this is the point where kidney stones frequently get hung up. This is yet another reason to rapidly hydrate yourself in order to flush out the stone or stones and to facilitate their passing through the potential bottleneck at the UVJ.

OTHER IMPORTANT SIGNS OF DEHYDRATION

1. Fatigue, especially fatigue that is disproportional to your exertion
2. Flushed skin that is red-appearing and dry to touch
3. Decrease in your quantity of urine.
4. Headaches are frequently caused by dehydration. Alcohol induced headaches (hangovers) especially are helped by lots of water. Something I had to learn in college the hard way.
5. Rapid breathing: Just like when a dog is panting, dehydration when severe in humans will lead to rapid breathing and if very severe will also be accompanied by a rapid pulse.
6. Mental confusion is another sign, especially when dehydration is severe. A little foggy head is the start of it. It often progresses to irritability and downright grumpiness. Dehydration, if severe, may progress to incoordination and falling.
7. Decreased skin turgor: Skin turgor means the elasticity of your skin. Normal skin is quite elastic and when you pinch a section of skin on a patient's arm for example, it should immediately snap back into place. In dehydrated patients their skin turgor will diminish and the skin will remain tented or folded when pinched.
8. Nausea is a frequent sign. Although if you are nauseous the last thing you feel like doing is drinking, it is essential to hydrate yourself if you have progressed to the point of nausea. Sometimes it will progress to vomiting which will only worsen someone's fluid status, so you have to take it slow. The best way to orally hydrate someone in this state is to have them take frequent sips of water.
9. Dizziness and vertigo
10. Loss of appetite
11. Constipation. When you are dehydrated your stools also become dry as your body desperately tries to conserve any remaining water. When your stools are dry they are hard to pass and your intestinal transit time goes up and you become constipated.

ELECTROLYTES AND DEHYDRATION

When you are dehydrated your body has lost a significant amount of its free water content; in addition it has lost key electrolytes like sodium, chloride, and potassium. For this reason hydration must look to replace those key electrolytes that have been lost. Most hydration fluids if commercially made will contain these electrolytes plus some sugar.

Since dehydration is such a common problem it is important that you learn to hydrate someone without intravenous access.

Sports drinks contain significant amounts of potassium and other electrolytes and are excellent when used to supplement water in order to provide all the electrolytes needed. One good thing to stock in your medicine chest is Gatorade powder, you can store a large quantity of it, it is very cheap, and kids love it.

Also keep in mind, as with most medical conditions, the very young and the very old are most vulnerable to becoming dehydrated. It is the old bell-shaped curve that I am more and more convinced is applicable to almost everything in life.

The very young are at one end of the bell-shaped curve and the elderly are at the other with the vast majority of us lying in the middle of the curve.

How to Make Fluids for Hydration

First of all, use clear fluids as the solvent to mix the ingredients into. Clear fluids are things like water, vegetable broth, Gatorade, sports drinks, and Pedialyte. Encourage the patient to slowly and steadily drink these fluids. If you drink them too fast you will become nauseous and vomit.

You can make your own with the following formula (make sure you are as exact as possible to maintain the correct ratios). Here are a few examples of mixes for rehydration that you can make at home:

Take one liter of water (a quart will suffice if you are weak on the metric system like most people) and add the following:

6 teaspoons of sugar

1 teaspoon of table salt (sodium chloride)

One-half teaspoon of salt substitute (potassium chloride)

A quarter teaspoon of baking soda (sodium bicarbonate).

A second, simpler formula can be used to make a small bottle of fluid for hydrating yourself if you suspect that you are starting to suffer with dehydration.

To one pint of water add a pinch of salt

A teaspoon of either lemon or lime juice

A teaspoon of sugar.

Sip this slowly until it is gone and repeat it as often as you need.

A third formula that is very easy to make is as follows:

Take 1 quart of water (950 ml).

One-half a teaspoon of table salt, which is approximately 2.5 grams,

6 teaspoons of sugar, which is approximately 30 grams.

OTHER METHODS FOR THE TREATMENT OF DEHYDRATION AND ITS CAUSES

One of the core principles to follow when treating patients with dehydration is to stop the loss of fluids, you need to get this part under control or you will never be able to rehydrate the patient.

Once the fluid loss is stopped by controlling diarrhea, vomiting, sweating, or frequent urination, then you will need to aggressively start your rehydration of the patient. If the patient is overheated, undress them and get them to a cool spot in the shade and out of direct sunlight. Cool them down with a cold facecloth or use rubbing alcohol to rub them down; this will cool them rapidly as it evaporates. If you are hiking somewhere and you start to dehydrate, then find a cool place, rest, and hydrate yourself. If you find yourself in an open area like a desert try to find a hill if possible and rest in the shadow of it, if no hill is available digging a hole and lying in the shade of the hole during the day and traveling at night will cool you off and stem your fluid losses from sweating.

If your dehydration is caused by diarrhea, once you are done with rehydration you can start them on the BRAT diet. This will help slow down the diarrhea by its bland nature and will slow intestinal motility (movement), thus slowing water losses. The BRAT diet stands for Bananas, Rice, Applesauce, and Toast. This is especially helpful in children. Other foods that you can substitute for these are soda crackers, Jell-O and potatoes. Jell-O and other gelatins are especially useful because they are primarily made of water and are very well tolerated by patients, as well as tasting good. If available, bananas are good because besides containing a high in potassium. Hydration can also be helped by giving foods that contain a lot of water such as strawberries, watermelon, cantaloupe, honeydew melons, pineapple, cucumbers, and celery.

Note: A gastrointestinal (GI) infection that causes diarrhea, nausea, and vomiting is often followed by a temporary (about two weeks) lactose intolerance. Therefore dairy products of any kind should be avoided for two weeks or so until the patient recovers properly. After the two weeks, dairy products should be very slowly reintroduced to determine a patient's tolerance. If it reactivates the diarrhea, then back off and wait another week or two before trying again.

Other factors that may contribute to dehydration are things such as caffeine. Caffeine is a diuretic which means it makes you urinate (pee). Caffeine is not only present in coffee, but is also found in black, white, and green tea (there is no caffeine in herbal teas). For this reason chamomile tea or any of the other herbal or decaffeinated teas are an excellent choice for rehydration. There is also caffeine in Mountain Dew, chocolate, Coca-Cola, Pepsi, and Dr. Pepper as well as unlikely places, such as in Excedrin.

Alcohol also causes dehydration, so never try to rehydrate yourself using alcohol like beer. The dehydration caused by alcohol is one of the reasons you get a hangover.

As I mentioned above, sport drinks like Gatorade are excellent for rehydration. A wonderful natural sports drink is coconut water, made from the largest seed on the planet, the coconut. Coconut water is naturally high in electrolytes. Coconut water has the same consistency as blood plasma and has even been used as a saline solution for IV fluid replacements in emergency situations, similar to Quinton's Marine Plasma! Coconut water is very high in both potassium and iron and low in sugar and works very well for rehydration.

Do not get confused between coconut water and coconut milk. Coconut water is really coconut juice; it is the liquid inside a young coconut that splashes around when you shake it. Coconut water is full of electrolytes, enzymes, vitamins, minerals, and phytonutrients. It is also sweet and clear in color. Coconut water also is a good source of vitamin C and also contains about 3 grams of fiber per cup. Young coconuts of five to seven months in age produce the most and the best coconut water. Coconut milk on the other hand is made by mixing coconut water with the coconut meat of the nut and then squeezing the mixture under pressure. Coconut milk is also a healthy drink full of minerals, vitamins, and medium chain triglycerides. Medium chain triglycerides are a type of fatty acid that is most easily utilized by the human body and is excellent for you.

Both yogurt and cottage cheese are good for rehydration since they both contain high levels of sodium and potassium and will help you restore your body's levels back to normal.

Another mix that works well for rehydration is to take one cup of yogurt and mix it with one teaspoon of fenugreek powder. Eating this mix several times a day will help rehydration. That is an old standby treatment for dehydration.

CHAPTER THIRTY

ARTHRITIS, JOINT PAIN, MUSCLE ACHES, LIGAMENT AND TENDON INJURIES, AND GOUT

INTRODUCTION

TABLE OF CONTENTS:

Chronic joint pain whether it is from osteoarthritis, rheumatoid arthritis, gout, injuries, or other causes is a condition/disease state that will often require treatment. One-half of all people will have some osteoarthritis by the age of sixty-five. Even more common are injuries from falls, pulled muscles, twisted ankles, bad knees, and bursitis problems that occur quite frequently. All of these will require variations of the same treatment protocols that I will cover in this chapter.

Certainly some arthritic pain is caused by gout and that is treated differently and for that reason it is covered at the end of the chapter separately.

Sometimes the cause of a severe isolated painful joint is due to an infection, but almost always that involves a point of entry, meaning a skin tear near the affected joint. Often times the point of entry cannot be found. That is a medical emergency of sorts and requires antibiotics and prompt medical care from a physician.

In this chapter I am not addressing that, but rather all the other causes of joint pain and chronic diseases such as osteoarthritis (by far the most common cause of arthritis), rheumatoid arthritis and gout. However, for you the reader, the most likely cause of your joint pain will be acute (short term) injuries from playing sports , gardening, lifting something the wrong way, falls and rough sex (you can only hope).

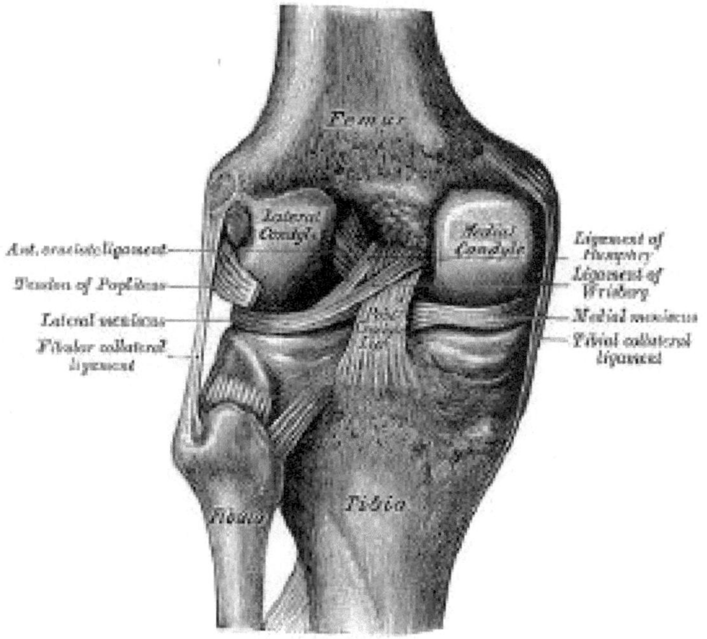

TREATMENT METHODS FOR JOINT LIGAMENT AND TENDON INJURIES.

This is a book on alternative medical treatments that basically means treatments that you do not have to go to a physician. Since I practice integrative medicine, which is combining the best treatments from western medicine (the kind of medicine practiced by almost all physicians in the United States) and over the counter and natural treatments. I only care about what works, I have no ax to grind, I want what is best for you as the patient and my reader. In this case for joint injuries many times the fastest way to get relief is from over the counter medications. For that reason, I will first describe those medications and then I will get into natural, nutritional and alternative treatments.

Here are some examples of nonprescription pain meds I would buy for your medicine chest:

1. **Aleve or Naproxen:** This is the longest acting of this group, will last 12 hours.
2. **Excedrin** (a combination of aspirin, Tylenol and caffeine)
3. **Ibuprofen** (also known as Advil or Motrin)
4. **Tylenol extra strength** (also known as acetaminophen)
5. **Aspirin:** both 81 mg baby aspirin and full dose 325 mg. Try to get the enteric-coated aspirin so it will pass through your stomach before breaking down in your intestines. The trade name for the enteric coated aspirin is Ecotrin. This prevents upsetting your stomach. The aspirin works very well for cardiac problems, fevers, and clots as well as pain. Note: Take all of these on a full stomach to avoid any GI upset. The only one you can take on an empty stomach is Tylenol.

Keep in mind that Tylenol is toxic to your liver in doses greater than 4 grams per day. (1 gram= 1,000 mg). Be very careful with the combination of alcohol and Tylenol. That combination will increase the toxicity to your liver much below the 4 gram a day threshold and should be kept in mind.

NOTE: All of the NSAIDS (non-steroidal anti-inflammatory drugs) and aspirin will bring down a fever, but this is not necessarily helpful for you. In fact in many cases bringing down a fever will be counterproductive. I do not want you ever treating a fever unless you are delirious or your temperature is in the 103 degree F range. Your body is an incredible machine and it does not do anything by chance. Fever is produced to kill any invading microorganisms such as bacteria and viruses which only live in a narrow temperature range close to 98.6 degrees F that is why they can colonize our bodies and make us sick. Raising your body's temperature with a fever literally cooks them.

Heat, Ice, Splints, And Slings

Your medicine chest should also include a good supply of ice and heat packs, duct tape, splints, and a sling or two. Slings can also be easily made with any long piece of cloth. Do not underestimate the usefulness of slings. Their purpose is to take the weight and the resulting muscle tension of your arm off of your shoulder. Once you remove this weight and tension, it allows the healing process to accelerate. Patients are always amazed by the immediate relief they feel when I support their elbow with my hand and remove the weight of their arms. You should also have a generous supply of ace bandages, which come in very handy to wrap areas for a variety of sprains and injuries.

Any acute (recent or short-term) joint, muscle, or bony injury should be immediately treated with ice or some cold compresses. After three days you can switch to heat or stay with ice. You will have to see which one works better for you. Heat usually helps when there are pulled muscles involved by relaxing them as well as increasing blood flow to them. Trial and error will be the best method to determine which modality works best for you. There is no right or wrong method. Another method is to alternate heat and cold, start with heat for about three minutes, then switch to cold, keep alternating them for twenty minutes.

Any minor sprain or strain type injury should be treated with the same protocol, RICES: This stands for ***Rest, Ice, Compression, Elevation, and Splinting.*** It is an excellent protocol and should be memorized and utilized for those injuries. You are learning to use acronyms like every medical student does. Acronyms help immensely to aid your memory and provide a checklist of the proper procedures to follow.

Rest: Once a joint is injured you need to not use it for a while. The repeated use of an injured joint will place excessive strain on that joint and greatly slow and even prevent proper healing. This is especially true of weight bearing joints like the hip, knee and ankle. The spine and back are also in this category. Stay off of that injured leg and don't use that arm with the injured shoulder, it will only make things worse and prolong the length of time you are suffering.

Anatomy of the Human Knee

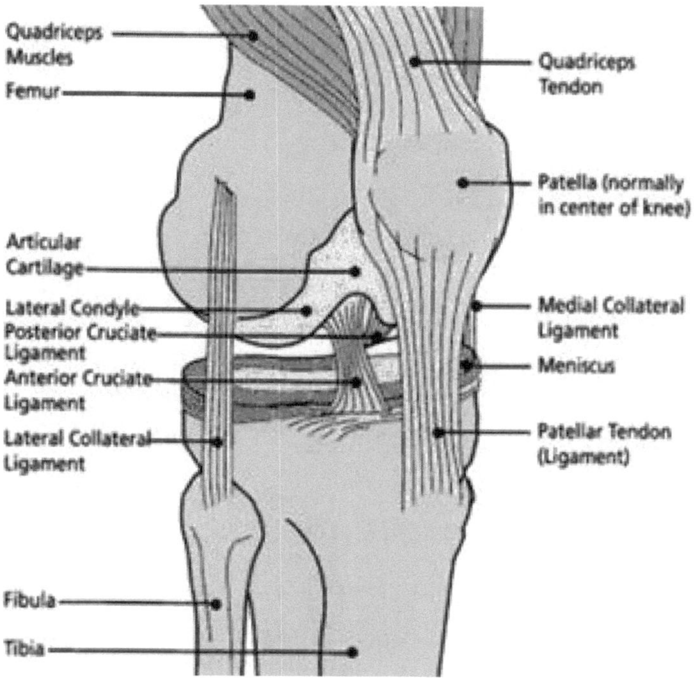

Front Side of the Knee

Ice: The use of ice and or cold compresses will significantly decrease pain and swelling. This ultimately will accelerate the healing process. You should apply ice or cold compresses for about a half hour (or as long as you can take it). Ice itself should probably be limited to about ten minutes or so. Never apply ice (or heat) directly to the skin, always place a thin barrier of cloth or other suitable material between the ice and the skin, this will prevent damaging the skin (you could even cause frostbite). Do this several times a day, especially for the first two days. This is the most important time to use the ice/cold compresses. Injured joints and soft tissue causes blood vessels to leak, pouring out fluids into the injured joint or muscle. When this occurs in your muscles and adjacent tissues this results in what is known as soft tissue swelling. The idea of ice is to constrict (shrink) these blood vessels and thereby decrease the release of those fluids and decrease the swelling.

Compression: A compression bandage is just simply a snug bandage applied starting below the affected joint and continuing over it and above it. An ace bandage will work very well for this. What you are attempting to do here is to apply external pressure that will diminish the soft tissue swelling.

What you don't want to do is to cut off adequate blood flow to the area. If it is too tight, you will get numb feeling or a tingling sensation like the area has "fallen asleep". If the area beyond (downstream) the compression bandage is blanched white in color or cyanotic (blue), then you have cut off blood flow and you have to loosen the bandage or you will cause permanent damage. Strips of cloth will work just fine for this, you should have a good supply of ace bandages in your medicine chest. They have many uses and are very inexpensive. In a pinch, duct tape can be used, but place a thin piece of cloth between the duct tape and the skin to prevent the tape from sticking to the skin.

Elevation: If possible the sprained or injured joint should be elevated above the level of the heart. Any elevation will help gravity decrease the edema (fluid accumulation) in the area, this in turn will accelerate the healing process.

Splint: This means immobilizing the injured joint in an attempt to prevent further injury to it. This can be done with a sling, brace, or splint. The compression bandage will also contribute to this stabilization. If it is an arm or leg, use anything that is unbendable.

A few thick branches will suffice in an emergency situation. Place them on either side of the injured arm, leg, or neck. Get creative, anything stiff and of the proper length will suffice; broom handles, lengths of wood, even PVC piping. As the saying goes, "necessity is the mother of invention", nothing could be truer for people interested in alternative medicine; you will learn to be resourceful and you will learn what treatments work for you and which do not. That is the beauty of this book. I have tested all the treatments listed here and only give you the ones I know to work.

WEIGHT LOSS, EXERCISE, AND NUTRITION

Every medical textbook will stress weight loss and exercise as two very important treatment strategies to use with arthritis, especially the most common type of arthritis known as osteoarthritis.

In this book I will teach you how to use nutrition to strengthen your body and nourish it from within, rebuilding your body into a robust disease resisting machine. Remember, carbohydrates are what make you obese, not fat (unless you are living on a really high fat diet). Americans have proven this in the largest nutritional experiment in history. Since the 1980s America has been on a low-fat obsession only to find the rates of obesity sky rocket. The reason for that is simple. Our diets have become increasingly laden with carbohydrates such as the notorious high fructose corn syrup that has entered most processed foods. Carbohydrates break down to glucose (a type of sugar) and this triggers the release of insulin. Insulin has many roles in the body, most people are aware that it is used to lower blood glucose levels in diabetics, and that is true, but it has other more ominous functions as well. Since man developed in an environment that was boom or bust when it came to food supplies, the body became very adroit at using the calories it was provided in the best way to insure long-term survival. If early man had an abundance of sweet fruits to eat their bodies converted these excess calories into glycogen in their muscles and liver and fat for storage for a later time when they possibly would be starving.

Glycogen is just glucose folded up into a more easily stored form. Insulin also protects the fat you already have and promotes the production of new fat. As you can see insulin is primarily a fat promoting hormone and thus is the cause of most of our current obesity problem. People are grazing all day, eating little sweet snacks, drinking soda and juices laden with sugar, eating carbohydrates like chips, cookies, muffins, and other snack foods all day long. This constant input of carbohydrates leads to chronically high insulin levels and the resulting metabolic disaster of obesity and eventually insulin resistance and the development of type II diabetes.

Is it any surprise that we are seeing skyrocketing levels of both obesity and now diabetes in children as young as elementary school! Therefore a low carbohydrate diet will always lead to weight loss; the thinner you are the less strain on your joints.

PROPER NUTRITION FOR HEALTHY JOINTS

I always stress to my patients that a healthy body provided with all the proper nutrition will easily ward off most illnesses and even chronic diseases. It is never too late. If you are suffering with arthritis and joint problems the time to start eating better is now. I believe many diseases can be cured by rebuilding the body from within by providing it with all the tools it needs, especially vitamins, minerals and trace elements. Growing your own nutritious food is the easiest, most inexpensive way to reach that goal. Growing your own food in enough abundance will be problematic unless you are a farmer or a master gardener. I am an avid gardener and even built a permaculture orchard on my property in addition to my large garden. Despite my most valiant efforts, both had fallen prey to an army of rabbits, chipmunks, squirrels, woodchucks, birds, and deer, to name a few. If we had to survive on the food I attempted to grow, by winter's end we would be starving. I think that growing your own food is an excellent start to a good diet that will promote weight loss. If you live outside of a city, even in the suburbs, there are abundant sources of wild foods readily available which are organic and quite healthy.

A good book on edible and wild plants in your area of the country will be invaluable for recognizing food sources that we otherwise would have written off as weeds. A few dollars spent on a couple of books of this type I believe is money well spent. The grandfather of foraging for natural sources of foods is Euell Gibbons. He has written a series of wonderful books on the subject that are very comprehensive. Another author of note on the subject of edible wild foods is Samuel Thayer; he has written two books on the subject, *The Foragers Harvest* and *Nature's Garden*, both of which I highly recommend.

The germ theory is just that, germs or various types of infectious organisms like bacteria, fungi, and viruses are responsible for the various diseases that infect humans. I certainly agree with the germ theory, but with an important caveat. All the trillions of cells that comprise the human body are suspended in a small sea of surrounding extracellular (outside the cell) or interstitial fluid. This is the "terrain" of the body. It is very similar in chemical composition as well as distribution to sea water. It has all the same minerals and trace elements that sea or ocean water contains. Our bodies are able to absorb these inorganic minerals only after they are made into organic compounds by microorganisms in the soil. Only live soils not poisoned by current farming practices that just use NPK (nitrogen, phosphorus, and potassium) fertilizer, pesticides and herbicides are capable of the conversion of inorganic substances to organic. These chemical farming practices have depleted all of the minerals and trace elements from our soils. The United States Congress in a report from the 1930s already recognized this as a significant problem and was sounding alarm bells. That is why I am such a big proponent of utilizing rock dust and Azomite to put back all of the minerals and trace elements that plants and ultimately humans so desperately need for good health. Azomite is a highly mineralized complex silica ore mined from an ancient sea bed in Utah which was filled by an eruption of a nearby volcano. Azomite contains over 70 minerals and rare trace elements and is a wonderful way to re-mineralize any soil. I also am a big fan of using sea solids but these are harder to find than rock dust or Azomite. Following organic farming practices as well as adding minerals and trace elements to the soil and mycorrhizal fungi, will greatly enhance the beneficial microorganisms in the soil. They will thrive and the soil will be alive the way it should be. These enlivened soils will be chock- full of minerals and trace elements that have been converted from inorganic to organic by these beneficial microorganisms. Once in organic form they then can be ready for our bodies to absorb and properly utilize. Plants grown in such soils will be large and robust, with thick stalks and branches.

They will be healthy and will not require pesticides or other interventions. There is even a way to do this with solids from sea water, but that is a whole other book. My belief is that just like plant life will be robustly healthy when provided with these minerals, so will humans.

After over twenty-five years of researching diseases and their causes, I will have to agree with the late Nobel laureate Dr. Linus Pauling. Dr. Pauling felt emphatically that all diseases had their roots in a deficiency of some mineral or trace element. These deficiencies affect the terrain and in turn the cells that are completely covered by it. The cells get all of their nutrition through the extracellular fluid. It is my belief that if this fluid or terrain is supplied with a full set of minerals and trace elements that it will lead to homeostasis (getting the body back into balance) and robust good health. It does not work overnight, but I have had wonderful results in alleviating the pain and inflammation of arthritis in my patients by replenishing their minerals and trace elements.

Basically you can re-mineralize your body by mineralization of the soil you grow your food in, they will uptake the minerals in organic form and make them available to your body. Or, you can circumvent the plants and mineralize your body directly. Here are my two favorite ways to do just that.

Quinton's Marine Plasma

One of the greatest nutritional sources ever is produced in the world's oceans by plankton. The plankton grows into giant schools that are shaped like a vortex (tornado) with a mouth many miles in size. Into these life-filled vortices come all types of microscopic sea life up to whales to feed on this nutritious plankton. They truly are fountains of life, filled with three kinds of plankton. Zooplankton are animal plankton, the phytoplankton are plant plankton and you guessed it, the bacterioplankton are bacterial plankton. The zooplankton eat phytoplankton, bacterioplankton, both of whom live on the upwelling nutrients carried by these vortices from the ocean floor and are responsible for re-mineralization. The human body cannot absorb or assimilate inorganic compounds. There is no nutritional value to you at all in chewing a rock which is inorganic.

Waters harvested in these constantly evolving and moving vortices of life are chock-full of amino acids, minerals, and trace elements of all types. It is no coincidence that these are exactly what our body needs to ideally function. There is a wonderful current product that collects such rich water. They cold-filter it and remove all of the plankton but leave all the wonderful milk. It is called milk, but it is clear and not white at all. The product is called Quinton (Quinton's Marine Plasma). It is expensive but if you have the funds, I think it is a worthwhile item to have. If you have enough, drink an ounce of it daily to maintain good health. What this will do is essentially provide all the minerals and trace elements in an organic form that your body can assimilate. After a few months of replenishing your depleted extracellular fluid you will have transformed your body's "terrain". Now your cells will be awash in a sea of health-promoting fluid that will nourish your cells with all of the minerals and trace elements and amino acids that it needs. You see, cells do not touch each other; they are very close but are awash in this extracellular fluid. With the proper electrolytes in this fluid the cells are better able to communicate. This fluid at the proper pH will also facilitate cell function and removal of waste products. This in turn will go very far in healing many diseases that have a basis in deficiencies of many minerals and trace elements.

Replacing just one mineral or trace element will cause an imbalance of others. For example, taking in too much zinc will result in a copper deficiency. Quinton's Marine Plasma has the same balanced blend of nutrients and minerals that the sea and our blood have. It was previously a military secret that the French army, during WWII, ran out of plasma and used Quinton for blood transfusions for their troops with great success and no harmful side effects. By the way, I am not suggesting you do this, but I am just noting how wonderfully it worked due to its composition. By using the same natural balance of minerals and nutrients found in these plankton- rich areas of the sea, you are essentially duplicating the same primordial sea in which the same unicellular organisms that started life developed.

Those same seas provided these simple organisms with all of the salts and minerals they needed for life. Over the course of millions of years the life in those primordial oceans became more complex and eventually this variety of sea life made its way onto land. Once we left the sea and began to dwell on land we no longer had the luxury of this primordial soup of life. Our health then and now depends on us getting all of these minerals and trace elements that our bodies require. A deficiency of any one of these has far-reaching effects for your body's healthy balance or homeostasis. Once this equilibrium is disturbed it leads to the many diseases of which we currently suffer.

In addition, pregnant women are often lacking many of these minerals and trace elements or have depleted supplies of them. Their bodies will take what it needs for the developing fetus in order to insure proper mental and physical development. This only works if the mother has an adequate supply; if she does not, then the fetus starts life with mineral and trace element deficiencies. The consequences of these deficiencies have far-reaching effects upon the life of these unfortunate children. It is criminal in my opinion that all pregnant women are not given supplements containing these minerals and trace elements in an organic, easily assimilated (absorbed and used by the body) form. Medical studies on pregnant women are always fraught with challenges and thus are avoided as much as possible, thus showing once again the horrible effect our legal system has upon every day Americans, leaving us as prey to these horrible malpractice attorneys who pounce on every child not born perfect, despite the mother drinking and smoking or just eating horribly, it must be the obstetricians fault!

To illustrate to you how essential minerals and trace elements are for a developing fetus, let's take a look at iodine. Did you know that a pregnant woman who has insufficient iodine will give birth to a severely retarded child known as a cretin? The converse of that is that if you supplement with iodine during your pregnancy you will raise the IQ of your child by twenty points! Impressive as that is for one mineral, imagine how healthy our newborns would be if we supplemented every pregnant woman's diet with the full complement of minerals and trace elements.

The Secret Of The Soil; Fulvic Acid

There are two ways of treating arthritic pain and joint discomfort; one is preventing the inflammation from within, giving your body all of the building blocks it needs to not only build strong bones, ligaments, tendons and joints. The second way is treat the inflammation once it is established.

I much prefer the first method and that is why I use Quinton's Marine Plasma as outlined above and also another product called Supreme Fulvic. Supreme Fulvic is different than Quinton's Marine Plasma due to its fulvic acid and humic acid content. Both are outstanding products for you to build a strong body that has low levels of inflammatory chemicals circulating in your blood.

Fulvic acid is a virtually unknown product, it is produced by healthy microorganisms in organic soils, that are free of pesticides and herbicides and not poisoned by chemical farming practices. Fulvic acid and its brother humic acid are both types of "humic substances", they are both the major components of organic matter found in healthy soils. These humic substances are what make soil healthy by their biochemical activities. They contain natural sterols, hormones; fatty acids, polyphenols, and ketones. They also contain large amounts of phytochemicals (phyto means originating from plants) such as bioflavonoids and many other beneficial substances.

Man has evolved eating large quantities of plants since the very beginning of our appearance on Earth, and by doing so always ingested large quantities of fulvic complexes. Now, during the last hundred years we have adopted chemical farming methods that are producing foods devoid of this magical fulvic acid, and guess what has happened? We are ravaged by chronic diseases such as arthritis, hypertension, diabetes and cancers of all types.

Why is fulvic acid so good for us? First of all fulvic acid contains over sixty minerals and trace elements , amino acids and humic substances that are essential for proper nutrition and the growth of every cell in our body. Fulvic acid also attaches itself to the outer part of our cells, making them more easily penetrated by the nutrients that our cells need. How cool is that? Nature produces a substance that plants require and once ingested by humans not only provides those essential nutrients but also makes it easier for our cells to absorb them! Fulvic acid attaches to the cell wall and lowers its surface tension, thereby allowing water, nutrients to go in and waste products to go out, creating a vibrantly healthy cell.

Cells communicate by electrical and chemical signals. Fulvic acid aids in this by helping the cells maintain their proper voltage; it also soaks up free radicals and neutralizes toxins and other pollutants that are ravaging our bodies. Fulvic acid is a very strong antioxidant, helping our bodies ward off infections of all types.

What does this have to do with arthritis? I have been using Quinton's Marine Plasma and Supreme Fulvic for years to help my patients reconstruct their bodies from the inside, quenching inflammation and purging their bodies of toxins and free radicals while building strong cells that have all the amino acids (building blocks of proteins), vitamins, minerals and trace elements. After a few months of using these products they report that their "hot, painful joints" have cooled off and are no longer painful. I much prefer this method of rebuilding the body from within and preventing the inflammation that leads to arthritis over attacking the inflammation that has already occurred. I call this method "Remineralization of your body, you will be amazed at how well it works to cool down your arthritic joints, while building a body that is healthy, strong and disease resistant. Call me crazy, but as a physician those are the kind of medical treatments that really get me excited. I just love seeing happy, smiling patients that are no longer suffering with their arthritis.

The Importance Of Collagen For Healthy Joints

Nothing is more critical to the health of your connective tissue such as your joints, ligaments, tendons, bones and skin than collagen. Collagen is a family of structural proteins that make up your body's connective tissue. Connective tissue is what lies between and around your cells helping to connect them together, hence the name. Think of it as a matrix in which your cells are embedded. Connective tissue also supports body parts and connects them such as tendons, joints and ligaments. Think of connective tissue as the glue that holds your body parts together, and provides it with strength. The primary protein of connective tissue is collagen whose name originates from the Greek word for glue.

Collagen is a fascinating protein whose structure eluded scientists for years, but now is known to be a triple helix. A helix is a winding structure similar in shape to a metal coil spring. DNA is the best known example and is a double helix or two springs intertwined or braided together. Collagen goes one step further and is a triple helix or a triple-braided structure, as you can imagine this gives it significant strength, and nature exploits this structure by using it in ligaments, joints, ends of bones, and skin, thus the critical importance of healthy collagen for healthy connective tissue. The longer the chains of collagen fibers, the stronger they are, and the stronger the tissues that are made from them. Collagen also gives skin its ability to stretch, slide over muscles, and rebound to its original position and shape.

Collagen is made primarily from the amino acids proline, lysine, and glycine. The production of collagen is dependent upon vitamin C as a cofactor and various enzymes. A severe deficiency of vitamin C leads to scurvy. Scurvy is characterized by bleeding gums, loss of teeth, non-healing skin lesions and wounds, and discoloration of the skin, all the result of improperly made collagen.

An English physician, Dr. James Lind, was the first to indirectly realize the importance of vitamin C by providing fresh fruit such as limes to British sailors on long sea voyages to prevent scurvy. This worked wonderfully and prevented the epidemics of scurvy that had been incapacitating and killing so many sailors. This also led to the derogatory term Limey for the English.

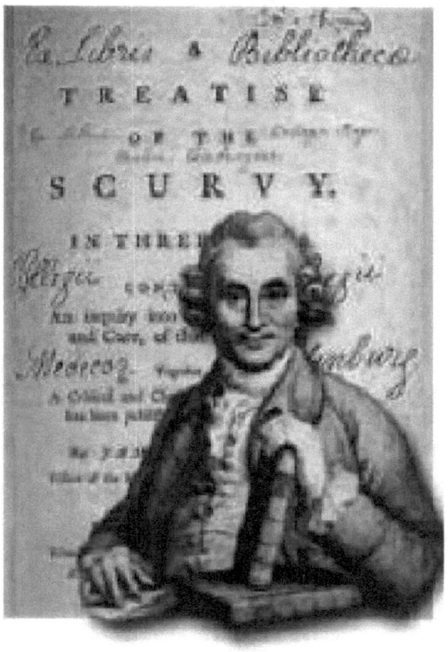

Dr. James Lind

When the fibroblasts in your body are forced to make collagen from a pool of nutrients that is lacking vitamin C, all the correct amino acids and minerals, it results in a structurally weakened triple helix. What does this mean in English? This means that your ligaments, tendons, joints, and skin are lax and not as strong as they should be. Your skin sag, your joints become inflamed and painful, your muscles hurt, and in short you act like an old man, getting up stiff and in pain. This also results in numerous sports injuries, slower growth, skin and joint problems, especially in children and adolescents. Ultimately as you age, this results in sagging skin, jowls, stiff joints, and eventually stiff blood vessels; since collagen also is in the wall of blood vessels. (Blood vessels also need healthy fats, magnesium, calcium, and vitamins C, D, and K2 to keep themselves pliable and healthy.)

How Do We Keep Our Collagen Healthy?

As humans we will need to keep ourselves strong and healthy; joint, bone, skin, and teeth are critical components of that healthy body, all of which depend upon proper collagen production and maintenance, for which supplying the proper amino acids and vitamin C are critical. Proper collagen formation is also critical for proper wound healing.

Vitamin C is very inexpensive and even the cheap brands work fine. Large tubs of vitamin C crystals or powder can also be purchased inexpensively. The amino acids are also easy to come by on an ongoing basis by making bone broth. Collagen in bones, cartilage, ligaments, and joints is similar in animals as in man. One of the main components of collagen are the glycosaminoglycan's. Two members of the glycosaminoglycan family are glucosamine and chondroitin. The same glucosamine and chondroitin found in glucosamine/chondroitin supplements. Glucosamine is able to resist digestion in the stomach and is absorbed in the intestines, and enters the blood and is taken up by connective tissue. Once glucosamine is taken up by cartilage it helps produce new healthy collagen and heals inflamed, painful joints; it also helps everywhere collagen is found, such as bones, ligaments, tendons, skin, hair, and even teeth. Chondroitin is one of the major components in cartilage, in which it helps absorb water keeping the cartilage smooth, flexible, and moist, thus avoiding drying and fraying of the cartilage. Chondroitin also inactivates enzymes that break down cartilage and helps the production of new cartilage.

Americans have been off traditional diets that nourished mankind since Homo sapiens emerged on the world scene. Since time immemorial man has cooked and eaten the entire animal, not just the meat as is currently done. Traditionally, a soup was made of chicken or beef bones, for example. This soup or broth was done by slow cooking the entire carcass of a chicken, including the feet, over the course of several hours the cartilage dissolves and the bones fall apart, releasing into the broth healing minerals such as manganese, magnesium, calcium, boron, and trace elements as well as proteins such as glucosamine and chondroitin, vitamins and enzymes...all of which made a stew of healing, nutritious substances that made people grow strong, tall, with straight teeth (no crowded overlapping teeth), symmetrical faces, square shoulders, and healthy joints. In the last several generations, especially in America and other western nations, we have industrialized our food production and have made food preparation an industry. Unfortunately, this has stripped our food of many of these essentials for bone and joint health.

We should follow the example of every "primitive" society that preceded us, and eat the entire animal, wasting nothing. The connective tissue of these animals contains all the ingredients our connective tissues need to be healthy. You do not need supplements, you need good nutrition. Even supplements like glucosamine/chondroitin have been isolated and processed and compressed into a pill, devoid of manganese and other minerals, trace elements, enzymes, amino acids, and other nutrients found in the animals' tissues. There is no case where the supplement is better than the natural source.

Bone broth will not only help your bones, teeth, skin, and joints, but it also helps your digestion and therefore your allergies, asthma, and immune problems, and will even help reduce cellulite. Cellulite has been shown to be fat deposits on an abnormal skeleton of collagen fibers; hence it is corrected not by reducing fat intake but rather by improving the health of your collagen! I am absolutely sure that I have now gotten the attention of my female readers! Glycine and other amino acids also help produce the neurotransmitter serine, which helps improve memory, mood, and alertness never a bad thing.

As patients we need to nourish ourselves and our growing children with all the nutrients we all need to maintain and grow healthy strong bones, joints, cartilage, tendons, ligaments, blood vessels, teeth, and skin. The answer for this is bone broth, minerals and trace elements, and vitamin C.

How To Make Bone Broth

The first thing to remember with making bone broth is to use either free-range animals and/or animals grazed on organic pastures, this will avoid the toxic chemicals concentrated in the tissues of animals raised in factory farms. Wild-caught fish can also be used to make bone broth. When you cook meat on the bone you are helping to extract all the vitamins, minerals, and trace elements along with amino acids, natural gelatins, phosphorus, and the all-important glycosaminoglycan's such as glucosamine and chondroitin, and your soup or stock is now chock-full of these nourishing substances that your body can recognize as food, absorb, and utilize.

Bone broth is also known as stock; different terms for the same thing. Bone broth is cheap to make, probably from parts that you previously would have thrown away such as the carcass of a chicken, and is incredibly nutritious for your body and tastes really good to boot.

Ingredients For Bone Broth:

2 to 5 pounds of bones (depending upon their availability, the size of your pot, and how much you want to make. You usually will need about a gallon of water for every 2 pounds of bones. If you are using cow bones or goat, horse, or other large animal, it helps to roast them in the oven first for about a half an hour or so, at about 350-400 degrees. This will remove some of their bitter flavor.

Add onions, carrots, celery, and garlic to add nutrients and flavor as per taste (add the garlic about a half an hour before it is done cooking). Other herbs and spices can be added depending upon your taste preferences.

Apple cider vinegar: Use about one tablespoon per pound of bones.

Sea salt: This is optional, but I like to use it to add minerals and trace elements.

You could also put a tablespoon of Azomite into the mix.

Take a large five-gallon pot and put your bones in and then add water to cover the bones. Now add the vinegar and let the bones, cold water, and vinegar sit for a half an hour or so. The acid vinegar will help leach out minerals from the bones. Now fire up the stove and let it heat up until it is boiling, then reduce the flame to a simmer and allow it to simmer. During the simmering many impurities will gather on the surface as a grey scum; just scoop this off with a spoon and discard it. The simmering is the long part and will take up to forty-eight hours for beef, twenty-four for chicken and eight for fish bones. When done, remove it from the heat and let it cool slightly then pour it through a strainer to remove bone fragments and other large particles, pour it into glass bottles and store it.

Note: It will form a gelatin-like consistency that is easily made into a liquid upon reheating. It will last about a week in the refrigerator, but will last a long time frozen. You can even freeze it and put it in ice cube trays and then empty the bone broth cubes into plastic bags and store them.

Alternative Methods For Treating Joint And Muscle Pain

Here is a list of other alternative treatments for joint, muscle pain, stiffness, and injury: See the appropriate areas in this book for full descriptions on how to use these treatments.

1. **Castor oil packs:**

   Soak a piece of flannel cloth with castor oil and drape it over the joint you want to treat then put a heat source (a heating pad or a hot cloth) over it for an hour at a time. It works wonderfully to penetrate the skin and soothe and relax underlying areas.

2. **DMSO:**

   DMSO stands for dimethyl sulfoxide .Rub it into the affected joint or painful soft tissue (muscles and fatty areas) several times a day. It penetrates the skin rapidly and will give you a garlic taste, as well as give your body a slight garlic odor. DMSO works very well for joint and muscle pain as well as being an excellent carrier oil (it is not really an oil) to transport other substances across the skin. DMSO is illegal in many states for use by humans; I disagree with this and think it is safe, especially for short-term use. That being said, it is sold by veterinarian supply houses and places like Tractor Supply, as well as on the Internet for use on animals (with a wink and a nod).

3. **Epsom salt baths and poultices:**

   Two cups of Epsom salt in the hottest bath you can stand, without burning yourself, for one-half hour. This is the amount of time it takes for the full transdermal effect of the magnesium sulfate (Epsom salt). Epsom salt is magnesium sulfate and readily crosses the skin, relaxing and soothing sore muscles and joints, decreasing inflammation. After taking an Epsom salt bath be very careful upon exiting the bathtub; since it relaxes muscles your legs will be rubbery and you will feel like Gumby, be careful not to fall.

4. **Glucosamine-chondroitin:**

   Glucosamine is a natural substance made by the body and not found in foods except for the shells of crabs, lobster, and shrimp and the bones of animals. Glucosamine helps heal the cartilage in your joints. Glucosamine is one of the structural building blocks of cartilage.

   Cartilage wraps around the ends of bones helping to form joints and allows for the smooth movement of bones and joints. Chondroitin is a natural substance made by the body and is part of the makeup of cartilage. Chondroitin works by helping cartilage to absorb water, thereby keeping it hydrated and reducing friction and wear and tear on the cartilage. Chondroitin also helps reduce the enzymatic breakdown of cartilage, and since it is a component of healthy cartilage it helps build new cartilage. The doses for both glucosamine and chondroitin are around 500 mg tid (three times daily) for both of them. A preferable way to get your glucosamine/ chondroitin is by making bone broth as outlined above.

5. **MSM (Methylsulfonylmethane):**

   At 1 gram a day this works wonders for joint pain and stiffness. It has both anti-inflammatory and analgesic (pain relieving) effects and is generally well tolerated. My wife, Lynne, suffered with joint and muscle aches that were almost completely alleviated by using MSM. It is an organosulfur compound that is very similar to DMSO. It provides a biologically active form of sulfur that helps the inflammation of joints.

6. **Sam-e (S-adenosyl-L-methionine):**

   This naturally occurring compounds first used to treat depression and it was found to have beneficial effects on patients' arthritis, but the mechanism of its action is unclear. It might lead to some GI side effects, but they are mild. It is often times included in glucosamine/chondroitin products. The dose is about 1200 mg/day (usually in three divided doses of 400 mg each).

7. **Oral hyaluronic acid (HA):**

   HA is a normal component of the synovial fluid that bathes joints. Previously it was administered to patients by an injection directly into the joints. Now an oral form is available and the usual dose is 200 mg/day. HA acts as an immune modulator, keeping inflammation in check and promotes healing of connective tissue and skin, thus its beneficial effects on inflamed joints such as in arthritis.

8. **Omega-3 fatty acids:**

   Fish oil, walnut oil, and flaxseed oil. These work surprisingly well to squelch inflammation in joints. Many patients whom I have placed on omega-3 fatty acids for other reasons have repeatedly reported to me how good their joints feel. A good dose is 4 grams a day, either divided into four individual, two twice a day, or four once daily. If you can take them before you eat, eat immediately after taking them, this way the food will block any regurgitation of the fish oil and its resulting nasty fish taste in your mouth!

9. **Curcumin,**

   Curcumin is contained in turmeric, is a popular South Asian spice which is a member of the ginger family. Turmeric is what gives the curry in Indian food its characteristic color and flavor. Curcumin has strong anti-inflammatory effects and is an antioxidant as well. It also stimulates the gallbladder to empty its bile into the small intestine, helping digestion. It is not very soluble in water and needs alkaline conditions to increase its solubility and its bioavailability (its absorption and uptake by the body resulting in higher plasma or blood levels). A good trick is to add a pinch of baking soda to alkalinize the curcumin and thus increase its bioavailability. Curcumin comes in various forms. Here are the doses of the different forms available currently

   Dried root, 2 to 3 grams daily

   Fresh cut root, 1 to 3 grams daily

   Standardized powder in capsules 500 mg tid (Three times daily)

   Tincture approximately twenty-five drops tid

10. **Essential oils such as: Lavender Oil , German Chamomile Oil, Everlasting Oil and Peppermint Oil**

    Note: I strongly recommend diluting these oils in a carrier oil (also called a base oil). Carrier oils are thus named because they help carry or transport the essential oil across your skin to their target areas such as joints, ligaments, and tendons as well as sore muscles. Diluting essential oils will not dilute their effect at all, in fact on the contrary, these carrier oils will potentiate (make them more potent) the essential oils dissolved in them. In their pure undiluted forms many essential oils are sometimes too strong and are irritating to the skin, causing burning and redness and sometimes rashes to develop at the site of their application.

    Most seed oils can be used as carrier oils such as sesame, hazelnut, almond, for example. See the section on essential oils and seed oils for full details. Seed oils such as these and others should be kept in ample supply in your alternative medicine chest, they can also be used as food if you need them, which doubles their usefulness in an emergency.

    A simple, reliable way to mix essential oils with a carrier oil is to mix 2 ounces (or two tablespoons) of your carrier oil with three or four drops of the essential oil. This will make an appropriate blend that will readily cross your skin and reach its target more effectively than using the essential oils undiluted. I highly recommend an outstanding book on this subject by Dr. Kurt Schnaubelt entitled The Healing Intelligence of Essential Oils. In this book he does an excellent job of educating you on the uses of essential oils and the science behind them.

11. **Astaxanthin:**

Astaxanthin is a very powerful antioxidant and consequently an anti- inflammatory agent. Astaxanthin's antioxidant capacity is the strongest yet found in nature and has been measured to be 6,000 times stronger than vitamin C!

It is a carotenoid or organic pigment made by plants like that found in carrots, and thus gives an orange/red/pink color to foods such as carrots but astaxanthin is a carotenoid that only comes from the sea. In fact, there is a single micro-algae called Haematococcus pluvialis that is known to produce astaxanthin, these algae are in turn eaten by krill, salmon, and shrimp, giving them their pink color. Farm-raised salmon get their pink color from synthetic astaxanthin. Avoid this, stick with the natural form which has been found to be twenty times as powerful. Astaxanthin is also fat soluble and will need to be taken with a fatty meal. If you want to get it from wild salmon then you will need to eat about 4 ounces daily.

In supplement form the dose is 4 mg daily with fatty food. You can also get your dose of astaxanthin from fish oil, getting the other benefits of the omega-3 fatty acids at the same time. Krill are interesting tiny shrimp-like crustaceans that swim in massive dense schools up to several miles across that migrate vertically. After feeding on algae deep in the oceans they migrate towards the surface where they are eaten by other fish such as salmon, thus cycling nutrients from near the ocean floor to the surface. Since they live mostly in very cold arctic waters they have developed a high phospholipid content that keeps their cell membranes nice and flexible, and it does the same for your joints. The usual dose of krill oil is about 300 mg daily, however with arthritis, especially if you want to use it instead of Aleve or Naprosyn, then you should take about 1,000 mg daily, or 1 gram.

12. **Resveratrol:**

Resveratrol is a plant-derived polyphenol (phenols are almost always good for you) that is found naturally in the skin and seeds of grapes and other plants.

Resveratrol is a strong antioxidant, and also decreases the stickiness of platelets (which is important for heart disease and blood clots), has been touted to lower cancer rates and even help weight loss. In some studies it even helped in diabetes by lowering insulin resistance, which is the primary cause of the current epidemic of type 2 diabetes.

Resveratrol is found primarily in red wine because red wine is fermented with the grape skin whereas white wine is not. Hey, look at it this way; at the very least it is a good excuse to drink more red wine! Resveratrol is also found in sprouted peanuts and in my all-time favorite plant, the mulberry. Mulberries contain significant amounts of resveratrol. Mulberry trees are one of the easiest fruit trees to grow and do not require any special spraying since they rarely suffer with any of the usual diseases of fruit trees. I grow over fourteen varieties of mulberry on my Connecticut property. The dose of resveratrol is from 200 to 500 mg daily, but for arthritis it is better to use the higher dose of approximately 2,000 mg daily, or 2 grams.

13. **Boron:**

Boron is a trace mineral found in most plants. As with all minerals and trace elements it is becoming progressively depleted in our soils, resulting in lower plant levels and in turn lower human levels. A plant- based diet grown on fertile organic soils will usually deliver between 2 to 5 mg of Boron daily, but studies show that our western diets deliver considerably less, more like 0.25 to 2 mg daily The overcooking of foods, phytic acid in many foods, and candida infections all further lower levels of boron in many patients.

Boron is essential for bone and joint health and is also responsible for maintaining the integrity of cell membranes in humans and the cell wall of plant cells. Boron is strongly antifungal (soaking your feet in a solution of Borax and water will rapidly kill the fungus causing athlete's foot), antiviral, but with little antibacterial effect. In the body boron has its highest concentration in the parathyroid gland, dental enamel, and bones. Boron is responsible for giving both the enamel of your teeth and your bones their characteristic hardness, thus one of the reasons I suggest taking this daily, especially if you have osteopenia (the stage before osteoporosis) or osteoporosis.

Boron works by regulating the absorption and metabolism of the key minerals that are players in bone development; calcium, magnesium, and phosphorus through the actions of the parathyroid gland. As I have said in the past, minerals are essential for the functioning of enzymes and vitamins. Iodine for example is essential for proper thyroid function, and so is boron for proper parathyroid function. When you have a low boron level, it causes an increase in parathyroid gland activity, which causes bones and teeth to release their stored calcium, leading in turn to tooth decay, osteoporosis, and arthritis. Many studies have shown a direct correlation between arthritis levels and the boron levels of a country's soil. Jamaica, for instance, has a very low level of boron in her soil and their arthritis rate is over 70 percent! Boron will also work for rheumatoid arthritis juvenile arthritis, and SLE (lupus).

When you supplement with Boron the usual dose is 3 mg daily, but double or even triple that if you have arthritis, joint pain and/or osteopenia or osteoporosis. Once your pain and inflammation is under control then you can lower it to 3 mg daily once again. Boron supplementation helps activate vitamin D which in turn increases the absorption of calcium into bones and teeth where it belongs. Boron is also involved in the production of other steroid hormones like estrogen in women and testosterone in men, it raises both and thus can be used in women who are suffering with hot flashes and men with low testosterone levels (also give zinc to help raise testosterone). Supplementation with boron was shown in several studies to be as effective as hormone replacement therapy, and for a hell of a lot less money!

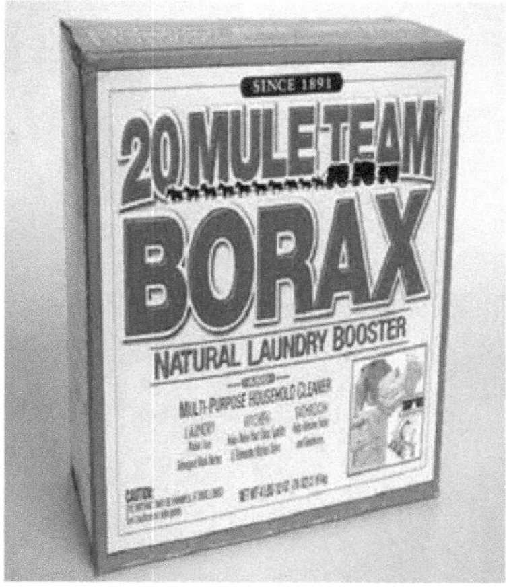

The common laundry detergent Borax is an important source of boron; it is a mineral and a salt of boric acid. There is no synthetic version and it is mined from dried salt lakes primarily in Turkey and the western United States. It is 99.5 percent pure and pharmaceutical grade borax is no purer than the 20 Mule Team Borax you buy in your supermarket. I still have fond memories as a child of 20 Mule Team Borax sponsoring some of my favorite westerns. There was a discovery of a large deposit of Borax in 1881 in Death Valley and the nearest railroad was located 165 miles away. The mine owners built huge wagons with rear wheels seven feet high and the bed of the wagon was sixteen feet long; these wagons carried twelve tons (24,000 pounds) of Borax each and the twenty-mule-teams pulled two wagons at once along with a 1200 gallon water wagon which was essential or the mules were going to die in those hot desert conditions. These mule teams were tethered to those wagons on 120 feet of equipment and ropes, pulling a total of 36.5 tons with each load.

You can use Borax safely and without problems if you follow these instructions carefully. The best way to use Borax is to make a concentrated solution by mixing a teaspoon of Borax, which is 5 or 6 grams, into a liter of clean, unchlorinated water. Use this as your "medicine bottle" take a teaspoon of this daily which will contain about 3 mg of boron. You can go as high as three teaspoons daily to treat your arthritis until it is under control, then lower yourself to one teaspoon daily of the concentrate as your maintenance dose.

Boron and Borax are very alkaline and as such are very effective in treating both topical and internal yeast and fungal infections. The reason for this is that yeast and fungi can only live in a very acidic environment and thus are readily killed by the elevation of pH caused by the very basic or alkaline boron and Borax. A moist powder made from Borax will work rapidly to relieve the discomfort of jock itch as well as that of athlete's foot, just rub the solution on the affected area.

For internal fungal infections such as candida you have to use a different ratio of Borax to make your solution. For the treatment of candidiasis you mix an eighth of a teaspoon of Borax in a liter of water, and over the course of a day drink the entire liter. It may have a soapy taste and you can make it sweeter with some lemon juice, orange juice, or even vitamin C crystals. You can use this until your symptoms of candida and its resulting leaky gut resolve.

Boron is very nontoxic, despite rumblings to the contrary which were based on flawed studies with incredibly high doses that would never be given if you follow my directions, in which there is ample room for error without any significant side effects. You can also use the same more dilute solution that you use for candida to treat oral thrush, just gargle with this several times a day.

14. Avocado soybean unsaponifiables (ASU)

ASU are natural vegetable extracts derived from avocado oil and soybean oil. ASU is touted to work to help the pain and inflammation associated with arthritis and indeed this has been verified by several different studies. The best dose is 300 mg daily. According to these studies patients used less pain medications and nonsteroidal anti- inflammatory meds after being treated with ASU, however you have to wait two months for it to take effect. The good news is that its residual effects last two months after you stop taking it, so it's a wash if you are a patient person.

Since only a small fraction of either avocado or soybean oils are unsaponified, you will not be able to eat enough of either soy or avocado to get a beneficial effect on your arthritis. Unsaponifiable means that it cannot be easily changed into soap.

ASU seems to work in the exact same fashion as painkillers and anti- inflammatory medications, that is, by suppressing prostaglandins and cytokines. ASUs have been shown to not only protect your existing cartilage, but also to promote the growth of new cartilage. As you remember, osteoarthritis, which is the most common type of arthritis that you will encounter, is painful due to the destruction of cartilage, so anything that promotes its healing and growth will work wonderfully as a treatment.

15. **Pectin and Grape Juice;**

Pectin is a water soluble carbohydrate found in the cell walls of plants giving them their support and strength. Commercially it is mainly extracted from citrus fruit, and is used as a gelling agent in jams and jellies. It should be taken mixed with grape juice in a ratio of one tablespoon of liquid pectin to eight ounces of grape juice. Take this twice daily, it usually takes a few weeks to work. It helps arthritis by helping increase the elasticity in joints, lubricating them and decreasing their pain and inflammation.

16. **Organic Apple Cider Vinegar;**

I prefer to use the brand Bragg's; it is organic and readily available in stores or online. Not only is it bursting with helpful enzymes and microbes but it also has an alkalinizing effect and is high in calcium, magnesium, phosphorus and potassium. Take it by mixing two or three teaspoons of apple cider vinegar in warm water, add honey so it tastes better.

Drink this three times a day.

17. **Fenugreek (Trigonella foenum -graecum)**

Fenugreek is an annual plant in the pea family, grown worldwide, but primarily in the Middle East and India. It is a rich source of protein, fiber, iron and many other minerals. Fenugreek has both antioxidant and anti-inflammatory properties and therefore works well in patients with arthritis. For our purposes we are using finely ground seeds. The dose is one teaspoon of finely ground fenugreek seeds followed by a large glass of water. The seeds can also be soaked overnight to make them more palatable and eaten the following morning.

18. **Extra Virgin Olive Oil (EVOO)**;

Extra virgin means the first pressing of the olives, I prefer mine to be cold pressed and not treated chemically or with heat which destroys many of the beneficial properties of EVOO. Only EVOO contains Olecanthal which is a natural phenol which has strong anti- inflammatory and antioxidant properties, and is also a potent inhibitor of Cox enzymes similar to non-steroidal anti-inflammatory drugs (NSAIDS) which are the primary drugs used to treat arthritis. In fact a teaspoon and a half of EVOO is equivalent to 200 mg of ibuprofen! Olecanthal is the ingredient that gives EVOO its distinctive taste, and causes that slight burning in your throat after you swallow it. The usual dose varies but is approximately two or three teaspoons daily, since I am Italian I love EVOO and use quite a bit more of it and my joints love it. It can also be used topically by massaging it into a painful joint several times a day as needed.

19. **Licorice:**

Licorice is derived from the root of a perennial plant in the pea family known as Glycyrrhiza glabra. Licorice's active ingredient is glycyrrhizin which has potent anti-inflammatory, antiviral, antimicrobial effects, as well as being protective of the liver. It is so potent an anti-inflammatory agent that its effects are similar to corticosteroids (commonly known as steroids). It is believed it has this effect by blocking the enzymes involved in inflammation as well as increasing the release of the body's cortisol thus depressing the immune response involved in inflammation.

NOTE: if you have high blood pressure or swelling of your legs you should be careful with licorice since it may exacerbate (worsen) those problems. If you are taking whole licorice, follow the manufacturers dosing instructions. If you are using the DGL extract then take a half teaspoon of the powder or two of the capsules before each meal.

20. **Stinging Nettle (Urtica dioica);**

Stinging nettle as every gardener finds out at some point has very fine hairs on its leaves and stems which cause a stinging , burning sensation and hive like swelling in areas of the skin that come in contact with it. However, when it is applied to painful areas of the body it has the opposite effect, scientists hypothesize that it does this by reducing levels of inflammatory chemicals as well as blocking pain pathways. For our purposes it has several other benefits beyond its pain killing effects. Stinging nettle contains calcium, boron, silicon and magnesium thus helping it build strong bones. It is easily found in most parts of the country or can be purchased online. Leaves can be applied directly to painful areas of the skin.

NOTE: pregnant women or women trying to get pregnant should not use stinging nettle since it may cause a miscarriage. It should also not be used by patients on blood thinners such as Plavix, Coumadin or aspirin. The plant is available commercially as dried leaves, tinctures, teas and capsules. Each manufacturer has their own dosage directions.

21. **Golden Raisins and Gin;**

This seems to be a favorite of many old timers in New England. Gin is made from juniper berries which are known to decrease the activity of white blood cells known as monocytes which are part of the inflammatory pathway. The golden raisins contain sulfides which help joint health and also decrease inflammation. Either way, it is a fun way to treat your arthritis, just don't drive after you take them! To make your potion take a cup of golden raisins and place them in a shallow dish and cover them with a half cup of gin, cover the plate with a cheese cloth and place them out of the way and wait a few weeks for the gin to fully evaporate. Eat about ten raisins a day , it is not a rapid cure and will take a few weeks to take effect.

22. **Juniper Tea:**

As state above juniper berries have potent anti-inflammatory effects and therefore help arthritis. Juniper berries contain significant amounts of terpenes which help mediate their beneficial effects. Take one tablespoon of dried juniper berries and mix them in one cup of water, add honey to make it more palatable and steep for an hour or so. Drink one cup twice daily.

23. **Dandelion (Taraxacum);**

Dandelion is probably one of the most easily recognized and most common of weeds found just about everywhere.

For our purposes it is overflowing with vitamins A,B,C and D, as well as the minerals iron, potassium and zinc. We will be using the leaves of the dandelion plant to make a tea, or fresh leaves can be used in a salad along with extra virgin olive oil. To make the tea take 3 teaspoons or fresh leaves or 1 teaspoon of dried leaves in one cup of water, bring it to a boil, strain it and drink the tea (you can add honey to help the taste as per your preference) twice a day.

24. **Blackstrap Molasses;**

    Blackstrap molasses is made from the third boiling of sugar syrup , reducing it to a thick black liquid. Produced this way the majority of the sucrose that started out has been crystallized and removed. The remaining liquid is concentrated and thus very high in potassium, calcium, magnesium, iron and manganese, as well as vitamin B6. For our purposes heat a mug of water to warm, not boiling and stir in one tablespoon of blackstrap molasses and take this once a day. **NOTE:** if you take it more than once a day it may cause diarrhea.

25. **White Willow Tea;**

    White willow or Salix Alba is a common tree in Europe and Asia and gets its name from the white color to the underside of its leaves. The active ingredient is salicin which is changed in the body to salicylic acid which is very similar to acetyl salicylic acid which is the active ingredient in aspirin. Fortunately for us the conversion of salicin to salicylic acid occurs in the intestines and thus does not cause an upset stomach. As with aspirin this should not be used by anyone with a bleeding problem, ulcers etc. It should also not be used by anyone already on a blood thinner of any type such as Coumadin or Plavix . To make a tea take two teaspoons of white willow bark powder and add it to one cup of water , add honey and lemon to taste and allow it to steep (to sit and soak) for about an hour and then drink it , once daily.

GOUT

Gout is another disease that will give significant joint pain and discomfort. Gout may strike any joint but in practice it commonly afflicts your feet, especially the base of your great toe (big toe). This foot or toe pain is known medically as podagra. The great toe will be swollen, red, hot and painful, any movement or touching of it will cause pain. Gout is caused by high uric acid levels in your blood. Uric acid comes from the metabolism of purines.

Purines are found in most meats, mushrooms, anchovies, organ meats such as liver and kidneys, herring, mackerel, sardines, scallops, and wild game. Purines are also found in beer due to its yeast content. Vegetables such as beans, lentils, asparagus, cauliflower, spinach, peas, and oatmeal also contain significant amounts of purines and thus may contribute to gout.

Treatment of Gout

Hydration

In clinical practice I have found that gout is most often caused by a combination of poor dietary habits combined with some level of dehydration. I use a Kool-Aid analogy to explain this to my patients. If you take a packet of Kool-Aid and mix it in a full glass of water, it will all dissolve and disappear.

Now if you take the same packet and mix it in a half glass of water what will happen is that the Kool-Aid will precipitate out of solution and gather at the bottom of the glass. Gout is the same situation, if your uric acid levels in your blood are elevated and you become dehydrated, this lowers your water content in your blood and at the same time raises the concentration of uric acid. It then precipitates out of solution and crystallizes in your joints, causing a gout attack. For that reason one of the simplest methods of treating an acute gout attack is to hydrate yourself, drink eight to twelve glasses of water a day and the attack will quickly disappear. You will probably need some painkillers until the pain lessens and so take Motrin or Aleve as needed (with food). During a gout attack you should also avoid meat and meat products and the other foods listed above to help drop your purine intake and subsequently your uric acid levels. You should also avoid alcohol during a gout attack; the worst offenders are beer, port, and other wines.

Uricosuric Medications

Typically we give uricosuric medications (meds that increase the excretion of uric acid by the kidney) such as colchicine and allopurinol, and these work wonderfully to quickly drop your blood levels of uric acid and subsequently your gout symptoms. Colchicine is derived from the bulbs of autumn crocus plants. I happen to really like growing these crocus plants here in New England, as you might have already noticed, I am a gardening fanatic and love growing just about everything.

Vitamin C

Vitamin C has been shown to help gout in two ways; it increases the excretion of uric acid by the kidney and at the same time decreases the reabsorption of uric acid by the kidney. Studies on vitamin C and gout were done with a 500 mg a day dose. Remember vitamin C is water soluble so it can be taken on an empty stomach.

Cherries, Blueberries, And Strawberries

Cherries have also been shown to have a uricosuric effect in a recent study. Ten to twelve cherries a day or the use of cherry juice or cherry extract will also work. Other berries such as blueberries and strawberries neutralize uric acid and help gout.

Over the years I have heard anecdotal reports from patients about soaking cherries in gin to help their joint aches. I was never quite sure if the cherries contributed anything or was the gin just working to numb their pain!

Lemons And Lemon Juice

Lemons and lemon juice have also been shown to help gout. Gout is also a cause of uric acid kidney stones ,and urologists for years have been recommending squeezing a fresh lemon into water daily and drinking it to prevent kidney stones. I have put many patients on this regimen with excellent results.

Celery Seed Extract

Celery seed extract has been shown to lower uric acid levels as well as having a potent anti-inflammatory effect. The usual dose is 450 mg two or three times a day.

Bromelain

Bromelain, which is an enzyme derived from the stems of pineapple plants, has also been found to be helpful in the treatment of gout.

The best dose for this is 500 mg three times a day on a full stomach. Bromelain has an anti-inflammatory effect and works well for gout and other causes of joint inflammation such as arthritis.

Fish Oil, Walnut Oil, Flaxseed Oil (Omega-3 Fatty Acids)

Fish oil also works very well for joint inflammation and gout. You should make sure that the fish oil you are taking has at least 480 mg of EPA and 360 mg of DHA.

Fish oil acts to quell or suppress the inflammation in joints. Over the years in my practice I have used fish oil in both over-the- counter and prescription strengths and patients have frequently remarked how their arthritis has improved. Walnut and flaxseed oils will also work very well in treating gout and other causes of joint inflammation.

Nettle Root

Nettle root is another agent that has uricosuric properties and helps gout. It is usually made from concentrated root extract and the dose is about 250 mg three times daily.

Drinking nettle tea is an old cure for arthritis, the“stinging” in stinging nettle’s name is from its high content of histamine which acts as an anti-inflammatory.

CHAPTER THIRTY-ONE

ORTHOPEDIC INJURIES: BROKEN BONES AND JOINT INJURIES

INTRODUCTION

TABLE OF CONTENTS:

This chapter on orthopedic injuries is for those cases where you are isolated and unable to reach proper medical care, and have to rely upon your own skills to help yourself or the injured party. In all other cases it is very much in your interest to go to an orthopedic surgeon. Orthopedic surgeons are very good at what they do and their skills and techniques cannot be replaced by alternative treatments. However, if they are not available and we have to rely upon ourselves we better learn something about bones, joints, tendons and ligaments and what to do when they are injured.

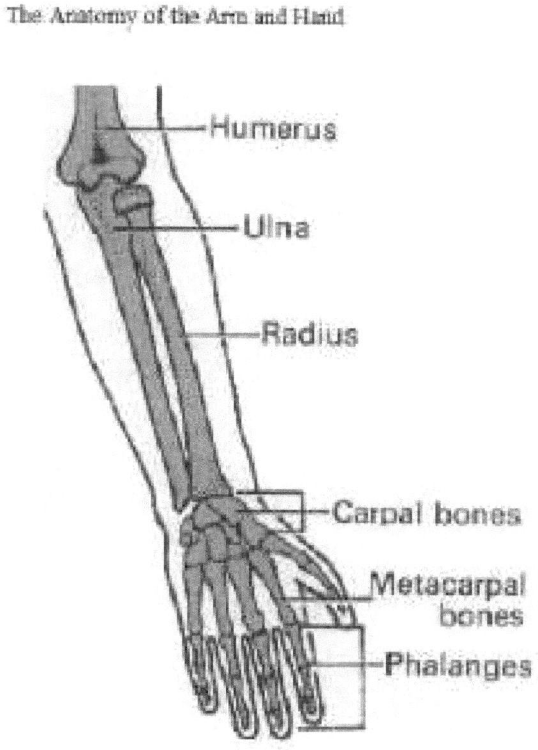

The Anatomy of the Arm and Hand

EVALUATING THE INJURY

When evaluating any potential broken bone or fracture, you must keep in mind the force that caused the injury.

Bones are rigid, but they do bend or "give" a little, when a force is applied against them they will bend a certain amount. Think of bones as a piece of long, brittle plastic, it will bend to a certain degree, after which it will snap. If that breaking point is just exceeded by the force applied to it, then it will just crack slightly, if it is largely exceeded it may break the bone right across, if it is wildly exceeded as in a car crash or gunshot, it might shatter the bone.

Fractures of bone are categorized in several ways but for our purposes there are two very easy ways to classify them, either as open or closed. Open fractures are of two basic types, one where the bone actually penetrates the skin and is sticking out and a second where the open wound extends all the way down to the surface of the broken bone. All other fractures are considered closed. Open fractures are more serious because once the skin is broken they are often accompanied by serious infections.

Here Is the Old Classification of Bone Fractures for Which You Need X-Ray Equipment:

Stable fracture: The bone is cracked and the broken ends of the bone line up and are barely out of their original position.

Open, compound fracture: The skin is either broken through by a piece of bone or the wound penetrates down to the broken bone. The bone may or may not be visible through the wound.

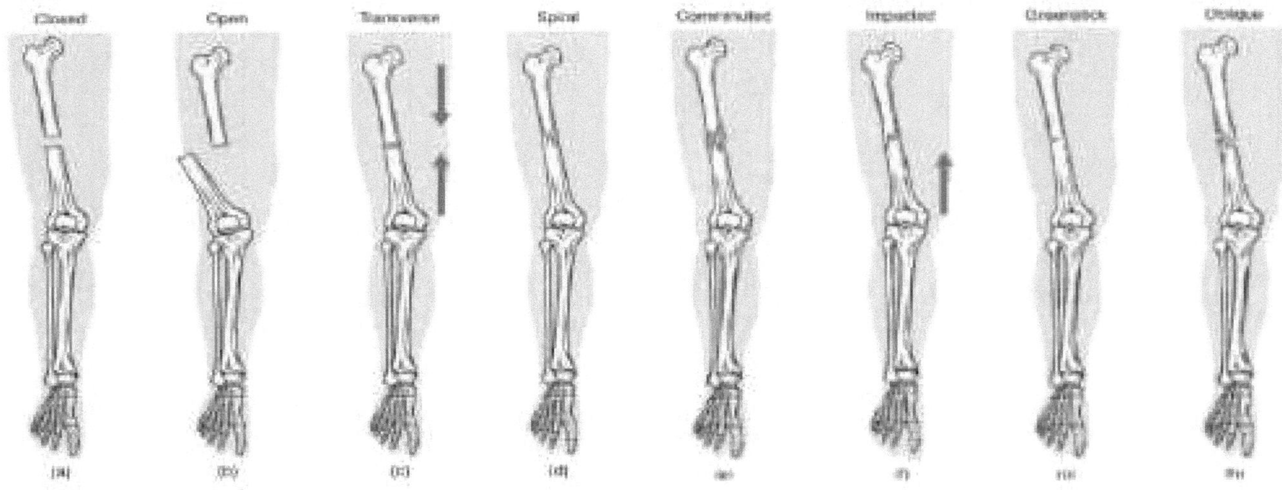

Types of Bone Fractures

Transverse fracture: It is a straight break perpendicular to the length of the bone or straight across the width of the bone. It has a horizontal fracture line.

Oblique fracture: Oblique means sideways, what you would have gotten with your Etch-a -Sketch if you turned both the horizontal and the vertical knobs at once…you would go between the two, that is an oblique fracture.

Comminuted fracture: In this type of fracture, the bone is shattered into three or more pieces.

WHY DO BONES FRACTURE (BREAK)?

Trauma

The most common cause of bone fractures is trauma and unfortunately you will probably be a victim of such trauma or witness it and have to immediately apply what I am going to teach you. What type of trauma is anyone's guess, but probably motor vehicle accidents, assaults, explosions, and gunshots would be high on my list of probable causes.

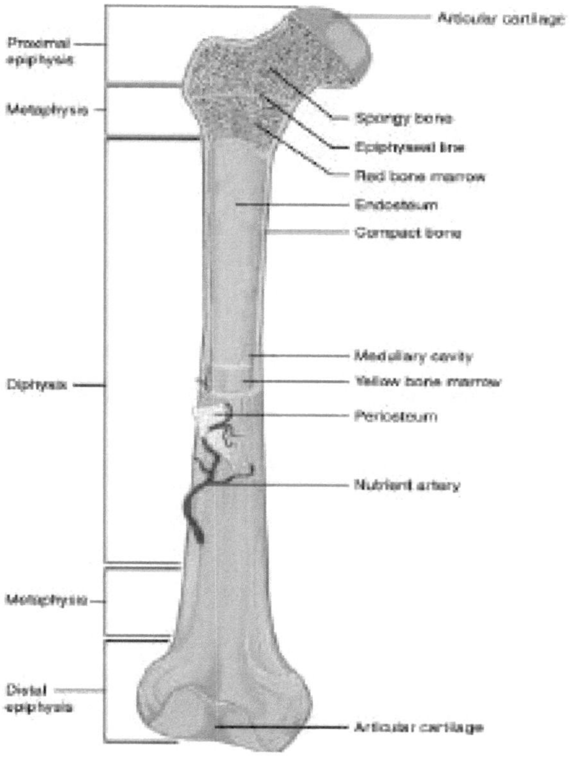

Anatomy of a Long Bone

Overuse Injuries

The second most common type will be due to overuse. This is the kind athletes are subject to. Repetitive motion causes muscles to tire and then weaken; this transfers much weight to the bones and eventually may result in a stress fracture.

Osteoporosis

Another cause, primarily found in the middle-aged and elderly, is osteoporosis. It also occurs in many patients who have been on chronic steroid therapy. Osteoporosis is a disease that causes bones to become thinned out as the minerals are leached out of the bone. These bones are therefore more brittle and tend to fracture sometimes just from the tension large muscles place on them. Classically this causes hip fractures. Many elderly patients just turn the wrong way and the muscular strain transferred to their weakened osteoporotic bones causes them to fracture, then the patient falls. The bone is broken before they even hit the ground. Several factors contribute to this but a few of the biggest are a sedentary lifestyle, poor diet lacking in calcium and Vitamins D and K2. Those three ingredients are essential for bone health and you need all three to build strong bones. Boron also helps to produce very strong bones. Exercise helps when you are younger, because as muscle pulls on bone, the bone responds by building more bone on the opposite side. This is why a sedentary lifestyle leads to osteoporosis.

Sunlight is also essential, because when your skin is exposed to sunlight it produces vitamin D. That has created a paradoxical situation in my practice where dark-skinned blacks and fair-skinned whites both have vitamin D deficiencies. Blacks (and other people of color) have evolutionally developed large amounts of melatonin or skin pigment and this served them very well in Africa, with the large amount of sun they were exposed to year round. However, when you take those same people and move them to a temperate climate like the United States or Europe they now have melatonin there genetically which is blocking the little sunlight they are now exposed to, resulting in vitamin D deficiencies. Fair-skinned whites, fearful of incurring sunburns and warned for decades by well-meaning dermatologists to avoid the sun, slather themselves in SPF 30 sunblock and therefore are hardly ever exposed to the benefits of healing, healthful sunlight. In earlier generations skin cancer was not a major problem even among northern Europeans who migrated to the United States, the reason being that they were outside all year round and had healthy, deeply tanned skin; they rarely if ever got burned. It is the recurrent burns that damage the skin cells and lead to skin cancers of various types.

Sunlight is wonderful for you and your body has developed evolutionally with large amounts of vitamin D available. This current worldwide epidemic of vitamin D deficiency is leading to multiple problems. Vitamin D is more of a hormone than a vitamin and is responsible for maintaining strong, dense bones, reducing rates of breast and other cancers, helping heart health, and a healthy immune system to name but a few of its benefits. If you want evidence of the immune-enhancing effect of vitamin D go no further than the flu virus. Vitamin D supplementation is eight times more effective at preventing the flu than a flu vaccine! That is very important to understand for your family's health, especially during the winter months when vitamin D levels are at their lowest due to a lack of sunlight and not so coincidentally the flu season peaks. As scientists and physicians study it ever more closely, they are finding more and more benefits associated with vitamin D.

What I advise my fair-skinned patients do is to get early morning and late day sun. You know the old saying, "only mad dogs and Englishmen go out in the midday sun". Start with about a half hour exposure at both ends of the day, with no sunblock at all. Avoid getting burned; if you feel it starting to burn, then stop for the day. Even the fairest skinned individuals will get a deep, healthy tan to their skin after a few weeks, after which they can venture out in the midday sun now that their skin contains healthy levels of melanin.

This will also give them a healthy, steady supply of free vitamin D and all of its associated health-giving benefits.

Symptoms Of A Broken Bone

Pain in or near the broken bone is the primary symptom of a fracture. The severity of the pain is subjective but in the vast majority of patients it will be severe. The patient may or not be able to use that limb for weight bearing or lifting, as for example in an ankle or arm fracture.

Note: Unlike a fracture, a patient with only a sprain will most likely be able to weight bear. That being said, some people are wimps and whiners and will complain bitterly of severe pain with only a mild sprain.

The swelling and bruising will be much more prominent with a fracture as compared to a sprain. A deformity of the bone…it looks broken, for example, a femur or thigh bone that is angled sideways is a dead giveaway even for a person without medical training. Or the bone has an angle where it should not be and is bent in unnatural ways. A deep, penetrating-down-to-the-bone gash or wound will very likely have an underlying fracture, especially if caused by a large force. A feeling of grinding along the shaft of a bone where there is usually none. This is the feeling that patients often describe as "bone on bone".

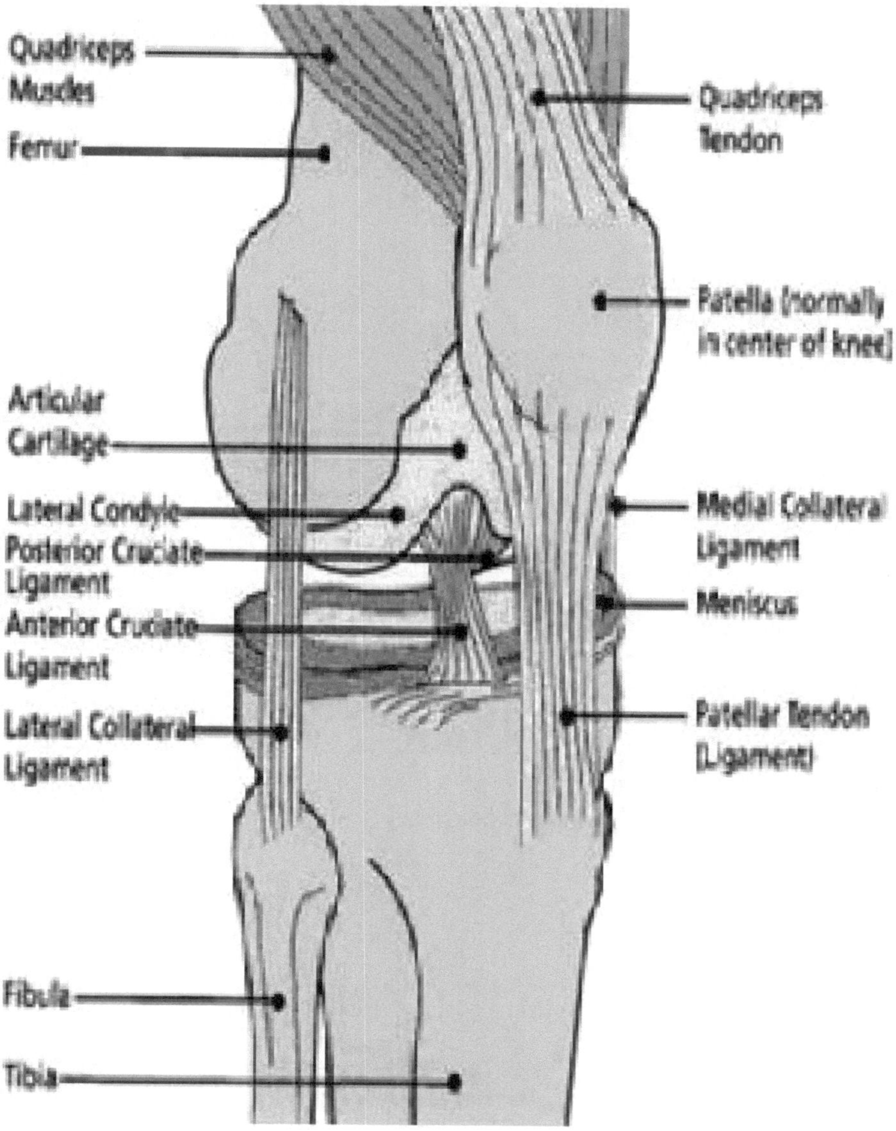

Anatomy Of The Knee
Front side of Knee

Ankle And Knee Injuries

Some of the more common bone fractures occur in both the ankle and the knee; here are some great tips in differentiating a sprain from a fracture without X-ray assistance:

Ankle Injuries

This advice was developed by a group of physicians in Ottawa, Canada, and is known as the Ottawa rules: they divided their rules into two sets, the first is to determine if you have a leg fracture, the second set determines if you have broken a foot bone. Let's first take a look at the anatomy.

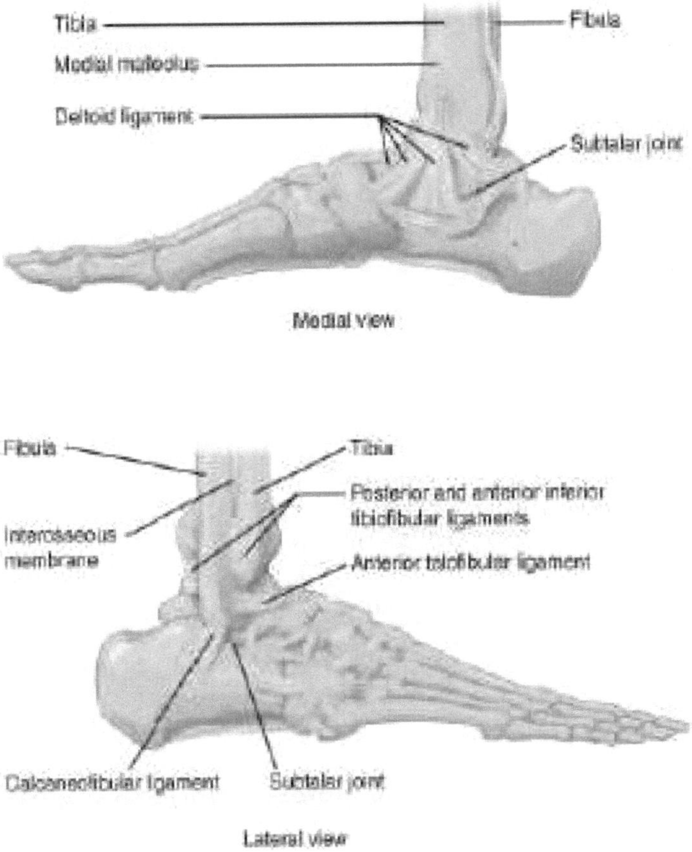

The Anatomy of the Ankle and Foot

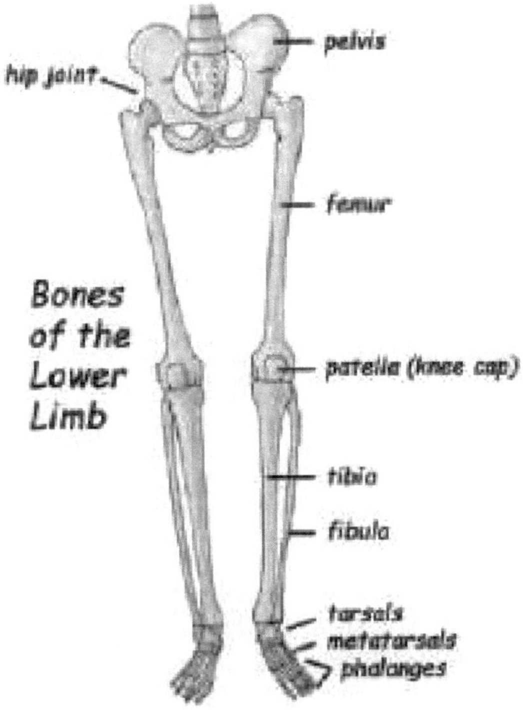

Let's first review some basic bone anatomy of your leg and foot. The lower leg has two bones, a large tibia and a smaller fibula. The lower end of the tibia is the large bony knob that forms the inside of your ankle. The lower end of the smaller fibula is the bony knob on the outside of your ankle. The foot contains the metatarsal bones (the hands are the metacarpals) that connect your tarsal bones to the phalanges of your toes. Those are the long bones of your foot. They are numbered one through five, with one being your big toe (the hand is also numbered one through five with one being your thumb). The navicular bone is the large bone of your foot and is diagonal to the underside of the bottom of your tibia on the inside of your ankle; you can feel it sticking out there if you feel your foot.

This first set of rules determines if you have broken your leg bones (tibia and fibula):

1. If you have tenderness upon pressing anywhere along the three inches above the end of your tibia.
2. If you have tenderness upon pressing anywhere along the three inches above the end of your fibula.
3. If you cannot weight bear at all. Note: If you limp, that is okay.

The second set of rules is to determine if you have broken any of the bones in your foot:

1. Tenderness when you press near the ankle along the fifth metatarsal. Note: the fifth metatarsal or little toe of your foot has a ligament connecting it to the ankle. Remember, tendons attach muscle to bone and ligaments attach bone to bone. If you roll your ankle or foot inward, this commonly causes the ligament which attaches your fifth metatarsal to your ankle to shear off and essentially break your foot.
2. Tenderness along your navicular bone at any point...along the top of it or the inner side.
3. Foot pain is keeping you from putting weight on your foot (weight bear).

Knee Injuries

Let's first do a quick review of the anatomy of a knee joint. The knee lies between the upper leg or thigh and the lower leg or shin. Nature uses the same bone distribution in a number of animals. It is one upper bone leading to two lower bones leading to five terminal bones. This is true in the arm and the leg in humans. In the human arm the upper arm has one bone, the humerus, leading to two bones in the forearm, the radius (on the thumb side) and the ulna (on the pinky or fifth finger side). The leg is no different, the upper leg has the large femur or thigh bone, the lower leg has the large tibia, which bears most of the weight and is situated directly below the femur, and the smaller fibula, which is on the lateral or outside of the leg and does little weight bearing.

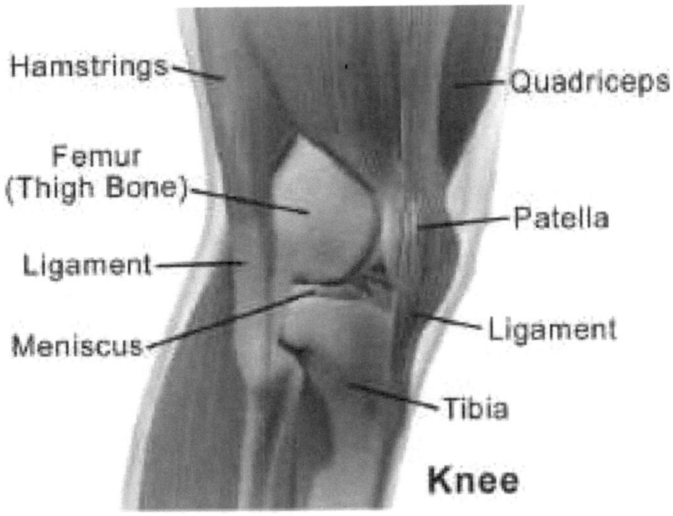

Note: The front of the body is the anterior surface, the back is the posterior surface, the sides are the flanks and the inside of the legs, for example, is the medial side and the outside is the lateral side. The palms of the hands are the anterior side with the thumbs on the lateral or outer part of the hand. There also is a knee cap, a small bone called the patella. There are ligaments (bone to bone connections) that stabilize the knee, the medial collateral ligaments are on the inside and the lateral collateral ligaments are on the outside. They prevent the knee from moving sideways, either to the medial or inside or the lateral or outside part. There is another pair of ligaments called the cruciate ligaments. There is a posterior cruciate ligament that prevents the tibia from sliding anterior or forward on the femur and an anterior cruciate ligament which prevents posterior or backwards movement of the tibia on the femur. There are also bursa sacs which keep bone from rubbing directly on bone and make the bones slide over the sac instead of each other. Inflammation of this bursa sac will cause what is known as bursitis. Finally, there is the meniscus of the knee, a thick cartilage that cushions the knee and prevents the upper thigh bone from crushing down on the lower tibia bone. Study the diagram above to help better understand this very important anatomy.

With what I am teaching you here, you should be able to at least make an educated guess as to the nature of any knee injury. You must be able to determine if it is a sprain, tendonitis, bursitis, fracture, or ligament tear. This is not very easy without the help of modern radiological equipment such as MRIs and CT scanners.

Since knee injuries are very common, being able to evaluate them and come up with a reasonable diagnosis is an essential skill to have. Let's try to make it easier with the following tips on evaluating knee injuries and complaints. Some are due to chronic diseases like osteoarthritis, others may be due to injuries, let's review it.

Chondromalacia Patella

In young patients like teenagers complaining of knee pain without trauma it may be chondromalacia patella. This is also known as patellofemoral syndrome. There is an inflammation of the underside of the knee cap or patella, with accompanying softening of the cartilage. It is also known as patellofemoral pain syndrome but technically this is without damage to the cartilage. This usually occurs in young people who are actively engaged in sports, but may also occur in middle aged folks who injure their knees by overdoing it. The weekend warriors who are not in shape and go out and play touch football or several pickup games of basketball are the ones I am referring to.

Osteoarthritis

Osteoarthritis is very common in middle-aged and elderly patients and is caused by long-term wear and tear on the cartilage as well as aging. It is the most common type of joint complaint in patients who suffer with osteoarthritis. It causes pain and swelling in the knee and stiffness.

Note: You can diagnose osteoarthritis from the presence of Heberden's nodes. They are caused by repeated trauma to the joint with the eventual development of spurs and enlargement of the joint. The distal joint of the fingers (the farthest joint right before the fingernails) will be enlarged and knobby. In the beginning there will just be a slight elevation to this joint and later, as it worsens, the nodes become larger and stiffer. Rheumatoid arthritis on the other hand (no pun intended) will cause Bouchard's nodes, enlargement of the middle joints or proximal joint (proximal means closer to the body, distal means further away) of the fingers with some ulnar deviation which means the hand deviates or bends towards the pinky finger side.

Examine the knee for an effusion, which is an outpouring of fluid into the joint space. This is your classic "water on the knee" and can be diagnosed by obvious swelling of the knee when it is severe, mild to moderate cases that can be diagnosed by a "bulge sign".

A bulge sign is on either side of the patella you will see swelling of the soft tissue. When you press one side, the other side will develop a pronounced bulging. Any form of arthritis or trauma to the knee may cause an effusion.

Meniscus Tear

A meniscus tear may occur with any violent twisting of the knee. The meniscus is the large cartilage that cushions the knee joint. A severe tear of the meniscus may cause a locking of the knee joint. A tear of the meniscus may occur with or without significant trauma.

Bursitis of the Knee

Bursitis is caused by inflammation of one or more of the synovial sacs or bursae. These bursae are all over the body at points where muscles or tendons slide over bones.

Bursitis is a very common form of knee injury and the knee is tender and warm to the touch and has edema or swelling. This is a common form of injury and also can be from overuse. If you place your hand on both knees at the same time, you will notice the warmth coming off the knee with bursitis, due to the inflammation.

Anterior and Posterior Cruciate Ligament (ACL and PCL) Tears

Both the ACL and the PCL (posterior cruciate ligament) are responsible for stability of the knee joint. Cruciate means a cross or X in Latin. These two ligaments cross each other and form an X in the knee. Injury to the front of the knee or ACL is much more common than injury to the back of the knee and the PCL. ACL injuries result in the knee "giving out".

Baker's Cyst

Baker's cysts are very common, especially in chronic injuries to the knee joint, like in osteoarthritis. A baker's cyst is a collection of fluid behind the knee. The patient will often complain that they are unable to bend their knee fully due to "something behind it". With the patient standing in front of you, compare the back of both knees and it will show the bulging of a baker's cyst on the involved knee.

Medial Collateral Ligament (MCL) Tear

A medical collateral ligament injury will produce pain on the medial or inside of the knee joint. These types of injuries commonly occur when a force pushes the knee in a medial direction (towards the other leg, not forward or backward).

Tendonitis of the Patella

In cases of tendonitis of the patella the tendons which hold the patella in place are inflamed and this occurs from recurrent trauma to the knee joint as in jumping in athletics. If you palpate (press) either above or below the knee cap or patella you will find this area to be very tender.

Gout

Gout can also cause knee problems. As you recall, gout is caused by uric acid crystals settling out into a joint, it causes pain and swelling in a joint and is difficult to diagnose without a blood uric acid level. Frequently the patient will have a history of previous gout attacks that may help you make the diagnosis. That is why whenever you evaluate a patient for any condition, ask them if they have ever had a problem like (fill in the blank with the problem) this before and if so, were they told what caused it? That may save you a lot of headaches.

Remember, common things are common, medical students often forget this as they get lost in multiple causes for every condition and are frequently tested on the exceptions to every rule. This has resulted in the old saying," a medical student hears hoof beats and thinks zebra". This phenomenon typically vanishes with a few years' experience under their belts.

Here are some tips from *Dr. James Hubbard "The Survival Doctor"*. He has an excellent website, *thesurvivaldoctor.com*, that covers various medical problems. One area on the knee aches, but the knee feels stable (this means when you move it back and forth it feels like it is normal, also hyperextending it or straightening the knee all the way and then pressing on the knee moderately) and there is no swelling...this is a sprain. Knee feels unstable...torn ligament. Knee locks up...torn meniscus. Sudden onset of significant swelling in the knee...this signifies a serious injury such as a fracture, tear, or dislocation and is probably not a sprain. You feel a lot of pain with weight bearing even when the leg is straight... bone fracture. Bones or knee joint appears distorted...fracture, dislocation, or both.

Knee looks distorted and at the same time you cannot feel a pulse in the foot...this is injury to an artery and is a medical emergency.

You need to get that knee joint or broken bone back in place or you may lose the limb. This is a major problem and if you don't get the joint repositioned you may have to put this in the Kiss-Your-Ass-Goodbye section. At the very least it probably will result in an amputation and without antibiotics in an emergency situation you can probably expect a twenty five percent mortality rate.

TREATMENT OF BONE FRACTURES AND OTHER JOINT INJURIES

The first thing you should do is make sure there are no active bleeding sites. If there are, you need to apply direct pressure with a sterile gauze, and if that is not available then a clean cloth or piece of clothing. See wound section for complete details. Bleeding has to be rapidly brought under control and this has to be your first priority. If you need to, cut away the patient's clothing to allow you better access to the bleeding point. Do this rather than making the patient move to avoid further bony injury.

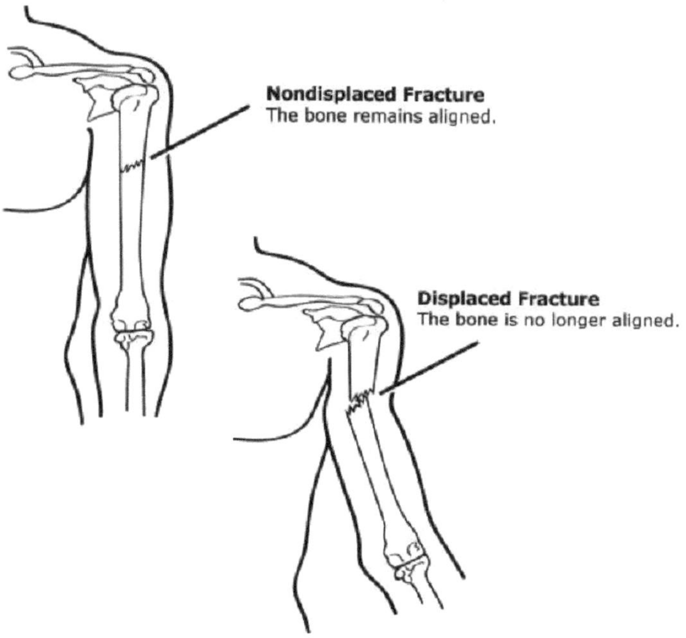

If you have the opportunity, apply a cold pack or ice to the broken bone to reduce the soft tissue swelling. Remember, never apply ice directly to skin without some cloth or other layer placed in between, otherwise you risk getting frostbite on top of everything else. Also give the patient a painkiller as soon as possible, if no narcotic analgesics (painkillers) are available, then use Motrin, Aleve, or Tylenol.

Keep the victim as comfortable as possible while you access the possible fracture. If you suspect a broken back or neck then the patient should not be moved. This is especially true if the patient tells you that they cannot feel their legs or arms or any part of their body. This usually signifies a major nerve injury and possible permanent paralysis. In an emergency situation this is almost impossible to treat without access to a hospital for specialized care. If you are outside you will have to eventually move him or her to a safe, secure location and out of the elements, however any movement may worsen their condition. Hence it has to be done as carefully as possible. The patient will have to be moved onto an improvised, stiff stretcher, which will limit their movements as much as possible. The head will have to be tied down with a strap or belt of some type securing the head in a rigid position, so the neck will not move. At least four people will probably be needed to move them a short distance indoors or to the safest location you can improvise. Herein lies the problem…what to do next? If you are in a wilderness area, someone has to go for help immediately, while someone else stays with the victim.

Fractures of long bones like the limbs may cause damage to the circulation. Also remember that a bent bone that finally breaks will have much more soft tissue injuries on the convex side than the concave side.

Note: A concave side is U-shaped with the open area upwards; concave…a cave holds water. Convex is the opposite. A symptom of this is the involved limb will be pale white, blue, or purple in color and pulse less…remember: Pale, purple, and pulseless. This is a medical emergency and that patient will die unless properly treated with joint reduction and or amputation. You will be hard-pressed to save this patient, but you may luck out after reducing (repositioning broken bones to their original positions) a fracture that was compressing an artery.

To check their circulation you can examine their fingers or toes with the capillary refill test. This involves applying pressure to the fingertips or toes until they turn white and then seeing if they refill with blood and turn red again. This should normally happen in two seconds. Examine the bone, if it does not look deformed, then placing a splint on the bone is your next course of action. Splints can be bought ahead of time and placed in your natural medicine chest or improvised on site. You will need any stiff, preferably flat piece of wood, an old board, even rolled up magazines can work and place them on either side of the involved limb and secure it in place with duct tape, ace bandages, or any rope or other method to tie it (bungee cords, Para cord, bandana, or strips of cloth, etc.). You can also wrap a pillow around a limb and duct tape that as securely as possible to improvise a splint.

The idea of splinting is to immobilize the bone in a position it might normally take, for example:

Fingers

Fingers should be slightly flexed (bent) as if they were holding something like a small ball or glass. Note: Fingers and toes can also be buddy-taped to the adjacent toe with padding in between if available, if not, then just tape them together, the uninjured finger will be straight and act as the splint. In my practice I use a cut-down tongue depressor; Popsicle sticks will work just fine.

Hands

For hand injuries a makeshift hand splint can be improvised. First, if available, take some cotton or gauze and put it between each finger and line the palm of the hand with it. The splint you need has to be the length of the middle of the forearm to the tips of the fingers. Next, take some newspaper or roll up an old magazine and use that, they are both very useful for this type of splint because they can be slightly bent to the underside or palm side of the arm/hand and are still rigid enough to provide support. Then wrap it in place with an ace bandage or some other bandages or strips of cloth or duct tape. Make sure the fingers are flexed (bent) and pink, not white or blue which would indicate that you are cutting off the circulation.

Wrist

A wrist should either be kept in a straight position or just slightly extended backward. Children will incur many of these fractures as well to their forearm and upper arms. This is because of children's natural tendency to put out their arms in front of them when they are falling. I can personally attest to this, I broke my forearm at the age of four when I bailed out off the top of a slide in pond when two other kids approached me from the front and back. The playground was built on concrete. New Jersey is a tough place, even at the tender age of four.

Arm

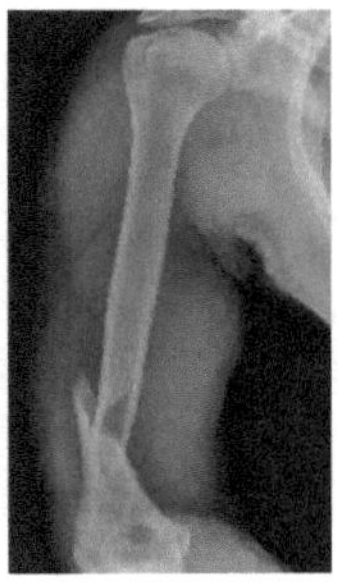

To splint an arm the elbow should be flexed (bent) at a ninety degree angle in relation to the upper arm, like an L. You can also make a sling for an arm. This can be done with a large piece of cloth (forty inches by forty inches), a pillowcase is ideal. Make sure the arm is well supported and slightly above its normal position with the pillowcase tied behind the neck.

Leg

The leg should be kept straight with a slight bend at the level of the knee.

Hip and Pelvis

If you suspect a hip or pelvic fracture to be the case, then strap their legs together with a towel or blanket between them and tape them or tie them securely in place and put the patient on a hard board to move. Note: An old door taken off its hinges would work very well.

Elbow

In cases of an elbow fracture you should fully straighten your arm and apply the planks or whatever objects you are using for the frame of the splint on either side of the arm and secure it as firm as you can.

TIPS:

Make the splints as tight as possible, but not too tight that it is painful for the patient. You should be able to slip two fingers under a splint but no more than that.

Save any splints, slings, crutches, walkers, wheelchairs or orthopedic immobilizers you or your family members have been treated with and put them in your medicine stockpile. I am very confident you will be thankful that you did, they do not take up much space (except for the wheel chair) and are hard to duplicate in an emergency. When making a splint, do not completely circumvent (wrap completely around) the involved limb, leave an open area along the length of the splint to allow for the inevitable soft tissue swelling that will occur.

REDUCTION OF BROKEN BONES

Reduction means repositioning back to as close as you can get to the original position of the fractured bone. Reducing a fractured or broken bone is one of the best things you can do for a fracture. It is also often very difficult to do even for trained medical personnel. There are a few techniques that I will cover here for the most basic of bone reductions that you will need as part of your knowledge base.

There are basically two types of bone fracture reduction techniques, open and closed. Open reduction involves opening up or surgically operating on the patient and that is well beyond your skills and the scope of this book, therefore we shall concentrate on the second method, closed reductions. Almost all closed reductions will require two people, one to hold the patient immobile while the other applies traction and manipulates the fractured bone. If possible the patient should be sedated or at the very least given the strongest pain medications you have available. Reduction of a fractured bone is very painful.

ARM FRACTURES OF THE RADIUS AND OR ULNA

The radius and ulna are the two bones of the forearm. The radius is on the thumb side and the ulna is on the pinky finger side. If there is a deformity of the bone, the first step is to bend the bone towards the deformity (making it worse momentarily) to exaggerate the deformity. Then push the bone back away from the deformity towards its original position before the fracture. The direction of the pushing should be done along the length of the arm, parallel to the long axis of the arm, not perpendicular to it or width-wise. Once it is back in its original position, splint it in place.

DISLOCATED OR FRACTURED ELBOW

With the patient lying on a bed or stretcher in a prone position (on their stomachs) with the broken elbow arm hanging down off the bed towards the floor, one person holds the patient in place while the second person applies steady traction towards the patient's hand, that is, pulling down on the arm. The next step is to flex the arm to a ninety degree angle (L-shaped) and reposition it here and apply the splint to keep it in place.

DISLOCATED OR FRACTURED SHOULDER

In cases of a dislocated or fractured shoulder, with the patient sitting up, one person takes a sheet and twists it to make it more like a rope.

Loop that twisted sheet under the patient's broken arm's armpit and take one side and cross his chest with it heading on a forty-five degree angle (towards the opposite side's ear). The second person takes the broken shoulder's arm and pulls it on a forty-five degree angle towards the floor. Note: The broken side's arm and the sheet should be in a straight line, with traction being applied equally in opposite directions, this should pop the shoulder back in place. The patient will be in a lot of pain but will know it when it is replaced in the original position.

An alternative method is to have the patient lie on his abdomen with his face down and the affected arm hanging down off the bed. Secure some weights for example from a barbell set to the arm and let it hang there for a few hours until the joint is stretched and then try to reposition the dislocated or broken shoulder.

DISLOCATED OR FRACTURED HIP

In cases of a dislocated or fractured hip have the patient lie on their back and relax as much as possible. If you have any means to sedate them, then now is the time to use it. Apply traction towards the involved leg's foot, pulling steadily and forcefully, then abduct (move it away from the body) the leg and internally rotate (back towards the body) the leg to get the hip back in its original position.

CHAPTER THIRTY-TWO
ASTHMA AND ALLERGIES

INTRODUCTION

TABLE OF CONTENTS:

This is one of those chapters that will come in really handy and I bet you will be coming back to often.

In this section I will first review the anatomy and physiology (the structure and how things work) of the respiratory system, then the various problems that affect it, and finally how to treat these problems without conventional pharmaceuticals.

ANATOMY OF THE SINUSES, NOSE, UPPER AND LOWER AIRWAYS, AND LUNGS

The Sinuses

The paranasal sinuses or just plain sinuses are a system of connected hollow cavities in your head. Paranasal means around the nose. They are hollow chambers, the largest sinus is only about an inch across; most are smaller. There are four different sinuses, all of which are connected, symmetrically arranged in pairs and whose job it is to warm and humidify air before it is sent down to your lungs.

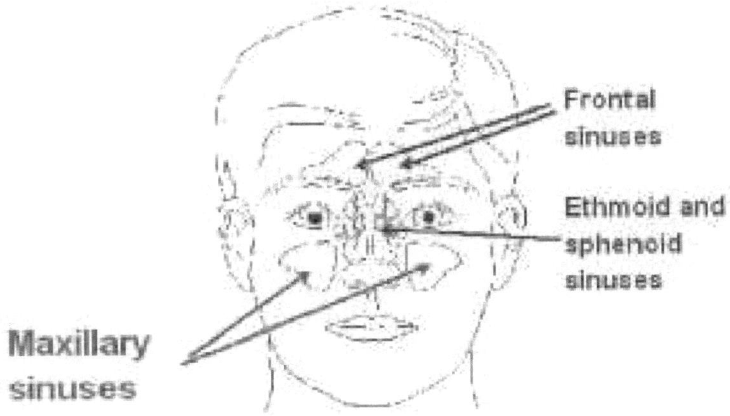

The four different sinuses are:

Frontal Sinuses: These are just above your eyebrows on the lower half of your forehead, in the frontal bone. There is one on either side.

Maxillary Sinuses: These are the largest and are located in the middle of your face between your eyes and your mouth on either side in the maxilla or upper jawbone.

Ethmoid Sinuses: These are located between your eyes at the bridge of your nose (where your nose meets your forehead) in the ethmoid bone.

Sphenoid Sinuses: These are located deep in your face behind your nasal cavity in the sphenoid bone; they are the least accessible of the four.

The Nose

The inside of the nose is lined by mucosal-covered, bony horizontal ridges that are called the turbinate's (or concha). There are three of these turbinate's that divide the nose into four horizontal channels. This serves to channel the air over the mucosa.

Nose and Nasal Cavities

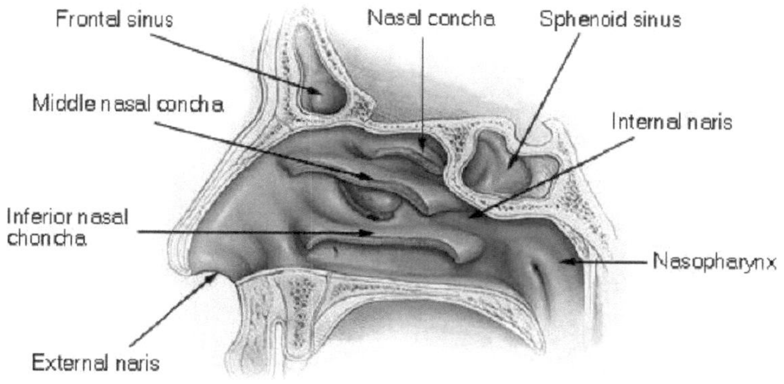

The mucosal lining of the nasal passages is the same lining that covers the respiratory tract, the gastrointestinal tract, and the urogenital tract.

It is composed of two layers, an outer layer known as the epithelium and an inner layer known as the lamina propria. The epithelium is involved with both absorption and secretion.

Since it is able to absorb substances it can be utilized to administer medications such as nasal sprays, and as every drug addict certainly knows you can also use it to snort powders and other substances. It secretes fluid to keep the nasal passages moist. When this goes into overdrive you have a runny nose or rhinitis. If it is caused by allergies it is known medically as allergic rhinitis.

The second layer or lamina propria is a thin layer of loose connective tissue, rich in various types of cells. The cells of the lamina propria perform many functions most of which involve immunity and allergic responses. It is the body's first line of defense in its various body cavities and thus is important in providing resistance to infections. It is also full of cells involved in allergy that release histamine when they are activated by allergens (pollen, dust, smoke, dogs, cats, etc.). Histamine is the chemical that triggers a cascade of allergic symptoms, hence our need to use antihistamines to block allergic reactions.

The nasal mucosa is also lined with fine hairs which help filter and trap dust and other particles and prevent their entry into the lungs. Very fine dust is able to pass over this barrier and enter the lungs. For example, in coal miners, coal dust is able to travel deep into the lungs, causing a condition known as black lung, named from the actual color of the lungs which are changed from their normal pink to jet black by the fine coal dust.

Air can enter the lungs either via the nose and nasal passages or through the mouth. There are advantages to both ways. The nasal route allows the air to be filtered, warmed, and humidified before being delivered to the lungs. The oral route allows for more air to enter the lungs quicker, since it is a larger bore opening than the nose and is closer to the lungs, but the air is neither filtered or warmed and humidified. You can experience this if you are ever in subzero temperatures and breathe deeply through your mouth; the cold air will almost be painful when it hits your lungs.

The nose has a thin partition in its center known as the nasal septum. If the septum is bent to one side it will restrict the air flow on that side and this condition is known as a deviated septum. Since the septum is very thin it can be easily perforated by trauma such as chronic nose picking or chronic drug use as is seen in cocaine and heroin addicts who use their noses as a portal (entrance way) to snort drugs. It can also become displaced to one side or the other by trauma to the nose; most boxers show this with their bent, distorted noses.

The Upper Respiratory Tract

The upper respiratory tract is comprised of the nasal cavity, the pharynx, and the larynx. The nasal cavity is the hollow space within the nose. The pharynx, or throat, is divided into three parts, the nasopharynx which lies at the back of the nose, the oropharynx, which is at the back wall of the mouth, and the laryngopharynx, which lies at the back of the larynx. The throat or pharynx is somewhat funnel-shaped. At the bottom of the laryngopharynx there is a flap of cartilage known as the epiglottis. The epiglottis acts as a switch between one side which goes to the trachea or windpipe, and the other side which goes to the esophagus which leads to the stomach. So, in essence the epiglottis is the switch that sends some things to your respiratory tract and others to your GI tract. When you swallow food the epiglottis slams shut over the trachea and prevents any food from entering it. When you choke on something and it "goes down the wrong pipe", this is the fault of your epiglottis. The larynx is the voice box. When it becomes inflamed or infected it is known as laryngitis, and the voice becomes hoarse like President Clinton's was quite frequently. The larynx contains two pairs of vocal cords and is essentially the airway that connects the laryngopharynx to the trachea.

The Lower Respiratory Tract

The lower respiratory tract consists of the trachea, the bronchi and bronchioles, and the lungs. The trachea or windpipe is about five inches or so in length and is made of a series of C-shaped cartilage rings stacked on top of each other. These C-shaped rings are on the posterior or back side of the trachea adjacent to the esophagus. The reason these C-shaped rings are open on one side is to allow the esophagus to expand when thick, large pieces of food such as meat pass down its length. The trachea connects the larynx with the bronchi and thus carries air from the neck into the chest (or thorax). The trachea has a mucosal lining that secretes mucous trapping dust and other solid debris preventing it from reaching the lungs, it also is lined by small hair cells called cilia that beat in unison in one direction, towards your mouth. The cilia with their layer of mucous and debris lying on top of the hairs is sort of like a mosh pit, where instead of people being carried along there is this mucous laced with debris being carried along back towards the mouth. The cilia line the entire respiratory system and are destroyed by smoking.

Once the cilia are destroyed they can no longer carry dust and debris out of the respiratory system. The goblet cells of the mucosal lining continue to make mucous to trap this foreign matter but it is no longer carried up and out of the lungs once the cilia are missing.

For this reason smokers develop a smoker's cough and are constantly hacking up the mucous that gravity carried down into their lungs, rather than up and out of the respiratory system.

The trachea enters the thorax or chest and divides into left and right branches known as the primary bronchi. Primary bronchi mean first bronchi; the respiratory tree ultimately divides twenty-three times before it ends in air sacs known as alveoli. The first three splits of the respiratory tree are known as the primary, secondary, and tertiary bronchi, after the tertiary bronchus comes smaller, airways known as bronchioles. The bronchi of the respiratory tree look just like a tree, dividing evenly in two each time. It always looked to me like a large cluster of grapes with the branches of the grapevine being the bronchi and the grapes themselves being the air sacs or alveoli. The bronchi also are lined with mucosa which has cilia as well. In the alveoli is where the gas exchange takes place and the body gets rid of its carbon dioxide and takes in life-giving oxygen. Carbon dioxide is a waste product of respiration.

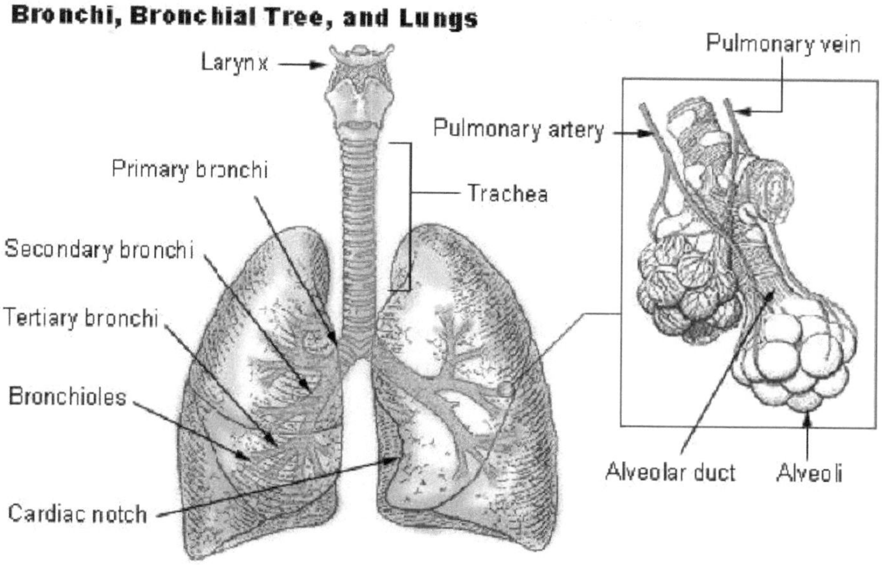

The lungs are not symmetric; the left lung has only two lobes or sections and is smaller than the right lung, which has three lobes.

The reason for this is the heart is on the left side of the chest and thus occupies some of the space which normally would be lung, that space is known as the cardiac notch. Both lungs are surrounded by a membrane known as the pleura. The pleura is a double membrane that has a thin layer of fluid between the two layers that allows them to slide over each other as the lung expands and contracts with breathing.

The pleura also protect and lubricate the surface of the lungs as we breathe. When this membrane becomes infected or inflamed the condition is known as pleurisy and produces pain upon respiration. Many times, when the pleura are infected by a virus or an adjacent pneumonia or tuberculosis, it will react by producing fluid that collects in the space between its two layers; this is known as a pleural effusion.

INFECTIONS OF THE RESPIRATORY TRACT

Any part of the respiratory tract can become infected. Infections lead to inflammation of the infected parts and consequently the names of the various anatomical areas infected all end in the suffix "itis", which means inflammation.

For example infection of any sinus is known as sinusitis, infection of the larynx is known as laryngitis, infection of the pharynx is known as pharyngitis, and infection of the bronchi as bronchitis. The only exception to that rule is an infection of the lung which is called pneumonia. At times when the pathogen or germ is known as the cause of an infection, it will precede the site of the infection, for example a strep pharyngitis (strep throat), a staph pneumonia, etc. Note the name strep is an abbreviation of streptococcus and staph is an abbreviation of staphylococcus.

ASTHMA

Asthma is derived from the Greek word for panting. Asthma is caused by chronic inflammation of the airways. Asthma typically is a reversible condition where the airways become inflamed and the mucosal lining swells and puts out clear mucous eventually plugging or mechanically obstructing the airways. The bronchioles are surrounded by smooth muscle and when they are stimulated by allergens, smoke, or other irritants, will contract and severely limit the size of the airways leading to what is known as bronchospasm.

Bronchospasm in turn causes chest tightness and often a high pitched whistling sound with inspirations (breathing in) known as wheezing.

Bronchospasm can be caused by drugs such as the class of blood pressure medications known as beta blockers, smoke, cold air, allergens (substances that trigger allergic reactions such as pollen, dust, dog and cat dander, grass, trees, mold), changing hormone levels in women, insect bites and stings in those people who are allergic to them. Perfumes are notorious for bringing on asthma attacks. Food allergies may also trigger asthma attacks, the worst offenders of this are peanuts, dairy, eggs, citrus, chocolate, and wheat products.

In children approximately 90 percent have allergies driving their asthma, this level drops to 70 percent in people between sixteen and thirty years of age and drops to 50 percent in adults older than thirty. These allergies are from all causes such as dust, pollen, dander, etc. however this shows the critical need to reducing exposure to these allergens to control asthma.

I should mention the "Hygiene Hypothesis" as an explanation of the skyrocketing levels of asthma, especially in the developed world. This hypothesis states that children who grow up in less hygienic, crowded, dirty conditions, especially with exposure to animals, have much lower rates of asthma than wealthier children who typically have fewer siblings and whose mothers are anal about cleaning and sanitizing many of the surfaces these children are exposed to. The theory is that the developing immune systems of these poorer children are exposed to many more allergens and pathogens (germs) at an early age and become stronger and more robust. The immune system seems to learn to differentiate between self and foreign matter and only attacks the allergens and pathogens and spares the child's lungs, thus avoiding the inflammation that leads to asthma. If you have allergies that are even moderately severe in nature, I highly recommend that you have several EpiPens in your medicine chest. EpiPens contain epinephrine (adrenaline) that will rapidly reverse any life-threatening swelling and spasm in your airways and may very well save your life. There is nothing else that will work as rapidly.

Epinephrine or adrenaline is a hormone involved in the "fight or flight response". We have evolved with this emergency response system of fight or flight. All the things that epinephrine does are to make you breathe better, raise your blood pressure, increase your heart rate to deliver more blood filled with oxygen to your muscles, sharpen your vision, etc. Epinephrine is essentially getting you ready for the fight of your life. Stress can lead to chronic adrenaline release and palpitations, tachycardia (fast heart rate), headaches, tremors, and hypertension (high blood pressure) as well as panic attacks and other symptoms.

Symptoms Of Asthma

Symptoms of asthma include shortness of breath, wheezing, a cough which typically is worse at night or early morning and usually dry (no phlegm or mucous produced, as opposed to a wet cough where there is mucous produced), chest tightness, and sometimes chest pain, especially with deep breaths. Coughing may be brought on by breathing in cold air and exercise frequently induces (brings on asthmatic symptoms.) Asthma can be brought on by a number of conditions, esophageal reflux (the splashing of gastric secretions from the stomach into the lower esophagus), sleep apnea, allergies, sinus, and lung infections. Many patients develop tachycardia or a rapid pulse; this is due to a drop in oxygen levels in their blood as a consequence of which the body has to deliver more blood to get the same amount of oxygen, hence the rapid pulse. The patient will be in various degrees of respiratory distress, some just breathing heavily, others loudly wheezing and coughing, and others may progress to the point where they become cyanotic. Cyanotic means they develop a blue/gray color to their lips, face, and tips of their fingers; this is a very bad sign and these patients are in extreme danger.

Treatment Of Asthma

Asthma is typically treated with inhalers and steroids and bronchodilators (substances that relax the smooth muscle that is wrapped around the bronchioles, allowing them to dilate or enlarge). Examples of bronchodilators are Albuterol, Proventil, Ventolin, and Xopenex. There are many others on the market as well.

For our purposes the best way to control asthma for you and your family members will be prevention. It is infinitely easier to prevent asthma than to try to treat it later, especially with little or no pharmaceuticals available such as steroids or bronchodilators. Avoidance of allergens, smoke, airborne toxins, animal dander (especially from cats even more so than dogs, but both allergies are very common), infections, dust and dust mites, and breathing in extremely cold dry air. Emotional upset will also trigger asthma attacks and should be avoided as much as possible, this one will be problematic for most of us.

Here are some other simple things you can do to minimize your asthma risk and decrease your exposure to allergens that trigger asthma:

Decrease your intake of animal proteins and switch to more plant-based protein sources. Eliminate dairy products like milk.

Most adults lose the ability to produce lactose and have varying degrees of lactose intolerance. Keep yourself well hydrated; dehydration can trigger asthma symptoms and also leads to thick mucus that sometimes causes plugging of airways and is difficult to expectorate, or cough up. Increase your intake of antioxidants like vitamin C which has a dual mechanism for helping asthma; it works as an antihistamine as well as helping neutralize free radicals and decrease inflammation. Increase your intake of omega-3 fatty acids (fish oil, flaxseed, etc.) to help decrease the inflammation of asthma.

Anyone with serious asthma problems might find themselves in a situation where they do not have access or run out of their medications thus here are some alternative ways to treat asthma:

Magnesium Sulfate

Magnesium sulfate (Epsom salt) is given in hospitals intravenously due to its relaxation of the smooth muscles of the bronchioles resulting in increased airflow and decreased wheezing. You will most likely not have intravenous access available but you still can increase your body's magnesium levels by several methods. Magnesium can be taken orally, the usual preparation available in pharmacies over the counter is magnesium oxide; it is inexpensive and only moderately absorbed. There is also magnesium oil available on the internet, which is expensive but readily absorbed across your skin, it sometimes causes a little burning sensation when applied to the skin. You can also drink Epsom salt, the directions are right on the box; this method is readily absorbed but may give you some diarrhea.

The dose of oral Epsom salt is:

Adults and children older than twelve: Two to four level teaspoons dissolved in an 8-ounce glass of water.

Children six to eleven years old: One to two level teaspoons dissolved in an 8-ounce glass of water.

For children younger than six years old it is not recommended. That being said, in a severe asthma attack with no other treatment available, I would give it a shot at half a teaspoon; it may just save your child.

Note: Do not mess around with an asthma attack, get yourself or whoever is having breathing problems to a medical facility asap, these attacks can easily become life threatening.

Antihistamines

Many times asthma is triggered by and driven by your body's reaction to a variety of airborne allergens such as dust, grass, pollen, trees, animal dander, cockroaches, and mold, to name but a few. Allergies cause the mast cells to release their stores of histamine, leading to a cascade of reactions in your body. Antihistamines neutralize and block the release of histamine and as such have a place in the treatment of asthma. Unfortunately most of the antihistamines with the exception of Benadryl are very expensive. Sometimes you can find stock bottles of Zyrtec or Claritin in buyers' club stores like Sam's Club or others, these are typically less expensive. Benadryl is very inexpensive, has multiple uses, and should be kept in large quantities in your medicine chest.

Benadryl 25 mg orally every four to six hours should block any allergy symptoms and help your asthma; it is, however, very sedating, thus explaining its use as a sleeping aid in a variety of over-the-counter medications like Tylenol PM. Remember, vitamin C also acts as an antihistamine, so keeping high levels of this all-important vitamin in your blood will help treat allergy-driven asthma. I would recommend about 1,000 mg (1 gram) of vitamin C two to four times daily; you may need to reduce the dose if you develop diarrhea (loose stools).

Natural and Alternative Treatments for Asthma

Lobelia: Lobelia (Lobelia inflate) is also known as Indian tobacco, due to Indians smoking this herb. It is also a nice plant and easy to grow in your medicinal garden. Use a tincture of lobelia, mixing it in a three to one ratio with a tincture of capsicum, or cayenne pepper, so for those of you who are math- challenged this means three drops of lobelia to one drop of capsicum. The dose is approximately twenty drops or one milliliter (ml) into a glass of water and drink it at the start of an asthma attack and repeat it every half hour or so until the attack is under control. No more than four times daily, and it should be avoided in patients suffering with hypertension and/or heart conditions.

Green Tea also has been shown to improve asthma. There is no real dose, but drinking it regularly may help to reduce the inflammation and bronchospasm that drives asthma. Adding honey to your tea to sweeten it will also help asthma. Use this tea/honey combination three or four times a day, with one teaspoon of honey in each cup of tea.

Astragalus (Astragalus membranaceus): Astragalus is an herb, the root of which is used to produce this medicine. It acts to strengthen and regulate the immune system and decrease inflammation. The typical dose is 500 to 1,000 mg twice daily. Avoid this herb if you have a fever.

N-acetylcysteine (NAC): This is a derivative of the amino acid cysteine. It is a good antioxidant and also liquefies mucus in the sinuses as well as the bronchial tubes. The dose is 500 mg two or three times a day.

Lycopene: Lycopene is a bright red carotene pigment found in tomatoes, watermelon, and other red fruits (although it is absent in strawberries, cherries, and red bell peppers). It is also an antioxidant and has been shown to help especially in cases of exercise-induced asthma. The dose is 30 mg daily of lycopene. An additional benefit is that lycopene has been shown to decrease sun damage to the skin caused by UV radiation.

Quercetin: Quercetin is a flavonoid or plant pigment found in many fruits and vegetables. Quercetin is an effective bronchodilator and also blocks the release of histamine, so is useful in both allergies and asthma. The dose is 1,000 mg three times a day.

Cordyceps (Cordyceps sinensis): Cordyceps is a Chinese medicinal mushroom which has been shown to reduce bronchial secretions and expand the airways. The dose is 800 mg twice daily. It is also used in Tibetan medicine where it is purported to be an aphrodisiac.

Turmeric (Curcuma longa): Turmeric is a perennial herb that is native to southern India. The rhizome or bulbous root is used as a source of this medicine. The resulting powder is deep orange/yellow in color and is used as a dye as well as a spice in Indian cuisine. A paste made from this powder also has antimicrobial properties and works well as a wound dressing. Turmeric also has strong anti-inflammatory properties and as such is useful in asthma. The dose is approximately one teaspoon of turmeric powder in 8 ounces of warm water three times a day. As a wound dressing it can also be applied several times a day to prevent wound infections.

Ginko Biloba: Ginko has both antioxidant and also anti-inflammatory effects and thus is very useful in the treatment of asthma; it also supposedly helps with memory problems. The typical dose is from ginko extract containing 24 percent flavone glycosides. Take between 120 and 240 mg daily depending on your symptoms.

Selenium: Selenium is a trace mineral that is also a powerful antioxidant, unfortunately like most minerals and trace elements; it is rapidly becoming depleted in our soils. This might in fact be one of the causes of the worldwide spike in asthma cases that continues unabated. There are many enzymes that need selenium to activate them, including glutathione peroxidase. This enzyme is key in protecting your lungs against free radical and oxidative damage. Studies have shown that patients with the lowest selenium levels have the highest levels of asthma. Low selenium levels are also associated with high cancer rates. A daily dose of 200 mcg is recommended. A cocktail of B6, magnesium, and selenium has been shown to be effective in the treatment of asthma. The recommended doses of vitamin B6 is between 50 and 200 mg a day, and magnesium is between 400 and 800 mg daily.

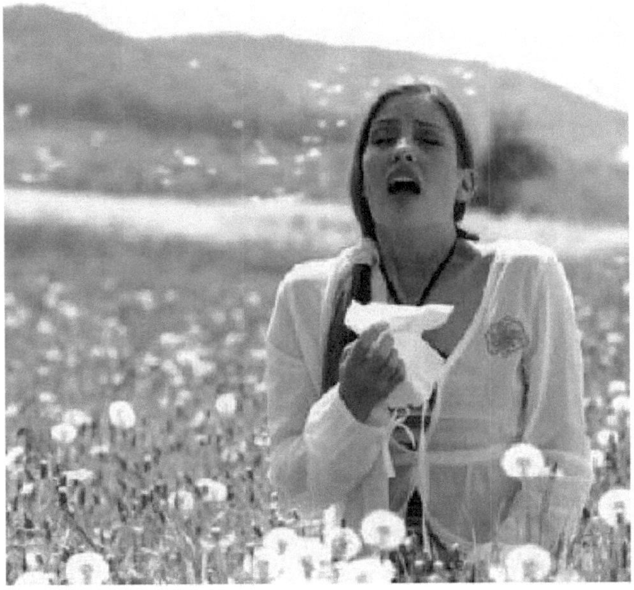

ALLERGIES

An allergy is a hypersensitivity disorder of the immune system. Hypersensitivity means an undesirable reaction by an otherwise healthy immune system. There are two types of hypersensitivity reactions, allergies and autoimmune disorders. Autoimmune disorders occur when the body fails to distinguish self from foreign invaders and attacks itself, leading to a variety of disorders.

Symptoms Of Allergies

Allergies usually manifest themselves with itchy, watery red eyes, stuffy, itchy nose and sinuses, hives, and eczema, and may trigger an asthma attack as I described above. If it is an asthma attack there will be additional symptoms of dry cough or one productive of clear sputum, wheezing, and chest congestion and tightness. Allergy symptoms with nasal, sinus, and lung congestion can sometimes be caused by foods such as dairy products, soy, and wheat, which are all mucus-producing foods. Dairy products are probably the worst offenders in this group, and excluding them from your diet might go a long way to decrease mucus.

Anaphylaxis

In some patients who are severely allergic to something, these symptoms may worsen and the person may have a full-blown severe allergic response that is life-threatening, or what is known as anaphylaxis. This is a medical emergency and any patient with these symptoms who you might even suspect has anaphylaxis needs to be taken to a medical facility ASAP. Once again, I am teaching you how to deal with it as best as you can under the presumption that you cannot reach a physician or a medical center.

Patients who develop anaphylaxis develop severe itchy rashes, hives, facial flushing (gets very red), facial and eye swelling, and throat closure that can be so severe that it may cut off their air supply and kill them. It may also cause low blood pressure.

Anaphylaxis is frequently caused by bee stings and other insect bites, but can also be caused by food, medicines, or other allergens. In cases of anaphylaxis the best treatment remains epinephrine administered by needle at a dose of 0.3 ml, or just use the EpiPen. That is why I am so emphatic about getting a supply of EpiPens, there is really no adequate substitute, and there is usually not much time to reverse these symptoms before a patient will die.

Once the blood pressure drops the body will attempt to compensate by increasing the patient's pulse rate making it rapid, or what is known as tachycardia. If the pulse rate and the respiratory rate slow down, this usually means impending shock and is a bad sign; these patients may develop blue lips and fingers from their low oxygen levels as well. The patient may develop gastrointestinal symptoms with nausea and vomiting and sometimes loss of bowel and bladder control.

Many patients get severe headaches from the dilated blood vessels; the same dilation causes the blood pressure to bottom out.

Typically, anaphylaxis is treated in an intensive care setting with IV fluids, epinephrine, oxygen, and other supportive care.

If you suspect a patient of becoming anaphylactic then you should immediately give 50 mg of Benadryl and repeat it, if needed. If you have any steroids like Medrol (usually comes in what is known as a Medrol dose pack, but may come in a bottle) or prednisone, then administer those immediately. If it is caused by an insect, scorpion, or snakebite then refer to the section on bites for complete details. The general idea is to decrease blood flow to the area of the bite, using periodic tourniquets, ice packs, elevation of the limb, etc. If you have any activated charcoal handy then immediately after flushing the bite, administer a generous amount of the charcoal to absorb any toxins that might not yet have entered your circulation.

One last word on anaphylaxis, if you have had it in the past, or if you have allergic reactions that are getting progressively worse, then you might want to consider getting desensitization shots at your local allergist now. Prevention is always the best treatment option.

Treatment of Non Anaphylactic Allergic Reactions

Antihistamines

Since most allergic reactions are mediated by histamine, therefore it makes perfect sense to treat them with an antihistamine. Antihistamines come in sedating and non-sedating varieties. Sedating means it makes you tired. The older antihistamines like diphenhydramine (Benadryl) and doxylamine (Unisom) are some of the most potent antihistamines, but both are sedating. Other more recent non-sedating antihistamines include Allegra, Claritin, Clarinex, Xyzal, Zyrtec, and others. The reason they are non-sedating is that they do not cross the blood-brain barrier and mostly work on peripheral tissues. However, very high doses may cross the blood-brain barrier enough to induce grogginess. Meclizine, which is also called Antivert (anti-vertigo, catchy name don't you think) is also an antihistamine, it is sold also as Dramamine and used for sea sickness.

Steroids

Synthetic steroids like Medrol (methylprednisolone) and prednisone can also be used to treat allergic reactions.

If you have any injectable steroids like Depomedrol or cortisone, then using them would be useful if a severe reaction is developing. Steroids cannot be used for long periods due to their numerous side effects such as osteoporosis, weight gain, diabetes, cataracts, and immune suppression.

Neti Pot

Neti pots were traditionally used in India to flush out inflamed, allergic sinuses and nasal passages. They are readily available in the United States now and are very useful to flush out and clear many allergens from the nasal passages. It sort of looks like a small Aladdin's lamp. A saline (salt water) solution is used and it is very effective.

I have many patients who use it and swear by it, including my wife, Lynne. They are available at any pharmacy. You can make your own saline solution by mixing a half teaspoon of sea salt into lukewarm water. Neti pots are used by leaning over the sink and cocking your head to one side. Put the spout of the neti pot into one nostril and allow the water to flow in and then out the opposite nostril. Use about half the water in the neti pot and then repeat it by cocking your head to the opposite side and use the other nostril to insert the neti pot, etc.

You do not have to use a neti pot, although it is inexpensive and very easy. You can simply fill your cupped hand with the solution and alternately snort it up each nostril. You can also use saline nasal sprays to flush out your nose. I have found that it is much less expensive to buy saline wound-flushing spray and use that up your nose, its bottle is large and a little inconvenient, but it works just as well and you can buy a whole lot more of these for the same price.

Use the neti pot two or three times a day, as needed. I would also use it to flush out and clean your nostrils before bed, so you don't wake up all congested.

Quercetin

Quercetin is a flavonoid plant product that has strong antihistamine and antioxidant effects. Its use for asthma is described above. The dose for allergies is much less, usually 1,000 mg daily instead of three times a day. However, if your allergies are driving you crazy use it three times daily until they quiet down. Quercetin helps stabilize the mast cells that are responsible for releasing histamine.

Foods that are naturally high in quercetin include citrus fruits, apples, broccoli, onions, tomatoes, tea, and wine. Quercetin should be taken between meals to help its absorption.

The addition of an enzyme that is derived from pineapples called bromelain helps potentiate (makes it more effective) Quercetin by increasing its absorption in the GI tract; the two seem to amplify the effects of the other and are useful together also for eczema. Try to use the same number of milligrams (mgs) of each when using them together. Do not take bromelain if you are allergic to pineapples.

Butterbur (Petasites hybridus)

Butterbur is a common European weed that has been found to have strong antihistamine activity. Interestingly, it derives its name from the practice before refrigeration of wrapping butter in its large leaves to prevent it from spoiling. The dose is 8 mg four times a day. Studies have shown it to be as effective as Zyrtec, but totally non- sedating. Zyrtec is supposed to be non- sedating but that is not always the case, many of my patients report that it sedated them.

Stinging Nettle (Urtica dioica)

Stinging nettle is a common weed in the United States; I have it in my garden in Connecticut. I can personally attest to the pain those little needle-like nettles cause when you grab them without gloves, so be very careful.

Stinging nettle has potent antihistamine effects without any of the unwanted side effects such as drowsiness and dry mouth. Stinging nettle slows down the body's production of histamine. It comes in various forms including tinctures, teas and a freeze-dried extract of the leaves. The dose of the freeze- dried extract in capsule form is 300 mg daily but this may not last long enough and may need to be repeated.

Vitamin C (Ascorbic Acid)

Vitamin C, besides being a powerful antioxidant, also has strong antihistamine actions. Since it is both water soluble and perhaps the least toxic substance on the planet (there have never been any overdoses with vitamin C, it is safer than water which can kill you if you drink enough), one need not worry about taking too much of it. For allergies everyone is different but approximately 1,000 mg (1 gram) between three to six times daily will work wonders for your allergies. You may have to back off a little on the dose if any diarrhea develops.

MSM (Methylsulfonylmethane)

MSM is an organic sulfur compound, also known as DMSO 2. It comes in a convenient capsule form, and is readily available over the counter. It works very well to reduce inflammation and is quite famous for its effect on painful joints and muscles. Presumably it works by providing sulfur that is biologically active and needed by the body. It has a lesser known effect on reduction of allergy symptoms. The effective dose of MSM for allergies is 3,000 to 5,000 mg daily. It is very well tolerated orally.

Omega-3 Fatty Acids

The source of these omega-3 fatty acids can either be land-based as in flaxseed oil or walnut oil, or can be from marine sources as in fish oil and krill oil. Krill oil has the added advantage of containing astaxanthin, which is a potent antioxidant 6,000 more powerful than vitamin C.

The effective dose for allergies using flaxseed oil is two tablespoons daily. For fish oil I recommend buying the best brand you can afford, due to mercury contamination with the cheaper brands, and take 4 grams a day. I also recommend eating after you take your fish oil, this way the food on top of the fish oil in your stomach will prevent any "burping up" of this fishy oil.

Eyebright (Euphrasia officinalis)

Eyebright belongs to a large family of flowering herbs that live at high altitudes in alpine and sub alpine meadows. Eyebright gets its name from its use for the treatment of eye infections. For eye infections eyebright is made into a poultice. It works very well for infections of the eyelids as well as the eyes, such as conjunctivitis (pink eye).

Eyebright also works very well to treat the congestion associated with sinus infections, colds, sore throat, hay fever, and other allergies. Its mechanism of action is via its anti-inflammatory effects. Besides being used as a poultice, it is also used as a tea and as an extract in capsules, as well as a tincture to be instilled into the eyes.

The dose of eyebright for allergies is one capsule three times a day. It can also be instilled directly into the eye in the form of a tincture. Mix five drops of the tincture in a half ounce of saline solution, and apply this to the eyes twice daily.

Serratiopeptidase

Serratiopeptidase is an enzyme that is produced in the intestines of silk worms and allows the emerging silk moth to dissolve its cocoon and escape. Serratiopeptidase contains protease enzymes, which are enzymes that dissolve proteins; the two other digestive enzymes are lipase to dissolve fats and amylase to dissolve starches. The substances that an enzyme specifically targets are known as substrates, and enzymes are very specific in their targeting and have zero effects on non-substrate substances. That is the beautiful part about enzymes, and is the reason they have so few side effects.

In allergies, there are the antigens, which are substances that trigger the immune response. The immune system sends in antibodies or immunoglobulins such as immunoglobulin E (or IgE) which bind to the antigen and form a complex known as the Circulating Immune Complex. These circulating immune complexes trigger additional responses from the immune system which attempts to neutralize and clear them from the body.

The theory behind taking protease enzymes is that these circulating immune complexes are primarily composed of proteins. We know from tagged studies that enzymes taken on an empty stomach are absorbed whole and intact in the intestines and enter the circulation. Thus if you take protease enzymes on an empty stomach they will be absorbed intact and enter your circulation and clear these unwanted circulating immune complexes and help with your allergies.

Another use of digestive enzymes is to take them with your meals to help better digest your food and prevent the absorption of large food molecules that will be absorbed into the blood and help form circulating immune complexes that will lead to food allergies.

Serratiopeptidase is available online; there is no typical dose, but usually two capsules at bedtime on an empty stomach should suffice.

Essential Oils

Several different essential oils are known to help loosen mucus and decrease its production. They are able to penetrate deeply into the sinuses and the upper airways if aerosolized by making a steam inhalation of them.

You can try eucalyptus, lemon balm, tea tree, pine, cedar wood, sandalwood, thyme, rosemary, and peppermint oils. They can be used individually or in combination; experiment with them and find the combination that you like and is the most effective at breaking up your mucus and congestion and clearing your allergy symptoms.

How you do a steam inhalation is to take boiling hot water and place it in a large bowl, add three or four drops of the essential oil you have chosen. Take a large bath towel and place it over your head and cover the bowl on all four sides like you are making a tent out of it. Keep your face about a foot above the bowl and inhale deeply through your nose.

Note: If you get claustrophobic remove the towel and breathe fresh air for a few minutes and you should be fine. Do not do the steam inhalation if you are asthmatic, it has the potential to worsen your asthma if you are allergic to any of the oils.

Local Honey

The idea behind eating local honey is that the pollen the bees use to make it all comes from local plants. If you are suffering with allergies it is due to some local pollen source. Eating local honey desensitizes your allergies to the local offending agent.

I have to say anecdotally I have seen it work many times in my practice, which is in a rural area with a huge variety of native and foreign plant life. Most patients just take a tablespoon of it daily. I tell most of them to take it at bedtime, which will help them sleep and lose weight at the same time. Taking honey at bedtime provides a source of glucose that will break down slowly over the course of the evening and prevent any nocturnal hypoglycemia (low blood sugar) which in turn leads to mobilization of glycogen (the storage form of glucose, in which it is folded like an accordion, in plants this form of glucose storage takes the form of starch). The breakdown of the glycogen to glucose spikes its level in the blood and results in a corresponding spike in insulin.

Remember, insulin has two roles, one to lower blood glucose levels and the other is concerned with lipid or fat metabolism. Insulin affects lipids in two ways, it takes the excess calories from the glucose and converts them to new fat, while at the same time protecting the fat you already have. Honey prevents the hypoglycemia thus avoiding the spike in insulin.

This in turn prevents the production of new fat and leaves the old fat unprotected. The old fat is then broken down by the body to meet its caloric needs. It is a win-win situation.

Another way to take local honey is to make a mix of one tablespoon of local honey in a cup of warm water along with two tablespoons of apple cider vinegar which will prevent any reaction to allergens in the local honey.

CHAPTER THIRTY-THREE

COLDS, FLU AND RESPIRATORY TRACT INFECTIONS

INTRODUCTION

TABLE OF CONTENTS:

Colds, flu and respiratory tract infections like bronchitis and pneumonia are some of the most commonly encountered problems that will strike you and your family members. The vast majority of these are viral in origin, not bacterial, and as such antibiotics have no role in their treatment, since antibiotics only work against bacterial infections. Since they are viral we have limited treatments available, and the most important thing we can do is to prevent these infections by using good hygiene such as frequent hand washing and making infected people wear masks to decrease the amount of virus they are shedding into your immediate environment.

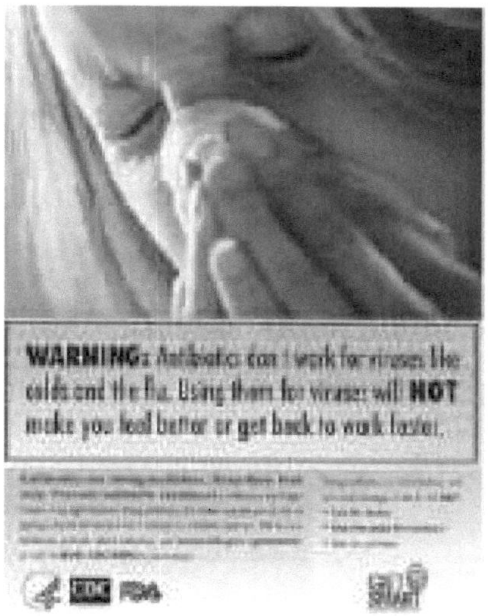

THE FLU VIRUS

The flu is a contagious respiratory illness caused by influenza viruses, it can cause mild to severe illness and frequently is fatal in those who are debilitated (weakened by other diseases), the very young and the very old.

There are three types of flu viruses that infect humans. Types A and B cause the annual flu epidemics that infect up to 20 percent of the population and are responsible for almost 50,000 deaths annually.

The third is type C and this causes a much milder form of the flu.

Type A flu is found in wild birds and humans and is the primary cause of the annual flu epidemics. Type B only infects humans and usually is not as severe, although occasionally it develops into a severe strain. Type C only infects humans and is very mild.

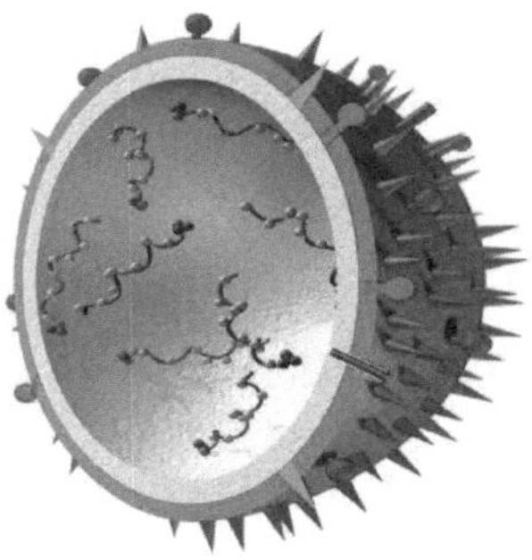

A person infected with the flu virus sheds viral particles (live virus) when they cough and sneeze and when they touch objects like doorknobs. The virus spreads by contaminating respiratory secretions like mucus that is coughed up, and can spread up to six feet from an infected patient. Thus the importance of making infected people wear masks and if no masks are available, they should be isolated from others to prevent spread of the virus. People should frequently wash their hands with soap and water or clean them with a fifty-fifty mix of hydrogen peroxide and water, they can also use alcohol. Remember, the clothes, bed linens, eating utensils, and dishes used by an infected person will also be contaminated. The good news is if you are washing these items they do not need to be isolated from the other non- contaminated items. The take home message here is that it is much easier to prevent catching the flu than it is to treat it once you are infected.

The medical establishment touts the power of your annual flu shot for preventing the flu, and it does work nicely most of the time. However, there is another school of thought that says that flu epidemics always happen in the fall and winter when our sun exposure plummets and the sun we are exposed to does not work very well on our skin to produce Vitamin D. Could the annual flu epidemic just be because our stores of fat soluble vitamin D are depleted and we become susceptible? A doctor in a western state who worked in a large prison thought so and as an experiment he put the entire wing of the prison he worked in on daily vitamin D supplementation.

As fate would have it a severe flu epidemic swept through the prison infecting inmates and guards alike. In the other wings of the prison, no vitamin D was given to the prisoners; in their close-crowded living conditions the flu spread like wild fire, infecting everyone.

In the wing of the prison where they were given vitamin D there were no flu cases! Vitamin D has been found to be eight times better at preventing the flu than the annual flu vaccine!

I am a primary care doctor and as such I am exposed to the flu as soon as it hits town, I have not taken the flu vaccine in over ten years, instead I take at least 5,000 international units of vitamin D3 daily (with a fatty meal), and I have not had the flu once. Remember, Vitamin D is fat soluble so you have to take it with a meal that contains some fat or oil to absorb it into your body. In fact all vitamins except the B vitamins and vitamin C are fat soluble and therefore must be taken with fat to absorb them.

Start supplementing vitamin D3 for you and your family as soon as the leaves drop in the fall and continue until the leaves return in the spring, very few of you if any will get the flu.

The incubation period for the flu virus after exposure is one to four days with an average of two days. One of the problems with the flu virus is that people who are infected begin to shed virus one day before they become sick and continue to shed virus for about another week. Many people infect others accidentally before they themselves become ill. Another problem is that some people with strong immune systems become infected and still shed virus particles infecting others and they themselves never develop symptoms. A person like that is more dangerous for your family's health than a sick person who can be easily identified and quarantined.

The flu is a fascinating disease. The reservoir for the flu virus is in the wild bird populations of Earth. As you may have noticed, the Centers for Disease Control (CDC) goes to Asia annually to obtain samples of the three most common current flu infections. The flu virus easily mutates and this causes a change in the antigens on its surface, these same antigens that your body recognizes and to which it develops antibodies. Every year through a process known as Antigenic Drift, which involves small changes in the viruses' surface antigens change and that is why the flu shot you got last year no longer works. Sometimes there is a major change in the antigens of the flu virus; if a major change occurs this can develop into a very deadly flu, this major change process is known as Antigenic Shift.

A major change or antigenic shift of the flu virus can result in a very deadly flu similar to the one that struck the world near the end of WWI which actually ended the war.

Millions of people died worldwide and some of our troop ships had major losses in troops as they crossed the Atlantic Ocean on their way to the front. At home so many people died that burying the bodies became a problem. A similar shift happened in 2009 with the H1N1 flu; it hit and spread over the entire world, causing a pandemic.

The reason the flu always emerges from Asia is due to the practice of Asian farmers keeping ducks and pigs together. Humans cannot get the flu virus from a bird, but they can get it from a pig. The wild ducks infect the domesticated ducks that farmers keep. A pig is able to get the flu from a bird and so the ducks infect the pigs and in turn the pigs infect the humans.

THE COMMON COLD

The common cold is a viral infection of your upper respiratory tract, which includes your nose and throat. There are over two hundred different types of viruses that cause the common cold and the rhinovirus is the most common culprit. A cold virus enters your body through your mouth, nose, or eyes and quickly spreads throughout your body. Just like the flu, the common cold is spread through droplets in the air, but is also caught by direct contact as in hand- to-hand contact, or from contaminated objects like drinking glasses, utensils, toys, telephones, and doorknobs. Once the virus is on your hands then it is easily transferred by you touching your head near your nose, mouth, or eyes.

Children are the most susceptible and the symptoms usually include a runny nose, sore throat, runny eyes, head congestion, and sneezing; the symptoms seem to vary from person to person. Infants and preschool children also have not developed the immunity to many of the cold viruses that adults have. The average child gets an incredible ten colds a year, and the average adult gets three colds annually. As a primary care doctor I have been exposed to every cold virus there is from contaminated patients, yet I have not had a cold in over fifteen years. I also am vigilant about hand washing and taking vitamin D and my antioxidant vitamins, especially vitamin C in high doses, which helps supercharge my immune system.

The incubation period or the length of time it takes to catch a cold after exposure to someone is about one to three days. Usually there is no fever and only mild fatigue and lasts for seven to ten days.

Signs that it may be turning into something more severe are development of a fever, persistence of the symptoms for more than two weeks, if the color of the mucus you are producing turns from white/clear to dark and green, new symptoms of severe headache, worsening cough, severe sore throat, swollen glands, stiff neck, vomiting, and abdominal pains and severe chills.

Children often go on to develop ear infections, strep throat, the croup, sinus infections, and in rare cases bronchitis and pneumonia.

HOW CAN YOU TELL THE DIFFERENCE BETWEEN A COLD AND THE FLU?

A cold is usually much milder than the flu, which makes you feel like you have been hit by a truck.

Flu symptoms are always much more severe and flu often leads to pneumonia, especially in the very young and the elderly. Colds are so named because your body temperature is low, you don't get a fever, or if you do it is very mild, whereas in cases of the flu you run a high fever of 100-102 F or greater, especially in children, with severe muscle aches and a dry hacking cough that just doesn't quit.

In my experience nothing illustrates the differences better between two illnesses as a table to compare them.

Symptom	Cold	Flu
Fever	rare and if present very mild	Fevers of 100-102 F are common and last 3-4 days
Headache	occasionally and mild	Commonly present and made worse by coughing
Aches and pains	occasionally and mild	Commonly and usually severe
Fatigued, weak	mild	Severe and can last up to 2 to 3 weeks or more
Exhaustion	never	Severe especially at the onset of the flu
Nasal congestion	frequent	Occasionally
Sore throat	common	Occasionally
Chest pain, cough	mild to moderate cough	Frequently severe, hacking cough and chest pain
Complications	sinus and middle ear infections	Bronchitis and pneumonia (life threatening)
Time of year	anytime	Seasonal from fall to spring annually

TREATMENT OF THE COMMON COLD AND FLU GENERAL RECOMMENDATIONS

The common cold and flu are viruses and as such antibiotics have no place, unless later on in the illness one develops a bacterial infection as a complication. Since there is no cure for the cold the goal becomes twofold, to boost your immune system to shorten the length of the cold and to treat the symptoms to make you more comfortable.

That being said, let's see what I have for you in my "bag of tricks". First of all there are some general principles that you need to follow to help shorten the length of your cold or flu, as well as making yourself more comfortable.

Keep yourself well hydrated, this will keep the phlegm (mucus) your body is producing nice and thin and runny instead of thick and obstructing. Any fever will rapidly cause dehydration from imperceptible water loss from your skin. Drink fluids in the form of green tea, organic vegetable broths, and chicken soup to help both with your hydration as well as providing additional nutrients to strengthen your body's immune system and provide antioxidants.

Get plenty of rest and sleep a lot; it allows your body a chance to rest and recuperate and saves your strength to resist the cold virus.

Avoid aspirin; especially in young children this has the potential to produce the deadly Reye's syndrome. Usually there is not a high fever with the common cold but many people immediately go to Tylenol for the mildest fever. Remember, your body does not do things randomly; it spikes a temperature in order to kill the invading viruses or bacteria, since they live in a narrow temperature range close to our body temperature this cooks them and kills them. If you have severe muscle aches or a headache take Aleve, Motrin, or Excedrin. Remember Excedrin has Tylenol, aspirin, and caffeine in it, so it may keep you awake if you are sensitive to caffeine and its Tylenol will also reduce your fever, so keep that in mind.

If you have a sore throat gargle with a combination of hydrogen peroxide and water in a fifty-fifty mixture, you can also use salt and water but hydrogen peroxide works better to kill pathogenic (disease-causing) organisms. In my practice whenever I recommend hydrogen peroxide almost universally people will wrinkle up their noses and make a face, they all think it has a horrible smell or taste.

I always take the time to uncap a bottle of peroxide and place it under their noses, always to their pleasant surprise. Hydrogen peroxide has no smell and therefore no taste, it is like club soda in that regard. One of the beneficial effects of vitamin C is that it naturally increases hydrogen peroxide production in the body's white blood cells, which those cells use to kill invading microorganisms. You can also mix an 8-ounce glass of warm water with one teaspoon of salt and gargle that deeply to soothe a sore throat. If your nose is sore from blowing it, apply some Vaseline petroleum jelly to the sore part on the outside of your nostrils and dab a little inside as well.

Rinsing your nose with store-bought saline solutions will help nasal congestion and soothe your nasal passages that are being ravaged by these viral invaders. You can make your own saline solution by dissolving a teaspoon of salt in a cup of room temperature or warm water. Do not use cold water; it could be painful and will not mobilize the mucus if it is very thick. Using a neti pot with a saline solution will also help drain your sinuses.

Using my mother's old favorite Vick's VapoRub on your chest at bedtime or during the day if you are bedridden. Vick's will help keep your sinuses clear from the menthol and camphor and help your cough and chest congestion. Rub it into your chest well and cover up, roll over and go to sleep.

For coughs and chest congestion heat a pot of water to a boil, shut off the flame, stand over it and place a towel over your head making a tent and inhale the steam to break up your chest congestion. An even more effective trick is to add a teaspoon of Vick's VapoRub to the hot water and place the towel over your head making a tent and inhale deeply. This works very rapidly to open up your chest and clear your head. Both methods should be done for about five minutes. Coughs will also respond to dextromethorphan which is an excellent cough suppressant and is found in over-the-counter medications like Vick's cough drops and Robitussin DM, both of which are over-the-counter so you can easily stock up on them. Mucinex (Guaifenesin) is also another excellent treatment for chest congestion and is an expectorant that will help you cough up that mucus by its thinning effect on the mucus.

Bad head congestion with a severe runny nose will also respond to Benadryl (diphenhydramine). The added benefit at bedtime is its sedative effects will help you sleep. Benadryl is over-the-counter and I recommend all my readers have a large supply of this handy in their medicine chest.

SPECIFIC TREATMENTS FOR THE COMMON COLD AND FLU

Vitamin C (Ascorbic Acid)

Linus Pauling and many other distinguished scientists have been proponents of vitamin C and its many health benefits. There are several books in the bibliography that are full of information about the use of vitamin C for various health conditions including any infectious disease as well as cancer.

Humans, other primates, guinea pigs, and the African fruit bat are the only animals that cannot make their own vitamin C. Presumably we lost this ability because of the huge amounts of vitamin C available from fruits and vegetables we were consuming. There is even a theory that our affinity for sweetness developed in us to insure we get enough vitamin C from sweet, ripe fruits. One of the pioneers of high dose vitamin C therapy was Dr. Frederick Klenner. Remember, vitamin C is water soluble and as such will be excreted in the urine (just like vitamin B, which makes your urine bright yellow) if there is any excess not utilized by your body, or it will give you diarrhea when given beyond your body's requirements. Dr. Klenner gave vitamin C intravenously in doses of over 100 grams daily to patients with infections and high fevers, only to find none of it excreted in their urine, and they recovered from very serious infections. What does that say about the vitamin C requirements when you are sick? In fact, another way to show your body's increased requirements of vitamin C is by its major side effect, diarrhea. When you are normal you may for example develop diarrhea at doses of vitamin C of 10 grams a day; now when the same person becomes ill they will not develop diarrhea at doses of 50 grams a day, thus demonstrating their body's new increased needs. For everyday use I would recommend 5 grams of vitamin C daily. All vitamin C is created equal, even cheap brands contain the simple compound ascorbic acid; synthetic or not it all works. Some people swear by Ester C but I don't think you need it. If you feel you are coming down with a cold then increase your intake of vitamin C in divided doses four times a day until you get diarrhea, then lower it until the diarrhea stops. Vitamin C is the least toxic substance known to man, it is less toxic than water; there has never been a case of fatal vitamin C overdose. Vitamin C boosts your immunity, it is an essential part of the water soluble arm of the antioxidant cascade and it supercharges your white blood cells which are your body's best defense against microbial invasion.

Echinacea (Echinacea Purpurea) And Goldenseal (Hydrastis Canadensis)

These two herbs both enhance immunity and help dry out mucus secretions. Echinacea also has antiviral properties and thus works well in cases of cold and flu; it is thought to reduce the length of colds as well as their severity. It works well when combined with goldenseal, but if you don't have any congestion or mucus production then skip the goldenseal. Echinacea and goldenseal each work on different arms of the immune system and therefore their use is not redundant but complementary to one another, hence the popularity of this combination in the treatment of colds and other respiratory tract infections.

Echinacea is also known as coneflower and grows wild in the United States and Canada and is also planted in many home gardens for its beauty. The entire plant is utilized and made into powder, tinctures, and teas. It is one of the most commonly used natural remedies in the United States. It is very easy to grow and I grow it extensively in my gardens; I recommend it for your medicinal garden.

Studies are contradictory; some showing little benefit and others showing that Echinacea can increase the total number of white blood cells (which are responsible for your immunity) and especially the all-important macrophages which help attack and digest foreign invaders. The name macro means large and phage means eater, thus big eaters.

There are few side effects from taking Echinacea and you have a greater chance of developing side effects if you are allergic to other members of the daisy family such as daisies, ragweed, chrysanthemums, and marigolds. The range of reactions includes everything from a mild rash to anaphylaxis (a life-threatening allergic reaction). That being said, most people tolerate Echinacea just fine, as evidenced by its widespread use.

Just like Echinacea, goldenseal has been used for centuries by American Indian tribes, especially the Cherokee. The potency of goldenseal is due to several alkaloids it has including berberine, hydrastine and canadine. All three of these alkaloids have astringent properties, meaning they dry out mucus membranes and eliminate that runny nose and sinus congestion. Goldenseal also is anti- inflammatory and has antimicrobial effects as well.

The dose is a 500 mg capsule (made of a mix of both goldenseal and Echinacea) four times a day until the cold ends. Or you can use the tincture at a dose of 2 to 4 ml four times daily.

Elderberry (Sambucus Nigra)

Elderberry is a commonly grown garden shrub that is easy to grow and will reward you with large crops of sweet black berries that also have wonderful medicinal qualities. The variety used medicinally is the European Elderberry (Sambucus nigra). Some of the benefits of using elderberry include its antiviral properties, making it ideal to treat colds and the flu, it also is anti-inflammatory, has antibacterial properties and is an immune enhancer (boosts your resistance or immunity). It is commonly used in cooked form as a syrup, juice, or tonic. It is sometimes added as a flavoring to foods. Both the dried flowers and the berries are utilized and are made into capsules, liquid extracts, or as a tea.

Commercially you can find sources of elderberry extract called Sambucol and Zand. The berries should never be eaten uncooked as they may cause severe diarrhea, nausea, and vomiting. A cooled infusion of elderberry can be used to soothe a sore throat. Doses of elderberry depend on the part of the plant used and its formulation:

Tea: Use the dried elderberry flowers; take two teaspoons or approximately 3 grams and pour a cup of boiling water over it and allow it to steep and then strain it. Drink five cups a day until your cold is gone.

Tincture: Take between 5 to 10 ml up to three times a day until the cold symptoms resolve.

Elderberry juice: Mix a teaspoon of elderberry juice in cold water four times a day until symptoms resolve.

Stems and leaves of the elderberry plant can be poisonous and should not be used. Elderberry, like almost everything should not be used in pregnant or nursing women.

Chicken Soup

No, I am not kidding, chicken soup -- often referred to as Jewish penicillin works wonders for the common cold and the flu. My mother is Italian but she also was a big advocate of chicken soup, and I must say it worked. Part of it could be the placebo effect of having someone who loves you doting on you and making you some soup, a little TLC never hurts anyone who is sick. I have found in my practice that some kind words and a little affection goes a long way in helping a sick patient, too many times these days doctors and nurses are busy staring at their laptops and not looking at the patients.

In my opinion that is not the art of the practice of medicine, which is an art that includes eye contact and other visual cues as well as concerns conveyed to a patient in a sincere manner. I am not opposed to hugging patients and kissing old ladies on the forehead. In this politically correct age that is frowned upon, but I couldn't disagree more. Genuine affection does wonders for patients and pardon the pun "is chicken soup for their souls".

There is some scientific evidence supporting the use of chicken soup for the common cold. Studies have shown that chicken soup slows the movement of neutrophils, this in turn decreases the inflammation since neutrophils are part of the body's inflammatory response. It also helps mobilize (speed up the movement) of mucus, helping to relieve congestion. It causes your nose to run but there is a school of thought that says this is good since it decreases the time the virus is in contact with your nasal mucosa and limits its ability to further invade your body. It also helps keep you hydrated and if warm enough will raise the temperature of your sinuses and help further mobilize those mucus secretions, as well as soothing a sore throat. Even something as basic as chicken soup can be improved upon, here are some ways to make yours an even more powerful brew.

Try adding some of the following ingredients to your next batch of soup.

Garlic: Fresh organic garlic adds wonderful flavor and the sulfa- containing compounds in garlic function as both strong antioxidants and anti- inflammatory agents. Garlic also boosts the power of the immune system.

Organic greens such as spinach, collard greens, kale, and swiss chard.

Organic onions, potatoes, turnips, and sweet potatoes will all add wonderful flavor and contribute their nutrients to the soup. A dash or two of sea salt will add some minerals and enhance the flavor.

When adding the above ingredients do so five minutes or so before the soup is finished so you retain most of the enzymes and minerals and flavor.

Lomatium Dissectum

Lomatium dissectum is a plant in the carrot family that grows in the Pacific Northwest and has been used there for centuries by the local Indians. Its common name is fern leaf biscuit root. It is a perennial herb that grows to about four feet tall with a thick, long taproot similar to a carrot. It has been shown to have strong antibacterial and antiviral properties and has shown activity against tuberculosis as well. Its antiviral properties have made it useful in the treatment of the common cold, sinus infections, throat infections, ear infections, bronchitis, and pneumonia.

It has also been shown to have antifungal properties and works well against Candida Albicans infections. Lomatium dissectum has been described as the strongest native antiviral plant in existence. That is reason enough for me to plant it in my medicinal garden, with no real antiviral meds to speak of this is a wonderful medicinal herb to have available. During the flu outbreak of 1918, the same deadly flu that put an end to WWI, the local white population in the Pacific Northwest was devastated, but most of the Indians used Lomatium and survived without any problems.

The plant is easily grown in any soil, its native habitat is rocky soil in sunny locations. The seeds are available on the internet and should be sown the previous fall and will germinate early in the spring. Lomatium has a low germination rate, so plant more expecting to have some losses.

Use of Lomatium may lead to a red, raised, whole-body rash which fortunately clears within twenty-four hours of its discontinuation.

Dose:

Tincture: Take 2 to 4 ml four times a day. Another alternative dosing is to mix the tincture in a cup of hot water, the dosing is to mix in a quarter of a teaspoon every four hours for five days.

Tea: Take one or two teaspoons of the dried herb and pour a cup of boiling water over it and allow it to steep for twenty minutes or so and then strain it. Drink this mix three times a day.

Capsules: Take a 500 mg capsule four times a day until the cold resolves. Many times it is used in a combination treatment with elderberry juice or oregano oil. I think it would be especially effective with the next medication that I describe below.

Andrographis Paniculata

Andrographis Paniculata is an annual herb that grows in Southern Asia mostly in both India and Sri Lanka. Due to its taste it is sometimes known as the King of Bitters. The herb has been introduced to many other countries such as Java, Indonesia, the West Indies, Thailand, and Malaysia. It is sometimes marketed under the name Kan Jang, for over a decade it has been the most popular cold remedy in all of Scandinavia.

The leaves and the roots are used to prepare the medicine. It has been used extensively in Ayurveda and traditional Chinese medicine. It has been used to treat colds and respiratory tract infections as well as rheumatic problems and ulcerative colitis.

NOTE: Pregnant women should not use Andrographis paniculata since it will cause miscarriages and terminate their pregnancies. The active ingredient in Andrographis is known as Andrographolide, which is responsible for its stimulation of the body's immunity. As well as being an anti-inflammatory agent, it has also been shown to protect the liver. Andrographis is not an antimicrobial agent, meaning it does not kill bacteria or viruses directly, but rather stimulates the immune system to eradicate them.

One of the wonderful benefits of Andrographis is that it works rapidly; levels peak in the blood within two hours of taking the medication.

Furthermore, it is rapidly removed from the body; 80 percent within eight hours, and 90 percent by two days' time. Other possible effects of Andrographis is to lower blood pressure, lower blood glucose levels, decrease inflammation, protect the liver from the effect of toxins, and inhibit the production of blood clots.

The dose of Andrographis in capsule form is 300 mg four times a day until the cold is resolved. In my opinion I think a combination of Andrographis Paniculata in order to boost your immunity together with the directly virocidal (virus-killing) Lomatium Dissectum would be a wonderful one-two punch that would knock out any viral infection. In effect the combination of those two would boost your defenses (immunity) and provide wonderful offensive capabilities (virocidal activity).

Zinc

Zinc is a mineral and a natural element found in many foods. Zinc is essential for good health and has antiviral properties that are beneficial when you are suffering with a cold or the flu. Zinc is the active ingredient in many cold and flu remedies. Unfortunately your body cannot store zinc and therefore needs a daily dose of zinc either in foods or supplements. Zinc is present in over 3,000 different proteins in your body as well as being essential for over two hundred different enzymes.

Zinc comes in various forms for the treatment of colds and flu. It comes as lozenges, liquids, sprays, and even as a gel. Zinc works by various mechanisms, one way in which it works is to prevent the adherence (sticking to the body's cells) of viruses and therefore blocks their replication, which is dependent upon entry into the cells in order to take control of the cell and begin churning out millions of replicas of themselves.

Zinc also decreases the duration of a cold and its symptoms. Zinc should therefore be started at the first sign of a cold or the flu. Zinc is also thought to have immune-enhancing properties, and as such helps your body fight off viral infections. It has been shown that zinc increases the production of white blood cells which help fight infections; for the same reason it is also thought to have cancer-fighting abilities.

Zinc is essential for many enzyme systems in your body as well as being responsible for your sense of smell and taste. Zinc is also known to promote healing and as such is given after surgery.

These same healing properties will help heal you from viral illnesses. Zinc is also essential for growth, insulin production, and for men, testosterone production.

Zinc deficiencies are common and are especially prevalent in the young and the elderly, making both groups even more susceptible to viral infections. Zinc deficiency comes from growing foods on zinc-depleted soils, plant-based diets, diets high in grains, and sometimes caused by certain medications such as diuretics, the blood pressure meds known as ACE inhibitors, and medications that interfere with acid production like Aciphex, Prevacid, Nexium, and Prilosec. The reason high grain diets impair zinc absorption is because they contain phytic acid which binds zinc, making it unavailable to the body. Phytic acid also impairs the absorption of calcium, magnesium, and iron. Animal proteins are known to increase the absorption of zinc, which is another reason that vegetarian diets lead to zinc deficiency. Foods that are high in zinc are legumes (beans and lentils), nuts, oysters, cacao (unsweetened chocolate) and meats, especially beef and poultry, especially the livers of these animals.

One of the easiest ways to diagnose zinc deficiency without a blood test is to look at a person's fingernails, when deficient there will be flecks of white on the pink nail bed. Other signs and symptoms of zinc deficiency include acne, poor memory, lack of smell and taste, growth retardation (slow growth), moodiness, and susceptibility to viral infections (lack of resistance to colds and flu for example).

Zinc is vital for our health and the health of our children. Zinc is also very important for women who are pregnant and/or breast feeding, in whom the requirements for zinc skyrocket in order to meet the demands of the growing fetus. If a pregnant woman does not get adequate zinc it can cause problems such as preeclampsia, low birth weight, growth retardation, and premature deliveries. Zinc is especially essential for children for proper growth mental alertness, mood, and memory.

You need to keep a very good supply of zinc supplements to insure to treat colds, flu, and other viral infections and especially if we have children, to ensure their proper growth and development.

Some of the other properties of this amazing essential mineral are as follows:

Sleep: Proper zinc supplementation helps the production of melatonin which is responsible for deep restorative sleep.

Skin Conditions like acne, eczema, psoriasis, and helping heal wounds. For acne zinc has been shown to be as effective as the antibiotic tetracycline.

Eye Health: Zinc helps prevent night blindness, macular degeneration, and the formation of cataracts.

Diabetes: Zinc is necessary for the production of insulin as well as its regulation.

Apthous Ulcers: Zinc lozenges will help heal apthous ulcers every time.

Male sexuality: Zinc is essential for the production of the male hormone testosterone, and as such if there is a deficiency of testosterone, zinc supplementation will help increase testosterone levels which helps raise libido (makes you horny) and helps erectile dysfunction. Zinc supplementation will also help cases of male sterility and BPH (benign prostatic hyperplasia or benign enlargement of the prostate gland).

As I stated above, zinc is best absorbed when it is attached to a protein. One way to get zinc in this form is to buy chelated zinc supplements. Chelated means that it is attached to something, usually a protein. Binding zinc to various substances makes it more absorbable. Examples are zinc acetate, zinc citrate, and zinc gluconate. These are all good ways to get your zinc. Zinc is also better tolerated when chelated than in its inorganic form such as zinc oxide and zinc sulfate. These inorganic zinc salts sometimes irritate the stomach and also interfere with the absorption of calcium. Certain substances like caffeine can interfere with zinc absorption and should not be taken at the same time as a supplement.

Long-term zinc supplementation can lead to iron and copper deficiencies and if you take it chronically (longer than three months), then you will need to supplement these two, especially copper. I like to supplement copper at the ratio of 1 mg of copper for every 50 mg of zinc daily.

The dose of zinc for colds and flu is 50 mg a day. You will have to check the percentage of zinc present in each pill to determine the exact zinc content. For example if your zinc citrate supplement is 250 mg and only 30 percent zinc then it really is a 75 mg zinc dose. Zinc is inexpensive and I recommend stocking up on it for your alternative medicine chest.

Sodium Bicarbonate (Baking Soda)

One of the most effective ways to treat any cold or flu is sodium bicarbonate or baking soda. How in the world can this help, you ask? It is quite simple; baking soda is an alkaline substance (opposite of an acid) and as such interferes with almost all viral infections. The reason for this is quite simple I go into it in a lot of detail in the chapter on Ebola, for those of you who like technical explanations). Viruses need an acidic environment to infect cells, the acid terrain facilitates (helps) the viral particles adhere (stick to) the human cells and fuse with them and then gain entry into the cell, where they replicate until the cell explodes and then spread. When you use baking soda you are making the area between the cells (where the virus is) less acidic and as such it prevents the viral particles from entering the cells and spreading the infection. This was one of the only successful treatments during the Spanish Flu of 1918. Sodium bicarbonate is very safe; once in the body it breaks down to water and carbon dioxide. That being said, there is one caveat, do not take sodium bicarbonate if you have a very full stomach, the production of the carbon dioxide can actually rupture your stomach!

Here is how they took it in 1918:

Day 1: One half-teaspoonful of sodium bicarbonate in a glass of cold water every two hours for a total of six doses.

Day 2: Same dose and interval between doses, but only four doses. Day 3: Take the same dose upon awakening and at bedtime.

Day 4 and after: Take it once daily in the morning until all the symptoms have resolved.

This formula will work for both colds and flu and also gives rapid relief for headaches.

CHAPTER THIRTY-FOUR
ANXIETY AND DEPRESSION

INTRODUCTION

TABLE OF CONTENTS:

Anxiety and depression are very common conditions that I treat daily in my medical practice. Over the years I have noticed several common denominators among these depressed patients. They oftentimes have no religion or God in their lives, many have been brought up without any religious training whatsoever. Do not misunderstand me, I am not saying that if you are religious you will never become depressed, that certainly is not the case. What I am saying is that without God in your life, your chances of becoming depressed are much greater than if you have a personal relationship with God. The other factor that I have noticed among these patients is their lack of direction or purpose in their lives. They seem to be drifting through life without any plan or even the faintest idea of what they are going to do next. These are just some of my personal observations that I have made over my long career as a physician.

Anxiety and depression are interesting in that they are twice as prevalent in the wealthier western countries and are significantly less than half as prevalent in the impoverished countries of the third world. That is exactly the opposite of what one would expect. We who have all of these luxuries and live lives that citizens of third world countries would never even dare to dream of, we are depressed in huge numbers and they seem to be oblivious to anxiety and depression. An explanation of this paradox might just be that people in poor countries are so busy struggling to scratch out their meager existences that they do not have the luxury of free time to be introspective and examine their lives.

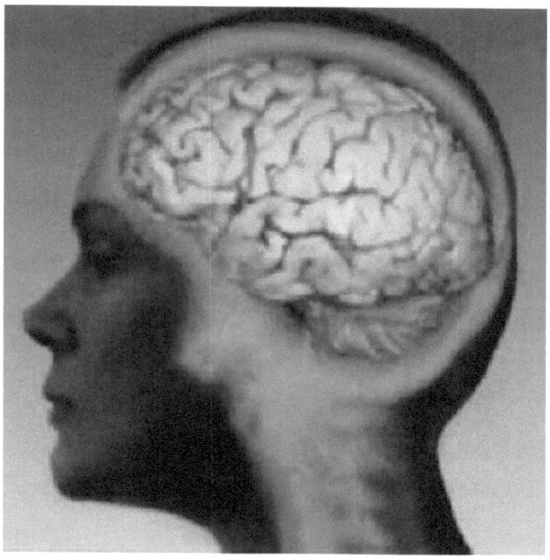

Anxiety and depression are undoubtedly different conditions, but there is considerable overlap between the two. Most of my patients who have depression also suffer with a certain degree of anxiety. I have found that many anxiety patients are also depressed but many have pure anxiety without any depression.

Currently there are large numbers of patients who are on Xanax and other anxiety medications, as well as antidepressants. Let's take a look at some healthier natural/alternative options for treating anxiety and depression.

TREATMENT OF ANXIETY AND DEPRESSION

Let's start with the simplest changes that could help your anxiety and depression.

DIETARY CHANGES THAT WILL HELP ANXIETY AND DEPRESSION

There are several changes that you can make in your diet and lifestyle that can help your anxiety. One of the best is to avoid hypoglycemia. Hypoglycemia means low blood sugar levels. When this occurs, the body releases adrenaline which is a stress hormone and this triggers the "fight or flight" reaction in your body, thus causing stress.

Hypoglycemia occurs from taking in simple carbohydrates. Simple carbohydrates are concentrated sweets such as sugar, soft drinks, candies, etc. These break down quickly when they are digested resulting in severe spikes in your blood glucose levels. These spikes in glucose are answered by similar spikes in insulin. In patients with hypoglycemia there is an excess of insulin produced and consequently the blood glucose levels drop below normal into the hypoglycemic range. It has been shown that caffeine and alcohol also contribute to hypoglycemia.

Caffeine has different effects on different people. You have probably noticed how some people can drink coffee at bedtime with no problem sleeping; others drink a cup late in the afternoon and cannot sleep that evening. The reason for this is genetic; most people metabolize caffeine normally, some people are slow metabolizers of caffeine and others are rapid metabolizers. If you are a slow metabolizer you burn up or metabolize your caffeine slowly so it lasts a long time, hence the insomnia after an afternoon cup of coffee. If you are a fast metabolizer you can drink a cup of coffee a few hours before bedtime without any problems. The metabolic rate is controlled by enzyme systems in your liver which are inherited traits.

Food allergies may also contribute to anxiety. Typically it is very difficult to nail down which foods are the culprits. The best method is to make a food diary and see if you develop anxiety shortly after eating certain foods. Sometimes these same food allergies are associated with migraine headaches, stuffy nose and head congestion, and even joint aches; that is why a food diary is so important.

B complex vitamins have been shown to be helpful in both anxiety and depression. B6, B12, and folic acid all are critical to the correct metabolism of the brain's neurotransmitters and thus to support overall brain health. You should take 50 mg B complex once or twice daily; since B vitamins are water soluble they do not have to be taken with food and any excess will be urinated out and will not have any side effects.

NUTRITIONAL SUPPLEMENTS AND OTHER TREATMENTS FOR ANXIETY AND DEPRESSION

Theanine And Gaba

Theanine is a non- protein amino acid found in green tea and the mushroom Boletus Badius. Non protein amino acid means that it is not one of the twenty-three amino acids that the body utilizes to make its vast array of proteins. Did you ever notice how green tea drinkers do not get "wired" on caffeine like coffee drinkers do? The reason is the calming effect of theanine which also improves mood and seems to impart an overall sense of relaxation. Green tea has been used in Asia for centuries with many benefits and no ill effects.

Theanine does this by blocking the binding of L-Glutamic acid to glutamate receptors in the brain. Glutamic acid is an excitatory neurotransmitter in the brain and as such leads to agitation and anxiety; blocking it leads to the opposite effects. Theanine also increases levels of dopamine in the brain and possibly serotonin levels as well, both of which help with anxiety and depression. Theanine also increases alpha waves in the brain which are associated with relaxation and lessening of anxiety. Theanine has been shown in several rat studies to also lower your blood pressure. Theanine has also been shown to be very effective as a muscle relaxant, helping patients suffering with injuries that lead to muscle spasms. Theanine also has been shown to be effective in treating insomnia.

Theanine also works by increasing production of GABA (gamma aminobutyric acid) which is an inhibitory neurotransmitter, meaning it does the opposite of excitation, so it relaxes you. GABA functions within the brain to inhibit emotions such as anxiety, panic, fear, depression, and even pain. GABA has also been shown to inhibit drug, alcohol, and tobacco cravings, and as such might prove very useful in those patients withdrawing from alcohol or addictive anxiety medications.

GABA is the most widely distributed neurotransmitter in the brain, which speaks to its many important functions, it is also found throughout the entire body. Giving both GABA and theanine together will work synergistically (they are more powerful together) to help decrease anxiety.

The dose of theanine is 200 mg a day, and if you want to increase its effectiveness you can add GABA 200 to 500 mg daily. In order to work effectively GABA needs both magnesium and vitamin B6. Both magnesium and B6 are required by your body to produce all the various neurotransmitters in our brain. Magnesium can be taken as a teaspoon of Epsom salt in water or soak in a hot bath for a half hour with two cups of Epsom salt dissolved in it. If you do this it is wonderful to do at bedtime, you will sleep like a baby and your entire body will become relaxed. B6 is readily available in pharmacies and I would take 50 mg daily that is more than enough to provide all the B6 your brain requires for neurotransmitter production.

Vitamin B-3, or Niacinamide

Niacinamide or vitamin B-3 is one of the members of the family of B vitamins known as B complex. It is related to niacin, and in fact it is a metabolite of niacin, meaning that when niacin is processed by the liver it produces niacinamide. The good news is it does not have any of the side effects of niacin like causing flushing; the bad news is it does not lower cholesterol like niacin. It also has been shown to help inflammatory skin conditions such as acne, and also has been shown to be beneficial in the treatment of Alzheimer's disease by improving memory.

For the treatment of anxiety niacinamide has been shown to have actions similar to benzodiazepine drugs such as Ativan, Valium, and Xanax.

One note of caution with the use of niacinamide is its potential for liver damage at doses greater than 1,000 mg (1 gram) daily. For this reason higher doses should be avoided. That being said, the dose you should use is 500 mg once daily.

Here is where the "art of medicine" comes in, for safety sake stay below the 1,000 mg maximum and add other nutraceuticals such as theanine, magnesium, or any of the others listed here until you get the anxiety under control. B complex vitamins should also be taken so you insure that you have all the other B vitamins that are essential for neurotransmitter production.

Magnesium and Calcium

The multiple and varied uses of magnesium never cease to amaze me. There are over 300 enzymes in the body that require magnesium to properly function! Anxiety can be triggered by a magnesium deficiency and such deficiencies are very common among Americans. Magnesium is known for its sedative effects, helping the body relax; it also helps leg cramps, constipation, and insomnia to name but a few.

Magnesium and calcium seem to function synergistically, each increasing the effect of the other. For this reason it is best to supplement both together to get that additive effect.

The dose of calcium is 600-1200 mg per day. Remember, calcium comes in various forms; you can also get calcium from Tums supplements which are made of calcium carbonate. Tums comes in various strengths, regular Tums has 500 mg of calcium carbonate. There are also 750 mg and 1,000 mg varieties. It is an inexpensive way to supplement calcium, while at the same time treating any heartburn or reflux.

Calcium also comes in OsCal which stands for oyster shell calcium. Certain foods may interfere with calcium absorption such as rhubarb, spinach, caffeine, and whole grains. There is no problem taking OsCal if you have a shellfish allergy that is typically caused by the proteins in the fish itself. OsCal is mined from ancient beds of oyster shells that have not had any contact with the actual animal for thousands of years, hence have none of the offending proteins that cause the shellfish allergy.

The dose for magnesium should be between 400-800 mg per day. Magnesium also comes in various forms including tablets of magnesium oxide, lactated magnesium, and others. It also comes in an oil as magnesium oil that can be applied topically. Magnesium oil sometimes causes a burning sensation when applied to the skin. To eliminate that you can add it to coconut oil as a carrier oil. Magnesium sulfate (Epsom salt) is another inexpensive form that can be drank mixed with water or applied topically. If you take an Epsom salt bath you need to stir two or three cups of Epsom salt into the hottest water you can stand (be careful lowering your genitals into that hot water!) and you need to remain in the bathtub for at least a half an hour; that is how long it takes for the Epsom salt to cross your skin and be absorbed which is known as the transdermal effect.

5-Hydroxytryptophan (5-HTP)

5-HTP is a naturally occurring amino acid and is important in the production of serotonin and melatonin. It is available over the counter and is used extensively in the treatment of anxiety, depression and is also used to suppress appetite and to treat insomnia. It is related to tryptophan, which is found in turkey and is responsible for that nap that you take every year on your couch after Thanksgiving dinner. Tryptophan is also released by heating up milk. That is why as a child your mother gave you a glass of warm milk at bedtime to make you sleep.

5-HTP is metabolized by an enzyme which is dependent on B6 (Pyridoxine) to the neurotransmitter serotonin. For this reason you should take a B6 supplement along with 5-HTP to better insure that reaction and to better increase your serotonin levels. Low levels of serotonin are responsible for depression. The most effective drugs for depression are a class of drugs known as the SSRIs, which stands for Selective Serotonin Reuptake Inhibitors; what they do in effect is raise serotonin levels in your brain.

The 5-HTP dose is 50 to 100 mg two to three times daily, along with vitamin B6. The usual dose of B6 should be about 25 mg once or twice daily or 50mg once daily. If you find numbness and tingling in your joints occurring then you should lower the dose of the B6.

Kava (Piper methysticum)

Kava is also known as kava-kava; its name is derived from the languages of the South Pacific islands where it is a native understory shrub that grows in sandy, well aerated soils with lots of rain, exactly what you would find in Samoa, Fiji, Hawaii, and other islands. Kava is one of those plants that have become dependent upon mankind for its reproduction, which is done almost exclusively by stem cuttings.

All plants give something in return for man's help, and in this case kava produces relaxation without sedation and therefore is very useful in the treatment of anxiety. At high doses it may have a slight inebriating effect and it is thus recommended not to drink any alcohol while taking kava.

The active ingredients in kava are known as kava lactones so far fifteen different varieties have been discovered. Kava is revered in Hawaii and the islands of Micronesia and certain strains that had significantly more kava lactones in it were used exclusively by their royalty. Kava affects various neurotransmitters in the brain including GABA, and increases levels of both dopamine and norepinephrine. Norepinephrine helps you relax but at the same time helps your ability to concentrate.

The dose of kava is 200 to 250 mg two or three times daily. There are different standardizations of the content of kava lactones, and the above dose is using a 30 percent kava lactone product. I recommend not buying kava with less than 20 percent kava lactones.

Do not use alcohol with kava and do not use it if you suffer with Parkinson's disease, hepatitis, or other liver problems. Do not take any other anxiety medicines while you take kava.

Rhodiola Rosea

Rhodiola Rosea is a perennial plant that mostly grows in cold mountainous areas around the world. It is also known as Russian Rhodiola and Golden Root. In both Russia and the Scandanavian countries Rhodiola Rosea has been used for centuries to help the local people deal with the harsh environment as well as the stresses of everyday life. Rhodiola Rosea is grown all over the world, but a recent study done in Korea showed that the Russian extract of Rhodiola was twice as effective as either the Chinese or the Tibetan extracts.

Rhodiola Rosea has also been shown to help relieve fatigue as well as simultaneously significantly increase attentiveness. Rhodiola has also been found to be a potent antioxidant and immune enhancer as well as improving sexual performance. The extracts of Rhodiola contain two active substances that are believed to make it so potent in the relief of both anxiety and depression, they are called rosavins and salidroside. You should look for preparations containing at least 2 to 3 percent rosavins and 1 percent salidroside; studies have shown that this concentration is the most effective.

The best way to take Rhodiola is to start slowly at 100 mg daily for one week. It may make you a little jittery in the beginning. You can keep increasing the dose until you have your anxiety under control with a maximum dose of 400 mg daily.

Valerian (Valeriana officinalis)

Valerian is also known as valerian root. Valerian is a perennial flowering plant native to both Europe and Asia and widely planted in the United States, where it has naturalized. It grows primarily in wet lands where it is tall and has a bad smell .Valerian root was used by the ancient Greeks and Romans as a sedative and to treat anxiety and insomnia.

Valerian root is processed and made into a tea or tincture or it is incorporated into capsules. The active ingredient in valerian has been somewhat difficult to isolate, and it most likely works by a combination of agents that it contains, such as volatile oils including valerinic acids and less volatile sesquaterpines and other esters. Many plants have their effects from multiple agents that act in concert; isolating one or two into a pharmaceutical many times does not work as well or at all. It is very difficult to mimic the effects of Mother Nature; plants are extraordinary chemists and are able to produce thousands of different compounds on demand.

Valerian is believed to have its sedative and anxiety reducing effects by its effect on GABA. Valerian seems to both increase the release of GABA by neurons (nerve cells) as well as inhibiting the enzyme that breaks down GABA, both means effectively increase the amount of GABA present. GABA, as you recall from my discussion above, is an inhibitory neurotransmitter, thus it has a relaxation and sedative effect on the brain.

Pregnant women and children under the age of three should not take valerian. You should also not mix valerian with kava, Saint-John's-wort and benzodiazepines. People with liver disease such as alcoholics should avoid valerian.

The dose of valerian varies as to the preparation. Valerian also takes several weeks to build up and get its full effect.

Here are some of the ways you can take valerian:

Tea: Take one teaspoon of dried valerian root powder and add a cup of boiling water and allow it to steep for ten minutes.

Tincture: Use one teaspoon (or maximum of one and a half teaspoons) of the tincture in a quarter cup of water.

Dry powder extract: Use between 250-600 mg. For anxiety it can be used at 250 mg three or four times per day.

Essential Fatty Acids

Essential fatty acids are fats that your body cannot manufacture and needs to function properly; therefore it is essential that these be obtained in our diets.

The brain is approximately 60 percent fats, and one third of that is composed of essential fatty acids, making it the fattiest organ in the human body. There are many types of essential fatty acids (EFAs), and omega-3 and omega-6 are two of the most important for brain health. The two most important types of omega-3 fatty acids are EPA and DHA. When there is a deficiency of these EFAs in the brain it many times will lead to abnormal behavior like Attention Deficit Disorder (with or without hyperactivity), addictions, anxiety, and depression.

Supplementing with these all-important EFAs treats all of those abnormalities, helping anxiety and depression, ADD, hyperactivity, and addiction problems. EFAs also help withdrawal from addictive substances like drugs, alcohol, and cigarettes. Nicotine addiction is one of the strongest addictions known.

Good sources of EFAs are cold-water fish and their fish oils. There are currently two pharmaceutical grade fish oils on the market, Lovaza and Vascepa. Both are only available by prescription and are many times more potent than the over-the-counter brands, and are mercury free. Mercury contamination is a major concern with taking fish oils, the cheaper brands tend to have more mercury. Buy the best fish oil supplements you can afford and keep them in a cool, dry place for storage. Like all oils they can spoil and become rancid if exposed to heat for any length of time.

The dose of EFAs that I recommend is between 1 and 4 grams a day. They typically come in 1,000 mg or 1 gram sizes. Take your fish oil and eat afterwards so your food lies on top of the capsules and there is less burping up of a fishy taste. If you develop diarrhea spread out your dosing of it over the course of the day.

Saint-John's-Wort (Hypericum perforatum)

Saint-John's-wort is a perennial flowering herb originally from Europe but now it is naturalized in meadows all over the world. Saint-John's-wort gets its name because it flowers on June 24th, which is St. John's day or the birthday of John the Baptist. Wort is the old English word for plant. The plant and flowers are traditionally harvested on June 24th. The seeds of this very useful plant can remain viable for decades in the soil and will germinate when the soil is disturbed. Saint-John's-wort has naturalized all over the world and in many places is considered an invasive, destructive weed and can be found growing on roadsides and abandoned fields.

Saint-John's-wort has been extensively used for depression, and is also very useful in the treatment of anxiety. It also has anti-inflammatory and antibacterial properties. The antibacterial properties have been exploited by using Saint-John's-wort to treat burns and other wounds to prevent infections as well as to promote healing. Saint-John's-wort is thought to work by raising serotonin, dopamine, GABA, and norepinephrine levels in the brain.

One of the possible side effects of Saint-John's-wort is photosensitivity, making the eyes very sensitive to bright light and giving patients who go in the sun rashes while on the medication. Ironically, the active ingredients in Saint-John's-wort are inactivated by light, so it should be stored in a dark bottle or kept in a cool, dark place. Saint-John's-wort should not be used in schizophrenics and patients with bipolar disorder.

Saint-John's-wort has also been shown to be ineffective in the treatment of ADD and ADHD; it does however work for menopausal symptoms. It should not be used in women who are pregnant or breast feeding; it also should be avoided in women who are trying to get pregnant since it might interfere with fertilization. Saint-John's-wort might also make the birth control pill ineffective by inducing liver enzymes that will increase the metabolism of estrogen. The two active ingredients in Saint-John's-wort are hypericin and hyperforin.

The dose of Saint-John's-wort is as follows: for anxiety and depression take 300 mg three times a day. For children under twelve use 300 mg once a day.

Inositol

Inositol is a carbohydrate that is found in all animal tissues and is present in the outer covering of our cells known as the cell membrane. It used to be included in the group of vitamins known as B complex and is still sometimes referred to as B8. It is known to help the liver process fats and also is an important contributor to the function of both muscles and nerves. Inositol has been found to be very low in the cerebrospinal fluid of depressed patients and it also helps the function of the neurotransmitter serotonin, low levels of which have been found to cause depression.

In nature many foods including nuts, beans, cantaloupe, seeds, whole grains, and especially citrus fruits contain a substance known as phytic acid which, when ingested, is acted upon by the bacteria in human intestines and converted to inositol. Americans ingest about 1,000 mg or 1 gram of inositol daily in our diets, once again depending on your intake of the above named foods.

Inositol has been found to be useful in the treatment of anxiety disorders, depression, premenstrual syndrome (PMS), polycystic ovarian syndrome, and even bipolar disorder. It has also been shown to help reduce high blood pressure and high triglycerides.

For anxiety, panic attacks, and depression the dose is 4 grams three times a day. There are no reported side effects from using inositol, but as with most treatments there are no studies in pregnant or breast feeding women, so as a general rule they should not be given inositol.

SAMe (S-adenosylmethionine)

SAMe is made in the body from an amino acid named methionine and its interaction with ATP, or adenosine troposphere. ATP is produced by the cells' mitochondria and is used by the cells for energy production. SAMe seems to work in the body by donating a methyl group after which it is converted to a compound known as S-adenosyl- homocysteine.

It has been reported to work for depression and also for osteoarthritis, which is the most common type of arthritis. In depression it has been shown to elevate the levels of the neurotransmitters dopamine and serotonin. The metabolism of SAMe requires the B vitamins B6, B12, and folic acid, so it is best to take a 50 mg B complex to provide those vitamins.

Studies have shown SAMe to be equal or greater than prescription strength drugs for depression. It has not been shown to be helpful in bipolar disorder.

The dose of SAMe is 200 mg twice daily on an empty stomach (take the enteric-coated form so it will not upset your stomach). If after several weeks you do not see enough improvement you can then increase the dose to 400 mg and you can go up to three times a day.

CHAPTER THIRTY-FIVE

DIABETES

INTRODUCTION

TABLE OF CONTENTS:

Diabetes is one of those chronic diseases whose prevalence is sky-rocketing due to the perfect storm of the standard American diet (SAD) which includes approximately 150 lbs. of sugar annually and a very sedentary lifestyle which comprises of many hours a day either on computers, video games or television. The age of the onset of diabetes has also dropped dramatically in the last several decades to the point where it is not uncommon to find school age children who are diabetic. The pharmaceutical industry has responded with a never ending array of new and improved medications to treat diabetes which is never a bad thing, however our focus is trained on finding natural/alternative ways to combat this scourge.

Let's take a look at some wonderful alternatives to traditional diabetic treatments, but first let me teach you all about diabetes so you understand what you are dealing with.

TYPES OF DIABETES

For our purposes there are basically two types of diabetes, cleverly named Type 1 and Type 2. Type 1 is genetic and strikes younger patients, in whom there is a lack of insulin production by their pancreas. These patients usually have a thin build. Type 2 diabetics are the majority of diabetics and this type is not the result of a lack of insulin but rather is due to insulin resistance. This usually comes on as we age but recently due to our poor diets this is appearing in grammar school age children. Many Type 2 diabetics eventually burn out their pancreases and do require insulin. How this comes about is due to chronically high levels of insulin in our blood as a consequence of eating large amounts of carbohydrates, which trigger insulin production in order to drive this high glucose into our cells.

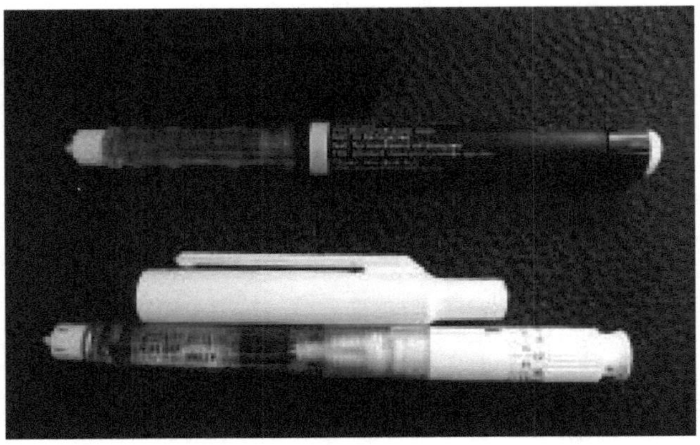

Insulin "Pens"

This chronically high level of insulin promotes the production of new fat and protects your old fat. Don't forget that insulin has two purposes, control of blood glucose and storage of excess carbohydrate calories as fat. That is why I describe insulin to my patients as a fat storage hormone. Once you understand the physiology of how this works then it immediately becomes clear to you that obesity is not a dietary fat problem, but is caused by dietary carbohydrates. Americas collective forty-plus year war on fat in our diets has skewed them towards carbohydrates (sugars) and salt for flavor. As you can see by looking around you, we have lost this war miserably; Americans are considerably more obese now than forty years ago.

Our standard American diet (appropriately called SAD) is now so heavily laden with starchy carbohydrates like bread, pasta, potatoes, and rice, as well as simple carbohydrates like sugars, candies, and high fructose corn syrup, that it results in the almost continuous need for insulin release in order to process all this sugar. Collectively as Americans, our sugar ingestion has skyrocketed one hundredfold in the last century. This is unprecedented in human history and our bodies are not designed to process all of this sugar, so much of it is converted to fat, hence our obesity epidemic.

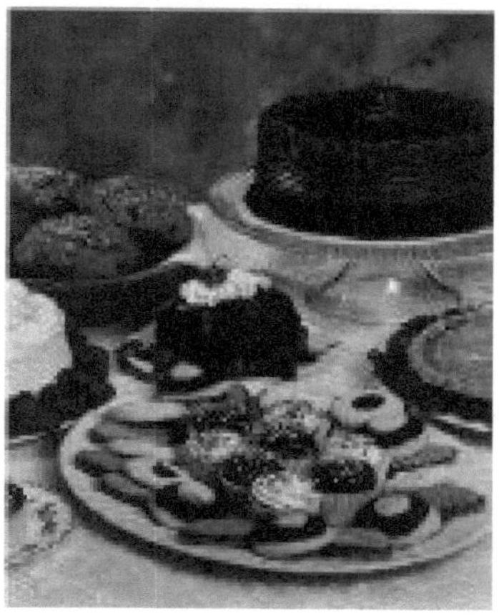

If you look at the Paleolithic (cave man) diet, you will see how low it is in carbohydrates, high in proteins and fat when they could get them. It primarily was plant based, augmented by meat and fish from game or shellfish when they were able to get some. The plants especially the fruits did have sugars, but these were packaged with lots of fiber and phytonutrients (nutrients that originated from plants) and thus were released slowly into the blood, thus avoiding the spikes in insulin that our modern diets have. The Paleo diet is extremely healthy for us, and is one that I would strongly suggest you adopt if you are looking to lose weight and also to get healthier.

Any bones found of cave men that have been carefully examined showed little or no tooth decay and the ones lucky enough to reach an old age showed little signs of the chronic diseases that ravage we "modern" men.

There are other types of diabetes such as gestational diabetes, which develops when a woman is pregnant, most likely in a woman who is already on the brink of diabetes herself in whom it is "unmasked" by the pregnancy. Most patients with gestational diabetes will revert to normal after their deliveries, but 20 to 50 percent of them will go on to becoming Type 2 diabetics.

Here is a little background information on fasting blood glucose levels and what they mean clinically:

Normal is a fasting blood glucose of 99 mg/dl or less.

Prediabetic is a fasting blood glucose between 100 mg/dl and 125.

Diabetic range is 126 mg/dl and above.

Progress is not a bad thing; in Roman times physicians would taste the urine of their patients to diagnose diabetes. Those with sweet urine were diagnosed with diabetes mellitus (which means honey-like in Latin). Boy, it sucked to be a physician in Roman times. Even Obamacare has not stooped that low yet; although they might, given their propensity toward torturing physicians with every kind of harebrained idea they can dream up. But alas I digress, let's get back to diabetes.

SYMPTOMS OF POOR DIABETIC CONTROL

The vast majority of diabetic patients will have a "blood sugar reaction" at one time or another, and most will have many occurrences The most common reaction is one of hypoglycemia (low blood sugar -- in medicine any hypo prefix means low and any hyper prefix means fast or high) which includes the following light- headedness, vertigo (dizziness), headache, nausea, diaphoresis (sweating), and palpitations (you feel your heart pounding).

Hypoglycemia is easy to diagnose if you have a glucometer to measure your blood glucose (sugar) level. Hypoglycemia is a blood glucose level of less than 70 mg/dl. If you don't have a glucometer handy the only way you can tell you are hypoglycemic is to quickly eat something sweet or take a teaspoonful of honey or sugar and see if within five minutes you feel relief of your symptoms.

Hyperglycemia or high blood glucose usually is not symptomatic and when it is the symptoms are mild such as frequent urination and increased thirst. Blood glucose levels that qualify as hyperglycemic are usually greater than 200 mg/dl.

NUTRACEUTICALS USEFUL IN THE TREATMENT OF DIABETES

Chromium

Chromium is so useful in controlling diabetes that it is often referred to as Glucose Tolerance Factor. It is a mineral and is considered an essential trace element. It helps the body process sugar better and therefore helps treat diabetes. The mineral chromium works by activating the enzyme tyrosine kinase which helps insulin attach to the insulin receptors found on the surface of cells. The insulin thus activated can do its job and allow glucose to enter the cell, thus lowering its level in the blood. This keeps insulin functioning well and in turn blood glucose is controlled and insulin levels are low, preventing the development of insulin resistance which is the hallmark of Type 2 diabetes.

The dose of chromium is 1,000 mcg a day but some experts recommend up to three or four thousand micrograms daily, for those patients who are difficult to control. It is inexpensive, so get a good supply of it if you are diabetic or there are diabetics in your family. It is also found in brewer's yeast and liver. Beer also has chromium but the other carbohydrates in it will be counterproductive to your quest for control of your blood sugar.

Cinnamon

The spice cinnamon contains phytochemicals (chemical made by plants) that vastly increase the metabolism of glucose by the body. It does this by mimicking the function of insulin and fooling the human body. It has no significant side effects and is inexpensive. In addition to which, it also helps lower total cholesterol levels, bad LDL cholesterol, and triglycerides. It has been touted to lower blood glucose from 18 to 29 percent. It also lowers blood pressure and insulin levels, both of which are very good things.

The dose of cinnamon varies in different studies. Some patients take it by capsule and some by making a tea with it. The tea can be made by mixing three tablespoons of cinnamon with one half to one teaspoon of baking soda in a quart of boiling water and place it in a jar (32 ounce), let it steep and then strain it through a cheesecloth or other filter. You can drink it cooled or hot, drink 8 ounces two or three times daily.

You can also take cinnamon in capsule form; take 500 mg twice daily. Other studies show up to 6 grams a day. Remember a gram is a thousand milligrams. The most potent form of cinnamon is called cassia cinnamon also known as Chinese cinnamon; this is easy to find and no different in cost. The studies on cinnamon were done on this type so I would recommend this kind over the others.

Enzyme Therapy

The use of the three digestive enzymes, proteases, lipases, and amylases, have been shown to be beneficial in diabetes due to poor digestive enzyme production by the pancreas in diabetics. These are to be taken with meals to aid in digestion of foods. There are two prescription brands currently on the market named Creon and Zenpep, both of which are excellent for this purpose. You can also purchase these in nonprescription strength. There are other enzymes involved in the metabolism of carbohydrates, especially starches that can also be utilized to prevent their breakdown into glucose, see transglucosidase below.

MAGNESIUM

Magnesium is an essential mineral for human health and contributes to glucose control in diabetics via some of the 300 enzyme systems that are dependent upon magnesium for their activation.

Magnesium helps lower blood glucose levels and also is involved in glycolysis, which is the breakdown primarily by muscles of glucose to lactic acid. It is not clear which came first the magnesium deficiency or the insulin resistance, but diabetes causes increased urinary loss of magnesium, only worsening one's blood glucose control. As I have stated many times in this book, magnesium is the most important mineral you can take due to those 300 enzyme systems that require it to function properly. Magnesium is sometimes called the "Spark of Life" due to its multiple functions in the body and its indispensability for life.

The dose of magnesium ranges from 300 mg to 1,000 mg of magnesium daily. If you also have high blood pressure or migraine headaches or are prone to muscle cramping I would take the higher dose range. Magnesium will also help constipation, palpitations, cardiac arrhythmias, insomnia, restless leg syndrome, and any muscle sprains.

I have also found it useful in ADD and ADHD where it seems to have a calming effect on the brain similar to its calming effect on the heart helping to quench cardiac rhythm disturbances.

Fish Oil Or Omega-3 Fatty Acids

The omega-3 fatty acids in fish oil are what is known as essential fatty acids. Essential means that they cannot be produced by the human body from scratch from other fats or raw material and must be obtained in your food. In our diets we get omega-3 fatty acids from fish oil from cold-water fish, nuts, vegetable oils, flaxseed and flaxseed oil, and many other green leafy vegetables. Since they are so useful for multiple problems you should insure that they are included in your medicinal garden so they make their way into your diet. It is always best to get any nutrient directly from your diet as opposed to a pill or other concentrated forms, because in nature there is the totality of what you need provided by each plant in its most beneficial form that our bodies immediately recognize as food.

There are three main types of omega-3 fatty acids:

DHA or Docosahexaenoic acid, found in fish thus is known as a marine omega-3.

EPA or Eicosapentaenoic acid, also found in fish and is the other marine omega-3.

ALA or Alpha-linolenic acid is from land-based sources like plants, seeds, walnuts, vegetable oils, flaxseed, and animal fat from animals that have been grazed on open ranges. ALA is also found in legumes like kidney and pinto beans. Since the American diet is comprised mostly of these foods, ALA is the primary omega-3 eaten by Americans.

Omega-3 fatty acids originate in two places in the food chain. In the world's oceans omega-3 fatty acids come from marine algae and on land from various plants. In the oceans the marine algae are eaten by shellfish and cold-water fish such as herring, sardines, anchovies, mackerel, and salmon and consequently are concentrated in the fat of these fish. On land, animals eat these plants by grazing such as "free-range" and "grass fed" beef. They are more nutritious due to these omega-3 fatty acids and also other phytonutrients, minerals, and trace elements from the soil; they also taste a hell of a lot better! Farm-raised fish have no omega-3 fatty acids because they are not eating algae but are fed fish food that is processed.

They are also dosed with large amounts of antibiotics and are exposed to many toxins that they unfortunately concentrate into their fat. Avoid farm raised fish at all costs.

That being said, I was reading Scientific American recently and there were some intriguing methods of fish farming that might come about in the near future, where a boat has a very large, deep net that allows algae and other smaller members of the ocean's food chain to enter to feed the fish. These nets can be transported to any area desired. Not a bad idea, but I do not believe it is currently being utilized except in small experiments.

Fish oil, like magnesium, is so very essential for maintaining good health. One of the prime reasons for that is fish oil's effect on the cell membrane. The cell membrane is the wall around each cell that has receptors imbedded in it that are specific for hundreds of different molecules. The cell wall is made up primarily of fats and nothing is better for those fats than omega-3 fatty acids or fish oil. Fish oil makes the cell wall function better and hence substances like insulin will find the cell wall more receptive and therefore it will be able to drive glucose right through that cell wall into the cell, lowering its level in the blood and helping improve patients' diabetes.

Fish oil also helps the heart and blood pressure by its calming effect on the cardiac (heart) cells, preventing them from becoming irritated and producing abnormal heart rhythms that could be potentially fatal. They also help keep the blood vessel walls pliant and flexible, helping to lower blood pressure, lower the heart rate (pulse) and lower triglycerides (bad fats). Fish oil also seems to have a calming effect on inflammation all over the body, including joints, helping arthritic complaints. In my more than twenty-five years in clinical practice many patients have reported improvements in their arthritis while taking fish oils. Fish oils have also been shown to help lower cancer rates and help improve moods in chronically depressed patients.

The dose of fish oil is between 1 and 4 grams a day. If you also have arthritis, fibromyalgia, depression, or ADHD in addition to your diabetes, then I would take the 4 grams a day. If you can afford it buy the best fish oil you can get so hopefully it will contain less mercury and other toxins. Also, eat as much fish as you can; it is very healthy for you, but you will be hard-pressed to eat enough fish to provide all the omega-3s your body could use. I always advise my patients to take their fish oil before a meal, eat on top of it to prevent the burping up of any fishy smell. Also, if this remains a problem then take the fish oil in divided doses over the course of the day.

Since fish oils are polyunsaturated fatty acids they can oxidize and become rancid, so store them in a cool, dark spot and if you can, buy fish oil combined with vitamin E which will give it a longer shelf life.

Krill Oil

I am not sure if krill oil can replace fish oil, and if it does, does it do so on a one-to-one exchange? I am not sure, and from what I can research it appears no one else is quite sure either. But, it does seem as if the two are interchangeable, the good news with krill oil is the smaller size of the capsules, so if swallowing a large fish oil capsule is problematic for you then go with the krill oil. Krill oil has a different mix of omega-3 fatty acids than fish oil as well as containing the very powerful antioxidant astaxanthin which also helps boost your immune system. Astaxanthin has been proven to be 6,000 times more powerful than vitamin C in its role as an antioxidant.

Alpha Lipoic Acid (ALA)

ALA is a very potent antioxidant and very useful in diabetes. Unfortunately both the land-based omega-3 fatty acid alpha-linolenic acid and alpha lipoic acid, have been abbreviated ALA by some authors, only adding to peoples' confusion. ALA is able to penetrate everywhere in the human body due to its versatile fat and water solubility, and is present in every cell in the body; this speaks volumes as to its importance for human health. Its primary role is as an antioxidant. As such it works to attack free radicals that are produced by the body's conversion of foods into energy. The other major antioxidants vitamins, A, C, and E are either fat or water soluble, ALA is so much more versatile than those others due to its dual solubility.

ALA both improves the body's sensitivity to insulin and also helps treat diabetic neuropathy (nerve damage caused by poor control of diabetes) which is found in up to a quarter of diabetics. Diabetic neuropathy causes burning and pain and ultimately numbness and loss of sensation in the feet and hands of diabetics. Diabetic neuropathy is very debilitating and is the cause of endless problems for diabetics.

In the aftermath of Chernobyl the Russians treated radiation poisoning successfully with a combination of ALA and vitamin E. The daily dose is between 300 and 1200 mg daily. Remember this is the only substance in the human body that is both fat and water soluble, so it crosses the cell membranes as well as the blood-brain barrier.

You can take it on an empty stomach or with food, but I would recommend taking it with food. Since it is so important to your health ALA is made by your body, but supplementing it to treat specific conditions like diabetes will assist your body by raising your natural levels.

Foods that contain some ALA are of little help because the ALA in foods is bound to the amino acid lysine and your body does not have the enzymes capable of breaking that bond and using the ALA. Supplements containing ALA are best when they are not protein-bound and thus in free form and available to your body.

Alpha lipoid acid is also the keystone antioxidant in the antioxidant cascade. What is the antioxidant cascade, you ask? The antioxidant cascade is how the body's antioxidants renew and regenerate one another. ALA is at the top since it is both fat and water soluble. It helps regenerate both legs of the cascade. On the water soluble side is glutathione and vitamin C which help regenerate one another, and on the fat soluble side there is vitamin E and CoQ10 which regenerate each other. Keeping this cascade in mind, the easiest way to boost your immune system and supercharge it is by supplementing the members of this antioxidant cascade, by taking vitamin C, vitamin E, ALA, and CoQ10. Most forms of glutathione are rapidly removed from your circulation by your liver and therefore cannot be supplemented; however nothing raises glutathione levels better than ALA. What this means is that ALA in a free form (unbound to a protein) is able to circulate everywhere in your body; as it does so it constantly is recharging and reenergizing the other antioxidants in this cascade revitalizing them and sending them back into action to neutralize free radicals and prevent disease as well as aging!

Vanadium

Vanadium is an essential trace element that has the effect of mimicking insulin and therefore lowers blood glucose levels. It is found in black pepper, dill seed, unsaturated vegetable oils, and grains. The daily dose is between 5 and 20 mg daily.

Zinc

Zinc is an essential mineral for glucose metabolism. Zinc is essential for the normal production of insulin, as well as having hundreds of other enzymes that require it for their activation. It is especially helpful with boosting your immune system, hence all the zinc-containing products for colds, etc.

Zinc is also essential for proper wound healing and for that reason is critical for recovering surgical patients or anyone wounded. I have also found zinc very useful in my practice for patients suffering from oral canker sores which are known medically as apthous ulcers and apthous stomatitis; holding zinc lozenges directly over them in your mouth several times a day will heal them rapidly. I had dinner one evening with a prominent local endocrinologist. Being the nerds that we are, our conversation hit upon apthous ulcers and their treatment. He lamented to me that he has suffered with them his entire life and has been to specialists in London, New York, and Boston, but no one was able to cure his "incurable" apthous ulcers. I explained how I have cured them for years almost without exception with simply using zinc lozenges. I could tell he was listening to me but not believing me and was just being polite, so I sent him a box of lozenges with a note on how to use them. About a month later he called me at my office, absolutely astonished that his apthous ulcers had come back as they usually did and he had used the zinc lozenges and in twenty- four hours they were gone! Hey, even a broken clock is right twice a day!

The dose of zinc is 25 to 50 mg daily, which will require supplementation with 1 mg of copper to prevent copper deficiency. The copper is only needed in long-term use of zinc, if you are taking it for a cold, wound healing, and apthous ulcers, you will not need to supplement with copper.

Coenzyme Q10

CoQ10 is also known as ubiquinone, due to its ubiquitous nature, meaning it is everywhere (in every cell) of the human body just like alpha lipoic acid. This speaks volumes to its clinical importance for good overall health; whenever the body has a substance in every cell you know it is not by accident. Coenzymes are thus named because they assist enzymes in their biochemical functions. CoQ10 helps the metabolic chain reaction that creates energy within the body's cells. For this reason it is heavily concentrated in cells that require energy like the heart and muscles. Statin drugs that are used for the treatment of high cholesterol levels block the body's natural production of CoQ10, and thus adversely affects those cells that require it, causing muscle aches and ultimately if not supplemented, will affect your heart. In diabetes it is essential along with vitamin E and zinc in the production of insulin.

The dose I would recommend is between 100 and 200 mg daily. This has to be taken with a fatty meal since it is fat soluble and will not be absorbed if taken without fat.

Amino Acids

Amino acids are the building blocks of proteins. Proteins are nothing more than a long chain of amino acids strung together. There are approximately 40,000 different proteins that your body has to make in order to function properly; these include enzymes, hormones, and neurotransmitters. A hormone like insulin contains fifty-one different amino acids, therefore the need for proper protein or amino acid intake to supply all these amino acids just for this one hormone becomes readily evident.

There is no dose for this; you will need to find a good source of amino acids in a powdered supplement form. There are many kinds on the internet so for many folks price will be the determining factor.

Another option to provide your amino acids is eating two eggs a day (free-range) should supply at least all the essential amino acids, or eating the "three sisters"; squash, corn (maize), and climbing beans that Native Americans ate will also provide all the essential amino acids. Remember that essential amino acids means that the body cannot produce them, therefore they need to be supplied in your diet. There are nine essential amino acids: histidine, isoleucine, leucine, lysine, methionine, phenylalanine, threonine, tryptophan, and valine.

Maintaining a good protein supply is essential for your nutrition, especially if you have children. Growing children need all the essential amino acids, essential fatty acids, vitamins, minerals, and trace elements along with adequate sun exposure, exercise, and clean, fresh water to grow properly and to be healthy and vigorous.

It is exceedingly difficult and probably impossible to get all the minerals and trace elements you need in your diet, hence the need to supplement with a broad spectrum mineral and trace element drink. My personal favorite is one that also contains fulvic acid. Fulvic acid is wonderful for your body and to maintain health. Fulvic acid is produced in the soil by soil microorganisms as they convert inorganic minerals into organic forms that our body can more easily assimilate. Fulvic acid increases the permeability of the cell wall, allowing these vital minerals and trace elements entry into the cell.

Remember, all disease is due to cellular dysfunction; the name of the disease changes according to the tissues or organs where the cells are located. In order to function properly all cells need proper nutrition, pH, and adequate hydration. In addition, all cells need the proper terrain to be healthy. You see, cells are not as connected to one another as we sometimes think, upon closer examination they are imbedded in an extracellular (means outside the cell) matrix.

Without a healthy extracellular matrix there can be no intracellular (inside the cell) health; that is why pH, hydration, and proper nutrition are so critical.

You should also make sure that your medicinal seed vault has several varieties of each of the three sisters (squash, corn, and beans) along with many other vegetable varieties. This is an indirect way of providing your diet with all the essential amino acids that it cannot make on its own. Remember to buy open-pollinated heirloom varieties that you can save the seeds from for the next growing season. The non-heirloom or hybrid varieties will not give you viable seed.

The art of seed saving and germination, along with plant propagation (reproduction of plants by a variety of means) as well as grafting should be a skill that we all have and if possible we should teach this to our children so that they can develop an appreciation of nature and food as our medicine.

I strongly advise all my readers to familiarize themselves with the principles and practice of permaculture. Permaculture means permanent agriculture. It is a very useful skill to have for unbelievable food yields from small parcels of land. Typically there will be standard-sized fruit or nut trees in a row with shorter medium-sized fruit trees in front of them, and a third row of dwarf fruit trees.

The second row will have large berry or fruit bearing shrubs, followed by a row of medium and then small-sized shrubs. Under all the trees will be edible ground cover like strawberries, so every space available is planted with plants that either produce fruit, nuts, berries, or vegetables. To provide meat and fish you can construct a chicken coop with spaces between the floor boards with a fish pond below the coop. The chickens lay eggs and provide meat for you and their droppings feed the fish below, the water from the fish pond is used to flood an adjacent rice paddy where the fish droppings along with the water provides nutrients to grow the rice. The rice filters the water and removes the impurities and the sunshine's ultraviolet light helps clean the water as well…by the time the water exits the rice paddy it is potable (good to drink). This is an amazing system where on just a few acres you can produce enough fruit, vegetables, meat, and fish to not only live, but to earn a living as well. A permaculture system is done organically and provides fresh wholesome food, once the system is properly established it becomes an almost self-sustaining system.

Even if you are living in a suburban environment without acres of land to plant, you can plant edible plants on your property such as berry and fruit trees or even nut trees, any grass converted to gardens is one step closer to nature and healing our planet. You can also go vertical by planting stacked gardens.

One method I have done is to take large PVC tubing and cap both ends and drill large holes along the length of it, fill it up with potting soil and place strawberries or small vegetables in the holes and stack these next to each other, this allows you to go vertical and utilize space that previously was unavailable for food production. On YouTube there are videos of people draining their swimming pools and making them into gardens, great ideas for maximum food production.

I apologize for the digression, however there are some health practices that are essential and growing your own food organically is one of the most important things you can do for your health.

Vitamin E

Vitamin E along with Coenzyme Q10 has been shown to stimulate the production of insulin and hence help the control of diabetes. It also has other beneficial effects in diabetes by its anticlotting effect. This helps prevent the vascular complications of diabetes that affect many patients' eyes and kidneys. Vitamin E supplementation has lowered the insulin requirements of many diabetics.

The dose of vitamin E is 400 international units once daily with a fatty meal, since it is fat soluble and you will not absorb it without ingesting it with fats.

Vitamin E is composed of approximately ten lipid soluble (which means the same thing as fat soluble) compounds of which the tocopherols and the tocotrienols are the main components. Among the different types of vitamin E, the most common are the alpha and the gamma tocopherols. The alpha is more common in European diets due to the preponderance of olive and sunflower oils in their diet. The American diet by contrast is dominated by gamma tocopherols due to the abundance of soybean and corn oils in our diet.

Since vitamin E is fat soluble you will only find it in foods that contain fat like butter, vegetable oils, seeds, margarine, olives, olive oil, avocados, nuts, and nut butters. Sunflower seeds contain higher amounts of vitamin E than any other food; greens such as collard greens and spinach also are high in vitamin E. Sunflowers are very easy to grow and if you select the right giant-headed varieties they will produce a large, pie-sized head jam-packed with nutritious seeds as a reward for your efforts. Buy yourself a large quantity of these inexpensive seeds and keep them in your medicinal seed vault. Sunflower seeds are full of vitamin E, many minerals and fiber as well as containing phytosterols.

Phytosterols are compounds that are similar in structure to cholesterol but work in our bodies to lower cholesterol levels, enhance immunity, and lower our risks for cancer. Not too shabby from the seed of a plant that grows like a weed, requiring no fertilization or pesticides to thrive, only full sun.

As I mentioned earlier, the Russians used high dose vitamin E along with alpha lipoic acid to successfully treat radiation poisoning. Something to keep in mind with the Fukushima reactor number 4 still being so unstable; a critical meltdown or explosion of that reactor could contaminate the entire northern hemisphere of Earth making it uninhabitable for thousands of years, yet the world's politicians and the useless United Nations do nothing.

Fenugreek (Trigonella Foenum Graecum)

Fenugreek is an annual plant whose seeds are used in various countries' cuisines all over the world. Fenugreek seeds or defatted fenugreek seed powder can be used in the treatment of diabetes. It has been shown to lower blood glucose levels.

The dose for Type 2 diabetics is between 15 and 50 grams a day, depending on the severity of your diabetes. Fenugreek seeds can be bought for your medicinal garden and the plant is easily grown even under arid (dry) conditions.

Gymnasia (gymnema sylvestre)

This is an Ayurveda herb that has been used for centuries in India for diabetes. Gymnema Sylvestre is an herb found in the tropical forests of India and Sri Lanka. Traditionally in Ayurveda medicine, the leaves of this plant have been chewed to lower the sensation of sweetness. It has been reported to have beneficial effects in both Type 1 and Type 2 diabetes; the mechanism by which it works is by raising insulin levels and thus lowering blood sugar or glucose levels. The sensation of blocking the taste of sweetness in the mouth is thought to be secondary to blocking of sugar receptors on the tongue.

The dose is 400 mg daily for either type of diabetes.

Huereque

This is a plant-derived compound from the root of the Mexican cactus of the same name.

Huereque is very effective at lowering blood sugar. It will last for approximately six months and then you need to go off it a month and restart the cycle again, that works to reset the tolerance that invariably develops. Tolerance means your body gets used to it and it no longer is effective.

The usual dose is approximately 1200 mg daily, taken in three divided doses. Capsules come in various strengths and are readily available online some being 200 mg others being an odd 590 mg, which is close enough to 600 to just take two daily.

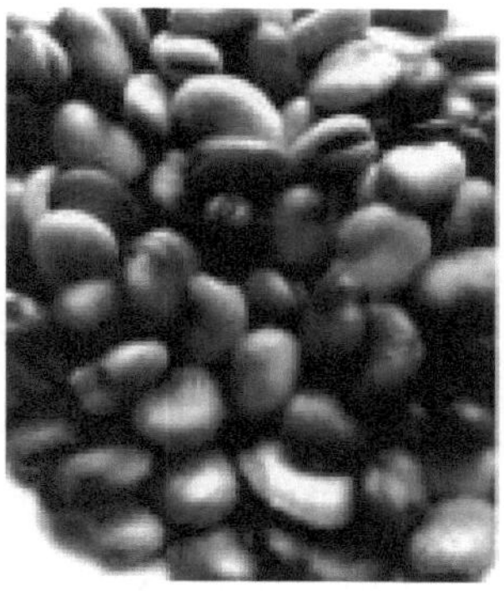

Legumes (Beans)

Beans, if eaten with every meal, will slow the absorption of glucose into the blood stream and eliminate the spikes in glucose that many diabetics suffer with. The effect supposedly will last through the next meal as well. I would recommend beans with every meal if you have them available. They are also very easy to grow in your organic garden. Beans are also an excellent source of soluble fiber, protein, and is one of the "three sisters" utilized by Native Americans.

One cup of cooked beans provides between 9 and 13 grams of soluble fiber. Beans are also very high in protein, complex carbohydrates, iron, and folate. Folate is one of the B vitamins sometimes known as B9. Folic acid is just the synthetic form of folate. Folate along with vitamin B 12 is necessary for DNA replication and many other bodily processes.

Beans also come in hundreds of varieties and flavors and are fun to grow. I would seriously recommend keeping a large supply of beans of various varieties that you can grow out and save from season to season. If stored properly the seeds last for many years. I would go online and buy a number of different varieties Try a source like the Seed Savers Exchange for wonderful heirloom varieties that are open-pollinated.

Other than some wicked gas they are well tolerated and very good for you, as well as being an inexpensive protein source. The reason why beans are so gas producing is because they contain a type of oligosaccharide or sugar compound (which is also found in cabbage). The human body does not make the enzyme necessary to digest these sugars hence the job falls upon the intestinal bacteria of the colon, or large intestine. These bacteria break down the oligosaccharides into gases, two of which are methane and hydrogen, which as every high school boy knows are flammable and can be ignited! Contrary to popular opinion, methane is not the odor-causing component of your flatulence (farts), the odiferous component comes from volatile sulfur compounds (VSCs).

Many cultures, especially in Africa, prepare their bean dishes by fermentation; the yeasts that produce the fermentation also digest these oligosaccharides and thus there is no flatulence with fermented beans. Enough of this; you have just learned more than you ever wanted to know about beans and farting.

Beans are a summer crop that needs warm weather and about two months' time to fully mature and be ready to harvest. As the bean pods mature they turn yellow and dry up and the beans inside turn from green to their final mature color, many of which are multiple colors when dried. Many bean plants are vines and will need cages or trellises to support them, the Native Americans used corn plants to support the bean vines and this worked very well with squash plants to shade the base of both. Shading of the bean and corn plants greatly reduced their water loss and reduced the amount of water needed to irrigate these "Three Sisters".

You should be aware that some kinds of raw beans, especially red and kidney beans, contain an odor-free, tasteless toxin that can only be removed by boiling the beans for ten minutes.

Fiber (Roughage)

Fiber is important to eat with every meal. Our present diets are very low in plant fiber, which is indigestible and helps slow the release of glucose into your blood, helping diabetes. That is why the sugar in fruits with its associated fiber content is not a problem for diabetics, but fruit juice which has no fiber is a major problem. Fruit juice just pours sugar into your blood and spikes your blood glucose levels, leading to an insulin surge, which starts the whole negative cascade of fat protection and new fat production all over again.

Eating a diet primarily composed of plants and plant products will provide more than enough fiber in our new diets.

There should be meat from fish, game, and from farm raised poultry and animals, but the rest of our diets will be eggs, fruit, nuts, roots, and vegetables of all kinds. In fact, it most likely will be a healthier diet than our present standard American diet which is lacking in fiber, vitamins, minerals, and trace elements.

You should become well acquainted with edible wild plants that you can forage for in your area. There are several books in the bibliography that are excellent sources of information for foraging. One of my personal favorites is *Nature's Garden* by Samuel Thayer.

Fiber is basically the indigestible part of the plants that we eat. Fiber comes in two types, soluble and insoluble. Soluble fiber is named after the fact that it dissolves in water or is soluble in water. In the colon, fiber is fermented into gases as well as various other biologically active compounds; soluble fiber slows the passage of food through the intestines. Soluble fiber also acts as a prebiotic or food for probiotics or good intestinal bacteria. Insoluble fiber does not dissolve in water and acts like a sponge in the GI tract by drawing in water and thereby softening the stool and allowing for easier passage.

Food sources for soluble fiber include beans, oats, rye, barley, plums, prunes, avocados, berries of all types, broccoli, carrots, and Jerusalem artichokes (a perennial native American sunflower; the root forms a tuber that is very healthy for you, containing inulin which helps lowers blood glucose levels) flax seed, psyllium seed husks, and nuts (especially almonds).

Food sources for insoluble fiber include whole grains, wheat and corn bran, nuts, seeds, legumes, potato skins, green beans, cauliflower, celery, avocado and unripe bananas, the skins of kiwi, grapes, and tomatoes.

Vitamin B Complex And Vitamin C

B complex is all the B vitamins together; the reason you take them all is that we ultimately will need them all. There are several B vitamins that are essential for adequate diabetic glucose control. One of the most important is niacin or vitamin B3 and another is biotin; both of which are in B complex and help control glucose levels as well as insulin resistance. Niacin works synergistically with chromium, the two being much more powerful together than either alone. B6 is also involved in good glucose control. Vitamin C has been shown to help reduce insulin requirements. It also prevents vascular complications of diabetes; however the mechanism of action (how it actually works) is currently unknown. These vitamins are inexpensive and should be well stocked in your medicine chest.

Vitamin C is a valuable antioxidant and supports many bodily functions including the immune system; it also acts as an antihistamine. There are several wonderful books on vitamin C listed in the bibliography.

Berberine

Berberine is a plant alkaloid found in the roots of goldenseal, barberry and Oregon grape. It is known for its potent antimicrobial (it acts as an antibiotic, killing germs) effects, but it is also a very potent medication used in the treatment of diabetes. Studies have shown it to be comparable in strength to Metformin which is the most popular pharmaceutical for diabetes, and is very effective. Metformin also has the ability to lower cancer rates but the mechanism is currently unknown.

Berberine has virtually no side effects and lowers hemoglobin A1C, fasting and postprandial (after meals) glucose levels identically to Metformin, but is better than Metformin in lowering cholesterol and triglyceride levels. Berberine also lowered insulin resistance by a whopping 45 percent.

The best dose is 500 mg tid (three times a day). If you are diabetic, now is the time to load up on a large quantity of this nutraceutical. Of all the plant-derived and natural medicines this one seems to be the most potent in the treatment of diabetes. Goldenseal and Oregon grape are both easy to grow in your garden and should be planted now if you are diabetic or there are any diabetics in your family, this will provide you with your own source of this wonderful nutraceutical.

Berberine also comes from the barberry plant, which is very common in the United States, having become an invasive bush that is covered in small red berries that are full of vitamin C as well as its roots, which contain berberine. If you have any woodland on your property in the northeastern United States there is a very good chance you have some wild barberry plants growing there; be careful, they are covered with sharp thorns.

I just would like to touch upon the role of berberine as a natural antibiotic, which has been used in both traditional Chinese medicine and Ayurveda medicine for over 2,500 years! Berberine is very potent against bacteria, fungi, and viral infections. The viral part is very significant since man-made antibiotics do not have any effect upon viral infections. Berberine has also been found to be effective against super bugs, like MRSA (Methicillin Resistant Staphylococcus Aureus), which are very resistant to most present day antibiotics.

Berberine comes as capsules, liquid, and tablets The dose as an antibiotic is much lower than the dose for diabetes or for lowering cholesterol which is 500 mg tid, as an antibiotic 400 mg per day works just fine.

One of the only side effects is constipation which can easily be remedied by lowering the dose. Berberine also works to lower total cholesterol, LDL cholesterol, and triglycerides; it also raises good HDL cholesterol. That being said, I am not so convinced of the horrors of high cholesterol levels, the original studies were quite flawed and sometimes the cure is worse than the condition, but that is for another book.

Syntra5

Syntra5 is an all-natural herbal mix that was formulated to treat diabetes. It also lowers both triglyceride and cholesterol levels. It is a proprietary (company secret) blend of the following nutrients: chromium,

Vitamin C, biotin, vanadium, hydroxycitric acid (the active ingredient in Garcinia cambogia), Gymnema sylvestre extract, bitter melon extract, cinnamon extract, banaba extract and fenugreek. It is very effective and is also a little pricey, but it does work well and should be considered for those with poorly controlled diabetes. It can be found online.

Transglucosidase Enzyme

The transglucosidase enzyme works to block the breakdown of starches into glucoses. Starches are the way plants store their excess glucose, by producing starches which are hydrophobic (repel water), which solves a storage problem for plants. If they stored glucose in cells without converting it to starch, it would absorb water, swell and explode the cells. Hence, the production of starch by plants which cannot absorb water, which therefore keeps the plant light and not waterlogged and weighed down. In animals and humans the excess glucose is at first stored as glycogen, ultimately most of which is converted to fat for long- term storage. Insulin is the primary hormone controlling this process. This is the reason that carbohydrates in your diet make you fat; they raise insulin, plain and simple.

By blocking the breakdown of dietary starches such as bread, pasta, potatoes, rice, and cassava to glucoses this makes them unavailable for absorption by your body, which lowers your blood glucose levels and better controls your diabetes.

The dose is one capsule with each starchy meal. It is currently available through Life Extension Foundation as Glycemic Pro, and can be found on line at their website. By the way, they are an excellent source of quality vitamins and nutraceuticals and have been on the forefront of nutritional research for decades, often bringing both ideas and products to market long before anyone else. They also make another enzyme-blocking agent for diabetics called Triple Shield, which I also recommend.

Bitter Melon (Momordica Charantia)

Bitter melon is also known as bitter gourd, bitter squash, and African cucumber. Bitter melon is a tropical vine that is in the same family as watermelon, cucumbers, cantaloupes, pumpkins, squash, and zucchini and is widely grown in Asia, Africa, and the Caribbean for its fruit. It is a very ugly, long wart-covered green fruit sort of looking like a skinny wart-covered cucumber. The fruit is most often eaten while green or just slightly yellow, at which point it has a crunchy consistency similar to a green pepper, but bitter in taste. It can be grown in North America where it flowers during the summer months of June and July but fruits later in the fall from September through November. If kept on the vine, the fruit will turn orange and soft and will split open, revealing seeds draped in a bright red pulp.

NOTE; Bitter melon should not ever be given to pregnant women in whom it may induce bleeding and contractions, and result in an abortion.

Bitter melon contains a substance known as Polypeptide-P that is plant insulin and has similar activity in lowering blood glucose levels. Bitter melon also contains another substance which helps diabetics known as charantin which increases the uptake of glucose by the cells and increases the production of glycogen by the cells of the liver, muscles, and adipose, or fatty tissue. These two substances act together to substantially lower blood glucose levels in diabetics.

Bitter melon is also a wonderful source of various phytonutrients (plant-based nutrients), vitamin C, vitamin A, healthy flavonoids such as beta and alpha carotenes, zeaxanthin and lutein, B vitamins, iron, zinc, potassium, manganese, and magnesium. But remember, as with all foods you grow, their vitamin and mineral content cannot be present in the foods if it is missing from the soils. Plants cannot produce these minerals without taking them up from healthy soils with good microbes. These soil microbes convert minerals from their inorganic state to a digestible organic state and also produce fulvic acid to help increase the permeability of cells to these nutrients.

For this very reason I keep harping upon the necessity to have healthy organic soils enriched with either rock dust, Azomite, sea solids to provide the wide variety of minerals and trace elements that will make a robustly healthy soil microbial community that will nourish your plants and in turn nourish you. Poor soils cannot support healthy plants, plain and simple. Bitter melon also helps in constipation and colitis as well as gastrointestinal problems (other than diarrhea) by its action on promoting peristalsis (the movement of food through the digestive tract) and its stimulation of digestion.

Bitter melon is contraindicated (not to be used) in patients with diarrhea and active gastric or duodenal ulcers.

Bitter melon also comes in a tincture, the dose of which is 5 ml two or three times daily. It can also be utilized as a juice or eating the flesh of the fruit directly. The dosage of the juice for diabetics is 50 to 100 ml of juice daily; remember, mls are the same as cc's. If eating the fruit the dose is approximately 900 mg of the fruit three times daily for diabetes. I would just round that off to a gram three times daily. These dosages are approximations only and there are widely varied opinions on the dosage needed. If you are a diabetic and find yourself without medications and relying upon bitter fruit, you should proceed cautiously, due to its potency.

Some diabetics have been known to combine berberine with bitter fruit to get the better diabetic control from the synergy created by the two plants together.

CHAPTER THIRTY-SIX

HYPERTENSION OR HIGH BLOOD PRESSURE AND HEART DISEASE

INTRODUCTION

TABLE OF CONTENTS:

Hypertension means chronically elevated blood pressure within your arteries. Arteries are the blood vessels that carry blood away from your heart to your lungs and your entire body. Think of the heart and blood vessels as a closed system, with the heart being the pump and the blood vessels being the pipes.

When the heart contracts (pumps) the blood pressure in this closed system is the highest; this is the upper number on your blood pressure reading and is known as your systolic blood pressure. The normal upper limit of which is 140, above which is considered to be hypertensive. The lower number is your diastolic blood pressure, or the pressure in your arteries between heart contractions (between beats). The upper limit of normal on the diastolic blood pressure is 90. Measurements greater than 90 are considered to be hypertensive. The arteries continue to branch out from the large aorta to ever smaller arteries called arterioles and eventually to capillaries.

Elevation in a patient's blood pressure can potentially cause these small arteries to burst and bleed. This primarily occurs in the delicate arteries of the brain, eyes, and kidneys, causing damage to your brain (stroke), vision, and kidney function, all of which are complications of chronically elevated or dangerously elevated blood pressures.

Patients with hypertension are advised to lower their salt intake because salt is osmotically active, meaning it acts like a magnet drawing fluid into the blood vessels from the surrounding tissues. Since the circulatory system is in effect a closed system, any increase in water or fluid within its walls will increase blood pressure, hence the reasoning for putting patients on a low salt diet.

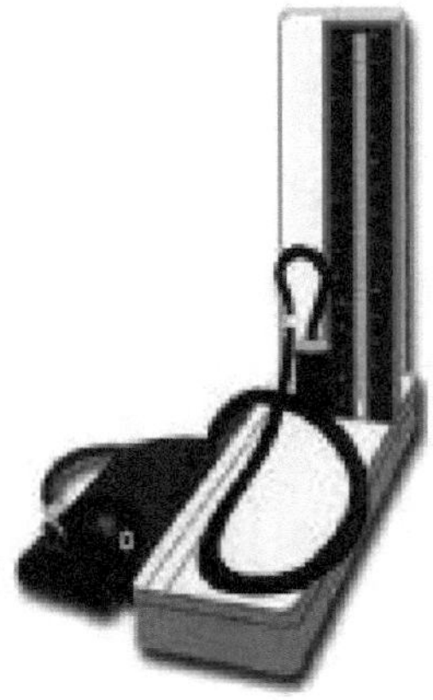

High blood pressure also damages the arteries themselves causing them to build up fat deposits within their walls along with calcium and other material and this leads to atherosclerosis or hardening of the arteries. These hard atherosclerotic arteries are very stiff, stretch less, and are more rigid and less flexible and this further elevates blood pressure.

A mixed blessing of the Vietnam war was the availability of nineteen year olds for autopsy. To everyone's surprise they showed early signs of atherosclerosis even at their young ages. So, from that we know that this is a lifelong process that culminates in hypertension and atherosclerosis and eventually heart disease. Controlling your blood pressure is critically important for your long-term health and also to avoid all the complications of hypertension cited above.

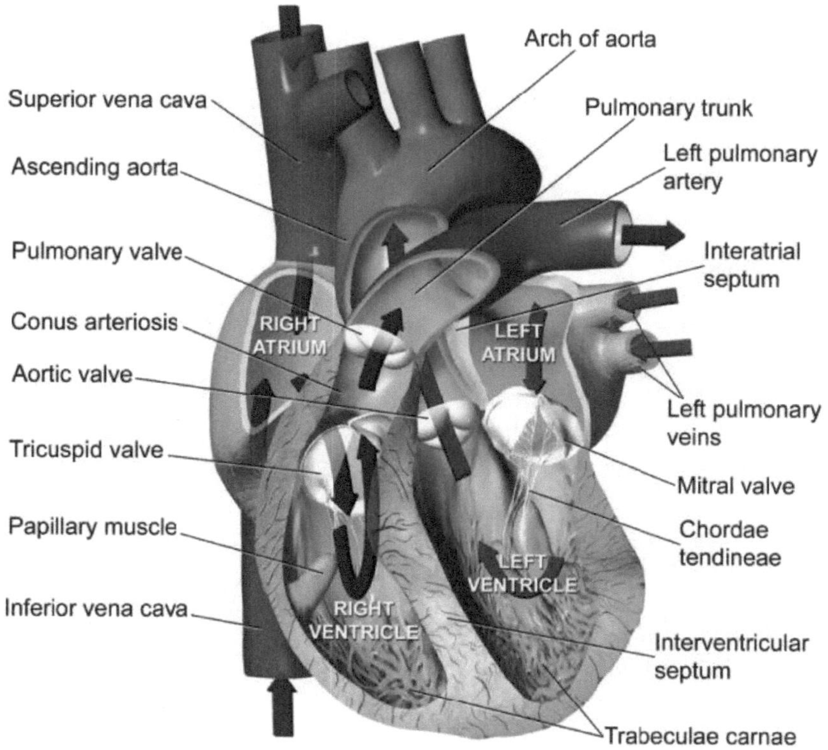

Sectional Anatomy of the Heart

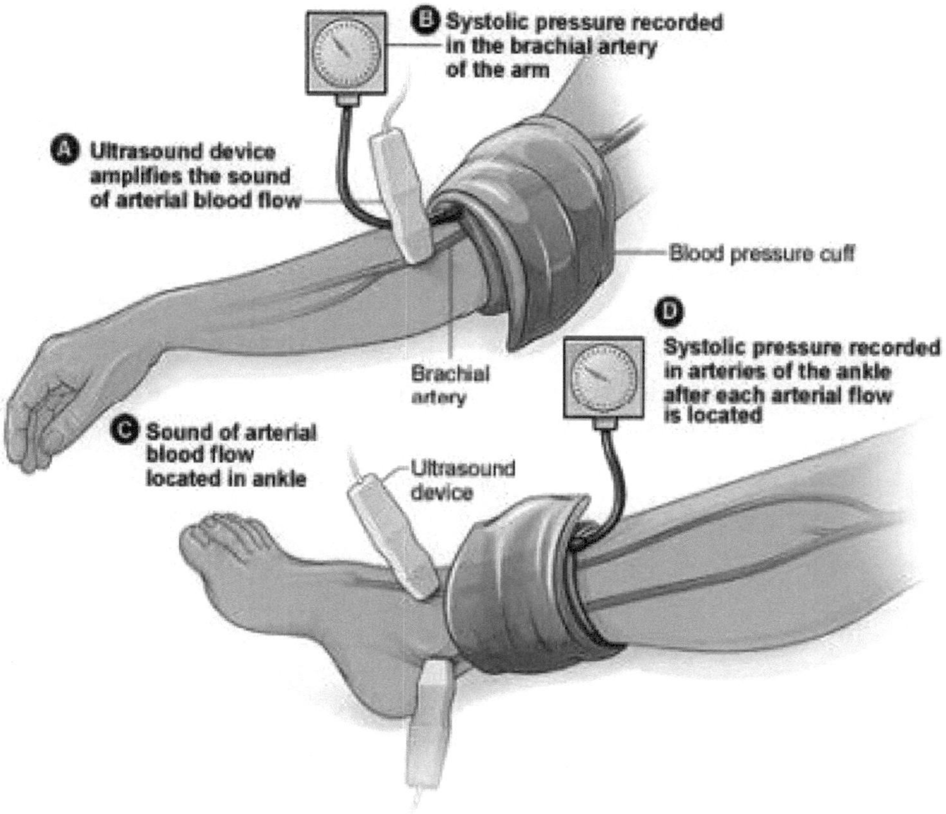

HOW TO MEASURE YOUR BLOOD PRESSURE

Heart disease and hypertension essentially respond to the same treatments, since they are essentially all part of the same cardiovascular system. Cardiac arrhythmias (abnormal rhythms of the heart) and angina or chest pain are different and there are really no alternative treatments available for any of the life-threatening arrhythmias such as ventricular tachycardia; although maintaining good levels of magnesium has been proven to be helpful in preventing some arrhythmias, as well as for lowering blood pressure. The same holds true for chest pain, other than nitroglycerin there is not much that can be done. Aspirin can be replaced by willow bark, but other than that there are no other options with any real effects.

Usually by the time a patient is suffering with advanced cardiac disease it is a consequence of a lifetime of dietary abuse, sedentary life-styles and/or smoking and that leaves us with very few options to treat this structural heart disease.

One of the few options you have is having the patients follow a Mediterranean diet, which is rich in monounsaturated fats like olive oil, high in fresh fruits and vegetables and antioxidants, and low in red meat and therefore is ideal for heart patients.

Have no fears my loyal reader, of course I am going to give you an entire range of natural treatments for your hypertension. You can use these alone or in combination depending on how high your blood pressure is to start with. Let's open our bag of tricks and see what we can come up with.

TREATMENT ALTERNATIVES FOR HYPERTENSION OR HIGH BLOOD PRESSURE

Use one or more from the list below. It may only take one or it may take several to get your blood pressure under control, but first let's look at some general measures that will help reduce your blood pressure, then we will get into the actual treatments.

Here are some life style changes that you can make that will lower your blood pressure: Weight loss of at least ten pounds will lower your blood pressure, naturally if you lose more, you will lower your blood pressure even further. Exercise will lower your blood pressure, but the catch is that you need to exercise for about thirty minutes a day, which will also give you some weight loss. Diet can also impact blood pressure. If you skewer your diet to more fruits and vegetables, that will lower your blood pressure. In addition a low sugar intake will help lower blood pressure more in the long term than short term. The presumption is that it does this by providing lots of potassium, magnesium and calcium which counteracts the negative effects of salt (sodium chloride). Alcohol intake gets a little complicated. If you just drink a little, on average less than one drink daily this will lower your blood pressure, however once you exceed this amount it causes your blood pressure to rise. That is a problem for a lot of folks, who like to have a few beers, or a cocktail or two every night. Once again like with most things in life, moderation is the key.

Okay, let's take a look at specific things we can do or take to lower our blood pressure without the use of synthetic medications that so often have unacceptable side effects.

Salt Reduction

One of the most important is to restrict your salt intake to no more than 2,000 mg or 2 grams of salt daily.

Any salt you are using should be sea salt if you have it available, since it provides a whole range of other minerals and trace elements that table salt or sodium chloride does not and has much less sodium chloride.

Avoid hidden sources of salt such as soy sauce, MSG, and canned foods which frequently contain a lot of salt. Caffeine also raises blood pressure and should be avoided as much as possible.

Other sources of hidden salt are cheeses, smoked meats, and naturally some foods like anchovies and sardines. Beer also contains significant amounts of salt and for that reason should be avoided in patients who are hypertensive.

Magnesium

Magnesium is the most vital mineral in your body and is used by over 300 different enzyme systems to work its magic. It is useful in the treatment of hypertension by its direct relaxation effect on the small arteries of the body, this causes them to relax and enlarge, thereby reducing your blood pressure.

The effective dose varies from individual to individual but is around 300 to 800 mg daily. It is frequently combined with calcium which also helps to lower blood pressure but not as much as magnesium. Patients with kidney failure should be careful taking magnesium and should use it sparingly.

Dietary sources of magnesium are dark green, leafy vegetables, nuts, and fish like halibut. Epsom salt baths can also be used since Epsom salt is magnesium sulfate and after a half hour in a bath will be absorbed directly through your skin. Milk of magnesia is also a form of magnesium known as magnesium hydroxide, also very useful for constipation.

Dark green leafy vegetables contain magnesium for the same reason they are green, chlorophyll. Chlorophyll is identical in its chemical structure to the iron-carrying compound in our blood called hemoglobin; the only difference between the two is the central element. In chlorophyll it is magnesium and in hemoglobin it is iron. All medical interns learn the usefulness of milk of magnesia for constipation by the saying, "If no b.m. in the p.m., give m.o.m. in the a.m.". Magnesium will also help treat cardiac rhythm problems by making the heart muscle less irritable and more steady and relaxed, especially when used in combination with CoQ10. Magnesium, calcium, and potassium deficiencies lead to many cardiac rhythm disturbances.

A further benefit of magnesium is that is has an alkalinizing effect upon the body, raising its pH and making it less acidic.

Foods that are high in magnesium besides nuts and dark green leafy vegetables are grapefruit, barley, rye, cherries, and apples. Epsom salt is another excellent and inexpensive source of magnesium. Epsom salt has multiple uses and a large supply of this should be included in your medicine chest.

Magnesium can also be taken as a supplement, usually available as magnesium oxide, which is not very well absorbed. As with most things you are much better getting your magnesium from plant foods.

Potassium

Potassium also has been shown to lower blood pressure, but just like calcium it does not lower it as well as magnesium. Potassium is also useful to take at bedtime to help you sleep and to help with cases of restless leg syndrome (magnesium also helps this). You should be careful taking this if you have kidney failure. Potassium deficiencies also lead to cardiac rhythm disturbances. Potassium, like magnesium, is readily available over the counter without a prescription. Potassium is an alkalinizing mineral just like magnesium. Remember that your body performs better and is healthier when it is alkaline most processed foods are acidic in nature and the typical American diet is highly acidic.

Foods that are naturally high in potassium are bananas, dried fruits like raisins, figs, dates, and prunes. Sun-dried black olives and a broth made of potato peels are both very high in potassium. Dulse, kelp, and Irish moss are all high in potassium.

Dulse is very good for you, providing iodine and other sea minerals as well, but the taste is hard to get past, at least in my humble opinion. Dulse is a red algae (a type of seaweed) that grows off the Pacific and Atlantic coasts and is eaten as a snack food by some cultures and is very popular in Iceland.

Other high-potassium-containing foods are apple peels, almonds, apple cider vinegar, beans, blueberries, carrots, fish, grapes, lettuce, sesame, soy milk, sunflower seeds, tomatoes, wheat bran, and wheat germ.

Once again I want to remind you to eat organic fruits and vegetables whenever possible, they do not have the toxic loads of non- organic foods that are grown in a toxic soup of chemical fertilizers, pesticides, fungicides and herbicides. It always horrified me that they are spraying fields of plants while wearing hazmat suits because the chemicals are so toxic, and we are eating these foods ingesting a toxic soup that our bodies have to detoxify.

Vitamin D

Vitamin D is very useful and little known as a treatment for hypertension. The mechanism by which it works to lower blood pressure is its effect on the lowering of renin, which raises blood pressure. When there is a lack of vitamin D, it has an effect on the gene that produces renin causing it to produce more renin than usual thus raising the blood pressure. Vitamin D allows this gene to work properly and to not overproduce renin, thus lowering both renin levels and blood pressure.

Vitamin D is fat soluble so remember it must be taken with a fatty meal or it will not be absorbed; once absorbed it is stored in adipose (fat) tissue. The dose varies depending on the weather and season. There are two sources of vitamin D for your body, food and sunlight; food such as egg yolks (twenty IUs per yolk) and wild-caught salmon (400 IUs per 5-ounce serving.

Remember, farmed salmon does not eat from the food chain and therefore has no omega-3 fatty acids, its color is artificial, and they are raised in a very toxic environment loaded with antibiotics, pesticides and other toxic chemicals.

The body can produce its own vitamin D if exposed to sunlight during the spring and summer months, other times of year the sun strikes the earth at a different angle and will not induce the skin to produce vitamin D. During the spring and summer months it is very healthy to be out in the sun, without sunblock, which will block sunlight and prevent vitamin D production. If you are outside for several hours a day this will give you all the vitamin D you need, then you will only have to supplement during the winter. Latitudes below thirty-four degrees north, approximately a line between Los Angeles and Columbia, South Carolina, will allow for vitamin D production from sunlight all year long. The amount of time you need to remain exposed to the sun depends upon your location, cloud cover, season, the amount of skin exposed, and skin tone. The fairer you are the less time you need exposed to the sun because your melanin (skin pigment) levels are low and are not blocking the sunlight. This is the same reason why blacks and other dark-skinned individuals living in the United States are almost all vitamin D deficient, since the large amount of melanin in their skin blocks the sunlight from stimulating vitamin D production. If they are in a tropical environment they have no problems due to the large amount of strong sunlight they are constantly exposed to, however when they move to a temperate environment such as Europe and North America they do not have this intensive sun exposure and thus almost all have low vitamin D levels.

How Much Vitamin D Do I Get from Sun Exposure?

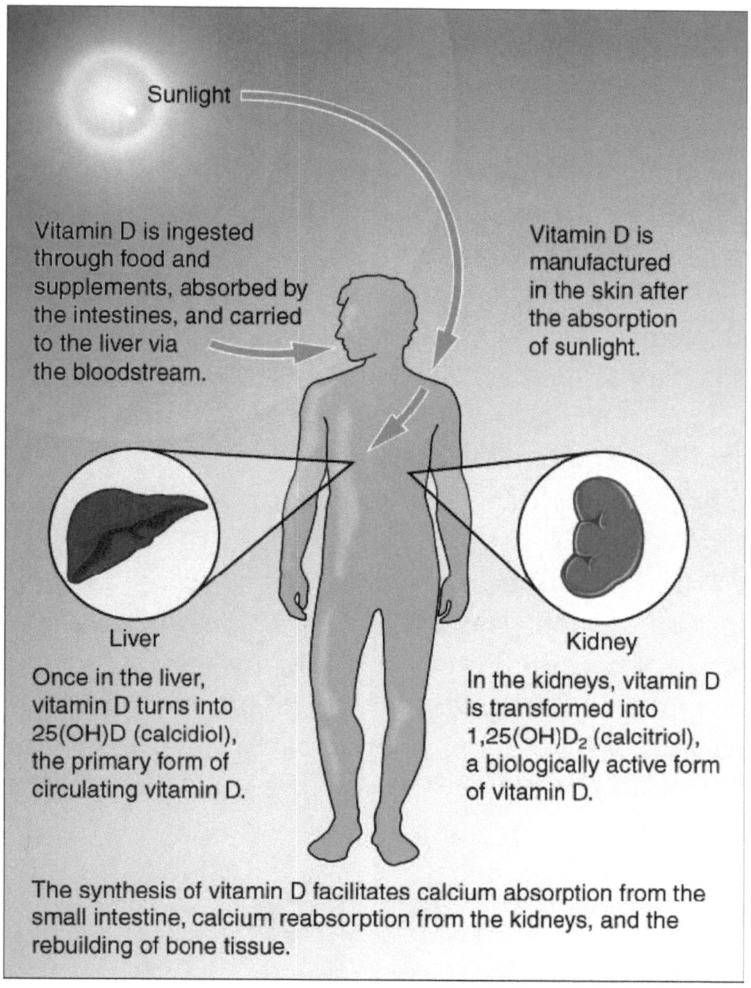

Under ideal conditions your body produces large amounts of vitamin D from sun exposure. Your body produces the active form of vitamin D which is vitamin D3 when exposed to the ultraviolet B radiation of sunlight. With your entire body exposed to the sun under ideal conditions, at the height of the summer you should be able to produce between 10,000 to 20,000 IUs of vitamin D in a half an hour. The most effective hours for vitamin D production are between 10 a.m. and 3 p.m. Under less than ideal conditions if you had to get your vitamin D from the sun you could go out and expose as much of your skin as possible for a half an hour three times a week, and this should enable your body meet all of its requirements for vitamin D.

The best form of vitamin D is D3. A good dose for individuals above the thirty-fourth parallel should be about 5,000 international units a day with a fatty meal.

Even up north this can be stopped during the summer months if you get enough sun exposure. Here in Connecticut where I practice, I typically advise my patients who are outdoors a lot to start taking their vitamin D when the leaves drop and stop when the trees leaf out. All my other patients who are not outside even in the nice weather I advise to take their vitamin D all year round.

People are inordinately afraid of the sun due to melanoma and other skin cancers, and this is a legitimate concern due to our modern lifestyles in which we are indoors the vast majority of the day. In earlier times even fair-skinned individuals had low rates of melanoma and other skin cancers because of their constant exposure to the sun. They were outside virtually from sunrise to sunset, working in fields without sunblock. Their sun exposure started in the spring and as the days lengthened they were already deeply tanned and thus protected from the sun when summer and its longer, hotter days arrived. Modern man gets skin cancer because of recurrent sun burns which repeatedly damage his skin leading eventually to malignant change (cancer).

Soaking up sunlight is healthy for a variety of reasons and there is a little known additional benefit of sunbathing to get your vitamin D level up…it will also lower your cholesterol. Since cholesterol is a precursor (a building block) for the production of vitamin D, when it is utilized to produce vitamin D its blood levels will decline. Not a bad way to lower your cholesterol while lying on the beach, a lot better than statins which I am not a big fan of, due to their side effects that are not often mentioned.

Tell that to your pale dermatologist next time he lambastes you for your tan. Always remember that vitamin D is a fat soluble vitamin (like all vitamins except B vitamins and vitamin C) and therefore will not be absorbed unless you take it with a fatty meal. You will need 5,000 international units of vitamin D3 daily with a dinner or another fatty meal.

Vitamin D also will help the intestinal absorption of calcium, magnesium, iron, phosphate, and zinc.

Sources of vitamin D in our diets are scarce and include all fish liver oils such as cod liver oil, many fatty fish such as catfish, salmon, mackerel, sardines, tuna, and eel. As you can readily see there are very few dietary sources of vitamin D other than fish, this is by design; we evolved as an outdoor species and thus had no great need for dietary sources of our vitamin D. Our current indoor existence as well as our non- organic diet are firsts in human history, and I think will be looked on in the future as a colossal mistake, that will have devastating long term consequences on our health as a species.

Celery And Celery Extract

Celery has been used in traditional Chinese medicine for centuries to lower blood pressure and treat hypertension. It does its work with as little as four stalks a day. Celery contains a phytochemical (plant-derived chemical) that works to relax the muscles in the arterial wall and therefore lower blood pressure. Celery also lowers stress hormone levels which will be very useful in our hectic, modern world. Stock some celery seeds of various types in your medicine chest.

I have not talked much about a medicinal seed vault but it is essential for you and your family. Grow things that you like to eat, but also make sure your diet has an excellent nutritional balance. Starting with the three sisters is one way and then add various vegetables that you like, that way you are assured you will get all the amino acids that you need. Make sure you buy open- pollinated (heirloom) seeds not hybrids, or you will not be able to harvest seeds for next year's garden. Buy them at the end of the garden season along with a good book on seed germination and other plant propagation techniques. For me working in my garden, on a beautiful sunny day with birds singing, and butterflies flitting around, with a nice breeze is such a peaceful and calming experience that it no doubt lowers my blood pressure and gives me a true glimpse of heaven on Earth.

Fish Oil Or Omega-3 Fatty Acids

Along with magnesium there are very few nutraceuticals that everyone can benefit from, including pregnant women and children. Omega-3 fatty acids are essential for both brain and heart health and have a modest role in lowering blood pressure. They also prevent cardiac arrhythmias (abnormal cardiac or heart beats) and lower the risk of sudden death. They are also useful for brain health and work well to help those with ADD (attention deficit disorder), depression, OCD (obsessive compulsive disorder) and bipolar disorder. They also help teens and others who are prone to violence.

Your medicine chest should be well stocked with as much of this as you can afford, as well as buying the best brand you can find to reduce the levels of mercury frequently found in the inexpensive brands.

The recommended dose is between 1 and 4 grams a day. I highly recommend taking it before you eat; eating "on top of it" will prevent you from burping up any fishy smell.

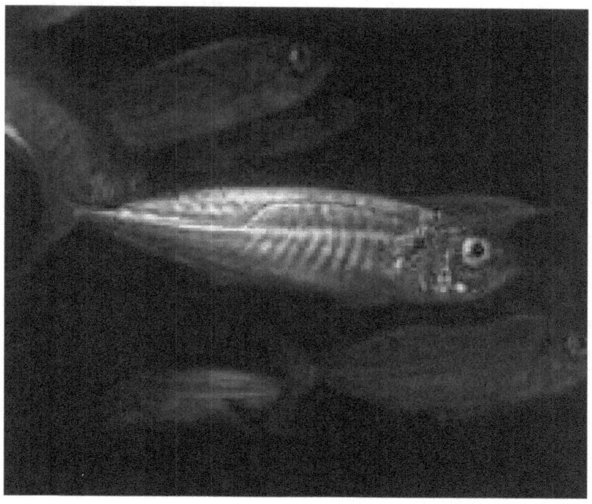

An often forgotten benefit of fish oil supplementation is its "cooling effect" on hot, inflamed joints such as in various arthritis conditions, fibromyalgia, joint aches of any type and diseases such as Lyme disease. I cannot count the number of patients who mentioned in passing that their arthritis or their fibromyalgia is doing wonderfully after a month or so on fish oil. Fish oil is a potent anti- inflammatory substance and by this effect it soothes inflamed joints. Krill oil also is helpful but contains a different mix of omega-3s and also contains astaxanthin which is one of the most potent natural antioxidants found in nature. The omega- 3s of krill oil are different from those of fish oil because the majority of the krill oil omega-3s are attached to a phospholipid (also known as marine lecithin) and are more easily absorbed by the human body.

Vitamin C Or Ascorbic Acid

The Framingham heart study which followed 85,000 women for almost two decades showed the value of vitamin C and heart problems. It was found that those women with higher levels of vitamin C either from supplements or diet had a 28 percent decrease in risk from cardiovascular disease.

Vitamin C works its magic in several ways; it prevents the oxidation of LDL (bad cholesterol) which lowers the damage this causes to the lining of blood vessels. Vitamin C also lowers the level of thromboxane (which is responsible for blood clots). Vitamin C also lowers the complication rate following an acute heart attack. Vitamin C also has a little known effect of working as an antihistamine, thus helping allergies.

Vitamin C is inexpensive and comes in various forms; plain old ascorbic acid is fine and the cheapest. Remember, it is water soluble so just like B vitamins can be taken on an empty stomach with no problems. There is absolutely no known toxic level of vitamin C, in fact it is less toxic than water, which can kill you if you ingest too much. If you take too much you will develop diarrhea. I would recommend that you stock a large quantity of vitamin C in your medicine chest for its many uses. Probably the cheapest form is to buy a large bottle of the vitamin C powder. For children, add it to a little Gatorade or Kool-aid and have them drink it daily, doubling your dose if you start to develop any illnesses.

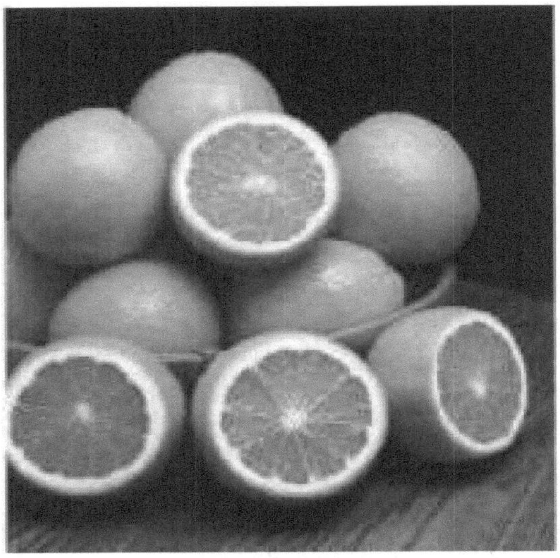

As a baseline for adults 1 gram (1,000 mg) daily should work just fine. Increase it also if you have allergies or need to heal a wound or if you have an infection.

In the bibliography I list several fine books on vitamin C use and its various benefits. The Nobel laureate Dr. Linus Pauling wrote an excellent work on vitamin C and cancer and studied the various wonderful beneficial effects of vitamin C for many years. Since Dr. Pauling there have been several others, the most recent being Dr. Thomas E. Levy, who has written several fascinating, books on vitamin C and its multiple uses and benefits.

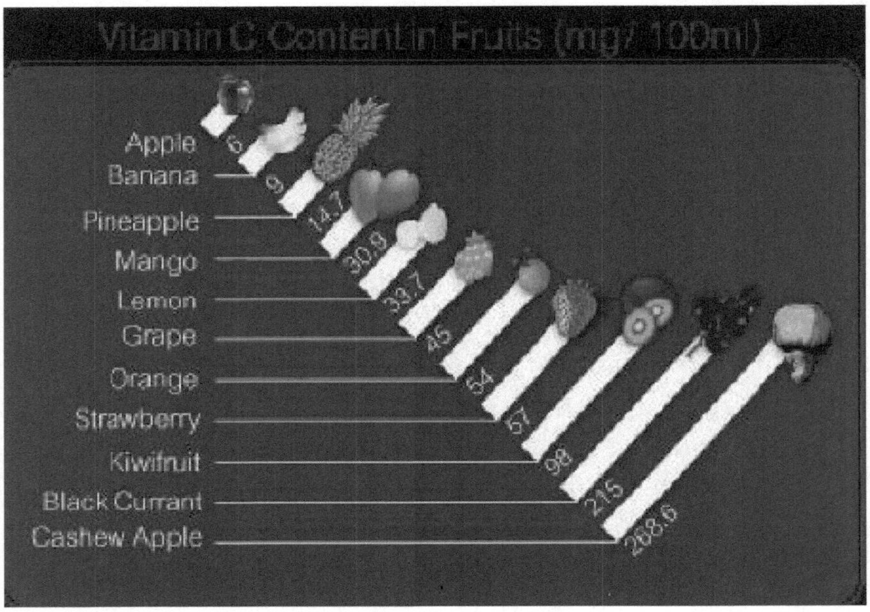

Vitamin C in the body is only found in its ascorbic acid form at a pH below 5; above 5 and in neutral solutions it is found in its ionized form and is called ascorbate. Ascorbate has the same functions in the body as ascorbic acid and is not weakened in its ionized form. A popular form of vitamin C is currently sold as Emergen-C which is a powder and an excellent way to get both vitamins B and C. The vitamin C in Emergen-C is in the form of mixed ascorbates and is readily absorbed and accessible by the body. Emergen-C is a wonderful product that comes in various flavors. I personally like the raspberry best, but my wife, Lynne, swears by the tangerine. This is a useful product to provide a strong dose of antioxidants as well as minerals and will also give you a nice energy boost.

Dietary sources of vitamin C are most fresh fruit and vegetables. All types of berries contain significant amounts of vitamin C. The recommended dose of supplemental vitamin C is controversial, in the interest of full disclosure I will say that I do believe in megavitamin therapy (large doses of vitamins) with vitamin C, therefore a minimum dose daily is 1 gram (or 1,000 mg), raising that to 5, 10, or even 20 grams a day or more when you are sick, backing off only if diarrhea develops. **NOTE:** Your body's vitamin C requirements go up exponentially with any illness, very ill people tolerate much higher doses than they normally would because their bodies need so much more. Analyses of the urine of patients who are very ill have shown no vitamin C present even after getting 20 grams intravenously!

Normally any excess vitamin C, since it is water soluble, will spill out into your urine. Keep this in mind when treating a very sick patient, keep pushing the vitamin C until they get diarrhea, and then cut it back until it stops, and then restart it at 25 percent less than the level that caused diarrhea.

CoQ10

CoQ10 as it is known stands for coenzyme Q 10 and is very important for heart health and your overall health. CoQ10 is intimately involved in energy production within the cell; hence cells that require a lot of energy like heart cells have greater requirements of CoQ10 than other cells. Muscle cells also have a great need for CoQ10. It is helpful in the lowering of blood pressure and preventing cardiac arrhythmias.

The recommended dose is 100 mg twice daily; double that if the patient suffers with congestive heart failure, along with selenium 200 mcg a day and magnesium as directed above. Keep in mind that Co Q10 is fat soluble so must be taken with a fatty meal to get absorbed, without a fatty meal it will pass right through your body unchanged and unabsorbed.

CoQ10 is also a vital part of the antioxidant cascade, which has two branches, a fat soluble branch where CoQ10 and vitamin E regenerate each other, and a water soluble side where vitamin C and glutathione help regenerate one another. Overlying both branches is alpha lipoid acid which is the only compound found in nature that is both fat and water soluble and therefore helps regenerate both branches of the antioxidant cascade. Supplementation with four of these substances will greatly boost your immune system by making you an antioxidant powerhouse. You cannot supplement glutathione since it is quickly removed from your circulation by your liver and is not available. For the above reasons you need to stock CoQ10 in your medicine chest.

Dietary sources of CoQ10 are primarily from organ meats such as liver, kidneys, heart, and also from muscles, so beef is a good source as is pork, chicken, and fish as well as oils such as sunflower, grape seed, olive, and soybean. It is also found in broccoli, parsley, spinach, grapes, and avocados.

Calcium

Calcium works synergistically (works better together than separately) with magnesium, potassium to lower blood pressure and help heart disease.

The dose of calcium is 500 mg daily. You can also get calcium from Tums supplements; crushed oyster shells are another source but they will need to be pulverized into a powder. Calcium, just like magnesium and potassium, is an alkalizing element and therefore has beneficial health effects and helps counteracts the high acid, unhealthy diet which most Americans eat.

Dietary sources of calcium are the well-known dairy products such as milk, cheese, yogurt, and others. Other lesser known sources of calcium in the diet include kelp and seaweed as well as spinach, chard and rhubarb, nuts, beans, blackstrap molasses, figs, quinoa, okra, and kale.

A great "hidden source" of calcium is dandelion leaves. Another great source of calcium that is easily missed are eggshells, these can be ground into powder and either added to food or dissolved in water and drank. Eggshells should never be wasted, crush them and sprinkle them in your garden, plants like goji berries need alkaline soil to grow and will flourish when eggshell powder is added to them.

Hawthorn (Crataegus Oxycanthae)

Hawthorn is a small tree or shrub, the extract of which dilates the walls of arteries and thus lowers blood pressure. The dose is 250 mg of the standardized extract tid (three times a day). Obviously the only source of hawthorn is from a hawthorn tree, the leaves, berries and flowers are used medicinally.

Hawthorne has wonderful cardiovascular benefits, lowering blood pressure, helping cardiac arrhythmias (abnormal heart rhythms), improving congestive heart failure and even helping atherosclerosis (hardening of the arteries). Hawthorne can also be used to treat intestinal tapeworms! Hawthorne's medicinal effect is presumably from a substance it contains called proanthocyanidin.

Garlic

Garlic has been shown to lower blood pressure and boost your immunity as well as add vigor and vitality to a tired body. You can grow it fresh quite easily and utilize it on your foods, I personally love the "stinky rose" and use it on many dishes. Or you can use the aged garlic extract at 600 mg bid or twice daily. Another benefit of the aged garlic extract is its lack of the pungent odor that the natural forms of garlic have due to their unique sulfur compounds that contribute greatly to their healthful benefits.

The most important of these sulfur compounds is allicin. Allicin not only promotes antioxidant activity but also has strong antibacterial and antiviral effects. These antimicrobial benefits come about by allicin's combination with vitamin C which helps kill these harmful microbes.

In order to get the most from your garlic it needs to be cut, minced, crushed, sliced, or chopped; this will produce allicin from the ruptured cells of the plant. Without rupturing the cells the precursor to allicin, called allilin, will not be exposed to the enzyme allinase, which produces allicin.

You need to let the newly chopped or minced garlic sit for ten minutes to allow the enzymes to produce the most allicin. The garlic is now ready to be cooked over a low heat for less than fifteen minutes to preserve the most allicin. If you cook garlic for any longer you will have substantial loss of enzymes and minerals, especially after forty-five minutes of cooking.

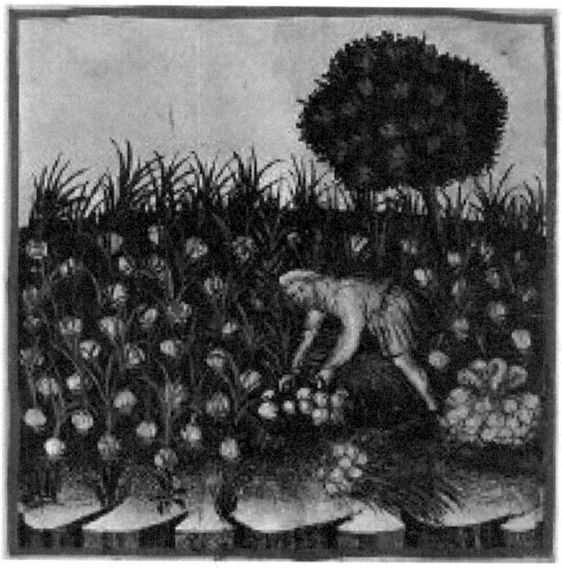

Do not attempt to store your garlic in oil at room temperatures, this may lead to botulism and could be fatal. If stored in oil it must be placed in a freezer and can be stored as such for several months.

To select the best garlic bulbs look for ones that are firm and plump and not soft, shriveled, moldy, or sprouting. Garlic continues to respire (breathe) after it is picked and should be stored in a vented, cold and dark place away from both heat and light, this will minimize its respiratory rate and thus extend its freshness. Either store your garlic braided and hung from some ceiling rafters to allow good air flow in the dark, net type bags work great if you don't braid it, never use plastic bags.

There is no set dose of garlic but one ounce or approximately three medium-sized cloves of garlic is a good daily dose. Cloves are the pieces that the garlic bulb breaks up into, similar to the way an orange breaks up into slices.

Valerian (Valeriana Officinalis)

Valerian is a perennial herb that is native to Europe and parts of Asia and is now naturalized in much of the United States. Valerian helps relax nerves and anxiety, which in some people is the trigger that drives up their blood pressure. If you are an "anxious" guy or gal with hypertension, then valerian is a good choice for your treatment. Depending if you have it in capsules or as a liquid, the dose is 300 mg tid (three times daily) or as a liquid use ½ to 1 ml tid.

I would recommend acquiring some seeds of valerian and keeping it in your seed vault and grow it in your garden as well and harvest its seeds and save them.

Passionflower (Passiflora Incarnata)

Passionflower works the same as valerian above; it calms frazzled nerves in anxious patients. Its dose is 250 mg tid or if in a liquid the dose is ½ ml tid (three times a day). Note: 1 ml = 1 cc, they are interchangeable.

Passionflower grows on a vine and is quite easy to grow; it is tender and will not live in the northern parts of the United States, but can be grown in your garden and overwintered indoors.

Taurine

Taurine is an amino acid or a building block to a protein. Like many amino acids it has a profound effect when used to target a problem. Taurine has been proven to lower blood pressure at the following dose: Six (6) grams daily between meals.

Taurine also has other beneficial effects within the body, such as maintaining cardiovascular health and helping with the development of skeletal muscles, acting as an antioxidant, helping the development of the retina and the central nervous system (the brain and spinal cord).

Dietary sources of taurine are seafood and meat and therefore a vegetarian or vegan diet would be severely lacking in taurine.

Dandelion Leaf (Taraxacum Officinale)

Dandelion functions as a diuretic (causes you to urinate) and thus lowers blood pressure. It is nice because it is also readily accessible on just about everybody's lawns.

Dose: 300 mg capsule tid (three times daily) or in liquid form 2 ml tid. A good guide to the preparation of herbal medicines should be part of your alternative medicine library; see the bibliography for some suggestions.

I would also recommend getting a book on edible wild plants for the area of the country in which you live. There are incredible amounts of edible plants right under our noses that can also be used as medicinal agents. In addition to which it is a lot of fun to go outside with your children or friends and find wonderful healthy wild foods that you can eat.

Olive Leaf

Olive leaf comes in the form of a powder; like many natural cures it will take several months to have its full blood pressure-lowering effect. Olive leaf extract and olive oil contain oleuropein which is a polyphenol that confers so many of their health benefits. Oleuropein not only lowers blood pressure but also lowers bad cholesterol, prevents cancer and aids in dementia as well as being a potent antioxidant and anti-inflammatory agent. Wow, that is quite a list of wonderful benefits from a single plant.

The dose for blood pressure lowering is 500 mg qid or four times daily. It is relatively benign with very few side effects.

CHAPTER THIRTY-SEVEN

FOOT: CARE OF YOUR FEET AND FOOT PROBLEMS

INTRODUCTION

TABLE OF CONTENTS:

If you are a reasonably active person, over the years you would have walked great distances on your feet; thus the importance of knowing how to care for your feet. Every one of us has had a foot problem at one time or another, whether it's a thorn in your foot, blister, heel spur or tendinitis. Anyone who had any of those problems will have the same memories as mine ......oooch, damn it, ooow..........let's face it if your feet are blistered, bleeding, infected or painful, it is exceedingly difficult to walk any significant distance.

FOOTWEAR

If you are reasonably active they you will require several types of shoes, depending on the environment, conditions you currently live in and also anticipating where you may wind up. At the very least you will need a good pair of hiking boots. As with all shoes, you should try these on at the end of the day when your feet are the largest. Try on all shoes before you buy them, due to differences between manufacturers' cuts and sizes. One foot is frequently larger than the other (this is very common) and both feet should fit comfortably. You should stand on your toes with the new shoe on and make sure there is a half inch between your toe and the tip of your new boots. Make sure they are comfortable day one, don't hope they will break in. You should, however, go on several long hikes or wear your shoes while you are working in your backyard to properly break in your hiking boots. Make sure they have nice thick soles with a nonslip type of cleat built into it. I once bought a wonderful pair of hiking boots that had round ball- like cleats. They were a disaster; I was sliding and falling over every wet leaf and rock I encountered. A backup pair would be ideal.

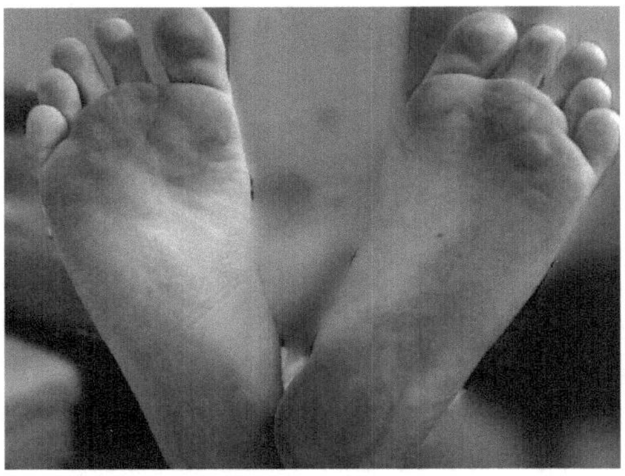

Photo of Friction Blisters on Feet

Improperly fitting boots or shoes will quickly produce blisters, bleeding, and severe pain and will change your pleasant hike into a nightmare. Also make sure you have an adequate supply of nice heavy cotton socks that will cushion your feet and keep them warm and dry.

I would also purchase some nicely insulated snow boots that are also halfway up your lower leg to prevent deep snow from entering the top of them. Look for snow boots that have a string or some other way to cinch the top of them closed to prevent snow entry. A few pairs of gaiters will help as well. These are the foot to eighteen-inch-long nylon devices with elastic at the top and bottom. These look like short pant legs. These are invaluable for fitting over the tops of your boots and keeping your legs dry. They are cheap and readily available at ski or mountain sports type shops or on the internet. Thank God for eBay and Amazon.com where we can find just about anything we need. Two pairs will more than suffice; they are very sturdy and will last a while. Some light cotton socks will also be needed for summer or warm weather use. I would also suggest a sturdy pair of sandals for hot weather. I personally love the ones that look like they are made from old tires. These are sturdy and will last years. A good pair of running shoes are always comfortable and nice to wear depending on what kind of activity you are planning.

FOOTCARE

In addition to the above advice about selecting proper shoes and socks, taking care of your feet is critical. At the end of every active day, , you should be doing a thorough examination of your feet. You should also use this same time to massage your feet. Good blood circulation is critical. Make sure shoes are not too tight or loose. They should just be snug.

Feel your feet as you rub them and feel for any painful areas. If you find a painful area, do a thorough examination of it to see what the problem is. Spread your toes and look for breakdown of your skin.

This is very important. Skin breakdown between your toes will look white and macerated (chewed up-looking). That often is the first sign of athlete's foot and/or might become the point of entry for other infections.

NOTE: After any washing or showering, spend the time when drying yourself to spread each toe and gently run a towel between them to soak up any moisture. This will also remove any dead skin, lint, dirt or other debris. If it is not too cold, allow your feet to "air out" for a few minutes. If you are outside in freezing conditions then dry your feet well as I instructed and cover them ASAP to keep them warm.

Look for any long toenails and trim them with a nail clipper, another indispensable item for your medicine kit. All of the literature on trimming toenails advises cutting them straight across but I disagree. After more than twenty-five years in clinical practice I have examined thousands of patients' feet. Ingrown toenails are a very common ailment. I can tell you unequivocally that almost all of them had a sharp edge that worked its way into the toe's flesh and eventually became ingrown. It makes total sense to me that a toenail shaped like a spoon will be much less invasive than one shaped like a knife. I have found that when you cut your toenails straight across you wind up with two sharp corners that frequently advance their way under the skin and produce painful ingrown toenails. Toenail clippers are curved; use this to curve the corners to prevent those sharp edges. I have had patients do this for years without any problems. Their toenail corners are now curved and it is more difficult for the nail to pierce the skin and become ingrown.

This is my opinion, but my method has helped countless patients with this problem. The experts do disagree with me, but oh, well, it is not the first time and won't be the last. As a doctor who is "in the trenches" doing patient care and not in an ivory tower spouting advice, my view of patients and their real life problems is often at odds with the conventional wisdom.

Diabetic patients should be especially vigilant about foot examination and care. Diabetics, especially those who are uncontrolled (have chronically high blood glucose levels) very often develop what is known as diabetic peripheral neuropathy. What this means is they get nerve damage (neuropathy) that often starts in a stocking and glove type of distribution (that is the peripheral part of the name). Diabetic peripheral neuropathy often starts in the feet of diabetic patients. NOTE: not just diabetics are prone to this. Many patients get peripheral neuropathies from nerve damage originating from spinal injuries. What basically happens is the nerves get progressively damaged and as a result don't work very well to provide the patient with sensation.

Hence they have feet that are either numb to the touch, or with overall decreased level of sensation; consequently these diabetic patients are frequently not aware of cuts and blisters and other foot problems; that is why it is recommended that diabetic patients be extra vigilant in their foot care and never walk barefoot, even indoors.

NOTE: If you are alone, or just prefer to do it yourself, a small mirror will be helpful in examining the soles of your feet.

After examining your feet and before you put your socks on is a good time to apply some foot powder liberally over your feet and especially between your toes. This will soak up any excess perspiration, especially in hot weather but also with heavy boots on. It will also cut down on friction and make your feet more comfortable. You can reapply it several times a day as to your personal needs and preferences. You should also sprinkle some on the soles of your feet and into your boots or shoes. It will also cut down on foot odor which is always a good thing. I personally like Gold Bond Powder; it is inexpensive and effective, but any talcum powder or baby powder will do. Keep a nice supply of it in your medicine chest.

COMMON FOOT AILMENTS

Athlete's Foot

Athlete's foot is by far the most common foot problem you will encounter. Athlete's foot is a fungal infection that will grow on moist areas of your feet. It most commonly is found between your toes, but may be anywhere on your feet. Athlete's foot is also called Tinea Pedis and is closely related to jock itch and ringworm. You will often see a flaking of the skin between your toes that is itchy, burning, or even painful. As with all fungal infections, athlete's foot thrives where it is warm, wet, and dark.

There are many antifungal creams on the market and I would advise getting several large tubes of these, either from a doctor you know or from a vet supply house. You will also need the same treatment for ringworm and jock itch.

NOTE: Ringworm has nothing to do with worms. It is a red, slightly raised ring of skin that is darker on the outside than the center and thus produces what appears to be a ring, or even horseshoe shape.

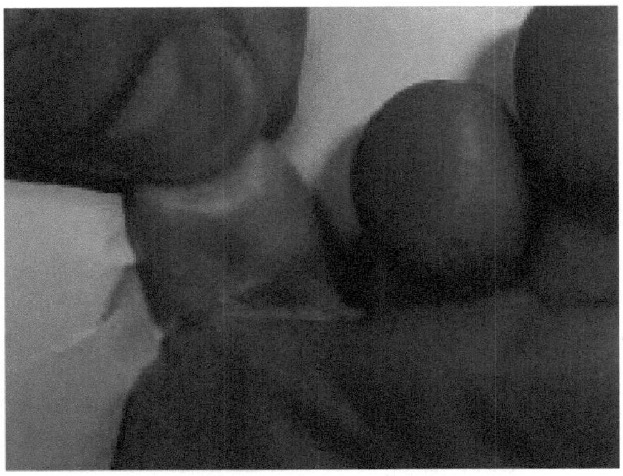

Photo showing athletes foot with its characteristic breakdown of the skin.

Having your shoes or boots constantly wet from immersion in water will make conditions perfect for athlete's foot. Athlete's foot frequently presents as a burning, itching, or stinging of your feet. There often are areas of peeling of your skin on the soles (bottoms) or other parts of your feet. It may develop into itchy blister-like areas. Many times a fungal infection of your feet will be on your toenails. This fungal infection of your toenails is referred to as onychomycosis, and it may develop with or without athlete's foot. The toenails will become very thick and yellow/brown in color. It usually has no severe clinical consequences and therefore treating it is a personal choice

NOTE: If for whatever reason you lose a toenail, especially on your big or great toe, you should save it. The reason being it is the perfect size for a cover for the now exposed, tender, underlying nail bed. It sometimes takes twelve to eighteen months for a toenail to grow completely back in, especially when it involves the big or great toe. During that time your very tender nail bed will be vulnerable to any trauma. All you need to do is drop something heavy on your toe, or jam your foot against something and you will scream in pain. What I have done for years is have my patients take their nail that has fallen off and simply tape it into its old position. It is a perfectly formed shield for your nail bed.

Athlete's foot is caused by mold-like fungal organisms called Dermatophytes. These normally are present on your feet but will not cause an infection unless the right conditions prevail.

Tight shoes that squeeze your toes together present one such condition. Plastic shoes or rubber shoes will also prevent aeration of your feet and predispose you to these infections.

Remember, athlete's foot, like many fungal infection, is highly contagious and can easily be spread by contact with infected shower floors, socks, shoes, and even bath towels. Athlete's foot left untreated can lead to the breakdown of the foot's skin nullifying it as a barrier, and thus allowing a secondary infection by bacteria. Another way these bacterial super infections are caused is by the athlete's foot fungus producing an antibiotic that kills off vulnerable bacteria (that might compete with the fungus). This leaves bacteria that are naturally resistant and therefore much more difficult to eradicate, thus the importance of treating fungal infections quickly and effectively. Different topical creams are useful to have for this such as Monistat, Lamisil, Lotrimin, or prescription Lotrisone cream. There are also different medicated powders such as Tinactin, Desenex, and Zeasorb, which work very well by also drying the area of the foot infected thus making it less receptive to the fungus.

NOTE: The same treatments will work on jock itch and ringworm. In a pinch zinc oxide diaper rash cream can be used. Athlete's foot will be more difficult to eradicate if it involves the soles or bottoms of your feet. The reason is that these areas have thickened skin that forms a barrier to treatment. Athlete's foot, when severe, can also be treated by oral antifungal pills such as Lamisil or Diflucan. However, I am assuming that you are interested in natural treatments.

Alternative Treatments For Athlete's Foot

One thing to keep in mind is that the pH of a fungus is very low, meaning they are acidic (acid like), they also secrete acids to dissolve food in their immediate environment, causing the area around them to also be acidic. I have frequently exploited this fact in my treatment of topical fungal infections like athlete's foot, ringworm and jock itch. If you apply a strong basic or alkaline substance (high pH) to a fungus, you will kill it.

For athlete's foot you can make a mix of baking soda (sodium bicarbonate) and water and soak your feet in it. Add three tablespoons of baking soda to a bucket of warm water and soak your athlete's foot in it. Alternately, you can add some water to some baking soda until it has a paste-like consistency and then apply that to the athlete's foot, ringworm, or jock itch. They all can also be treated in a bath of baking soda and warm water. This is less effective due to the dilution of the baking soda.

Another very effective treatment for athlete's foot is Borax laundry detergent. Borax exploits the same principle in treating athlete's foot as baking soda, its pH. Borax is very alkaline due to its high content of the mineral boron. Borax rapidly changes the pH to an alkaline or basic level and quickly kills off the fungus that causes athlete's foot. The best way is to take a cup of Borax and moisten it and then rub it into the entire surface of your foot, between the toes, the soles, and top of the foot.

Patients often remark about the quick relief that wet borax gives to a burning raw- feeling foot. It is not absorbed across the skin and has no side effects.

After you are done soaking the area, follow up with some topical iodine treatment with either Betadine, povidone-iodine, or tincture of iodine (iodine in an alcohol base). Iodine is a very potent antifungal treatment as well as being antibacterial and antiviral. Painting on some of these topical iodine mixes onto a fungal rash will kill off the fungus. Do it once daily until it is healed. Remember that Lugol's solution can be used as well but should be mixed with a little mineral or other carrier oils for two reasons. First to facilitate its transdermal (crossing the skin effect, secondly at full strength it frequently is irritating to the skin.

Remember: Topical iodine is also a very effective wound treatment and should be applied to any cuts, abrasions, skin tears, or open sores. It not only is wonderful at treating any bacteria, viruses, or fungi that may contaminate a wound, but also when absorbed helps correct our almost universal iodine deficiency.

Bunions, Corns And Calluses

A bunion is a bump on the outer edge of your big toe. Bunions form when the bone or tissue of the big toe's joint grow out of their usual place. The bunion is usually red, swollen, and painful. Frequently you will see them growing either on top of the big toe joint or on the medial (inside area between your feet) aspect of your big toe. They are frequently genetic (running in your family) and/or caused by tight, pointy shoes. This is why they are more common in women.

Frequently a callus or corn will develop over the bunion site or any other pressure point on the foot. A callus is flatter and wider, a corn is smaller and shaped like a kernel of corn and hence the name. They both are the end product of hyperkeratosis or a thickening of the skin produced by the body to protect the underlying area. Corns or calluses can be pared (cut) down with either a sterile scalpel or a sterile sharp small knife.

This should be done by using a motion that is as parallel to the bunion as possible, taking off small layers each time without cutting deeply into it. The callus will have a plastic-like feel to it. Ideally this should not cause any bleeding at all. As you get closer to the bottom of it the area will become softer and more tender...this is where you stop.

This can be repeated as often as possible. You can also use a bunion pad to cushion the area. **NOTE:** You should also purchase a nice supply of foot pads. These are inexpensive and very useful for many foot conditions. Pumice stones or emery boards can also be used. They are just dead skin and will not bleed and are usually not tender. If they bleed you went too deep.

Bunions, corns, and calluses can all be treated by soaking feet in Epsom salt. Place a cup of Epsom salt in the hottest water you can stand and soak your feet for a half hour. This repeatedly done will both soothe your painful, sore feet and also soften the thickened skin over all of these lesions. This skin softening will make it easier to pare down the dead skin by whatever means you choose.

Blisters And Other Foot Sores

Blisters on the feet are unlike other areas because they usually involve weight-bearing areas or pressure sensitive areas and have to be treated more aggressively. In areas other than the foot, if the blister is one inch or less, you can leave it alone and your body will usually heal it. This even holds true for blood-filled blisters. It will help immensely to apply a doughnut-shaped moleskin pad over it with the blister in the center opening. If it is very large you may need two or more moleskins applied over each other so that the blister does not protrude from the center. This will allow the moleskin to take the weight and not the blister. For those on the feet or larger than one inch you will need to treat them. First, make sure your hands are clean by washing them with soap and water. Then gently wash the blister and surrounding skin. Now take a small needle and sterilize it by immersing it in rubbing alcohol or hydrogen peroxide, or with a flame, and pierce the bottom of it. This will allow gravity to drain it. Usually you will also have to apply gentle pressure to the blister, going from the top towards the opening you made; this will allow you to drain the blister completely. Leave the overlying skin in place unless it is infected or filled with pus or dirty. In those cases gently cut it away. Leaving it intact will protect the tender underlying skin and provide a modest barrier to germs. If you have some, apply some antibiotic cream such as Bacitracin or triple antibiotic or Neosporin to the wound.

Also apply a small amount of the antibiotic cream to a rim of surrounding tissue. If you don't have any antibiotic cream, apply some Betadine or other topical iodines. Another option is to pour some straight hydrogen peroxide directly onto the blister site; by straight I mean undiluted with water at its normal 3 percent concentration found in stores.

Plantar Warts

Plantar warts are so named because they grow on the soles of feet or what is known as the plantar surface of the foot. They can be anywhere on the foot but are most frequently on the sole. The pressure of walking on them pushes them below the skin's surface and they frequently develop calluses over them. Warts have a central blood supply of capillaries that will appear to be a dark fleck in the center of it. As they get larger, patients will often describe the feeling like a pebble in their shoe. They are very annoying and can become quite painful.

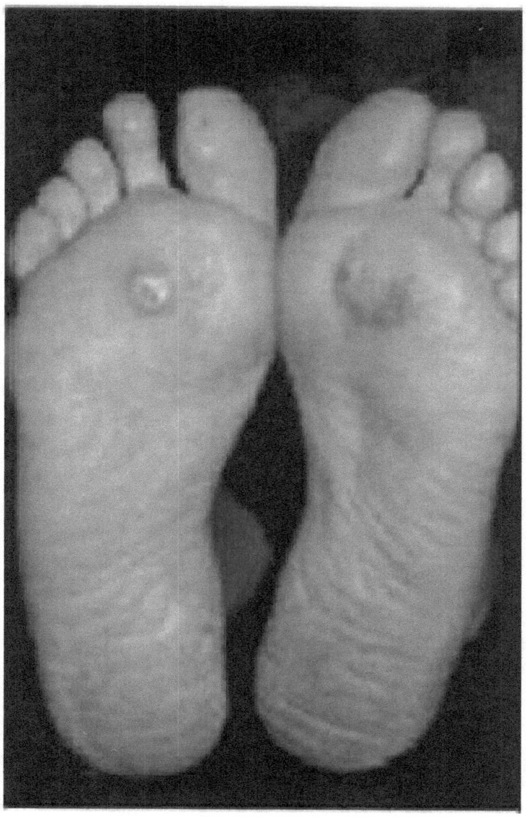

Treatment: Salicylic acid can be used. This will soften the surface and allow you to pare it down. This is the active ingredient in Compound W and Occlusal. Duct tape-covering a wart for a period of time will sometimes eradicate them, although this takes a while. The best treatment for them is paring them down the same way described in the section on calluses and corns.

Ingrown Toenail

An ingrown toenail is exactly that…when the sharp edge or corner of a toenail grows into the tip of the toe in front of it. It has been my experience that this is almost always a sharp edge; I have never seen a round corner grow into the toe in twenty-five years of practice. That being said, in the interest of full disclosure, the medical literature says just the opposite. Either way, what you have is a corner of your toenail under your skin. It almost always occurs on the big or great toe. The involved area will be painful, red, and swollen. This has to be removed or it will only worsen. Keep in mind, you do not want to remove the entire nail, but rather only the small wedge-shaped section up in that corner. It is best to also cut out a wedge of toenail below it to prevent its recurrence. I recommend rounding your toenail's corners to prevent a sharp leading edge from growing back.

Tight and pointy shoes and tight socks will also predispose to this condition. Before you do any cutting of the ingrown nail there are several things you can do to help yourself. First clean your clippers or scissors by sterilizing them as best as you can. You can use hydrogen peroxide or iodine to do this, also clean the toe with hydrogen peroxide or betadine before you proceed. With the clipper, scissor, or even a wooden pedicure stick, start on the section of nail closest to the ingrown part and grip it with the clipper and turn the clipper on its axis to turn the ingrown nail outward. This should free the nail from the skin of the tip of the toe. Then clip a triangle-shaped small wedge of toenail that was directly under the ingrown corner, removing that completely. After, clean your foot again with some hydrogen peroxide or some Betadine or other topical iodine preparation. Cover the toe with a Band-Aid.

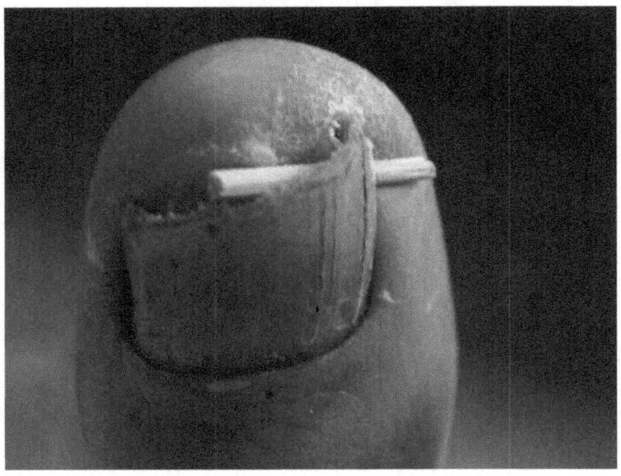

Photo of Ingrown Toenail Held up by Toothpick
(The toenail also has onychomycosis evident by its thickness and its yellow color.)

CHAPTER THIRTY EIGHT

URINARY TRACT INFECTIONS, HERPES, AND VAGINAL YEAST INFECTIONS

INTRODUCTION

TABLE OF CONTENTS:

Urinary tract infections (UTIs) are very common occurrences in clinical practice. Primarily they strike females to a much greater degree than males. This is due to the anatomy of the female genitourinary system (genitals, bladder, and kidneys).

THE ANATOMY OF THE URINARY TRACT

As always, I like to do a quick review of the anatomy. See the diagram below. The kidneys filter urine, it is their job to remove anything that the body can salvage from the urine to avoid waste. Primarily this means saving glucose (sugar) and protein. It also is responsible for the elimination of many soluble (dissolvable) waste products in a slurry, called urine.

The urine travels over the ureters to the bladder and from there it goes out via the urethra. Naturally in women this is a very short distance and in men, depending how lucky they are, it could be a long or a very short trip through their penises. This long urethra essentially protects males from most urinary tract infections because bacteria have to travel a long way to make it to their bladders, whereas in females it is always a short distance, hence the reason for women to have the lion's share of UTIs.

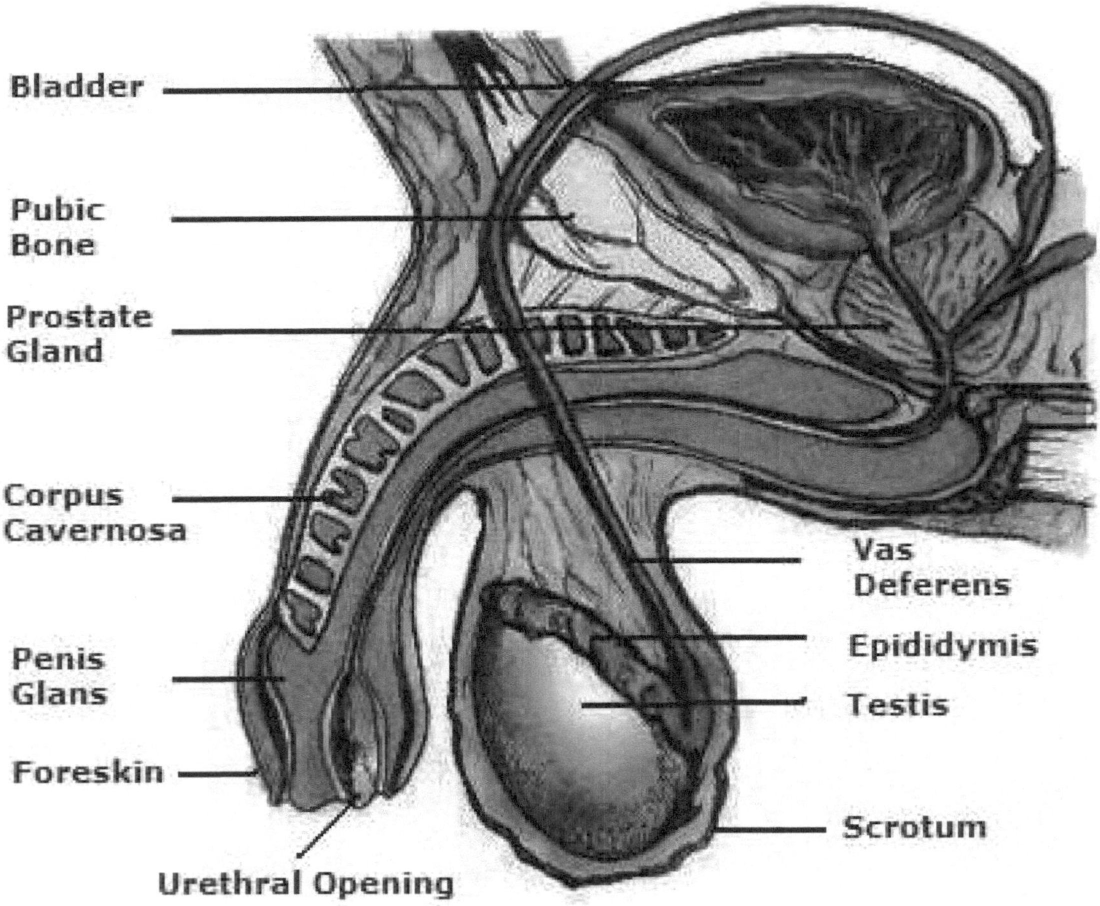

The Anatomy Of The Male Genitalia

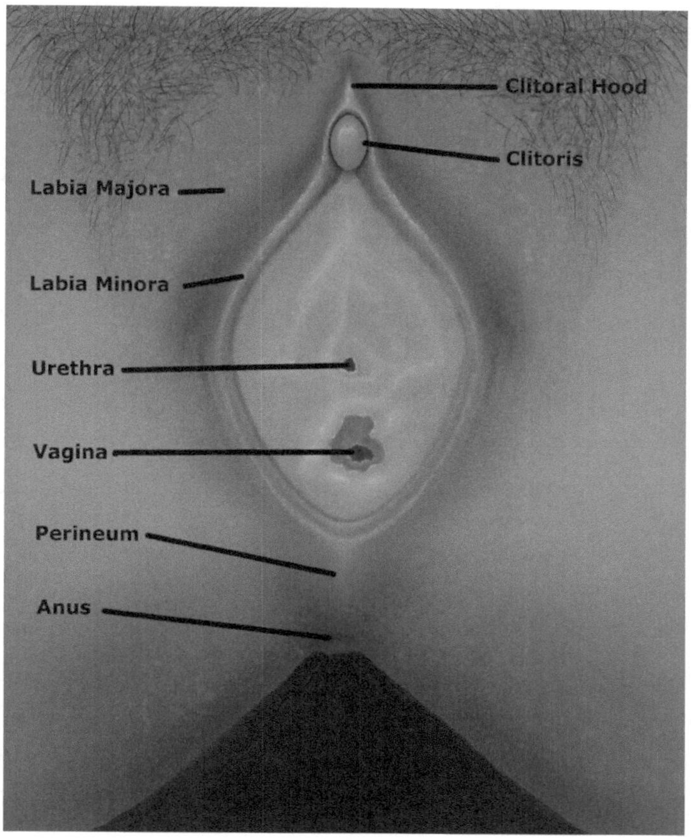

The Anatomy Of The Female Genitalia

The male genitalia are very simple. It involves the penis through which travels the male urethra. The urethra is the tube that carries urine and sperm. It exits the bladder and goes through a doughnut shaped prostate and out through the penis. The penis is responsible for carrying urine and sperm. The testes are a pair and contained within the scrotum. The testes are responsible for making sperm and producing testosterone, or male hormone. On the testes there is the epididymis, which is responsible for maturing, storing, and transporting sperm via the vas deferens to the urethra, through which the sperm exits the penis. The testes with the epididymis lying on top of them look sort of like an acorn with the epididymis the hood of the acorn. The prostate has an organ adjacent to it that is called the seminal vesicles, which secretes a mucous which is part of the discharge along with the ejaculation of male sperm, which travels on the spermatic duct which eventually joins up with the urethra.

The penis is made of three caverns or corpora…two of them fill with blood and are responsible for the penis enlarging into a full-blown erection. The third one lies in the center and is the soft underside of the penis called the corpus spongiosum (spongy). Through the center of the penis lies the urethra which carries both urine and sperm. The bulb-like head of the penis is called the glans penis and the straight part below that is the penile shaft.

The female genitalia are not complicated either. There are two ovaries, one on each side of the body in the lower parts of each side of the pelvis. The ovaries are responsible for the storage and the maturing of eggs which are produced each month from alternating ovaries. They also are responsible for the production of the two primary female hormones, estrogen and progesterone. The egg is then carried along the fallopian tube to the uterus. The uterus is connected to the vagina and the opening of the uterus is called the cervix.

The vagina is the internal female sexual organ, the external part is known as the vulva. The vulva has several parts; from top to bottom it is the clitoral hood with the clitoris encased below it. The vulva has two sets of lips, or labia; the labia minora (inner lips) and the labia majora (outer lips). The opening of the urethra in females is directly below the clitoris and is through which a female urinates.

Anatomy bonus: The G-spot, also called the Grafenberg spot after the German gynecologist who was among the first to note it to be an area of intense female sexual stimulation that would lead to female vaginal orgasm. It is approximately two to three inches inside the vagina on its "ceiling". Stimulation of this area as well as the clitoris will lead to intense orgasms. Stimulation of the clitoris leads to what is known as a clitoral orgasm and of the G-spot as a vaginal orgasm. I wonder what you would call a simultaneous vaginal and clitoral orgasm? I will have to have you readers submit suggestions....mine is a Ralphgasm (admittedly unlikely to catch on...LOL).

URINARY TRACT INFECTIONS (UTI)

These are very common in clinical practice and most women have had a few of these during their lives. It is more common in sexually active women. After sex women frequently have to urinate and this is a good thing, it helps flush out the urinary tract and with it any bacteria that might have entered. The urine is a sterile fluid meaning it has no bacteria growing in it. Infections of the bladder are known as cystitis and usually involve the urethra as well.

Men can get UTIs but they are much less frequent due to the length of their urethras, which makes it difficult for bacteria to travel along without being destroyed by the body's immune system or flushed out by urination. I am not going to get into the different types of bacteria which cause UTIs because you will have no way of identifying them at home, and the treatments I teach you will wipe out the vast majority of them. I am trying to keep this book as practical as possible and not wasting time on types of bacteria is one way to do that.

UTI Symptoms

Frequent urination, burning or painful urination (called dysuria), and sometimes bladder pain (the location of the bladder is just above the base of the penis, or in females inside your pubic hair triangle). Sometimes there will be what is known as frequency, meaning frequent urination and other times there will be hesitancy, where the stream of urine seems to hesitate before it comes out. Sometimes there will be a slight yellow discharge in women. Men may have penile discharge but this is an infection of the male urethra and commonly is from a sexually transmitted disease (STD) or a venereal disease such as gonorrhea, chlamydia, or syphilis.

NOTE: Sometimes a bladder infection may travel up to the kidneys in which case it is known as pyelonephritis. These infections are much more serious and will give different symptoms such as: High fever and/or chills, the urine may have a bloody or cloudy appearance, abdominal and more likely flank pain (pain on your sides) or in your kidney area (this is usually one sided or unilateral). The patient will seem much sicker than a simple UTI. This commonly occurs in the elderly and in these patients may also lead to confusion and disorientation. To determine if a patient is oriented, or with it, doctors typically ask about person, place, and time. Who am I, or who is the president, where are you, what is today's date.

Prevention of UTIs

I am sure you have all heard the old adage, "an ounce of prevention is worth a pound of cure. There are some easy things to do to prevent the majority of UTI's. As I stated previously, urination after sex is very important and helps flush out the bacteria. Also, hand washing before sex will remove a lot of bacteria on your hands before your transfer them to your partner.

Drinking large amounts of water will help continuously flush out bacteria and also dilute them. You can acidify your urine making it less receptive to bacteria by adding ascorbic acid or vitamin C daily. Cranberry juice also prevents the adhesion of bacteria to the bladder lining thus preventing infections.

Taking probiotics will help keep good flora (bacteria) in your vagina as well as your colon. Recent studies have proven that this helps your body's total immune function.

Using condoms if you are not in a monogamous (only one sex partner) relationship will vastly reduce your risk of catching both UTIs and sexually transmitted diseases (STDs).

If you experience vaginal dryness during routine intercourse it is advisable to use a lubricant to reduce any irritation caused by friction. This will only facilitate (make it easier) for bacteria to invade your vaginal wall.

When wiping yourself with toilet paper do so from front to back; this helps prevent bacteria from your feces from being transferred to your urinary tract. This applies primarily to women. I think most people go front to back anyway, but that could just be my own personal bias.

Wearing cotton underwear will help prevent UTIs by allowing good oxygen or air flow. Also take off any wet bathing suits after swimming and dry yourself well. The introduction of oxygen into any area of the body helps kill off most microorganisms.

TREATMENT OF KIDNEY INFECTIONS AND URINARY TRACT INFECTIONS

Both kidney infections and UTIs need to be treated with lots of water; you need to replace the water lost with frequent urination but more importantly you need to mechanically flush out your urinary tract and wash out the bacteria and dead white cells (pus) and other debris. Natural diuretics (substances that increase urination) such as celery, parsley, and watermelon will help flush out your kidneys. Eating them will help, but concentrating them into fresh juices will be even more powerful. Celery has many wonderful properties and has very few calories.

Cranberry (Vaccinium Macrocarpon)

Either in pill form (cranberry extract), take 500 mg twice daily or drink several glasses of unsweetened cranberry juice several times a day until the symptoms end.

Cranberry contains vitamin C and also prevents bacteria from sticking to the walls of the bladder and urethra. It also helps acidify the urine which is much less receptive to bacteria. Cranberry extract is much better at prevention than treatment of UTIs, so if you suffer with recurrent UTIs and urethral infections then use this daily or several days a week to prevent infections. If you want to use it long-term to suppress and/treat recurrent UTIs then take 400 mg of the extract in capsule form twice a day for three months or drink about 10 ounces of fresh cranberry juice daily

Cranberries are excellent sources of vitamin C and as such work very well to treat scurvy. The cranberry plant does not have to be grown in standing water as everyone seems to think, the advertisements showing cranberry farmers standing in knee high water with cranberries covering the surface is how the berries are harvested, by flooding the fields of cranberries and scooping the berries off as they float. I grow cranberries in my orchard and use them as a ground cover next to my blueberries. You do have to water them frequently just like their cousins blueberries, and like blueberries they like an acidic soil, so be generous with that peat moss and keep it wet.

Echinacea (Echinacea Purpurea) And Goldenseal (Hydrastis Canadensis)

Echinacea or coneflower gets its name from the Greek word echinos which means hedgehog, due to the head of the flower that bristles with little spines just like a hedgehog. Echinacea works to enhance the immune system and decrease pain and inflammation. Echinacea has been shown to have antiviral effects and as such has been used extensively to treat things like the common cold. The plant is beautiful and is easy to grow and should be included in any medicinal garden.

The entire plant is harvested for its medicine, using both the roots which make volatile oils and the above-ground parts of the plant which make polysaccharides which help stimulate the body's immune system. It has been shown to be helpful in the treatment of UTIs.

Echinacea can be taken in various forms such as a tea, dried extract, standardized capsules, and as a tincture.

Here are the doses of Echinacea:

Tea: Mix 1 or 2 grams of the tea in hot water, steep for ten minutes and then drink hot or cold once daily.

Tincture: 2-3 ml daily

Powdered extract: 300 mg once daily

Goldenseal when given together with cranberry is much more potent than either given separately. There is little evidence for goldenseal's medicinal effects, especially when given alone; and for that reason most of the time it is given with cranberry. It is reported to have antimicrobial effects and has been used to treat UTIs, vaginal infections, colds and flu, eye infections, canker sores (apthous ulcers), and diarrhea.

In combination goldenseal and cranberry can be taken either in capsule form (500 mg) or take about 4 ml of their tincture form, either one four times a day until the symptoms resolve.

Horsetail (Equisetum Arvense)

Horsetail is an ancient herbal remedy used to stop bleeding, treat tuberculosis, wounds, ulcers, and kidney infections. It also has some diuretic effect and will flush out the kidneys. Horsetail also contains significant amounts of silica and as such has been used to treat osteoporosis.

The plant is related to ferns and is a perennial found all over the world. On my property in Connecticut it is one of the most common weeds. The silica crystals that form on the hollow stems and leaves gives the plant an abrasive effect and as such was used to polish metals in ancient times. The leaves and stems are used, not the roots.

Horsetail should not be used by pregnant or breast feeding women, and people with chronic kidney disease. Do not drink alcohol while on horsetail; it lowers thiamine and may cause problems with alcoholics.

Horsetail comes in various forms but mostly the dried herbal form, tea, poultice, and as a tincture.

Here are the doses in the commonly used forms:

Capsules: 500 mg four times a day (standardized to 10 to 15 percent silica); take this for seven to ten days.

Tea: Two or three teaspoons full in hot water steeped for about ten minutes three times daily for seven to ten days.

Tincture: 2 ml of the tincture four times a day for seven to ten days.

External compresses: Mix about 10 grams with a liter of water

(use a quart if you are metrically challenged). Apply the compress to any infected area.

Oregano Oil

As I stated earlier, this has excellent antibacterial and antiviral properties and is useful in many kinds of infections that you may encounter.

It is worth keeping an ample supply of this in your medicine chest. Take 500 mg capsules four times a day until the symptoms are gone.

Uva Ursi (Arctostaphylos Uva-Ursi)

Uva-ursi is a small shrub the leaves of which are the source of this medication. As you can see from its Latin name, its common name is bearberry. Uva is Latin for egg and ursi means bear. Bears apparently like eating its fruit. The active ingredients are hydroquinone and its derivatives, especially arbutin, which is the primary active compound; however taking arbutin alone will not work due to its inactivation by the intestinal flora.

Uva-ursi has antimicrobial properties (kills germs) so it is excellent for treating UTIs. It is excreted by the kidney and acts as an astringent (drying agent) and also has anti-inflammatory properties so it soothes the inflamed mucosa of the bladder and urethra. It also is a diuretic and as such will lower your blood pressure and increase your urination; this works to flush out your kidneys and bladder, but diuretics also lower your potassium level so you should eat some dried fruit while taking this Uva-ursi has been shown to be effective against E.Coli and many other bacteria as well as killing candida albicans (yeast infections).

It also helps diarrhea from its tannin content, and can be made into a poultice for wound infections due to its antimicrobial actions.

Uva-ursi works best in alkaline urine, so in this case only, avoid vitamin C which acidifies your urine, and drink plenty of water. It should be avoided in children and pregnant and breast feeding women. High doses may damage your liver, take as directed.

Uva-ursi comes in various preparations, here are the doses:

Tea: Soak 3 grams of tea in 5 ounces of water for about twelve hours, then strain it and drink it hot or cold three or four times a day for five days maximum (due to potential liver damage).

Tincture: Take 5 ml of the tincture four times daily for five days maximum.

Capsules: Capsules come with a standardized dose of arbutin, take 250 mg capsule four times a day for five days.

OTHER THINGS YOU CAN DO TO HELP UTI'S

Another method I like to employ is to change the pH of the urine to more acidic. This prevents bacteria from sticking to the bladder and urethral walls as well as making a harsher environment for bacteria to live and thrive in.

This can be done by taking ascorbic acid (vitamin C). Take at least 1000 mg (1 gram) three times daily until the infection resolves. The vitamin C will also boost your immune system and help fight off the infection. Vitamin C is the least toxic substance known to man and nobody has ever overdosed on it. As you recall, it is water soluble and you will urinate out any excess, this fact plays right into our hands by having your body eliminate it through your kidneys and right into your infected bladder and urethra, lowering the pH of the urine making it more acidic.

An alternative strategy using the same concept is changing the pH of the urine to more alkaline or basic using sodium bicarbonate or baking soda. Use a half-teaspoon of baking soda in a half-glass of water ever four hours for two or three days. Do not use it for longer due to its pH effects on the rest of the body. The take-home message here is that bacteria and other microorganisms survive not only within a narrow temperature range, which is why fevers are so effective, they also live within a narrow pH range, thus manipulating it in either direction will make it incompatible for them.

A sitz bath or even hot compresses over your bladder area (over your pubic hair) will help soothe an irritated bladder. The addition of a few drops of tea tree oil, lavender oil, chamomile oil, or bergamot oil to your hot bath will help UTIs due to their antiseptic effect. Even a heating pad or a hot water bottle to the bladder area will help any cramps associated with the UTI as well as soothe the irritated bladder.

AZO, which is a urinary tract analgesic, can be bought over the counter. This gets excreted by the kidneys and numbs up the bladder as it passes through, it also will turn your urine bright red. AZO is something you might want to consider for your medicine chest if bladder problems are a constant lament for you. Many patients think they have UTIs but their urine is fine on dipstick analysis, they are urinating every few hours in small amounts, this is not a UTI but rather is known as Irritable Bladder Syndrome and is treated with hydration and AZO.

If you prefer to go the natural/alternative route rather than taking antibiotics then your best bet is to try to boost your immune system and alter your urinary pH with vitamin C, which will be part of boosting your immune system as well. The antioxidant cascade will have to be employed to get maximum benefit, this involves four different nutrients/vitamins:

Vitamin C: 1 gram or 1,000 mg four time's day (you can double it if no effect after 1 week). Note: if you get diarrhea cut the dose in half until it disappears and then raise it by 500 mg/day until you reach 4.000 mg or 4 grams/day.

Vitamin E: 800 international units twice a day, with a fatty meal or you will not absorb them.

Co Q10: 200 mg twice daily; same as vitamin E, it is fat soluble so take it with a fatty meal.

Alpha-Lipoic acid: take 600 mg twice daily, also with fatty food, although this is not as important as the Vitamin E and CoQ 10, since alpha-Lipoic acid is the only substance known that is both fat and water soluble.

Alter the pH, boost your antioxidants as much as you can and do all of the above-mentioned treatments for UTIs such as vastly increasing your water intake, etc. Employing all those tactics will eradicate all but the most resistant bacterial infections. If you are not getting any better, and or if you are worsening, it is a good time to get a second opinion from your doctor. A severe kidney infection can be deadly, so if you have any doubt (and this holds true for any medical condition you are trying to treat), err on the side of caution and have your doctor check you out. If the kidney infection spreads into the blood and the patient gets what is called septic (meaning blood poisoning from the spread of the bacteria), then even with antibiotics the mortality (death) rate is very high and without antibiotics the patient will very likely die.

HERPES VIRUS FAMILY INFECTIONS

Also known as herpes simplex; herpes family of infections come in various types:

Herpes labialis (on your lip) or oral herpes: These are the cold sores that many children and adults suffer with. This is caused by herpes simplex type 1. They can be anywhere on your face or head.

Herpes genitalis (on your genitals) This is the dreaded herpes that all sexually active adults fear with dread and is also called herpes simplex type 2. It is a sexually transmitted disease. (**NOTE:** Either type can be transmitted from the lips to the genitals, for example, or vice versa). Herpes of this type will manifest as a tingling or burning sensation at first that eventually will form small, clear-fluid-filled vesicles (blisters) that are very painful. They eventually break down into small open sores. These are very contagious and are shedding large amounts of virus.

Chickenpox (Varicella): Chickenpox mostly strikes children and will cause them to feel ill with a fever and malaise (they feel sick) and then fluid-filled itchy blisters will develop that will crust over. If you pick them they will leave holes and scar you where the blisters were. A patient is contagious from two to three days before the rash develops until the scabs resolve.

The primary treatment is to soothe the rash and prevent the itching. The combination of calamine lotion and Benadryl does the job quite nicely.

Herpes zoster (shingles): This is essentially an adult recurrence of an old chicken pox infection. You can only get shingles if you had chickenpox, and the lesions will be in the same area that you had the original outbreak. Since all herpes family viruses are stored in sensory nerves forever, shingles comes out when a person's immune system is weakened, either by another illness or exhaustion or other factors. The key fact with diagnosing this is that shingles DO NOT CROSS THE MIDLINE OF THE BODY. This is an absolute rule. The reason is as stated earlier it is stored in the nerve and will follow the path of that nerve, giving you a strip of lesions on one side of your body or the other. It usually only arises in one dermatome (distribution pathway of a nerve) and if it comes back will be in the same spot.

General Information and Treatment of Herpetic Infections

What all herpes family viruses have in common is that after the initial infection they become dormant (sleeping, or not active) and lie in a sensory nerve, and are there for the rest of your life. That is why the old joke about herpes is so poignant: What is the difference between love and herpes? Answer: herpes is forever. Any of us who are divorced can relate to that joke.

The herpes virus awakens or comes out of dormancy whenever the immune system is compromised, either by another infection, severe cold, too much sunlight, menstrual periods, or even depression.

Another fact that all herpes infections have in common is that they require the amino acid arginine to thrive and replicate (reproduce themselves). Structurally arginine is very similar to another amino acid named L-lysine (or just plain lysine). A very good strategy I have utilized over the years is to treat all herpes infections with L- lysine and also with vitamin C to boost their immunity and help shorten the infection. I usually give L-lysine 500 mg or 1,000 mg three times a day between meals along with vitamin C 1,000 mg. The L- lysine floods all the receptors on the cells' surface and blocks the uptake of arginine and consequently blocks the herpes virus from reproducing.

NOTE: There is no cure for herpes, this only forces it back into remission. Also remember that antibiotics only work against bacteria; for herpes you need antiviral medications such as Zovirax, Valtrex, Famvir, and Acyclovir. Certain energy therapies work as well against infections such as ultraviolet, photoluminescence, etc. but they are beyond the scope of this book (or it will have to be 2,000 pages).

Lemon Balm (Melissa Officinalis)

Lemon balm is a perennial herb and a member of the mint family and gets its name from the mild aroma of lemon emitted by its leaves. It is considered a calming herb and as such has been used to calm nerves and also as a sedative to help sleep. It has also been used extensively to treat the lesions of herpes and has been shown to prevent recurrence in the first outbreak of herpes and also soothes the swelling and redness and decreases the length of time of the outbreak.

The leaves of the plant are used to produce the essential oil of lemon balm; it is supposed that their tannin content has antiviral properties and for that reason helps heal herpes.

Lemon balm leaves can be bought in bulk and used as a tea or made into a poultice; it also comes as a topical cream, tincture, extracts, and in capsules.

Lemon Balm extract made into a topical cream will help heal cold sores or herpes labialis. Apply the cream about four times a day until healed.

Zinc

Zinc helps heal genital as well as lip lesions of herpes. Take about 30 mg twice a day, along with 3 mg of copper once a day, since zinc will lower copper levels. Alternatively, you can use zinc oxide cream topically (on your skin or surface) three times daily.

You can also make your own zinc oxide-containing cream by adding it to your skin lotion. Zinc oxide comes in a powder, which I recommend, and also a nano-sized powder which I want you to avoid. The nano particles are so small they readily enter the body and eventually the bloodstream, their long-term toxic effects are not currently known or understood. They are used because when they are applied to skin they enter it and disappear altogether without leaving a white film, which the non-nano zinc powder does.

B Complex

B complex (all the B vitamins together in one pill) will help shorten the length of a herpes outbreak of any kind. Take a 50 mg tablet twice a day until the lesions resolve. Remember, B complex like vitamin C is water soluble, so you can take it on an empty stomach. **NOTE:** It will also make your urine bright yellow.

Echinacea

Echinacea is well known for its antiviral properties and it also helps support the body's immune system. Take either 500 mg capsules three times a day or use it in tincture form, 2 to 4 ml of the tincture three times a day. See the section earlier in this chapter on kidney and urinary tract infections for a complete discussion on the uses of echinacea.

Propolis

Propolis has been shown to be very effective in treating herpes lesions. Propolis is a resinous mixture that honey bees collect from tree sap, tree buds, and other floral sources. Propolis is what the bees use to fill gaps and seal areas of their hives. Propolis is used for small gaps and large gaps are filled with beeswax. Even the venerable National Institute of Health (NIH) says that propolis is possibly effective in treating herpes infections of the mouth, cold sores, and throat infections. Use either the tincture or the ointment four times a day until you are healed.

Capsaicin

Capsaicin cream for the pain of shingles lesions has been shown to work well. Use a strength from 0.025 to 0.075 percent extract four times a day.

NOTE: You will get a burning sensation that might be severe if the skin is broken. The only way to neutralize this burning is with milk or dairy cream. Nothing else works; capsaicin is made from pepper of the same name and can cause severe burning.

Olive Leaf Extract (Olea Europa)

Olive tree leaves contain a polyphenol known as oleuropein which is responsible for many of the health benefits of olive oil and the extract of its leaves, it also gives olive oil its unique taste. Olive oil and extract have many anti- inflammatory and antioxidant and disease-fighting properties.

Olive leaf extract (olea europa) is known for its antiviral potency (strength); take 500 mg four times a day until the outbreak resolves.

VAGINAL YEAST INFECTIONS

Vaginal yeast infections are also very common in clinical practice, however most of these are side effects of antibiotic usage and can be prevented by eating yogurt while on antibiotics to continuously replenish the good bacteria or probiotics your body needs

Symptoms Of Vaginal Yeast Infections

Most women complain of a vaginal itching that may be severe at times, along with soreness to their vaginas that may make sexual intercourse painful. These patients oftentimes have a classic cottage cheese-like discharge from their vaginas. Anyone with a compromised immune system such as patients with HIV, cancer, or other severe infections will be more prone to Candida Albicans infections. Candida A. is the fungus or yeast that causes these vaginal yeast infections.

When these infections occur in the mouth you will see a thin net of white lesions either on the tongue or the mucosa (the lining of the cheeks and throat) and this is commonly known as thrush. Oftentimes patients have associated enlarged lymph nodes in their necks.

Treatment Of Vaginal Yeast Infections:

The first thing you should remember when treating a yeast infection is that fungus and yeasts love sugar, so the more you can limit your intake of sugars the better. Sugar also suppresses your immune system and allows these infections to flourish. Also avoid foods that are high in yeast and molds such as aged cheeses, nuts, alcohol, and dried fruits. Fermented foods usually are great for you, but yeast infections are the exception to that rule: avoid vinegar, pickles, and soy sauce. Also avoid sexual intercourse until the infection has healed, this will avoid further irritation and reinfection. Avoid tight clothing and wear loose-fitting cotton clothes that will allow the genital area to breathe. If you go swimming or your clothes get wet for some reason, change into dry clothing quickly and dry your vaginal area well. Also dry it well after a bath or shower.

Let's Take A Look At Some Effective Alternative Treatments:

Flaxseed: Take one or two tablespoons of flaxseeds with 10 ounces of water twice daily. Flaxseed has antifungal properties.

Garlic and onions: both have antifungal properties, and if you have a vaginal yeast infection you should consume large amounts of both of these. The sulfur they both contain is very healthy for your body and have antibacterial and antifungal effects.

Lactobacillus Acidophilus: Insert one capsule intravaginally (inside the vagina) every night for one week. It may very well lead to a vaginal discharge as it kills the yeast, so it is wise to wear a pad of some type.

You should also take L. Acidophilus orally at least twice daily. The strength of these probiotic bacteria is measured in organisms since they are alive. I would recommend at least 5 billion per capsule. I also recommend a mixture of several types of probiotic bacteria together, another excellent one is Bifidobacteria.

Boric Acid: Use 600 mg boric acid capsules (NEVER TAKE BORIC ACID ORALLY) and insert them in the vagina twice daily for one week. Just like with the Lactobacillus A. wear a pad to catch all the dead debris along with the vaginal discharge. Frequently it will cause burning of the genitalia; this can be treated either with vitamin E oil or with zinc oxide or Calmoseptine. Calmoseptine is wonderful for any anal itching or burning and contains zinc oxide with menthol which has a very nice cooling effect. You can use calmospeptine around your anus and genitals with no problem, it is soothing and will put out the hottest inflammation.

Oregano Oil (Origanum Vulgare): Take 500 mg capsule twice daily for ten days or you can use it in liquid form of 0.5 ml, also twice daily for ten days. Oregano oil has a potent antifungal effect and works very well for these infections.

PART FOUR

ODDS AND ENDS

CHAPTER THIRTY-NINE

EBOLA

INTRODUCTION

TABLE OF CONTENTS:

Ebola is a virus that originated in Africa. It is a deadly viral hemorrhagic fever, currently having a morality rate that averages about 70 percent. There were five subtypes or species in the Ebolavirus family or genus, four of which infect humans, the worst being the Zaire Ebola virus (now known as Ebola virus). The Ebola virus is related to other hemorrhagic viruses such as the genus Marburgvirus which includes Marburg virus (MARV) and Ravn virus (RAVV), LASSA fever, Rift Valley fever, Yellow fever, and Crimean Congo Hemorrhagic virus. The genus Ebolavirus and the genus Marburgvirus are very similar and seemed to have diverged genetically several thousand years ago. The bad news is that the genus Ebolavirus easily mutates, similar to the flu virus; the good news is that the mutation rate is only about a quarter of that of the flu. That being said, the flu virus is infamous for its mutations, so much so that the flu vaccine is only good for one season and the Center for Disease Control needs to go to Asia annually to get the three most current flu species to concoct a new vaccine. The mutation rate of the flu virus also occasionally mutates into an extremely deadly form such as it did in 1918 wiping out millions upon millions of people and effectively ending World War I.

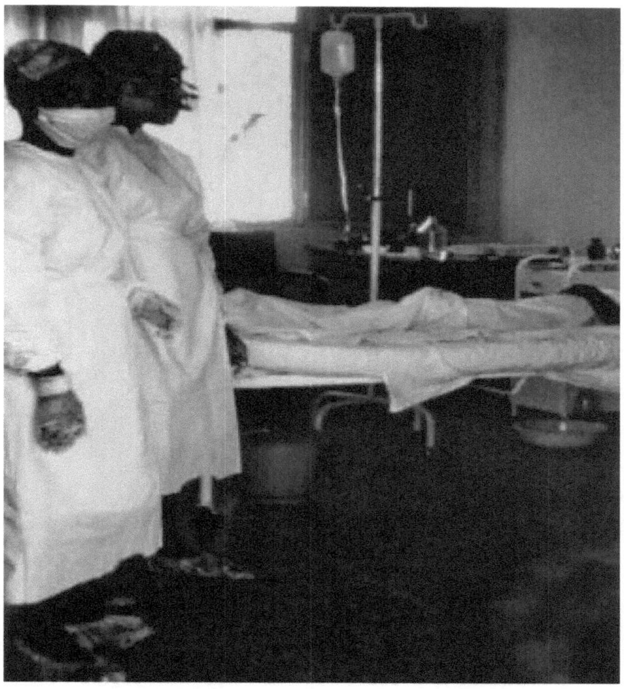

WHAT ARE VIRAL HEMORRHAGIC FEVERS?

The viral hemorrhagic fevers are a group of five RNA viruses that infect both humans and animals. As the name implies, these viruses lead to high fevers and bleeding or hemorrhages. They are very easily transmitted between host animals such as the fruit bat and humans. The genus Ebolavirus is included among the viral hemorrhagic fevers.

Signs of a hemorrhagic fever include flushing of the skin (skin turns red like you were embarrassed), petechiae (small red or purple spots from bleeding into the skin), outright bleeding such as from the nose, anus, or other areas, high fever, low blood pressure, shock, and death. Other less ominous signs are fever, muscle aches, lethargy (patient lays around tired and listless), nausea, vomiting, and diarrhea.

HOW IS EBOLA TRANSMITTED?

There are five species in the genus Ebolavirus known so far, and are named from where they were discovered. Ebola Zaire was originally discovered along the Ebola River in Zaire, which is now in the Democratic Republic of the Congo. It has since been renamed Ebolavirus (EBOV). The other four types are Reston (RESTV), Tai Forest (TAFV), Sudan (SUDV), and Bundibugyo ((BDBV). The Reston subtype infects primates but surprisingly has not been shown to infect humans. The genus Ebolavirus seems to be in the Philippines and Bangladesh as well as in Africa. This latest epidemic that is ravaging western Africa and is now in the United States is a new strain named Guinean Ebola Virus, named after the place of its outbreak in Meliandou, Guinea, in November of 2013. This new strain is related to previous strains but is genetically distinct, and for that reason it appears that it might very well have a different mode of transmission, possibly airborne. The University of Minnesota's Center for Infectious Disease Research and Policy recently published an article where they described the current strain of Ebola's mode of transmission as "unclear". The same article warned of transmission of this most recent strain as possibly from infected aerosol droplets that could spread it both near and at a distance from patients, suggesting that healthcare workers should be wearing respirators, not facemasks. That is hardly reassuring, and contradicts the CDC's public statements. If you take into consideration that the human pool of Ebola victims is currently the largest it has been in history, then the chance of further mutations in this latest strain of Ebola is enormous.

The epidemiology team tracking this latest outbreak already has found over 100 mutations in the first six months!

In a recent article in Science, of the fifty-eight members of the original science/ medical team tracking the virus, five died before the article was even published.

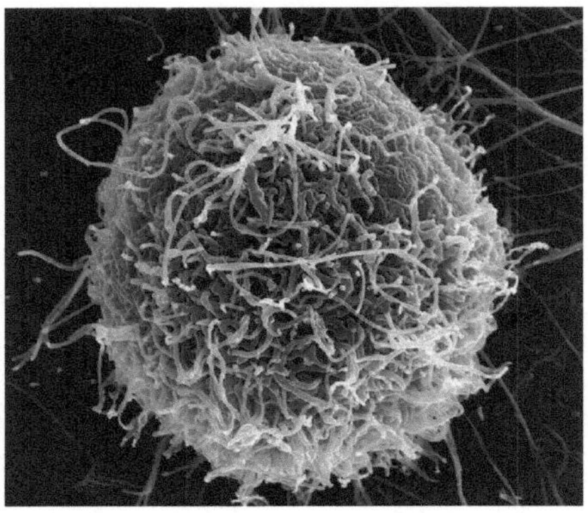

Photo of Ebolavirus particles on the surface of an infected cell.

Epidemiologists determine how far and wide an infection will spread through any population by using the "basic reproduction number", often abbreviated Ro (pronounced R naught). If one infected person spreads the virus on average to ten others, the virus (bacteria or fungi) has a basic reproduction rate or Ro of 10. If it only spreads to one other patient then it is stable and not spreading, or in decline. If the Ro is less than one, then the epidemic is dying out. Here in the United States, Ebola currently has a Ro of 2; no one knows what it is in Africa, but it appears to be much higher. The predictions for the number of new cases of Ebola in western Africa by the World Health Organization (WHO) made in September, 2014 for the month of October was 3,000 new cases, by October 7th they had already reached 8,376! The Ro seems to be rising much higher than the 2.1 they predicted for Sierra Leone and the 1.71 for Guinea. The WHO has now made a new prediction that this new strain of Ebola will probably become endemic among the human populations of western Africa .The CDC has also revised upward its earlier predictions that there will be 1.4 million new cases by the end of January, 2015. Overall, the trend is not good; a bad outbreak under ideal conditions could become a pandemic (an epidemic that spreads to many continents or even around the world).

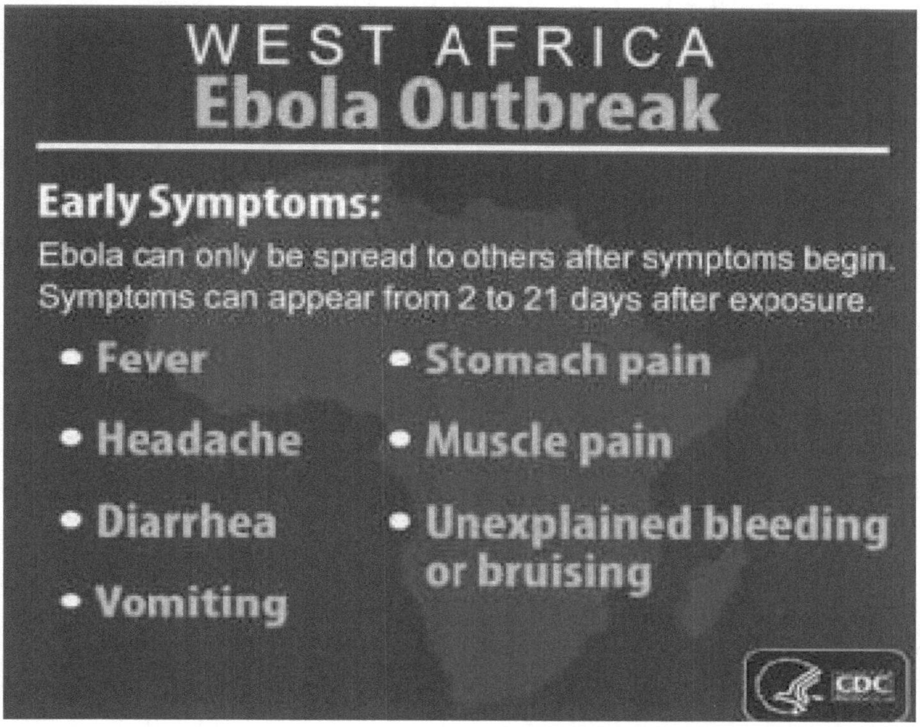

Nobody is quite sure, but it appears that Ebola originated either in fruit bats or monkeys, transferring the virus to humans by biting or exposure to the animals' blood or body fluids. Many Africans hunt wild animals for food. Their meat is referred to as bushmeat; the blood and body fluids of bushmeat can also be a source of disease transmission. The genus Ebolavirus only infects mammals, but seems to only be infecting primates such as monkeys, chimpanzees, and apes; so far no dogs, cats, etc. have been infected, even in Africa where the epidemic is currently raging.

Humans infect each other by exposure to body fluids, blood; sexual intercourse also can transmit the disease. When I say body fluids this includes sweat, tears, semen, feces, urine, saliva, vomit, and breast milk. Naturally you can also get Ebola from infected syringes, bloody gauze, etc. The WHO reports that even in patients that recover, the virus will survive and can be transmitted by their sperm for up to seven weeks after they seemed to have recovered. Recently there have been some reports of transmission through the air. This might explain some of the early cases like an American cameraman getting Ebola while on assignment in Africa. The official explanation was rather lame, saying he somehow got it from washing the car of an Ebola victim. Why would a cameraman wash an Ebola victim's car?

New evidence is emerging that Ebola can survive up to three weeks on a dry surface! Chlorine has been shown to kill the virus on surfaces, that is very important and I will come back to that shortly.

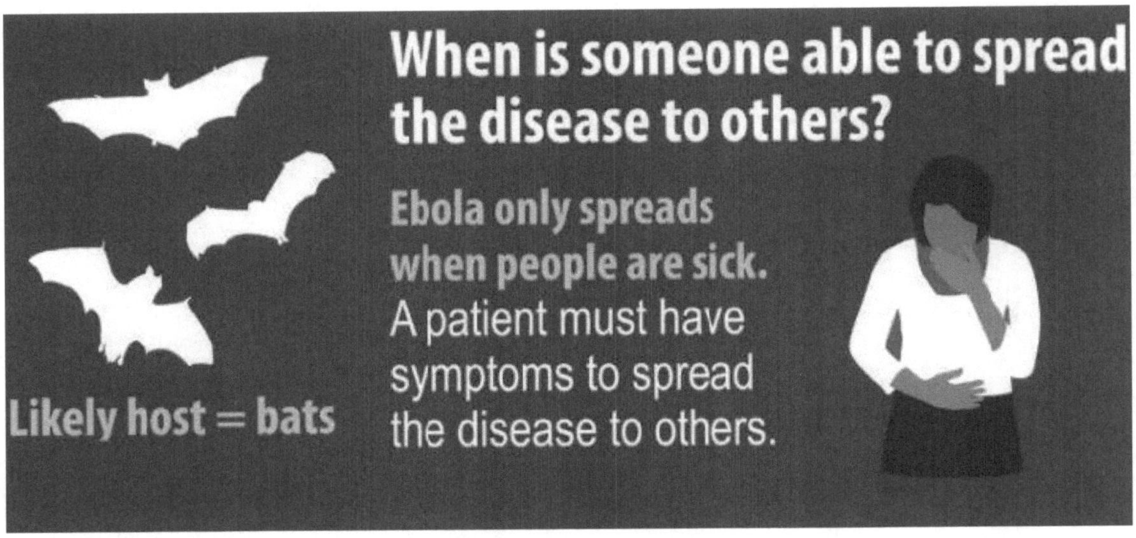

Not surprisingly, the United States government was not helpful at all, refusing to close our Southern border and prevent temporarily the admission of travelers holding passports from West African countries. They instead try to reassure us with ridiculous lies that the virus will not come here; one week later cases began to break out in the United States. Luckily we dodged that bullet during the last outbreak but how long will we remain lucky?

SYMPTOMS OF EBOLA

Ebola begins two days to three weeks after exposure. Many factors affect this incubation period, but primarily it is a consequence of viral load (the amount of viral particles in your blood), your immunity and your nutritional level, as well as the viral subtype with which the person was infected.

The Symptoms Of Ebola Come In Four Waves

1. The first wave includes fever, muscle aches, fatigue, sore throat and headaches.
2. The second wave involves vomiting, diarrhea, and rashes. At the same time the main organs of the body begin to fail, such as the liver and kidneys.
3. The third wave involves bleeding, both internally and externally. (inside the body and outside of it).
4. The fourth wave takes another one to two weeks and involves multiple organ failure, bleeding, shock, and ultimately death.

As you can readily see, the initial symptoms of an Ebola infection are common symptoms of many infections; that is the major problem with preventing its transmission, that is also a nightmare for healthcare workers such as doctors and nurses, who are on the frontline and undoubtedly many will become victims of this dreaded disease. How can I and my staff in my medical practice going to be able to do our jobs while at the same time protect us from this easily transmitted, deadly disease? The first cases in the United States were treated by doctors and nurses in hazmat suits, fully gowned and masked, and yet there was still accidental transmission of the virus; we cannot work in hazmat suits, where does that leave us?

The Ebolavirus already has mutated over one hundred times. These mutations are changing the behavior of the virus, as evidenced by the symptoms of its victims. According to the Center for

Disease Control (CDC) only 18 percent of the current Ebola patients have developed any hemorrhages! There is something different about the last outbreak that is very ominous; for that same reason I am dubious about the CDC's claims that Ebola cannot be transmitted through the air. No one has been able to explain many of the cases and it appears that some other form of transmission might very well be occurring.

Does Everyone Who is Exposed To Ebola Become Infected?

Here is where the entire Ebola epidemic becomes interesting. Depending on many factors, the death rate from Ebola is now hovering around 70-80 percent of those infected; the absolute numbers vary from country to country. Let's face it; relying upon poor third world countries such as those in western Africa for public health statistics is going to be problematic from the onset. Given that fact, let's try to look at this infection from the point of view of someone who is trying to avoid an infection and also if infected, how am I going to survive this nightmare. As a physician who has spent his entire life studying both conventional and alternative medical treatments, I often find myself looking at things from a radically different point of view. When I look at the Ebola epidemic, I first and foremost am looking at ways to prevent the transmission of the virus, and this means the people who were exposed to the virus and never contracted it.

We know they were exposed because we found IgG and IgM to Ebola in their blood; in other words, your body only makes antibodies to something it has been exposed to, no antibodies, no significant exposure.

Medical researchers are currently using the blood of patients who have recovered (survived) an Ebola infection. They take their blood and centrifuge it, separating the plasma (straw-colored fluid that contains the IgG and IgM antibodies) from the red blood cells. They then infuse this "convalescent serum" into the blood of current patients, thus providing them with valuable antibodies. One man who recovered, named Kent Brantly, has already donated more than a gallon of his blood to current Ebola patients. It is not clear if this strategy will work, it is further limited by compatibility issues, meaning the donor and the recipient need compatible blood types.

Secondly, I am looking at the 20-30 percent of Ebola patients who survived the infection, asking myself, why did they live and most of the others died? For me, those are the two questions that most need to be answered. Modern medicine seems to be walking lock-stepped, doubling down on finding a vaccine and treating already infected patients. They are using blood transfusions from survivors to treat the most recent infections. That is going to be problematic if a full pandemic develops because of loss of medical personnel from the infection, and the rate of infection is always going to outpace the survivor rate, thus making transfusion impractical. We need to find alternative approaches; that is where I am focusing my attention as the best approach for us.

In 1996 there were two outbreaks of Ebola in Gabon, Africa, both of which had an approximately 70 percent mortality rate. Scientists from Gabon's Franceville International Center for Medical Research studied both the victims and their families. Many of the family members had intimate contact with patients and presumably their infected body fluids while caring for them, yet many of them did not contract the disease. They found that over half of the symptom-free family members did have both IgG and IgM antibodies to Ebola, but never developed symptoms. Keep in mind, these friends and family members had contact with symptomatic patients and their bodily fluids -- only symptomatic patients can transmit the disease -- yet they never got Ebola! What is not yet clear is whether these patients have developed immunity to the species of Ebola they were exposed to, or are they immune to all species of Ebola?

During epidemics of every kind all throughout human history, there were always people who, despite significant exposure, did not contract any illness and seemingly sailed through unscathed.

The reason they did not become infected is that their cells and tissues were healthy enough that they vibrated at very strong frequencies, their extracellular and intracellular areas were bathed in fluids of not only the correct pH but also full of oxygen and life-giving nutrients, minerals, and trace elements, thus providing their bodies with the optimal "terrain". This optimal terrain enables them to resist most infections due to vibrant good health. Whenever this did not suffice they had their healthy, robust immune system response that, through various means including making antibodies such as IgG and IgM, was able to overcome any infection and contain it and then eradicate it. These antibodies serve as an immunological memory for the human body, thus if ever exposed to a similar microbe, it will remember it and quickly and effectively mount a robust defense and eradicate the invader.

Another interesting fact was that these same individuals also mounted a very strong anti- inflammatory response involving both cytokines and chemokines, both of which enhance the body's ability to eradicate these viral invaders. Cytokines are a family of proteins that are released by cells, that affect the behavior of other cells and sometimes even of the cell that released them. Cytokines are very important for cell signaling. Chemokines are a type of cytokine that causes chemotaxis, or the movement of cells towards a chemical.

TREATMENT OF EBOLA

Let me say emphatically from the outset, THESE ARE NOT CURES FOR EBOLA. However, there are many things we can do that if we get exposed to Ebola can either prevent us from becoming infected, or if we get infected will hopefully put us into the survivor category.

In my humble opinion, we have three opportunities to intervene with an Ebola infection. The first opportunity is in the prevention of exposure to the virus. This is by far the easiest point of intervention and the most effective. If that fails, we still have a second shot at bat. If we are exposed to the virus and it has now invaded our bodies, then our second opportunity is to prevent adherence to the cell and its subsequent invasion of the cell and spread to adjacent uninfected cells. That is more difficult than prevention, but easier than our third opportunity, which is treating an already established Ebola infection. Fail at this third opportunity point and there is a good chance you are going to die, in fact a seventy percent chance on average during an Ebola epidemic.

The Importance Of Lectins

When the body's immune system cells release these cytokines and chemokines, they travel in the blood to the liver and act as an early warning system, sounding the alarm that an infection is taking place. The liver responds by producing what is known as Acute Phase Reactants. These acute phase reactant proteins attack the invaders and further activate the immune system, as well as causing clotting of blood proteins around the invaders, walling them off and preventing any further infection by them. One type of these acute phase reactants are known as Lectins. Lectins are carbohydrate-binding proteins that form part of the innate immune system. These fascinating proteins are capable of pattern recognition, meaning they recognize the specific type of glycoproteins (a mix of glycol, or sugar, and protein shells) that are on the surface of various microorganisms such as fungi, bacteria, and in this case, viruses.

It is slowly emerging that one of the most important lectins produced by the body for its defense against viral and other invaders is Mannose Binding Lectin or MBL (also called Mannose Binding

Protein). MBL uses pattern recognition to identify these invaders and then attach themselves to the glycoproteins on their surface; once bound other members of the immune system destroy this MBL-microorganism complex, thus preventing an infection. Pattern recognition means exactly what it sounds like, every microorganism produces a glycoprotein coat or shell that is different, MBLs are able to determine the exact pattern these glycoproteins present and therefore recognize one microorganism from another. All of this technical information above was to demonstrate to you the importance of a healthy, robust immune system that is capable of producing large amounts of these MBL proteins, thus enabling the body to resist infections of all kinds, including Ebola. The flip side of this argument is that humans who are malnourished, exposed to environmental and other toxins, produce less of these MBL proteins and thus are more susceptible to infections of all types, especially Ebola.

MBL Protein And Red Algae

We fortunately have two ways to increase our MBL protein levels in our bodies. The first is to clean up our "terrain", limiting our exposure to toxins and pollution, correcting our acidic pH, making ourselves more alkaline, increasing our intake of healthy, organic, nutritious foods that provide the microRNA our bodies recognize, thus turning on our good health-promoting genes, providing a full spectrum of amino acids, fatty acids, enzymes, vitamins, fulvic acid, minerals, and trace elements. All of these along with adequate hydration with clean water, along with excellent oxygenation will make our bodies strong and capable of producing large amounts of MBL proteins as well as strengthening our entire immune systems.

The second way to increase our pool of MBL proteins is from sources outside of our bodies; fortunately for us there are other organisms that produce these, such as red algae. Red algae live in the world's oceans, where every drop of sea water contains copious amounts of viruses of all types. In order to survive in this viral pool the algae need to produce lots of MBL proteins to prevent themselves from becoming infected. There are over 6,000 species of red algae, some produce more than others, several of the superstar producers have been identified by scientists; they are currently feverishly working to produce these via recombinant DNA pathways in order to be able to patent their discovery. We on the other hand will use the natural source.

Red algae supplements are widely available and can be found online at Amazon, etc. Red algae also contain significant amounts of iodine and can be used for iodine supplementation; iodine supplementation benefits almost everyone but especially those who are hypothyroid.

L-Lysine

Another good idea is to supplement with L-lysine. L-lysine is an essential amino acid, meaning you have to get it in your diet. Diets high in sugar also lower L-lysine levels. L-lysine is known to help treat viral infections of all types, especially herpes simplex, the virus that causes cold sores. It works by blocking the receptors for arginine (another amino acid), which is essential for the replication of the herpes virus. It is less effective against genital herpes, but is thought to have overall antiviral activity and therefore might be useful in the treatment of Ebola; it certainly has no downside.

L-lysine is also helpful in the absorption of calcium, production of collagen, building muscle mass, production of enzymes, hormones, and antibodies of all types. L-lysine cannot be used in those who have renal impairment, and should be taken on an empty stomach. If you are going to take red algae supplements then I would take L-lysine as well as other immune boosters that I have outlined previously. Everything we can do to optimize our terrain will be helpful.

Sodium Bicarbonate And The Benefits Of An Alkaline PH

Someone who has been on the forefront of natural medicine treatments is Dr. Marc Sircus. He recently wrote a very interesting book entitled, *Treating Ebola and other Infectious Diseases with Natural Allopathic Medicine.* He also wrote an earlier book on sodium bicarbonate entitled *Sodium Bicarbonate: Rich man's, Poor man's Cancer Treatment.* Both are very interesting books chock-full of insights into both diseases, and I recommend both. He has a website, DrSircus.com and he calls his organization the International Medical Veritas Association. Veritas is Latin for truth.

Since Ebola appears to be mutating rapidly, and we do not currently have any effective treatment or a vaccine, we will need to find alternative methods of treatment. We need to exploit any weaknesses viral infections may have, finding their Achilles heel so to speak; one method is pH. It appears the vast majority, if not all viruses, depend on an environment that is moderately acidic.

Here is how it works in a nutshell. Viruses are the smallest living life forms on Earth, they are also parasitic and can live outside of a cell for some time, but eventually will die unless they gain entrance into a cell. Once inside a cell the viruses can either remain dormant or more commonly reproduce until they explode the cell and spread to adjacent cells. Remember the glycoprotein shell on virus particles that I described above; that same coat is how the virus gains entry into our cells. The glycoprotein coat attaches to the cell membrane (the envelope that surrounds all cells) and fuses to it; once fused, this allows the virus to enter the cell, where it takes over the cell's nucleus and begins to direct it to reproduce itself in great numbers. This fusion of the glycoprotein coat and the cell wall is pH dependent and usually requires a pH of less than 6. The hepatitis C virus, for example, requires a pH of between 5.5 and 6.3 to be able to fuse to the cell membrane. The Ebola virus also uses the same pH dependent fusion to gain entry into human cells, as does the common cold viruses and influenza (the flu).

Historically there is very credible evidence that changing the intracellular (the area between cells or what I described earlier as the terrain) pH to a more alkaline condition helps to prevent viral invasion of human cells. The Arm & Hammer company, which makes baking soda, reports that baking soda was used by some doctors quite successfully during the Spanish flu of 1918, which killed millions of people worldwide.

I think it is a very wise method of both preventing and treating Ebola, given the current lack of any treatment for Ebola and the fact that alkalinizing your body is quite safe, especially for short-term treatment of infections.

Sodium bicarbonate (baking soda) is very safe, however there are some precautions that you must do. The most important is never taking baking soda if you have a really full stomach; believe it or not, this could burst your stomach from the additional gas production. If you decide to take it for a long time to alkalinize your body then you should follow your pH with urinary pH strips, to ensure that you do not overdo it and become too alkaline, which is just as dangerous as too acidic. Your body flourishes at the correct pH, moving it in either direction is harmful.

During the 1918 Spanish Flu epidemic doctors used sodium bicarbonate to treat flu patients with the following dosages:

Day 1: Dissolve one-half teaspoonful of baking soda in a glass of cold water and drink it every two hours for a total of six doses.

Day 2: Using the same mix take four doses at two hour intervals.

Day 3: Take the same dose morning and evening.

Day 4 and after: One dose every morning until the cold is healed.

Vitamin C

Vitamin C has a long history of use as a treatment for everything from the common cold to high intravenous doses to cure otherwise hopeless cases of cancer. Any stress, including infections, causes the body to consume its vitamin C by utilizing it in its role as a powerful antioxidant. We know this indirectly because normally if you take a high dose of vitamin C, since it is water soluble and is not stored in the body in any appreciable quantities, you will urinate out any excess that your body did not use. If you have an infection, cancer, or any other severe stress, your body's needs for vitamin C skyrocket. Once again, we know this by giving huge doses either orally, intravenously or both; as the infection worsens the body's needs go up hand in hand, and even after huge doses there is no vitamin C found in the urine.

According to *Cecil's Textbook of Medicine*, one of the proposed mechanisms for the hemorrhages caused by the family of hemorrhagic viruses is capillary fragility. Capillary fragility is known to be caused by vitamin C deficiency, and is corrected by its administration (taking vitamin C).

A severe deficiency of vitamin C is known as scurvy. Some of the hallmarks of scurvy are bleeding into the skin and bleeding from mucous membranes such as the mouth and gums.

Vitamin C is also an essential part of the antioxidant cascade that is known to protect the body from infections. As part of the water soluble arm of this cascade vitamin C and glutathione help to both regenerate each other and alpha lipoic acid also regenerates both of them. On the fat soluble arm of the antioxidant cascade there is vitamin E and CoQ10 which also regenerate each other and also are regenerated by alpha lipoic acid (which is unique in it being both fat and water soluble). You cannot supplement glutathione, since it is removed and destroyed in the digestive tract, but I would supplement the other four -- alpha lipoic acid, vitamins C and E, and CoQ10 -- along with a good mineral and trace element supplement such as Supreme Fulvic. Glutathione is dependent upon selenium, sulfur for its production so it is important to make sure these are well represented in your diet.

Many of the victims of Ebola in Africa are malnourished from poverty and poor diets, their intake of vitamin C is quite seasonal, depending on the local fruit and vegetable production, and as such they are presumably much more vulnerable to infections such as Ebola. Either way, even if they had adequate vitamin C levels, the supplementation of vitamin C in infected patients has absolutely no downside and may very well save their lives. The family of hemorrhagic viruses which includes Ebola has been shown to rapidly consume large quantities of vitamin C, thus requiring unusually large quantities to treat the infection.

As a baseline, before you are ill, I would take between 1,000 and 2,000 mg of vitamin C daily, in divided doses. Vitamin C is water soluble so you do not need to take it with food. There is a fat soluble form of vitamin C called liposomal vitamin C. If there was an outbreak of Ebola anywhere near you I would immediately raise the dose of your vitamin C intake until you develop diarrhea, then back it off by 25 percent or so and see what happens, if you still have diarrhea reduce it another 25 percent.

The diarrhea or bowel tolerance is a good sign of how much vitamin C your body is consuming; it is not a fixed number and will rise and fall as your immune system wins or loses its battle with the virus. All viruses are susceptible to large doses of vitamin C; the trick is finding the correct dosage.

For our purposes I would keep a large supply of vitamin C handy, it is very inexpensive and is absolutely essential for your long- term health, especially in the wintertime when your supply of locally grown fresh fruit and vegetables will be exhausted.

Lomatium Dissectum

Lomatium dissectum is a plant in the carrot family and grows wild in the Pacific Northwest of the United States; there it has been used locally by Indian tribes for many centuries. It is an amazing plant, having antibacterial, antifungal, and antiviral properties. In fact, it is one of the strongest antiviral medicinal plants known, and was instrumental in saving many people who were wise enough to use it during the Spanish Flu of 1918. See the chapter on colds and flu for a more detailed explanation.

There are various ways of taking Lomatium dissectum:

Tincture: Take 2-4 ml four times a day.

Tea: Take one or two teaspoons of the dried herb in a cup of boiling water, allow it to steep for twenty minutes or so, strain it and drink this up to three times a day.

Capsules: Take 500 mg up to four times a day, until symptoms resolve.

It is oftentimes combined with elderberry juice and/or oregano oil; this combination potentiates it (makes it stronger).

Minerals To The Rescue: Zinc, Selenium

Zinc is helpful in the treatment of all viral infections. As far back as 1974 zinc supplementation has been shown to inhibit the reproduction of rhinoviruses, which are the viruses responsible for many colds. Zinc has been shown to have antiviral activity but the exact mechanism remains unknown.

Many of the enzyme systems in the body, as well as the immune system, require zinc to properly function, and this may very well be the mechanism by which it exerts it antiviral effects, but this is pure conjecture on my part (I am guessing). One of the known mechanisms for zinc's antiviral function is it prevents the adherence of viral particles to the cell membrane, so supplementing zinc acts similar to alkalinizing the pH. Zinc also has been shown to increase the production of white blood cells which are the most vital components of your immune system. Zinc is present in over 3,000 different proteins in your body as well as being essential to activate over 200 different enzymes. Your body cannot store zinc in any appreciable quantities and therefore must be taken daily.

Like most minerals, zinc is best absorbed when bound to a protein or chelated, try to buy your zinc supplements in this form for best absorption; otherwise you are just wasting a lot of zinc. Examples of chelated zinc are: zinc acetate, zinc gluconate, and zinc citrate. Caffeine also interferes with zinc absorption so do not take any zinc supplements with coffee, tea, or caffeinated products.

However, given the lethality of the Ebola infection and the almost total lack of side effects from supplementation with zinc, the multitude of benefits including antiviral activity, it would be stupid to not add this to our treatment protocol.

I would supplement with 50 mg of chelated zinc once a day; if an outbreak of Ebola occurs in your area I would double or triple this dose.

NOTE: If you use zinc supplements for a prolonged period (months), this will eventually lower your copper levels and you will need to supplement copper as well; short-term treatment will not need copper supplementation. As I have stated several times earlier in this book, for long-term zinc supplementation, the dose of copper should be 1 mg per 50 mg of zinc daily.

Selenium is a mineral with known antioxidant as well as anti-inflammatory effects, and being an important part of the immune system. Like many minerals, selenium is becoming progressively more deficient in our soils, consequently human selenium levels are decreasing around the world. Areas with the least selenium in the soil have the highest cancer rates. Also like many other minerals there are many enzymes that are dependent on selenium to properly function.

Selenium helps the immune system in many ways, one of which is the family of enzymes dependent upon its function known as the selenoproteins, which are responsible for the prevention of oxidation, without which viruses are better able to mutate and their infections last longer! That sentence alone should be enough to make you supplement with selenium when there is a local outbreak of Ebola or any virus for that matter.

AIDS patients showed a dramatic improvement in their immune responses when supplemented with selenium. Once again, selenium supplementation is a win-win situation, it helps prevent and treat viral infections, helps prevent cancer, and helps support your immune system, with no downside.

Selenium And Glutathione

Glutathione is dependent upon N-acetylcysteine, magnesium, sulfur, and selenium for its production, supplementation is difficult because it is destroyed in the digestive tract.

Garlic and cottage cheese are wonderful dietary sources of easily absorbed sulfur, and probably explains many of the health benefits of garlic recognized as far back as ancient Egypt. Sulfur also is found in large concentrations in onions, garlic, scallions, and leeks.

Glutathione is a very important link in the antioxidant cascade and is essential to fight off any viral infection, especially Ebola. Every cell in the body produces glutathione, and its level in our cells is predictive of how long we will live!

Without adequate levels of glutathione our bodies cannot chelate and remove many of the toxins and heavy metals that modern man is so exposed to; acid residues, toxins, and heavy metals thus accumulate in the cell and result in disease and cell death. This acidic environment is also conducive to viral infections such as Ebola. Glutathione acts as a natural scavenger, circulating through the body, attaching itself to anything foreign like toxins and most importantly virus particles (as well as bacteria and fungi) and eliminates them from the body.

There is a family of enzymes that are selenium dependent and acts similar to glutathione called glutathione peroxidase. These enzymes are antioxidants and also act as strong free radical scavengers. This family of enzymes has eight members; some are found in the entire body, but most are tissue specific, for example found only in the intestines. One type is found in sperm and protects the delicate sperm from being oxidized and thus damaged, for this reason a selenium deficiency often leads to male infertility. The good news is that most freshly grown, organic fruits and vegetables are high in glutathione peroxidases.

Recent studies on the highly infectious Zaire form of Ebola has shown the virus to ravage patients who are selenium deficient. The mechanism for this is somewhat confusing and beyond the scope of this book, but there is a lengthy very technical explanation of it at Orthomolecular.org, the website of the Linus Pauling Institute. Treatment with selenium has been shown to help the severe cytokine Under normal conditions the recommended dose of selenium is 60-75 mcg (micrograms or a millionth of a gram, whereas milligrams are a thousandth of a gram) daily, or 1 mcg per kg (a kilogram is roughly 2.2 lbs). Selenium is toxic at doses greater than 500 mcg/day.

I would recommend taking 200 mcg/day for protection from cancer and for general health reasons; if there is an Ebola outbreak I would double that to 400 mcg/day (in two divided doses).

The above doses are primarily for inorganic selenium. As I have said many times in this book, it is much better to get organic forms of minerals and vitamins so your body can absorb them better. The same holds true for selenium; its inorganic form is difficult to absorb and minimally raises selenium levels in patients. Examples of the inorganic forms are sodium selenite and sodium selenate. Examples of the organic form are selenium methionate (selenomethionine), selenocysteine, and brewer's yeast grown in a high selenium culture. Brewer's yeast (Saccharomyces cerevisiae) grown in such a culture naturally chelates and incorporates the selenium in an organic form, making it readily accessible to the body, along with B vitamins, enzymes and amino acids. Spirulina is also grown in ponds that are enriched with selenium and they too chelate it, just like brewer's yeast, making it organic and readily absorbable. Both brewer's yeast and spirulina chelate selenium with sulfur-containing amino acids (building blocks to proteins) such as methionine.

Four Thieves Vinegar Or Master Tonic

Four thieves vinegar or master tonic is always a good choice whenever you are suffering with a viral, bacterial, fungal or parasitic illness, since it has activity against all of them.

If you are very ill then I would take one tablespoon of master tonic every four to six hours until I fully recovered. If you are not improving I would take two tablespoons every 6 hours. This has great broad spectrum coverage as well as immune boosting properties that make it ideal for almost any infection.

Chlorine And Miracle Mineral Solution

Miracle Mineral Solution uses the chemical chlorine dioxide as its active ingredient; it is very different from chlorine. Chlorine is an element with the atomic number of 17. It exists as a yellow-green gas when pure, however it rarely if ever is pure in nature and frequently combines with other elements to produce a more stable form, many times forming salts such as sodium chloride which is table salt.

Chlorine dioxide on the other hand is also a yellow-green gas, but that is where any similarities between the two end. Chlorine dioxide is a powerful oxidant, and as such accepts electrons from other substances, for this reason it kills disease-causing organisms and also destroys some diseased tissues, but spares healthy tissue and normal cells within the human body.

Chlorine has been phased out over the last few decades as a water purification agent due to its production of cancer-causing agents known as Trihalomethanes (THMs); it has been replaced by chlorine dioxide, which does not produce THMs and is considered safe. Chlorine also reacts with nitrogen-containing compounds to form chloroform, but it does not produce bromochloromethanes, which are harmful compounds. Chlorine dioxide does not produce any of these harmful byproducts, and is now widely used in the food industry to clean foods and kill off harmful bacteria including E. Coli and others, and is considered safe.

To make Miracle Mineral Supplement (or Solution) you start with sodium chlorite which is very alkaline and also a very stable substance. You add citric acid to it to acidify it and this produces the chlorine dioxide (CL02) gas, which smells like chlorine or bleach, and is also yellow-green in color, but otherwise has no similarities to chlorine. This new chlorine dioxide is a very powerful antimicrobial agent as well as being antiparasitic (it kills parasites), but fortunately it does not kill friendly probiotic bacteria such as the lactobacillus species in our gut.

In medicine, we have been using chlorine dioxide to sterilize red blood cells for transfusion. It was even found that a 2.8 percent solution of sodium chlorite when activated with 15 percent lactic acid at a concentration of 1:100 killed all HIV in red blood cells!

Miracle Mineral Solution is a two part liquid that, when drank mixed in water, releases chlorine dioxide into the blood, disinfecting it of any microbes. MMS was developed by an American miner in South America named Jim Humble, in a desperate attempt to save him and his friends who were coming down with malaria. It worked beyond his wildest expectations; he even wrote a book about it called *Breakthrough, The Miracle Mineral Solution of the 21st Century*. In his book he claims to have successfully treated malaria on 75,000 patients in Africa. The presumed mechanism is that chlorine dioxide kills the malarial parasites by oxidation of its vital antioxidants, including glutathione, coenzyme A, and alpha lipoic acid. If MMS is capable of entering into a parasite and killing off its antioxidants, it most likely is doing the same thing in our bodies, to a limited extent, for that reason it is important to supplement with antioxidants while using MMS.

Since oxidants and antioxidants cannot be mixed without negating each other, you should not take any antioxidants such as vitamins A, C, and E, CoQ10, alpha lipoic acid, grapeseed extracts, etc. for three hours before or after MMS.

MMS is not approved for use in the United States, except to disinfect water, and is sold as such with a wink and a nod on the internet. As of October 2014, it has been banned in Canada and any supplies of it have been seized by the government, citing safety concerns.

In a scenario where there is a rapidly spreading fatal pandemic such as Ebola, with no other viable options, this could be a game changer for you. I have used it several times on family and myself. If you can, get past the bleach smell -- it smells identical to bleach. But there are only thirty drops or less and you can mix it with another drink to mask the flavor. However, the new drink cannot contain vitamin C (like orange juice) or it will diminish its strength. The reason is that MMS is a strong oxidant, and vitamin C is a strong antioxidant, hence they will negate each other.

MMS is touted as having strong antibacterial, antifungal, antiparasitic, and antiviral properties. Most viral illnesses are effectively treated with MMS, however hepatitis C, Lyme disease, and HIV, although showing improvement, proved to be more resistant to its effects. It is important to note that very high dose antioxidants such as vitamin C have proven to be very effective against virtually all viral illnesses; the orthomolecular literature is replete with examples of successful treatments.

It may also cause nausea, and therefore you may have to start with a lower dose and work your way up. You can reduce the nausea by taking it with a meal, but this also will weaken the effect of the MMS. Another strategy is to take it at bedtime so you sleep through any potential nausea. I started with a high dose and fortunately did not develop any nausea or side effects. The good news is that it is absorbed rapidly and most times cures malaria, blood poisoning, and other acute infections in one dose. This rapid absorption through mucous membranes can be exploited for those who are having problems with nausea or even vomiting. Instead of drinking it down, swish it around your mouth and throat and hold it there for a few minutes, allowing it to absorb. It can also be used intravaginally for women suffering with chronic candida infections. If the acidity of the solution burns, you can add a little sodium bicarbonate (baking soda) before adding the water to the mix.

Since MMS is so powerful, sometimes a Herxheimer reaction may occur. A Herxheimer reaction is caused by rapid kill off of microbes that release their contents into the blood; this often results in a flu-like illness that lasts for several hours causing fatigue, fever, chills, diarrhea, joint, and muscle pain.

It is the antiviral properties that make it so attractive in the case of an Ebola epidemic. There are reports warning of its potential toxicity, but there were no people coming forth anywhere saying they were harmed by it. There are many anecdotal reports in Jim Humble's book, as well as many online, the vast majority praising it. In a situation where there is a major outbreak of Ebola, at least you will have something to take that very well may work to clear your blood of the virus.

Chlorine is used topically to disinfect for Ebola, and works quite well, so why not chlorine dioxide? Currently the only treatments being utilized on Ebola victims are IV fluid support, antibiotics in case there is a bacterial super infection, painkillers, transfusions, and some use of convalescent serum taken from survivors. We are working on vaccines, and one is in clinical testing, but it will not be soon enough, if an epidemic starts to spread rapidly.

We have no effective anti-viral therapies, yet we keep marching in lockstep, off the cliff of good intentions. We need to start thinking outside the box. We need to try new therapies like this and the others I named above. What do we have to lose? We have absolutely no standard effective antiviral therapies; why not enlarge our bag of tricks? Why limit ourselves to the same losing plan, is that not the definition of insanity, doing the same thing over and over again and expecting a different outcome? This Ebola outbreak might mutate and weaken and eventually die out, or just smolder in occasional hot spots, or it might go the other way, which is everyone's biggest fear. Recent outbreaks behavior has been described by epidemiologists as, "burning hot", meaning its symptoms arise quicker and are more severe, and in a shorter time frame. That is not a good portent of things to come.

I think if it were truly as toxic as some people warn, there would have been a large number of patients injured, with reports everywhere its name comes up, but there were none. I and many people I know have used it with absolutely no problems, and some success in eradicating some wicked viral colds and bronchitis. How it will work against Ebola is anyone's guess. But, I do know this. There are only four hospitals with level 4 isolation beds available in the entire United States; the recent debacle in a good hospital in Dallas emphasizes the ill-preparedness of almost all hospitals. With that being the case, what is going to happen to the system with 10,000 or 50,000 or 1 million Ebola cases?

The system will collapse, worsened by the large number of deaths of doctors, nurses, and other medical personnel. There is no way any medical system can remain viable with such a lethal disease cutting swathes through its ranks. What happens then? It is not easy at all to replace a physician; you are talking about usually a minimum of eleven years of training, plus countless years of experience honing their medical skills. Nurses are easier to replace, but I doubt there will be a lot of volunteers for what will practically be a suicide mission.

The dose of Miracle Mineral Solution is dependent upon the concentration of the mixture. The sodium chlorite part is always the same, but the citric acid activator can come as 10 percent or 50 percent. You can also use lemon juice or vinegar as an activator, but it is much less effective and will result in less chlorine dioxide in the end product. With the 10 percent citric acid activator you need to use a ratio of 5 drops citric acid to 1 drop of sodium chlorite, if it is a 50 percent citric acid mix, then you can mix them one to one.

Start off slowly to see how you tolerate it, but a mix of 3 drops of sodium chlorite to either 15 drops of the 10 percent or 3 drops of the 50 percent. Allow the chlorine dioxide to sit for three minutes and then mix it in a glass of water or juice, and drink it down. You can increase the quantity of the sodium chlorite to 12 to 15 drops at a time, always mixing it with the citric acid activator with the same ratio depending upon the percentage of the concentration. For viral illnesses that are severe like Ebola, you can take the mix many times a day, the chlorine dioxide only lasts an hour or so in your blood. For most other illnesses it will only take one dose or so to do the trick, such as flu and malaria. But, if you think it did not do the trick you can repeat it.

NOTE: I am not recommending its use; I am only describing to you how it can be used. It is not approved for use in humans by the United States or Canadian governments. This is for informational purposes only and should not be construed as medical advice of any type. This book is written with the assumption that either you do not have access to medical treatment or are totally against traditional treatments and want to know what other options are available to you. As such, many of the treatments I describe in this book would not ordinarily be utilized. However, in such a scenario with no other options available and no standard medical care available, these options mentioned, such as MMS, become more viable and might very well be your only option available. MMS should not be used by anyone until they consult their local laws concerning its legality.

CHAPTER FORTY

ALTERNATIVE MEDICAL DEVICES

INTRODUCTION

TABLE OF CONTENTS:

WHAT IS SCENAR?

Scenar is a Russian invention, developed by the Soviets for medical treatment of their cosmonauts without the use of drugs in space. Scenar is short for Self Controlling Energy Neuro Adaptive Regulator.

According to the company, Scenar is a short pulse electronic neuro- adaptive therapeutic stimulator or what they describe as a small but very effective compact device offering electrotherapy.

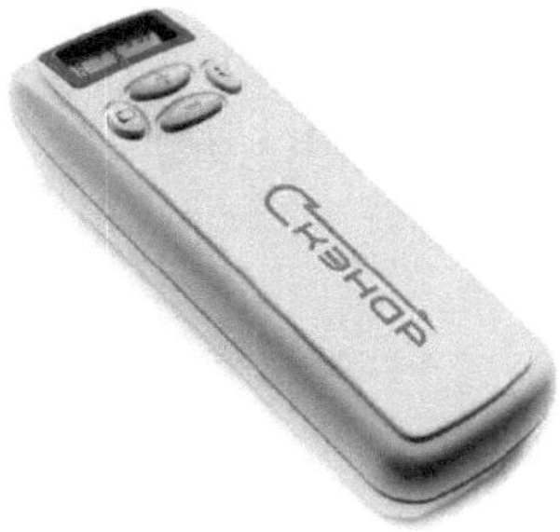

HOW DOES SCENAR WORK?

What the heck does this mean in English? Basically this machine measures electromagnetic signals from the body that are very similar to the signals emitted by our own nerves. These same nerve signals are carried along special nerves to the brain where they cause the release of neuropeptides which cause much more rapid healing to occur. Neuropeptides are small protein molecules released by neurons or nerve cells to communicate with other parts of the brain or other neurons. Scenar is able to read these signals and then mimic them by producing an electromagnetic signal that is almost identical to the original nerve signal. Basically, Scenar enters into a dialogue with your brain, transmitting and retransmitting electromagnetic nervous signals scores of times per second. Scenar does this along the original pathway used by the pain signals to your brain and modifies them, causing the release of those healing neuropeptides to the involved areas.

Scenar, when applied to a point of pain, also causes the release of endorphins which are the human body's own pain-killing chemicals.

Those two mechanisms in essence are the modalities used by Scenar to heal tissues and decrease pain.

SCENAR VS. TENS

Scenar does not involve any drugs and does not break the skin or cross it in any way other than by its electromagnetic waves. It does not hurt, and only causes a very mild tingling sensation at the site where it is applied to the skin. The Scenar is placed on the skin over a painful or injured area and the first thing it does is collect electromagnetic signals from the patient's body. Using its specially designed software, it modifies these signals and sends them back to the body. This biofeedback by the Scenar is what distinguishes it from other electrotherapy devices like TENS units.

TENS stands for Transcutaneous (crossing the skin) Electrical Nerve Stimulation and is essentially a device that creates electrical current that has been shown to interfere with the production of pain by the nerves of the affected area. The difference between a TENS unit and a SCENAR is like night and day.

A TENS unit only works by sending an electrical current along the involved nervous pathways and hopes to interfere with further pain production. A SCENAR on the other hand, first measures the electromagnetic waves being emitted by the body and then mimics those exact electromagnetic wave forms and sends them back to the body. It is much more specific and therefore much more effective.

SCENAR is very safe and can be used in combination with other types of treatment without any interference or problems of any kind. SCENAR however has not been tested in pregnant women, which is no real surprise when one considers the malpractice climate created in the United States by the legal profession. SCENAR also cannot be used on people with a cardiac pacemaker or who suffer with epilepsy (seizures); the reason for that is the electrical impulses might interfere with the pacemaker or stimulate a part of the brain that might lead to seizure activity.

HOW TO USE A SCENAR DEVICE

The typical session of treatment with a SCENAR takes about a half hour and involves repeatedly moving the SCENAR device (which looks like a TV remote control) over the involved area. Patients should not wash for two hours before or after a treatment and should not overexert themselves for the same amount of time.

If the area being treated is hairy, it might interfere with the contact made between the SCENAR and the skin, and if possible should be shaved. Acute problems (recent, not chronic) may resolve in three or four sessions, and usually continue to work long after each session is completed, chronic problems will take more sessions.

Since it is noninvasive and has no interaction with other treatments, there is no problem with using it for multiple treatments. Most patients report that they continue to improve for from three to five months after the treatments are completed. SCENAR may make the skin either red or pale and a feeling of "stickiness" has been described as the machine passes over an involved area that has been treated adequately, this is the body's signal that the treatment session is completed.

WHAT CONDITIONS DOES SCENAR TREAT?

The SCENAR can be used to treat any muscle, joint, bone, ligament, or soft tissue injury. It can be used to treat pain of any type, including migraine headaches and dental pain. It also has been reported to be useful for digestive problems when applied to the abdomen directly over the involved organ. I am not sure of the mechanism involved but it has been reported many times to be quite useful in shortening the length of infections of the respiratory tract and others, including some serious infections involving deep tissues within the body such as bone infections.

None of this is really surprising when you stop to think about the human body and how it functions. Every atom in nature vibrates at a certain frequency, every tissue of the body vibrates at certain frequencies, the brain and the heart are electrical organs generating endless electrical and magnetic waves. We use electrocardiograms (EKG or ECG), the K is from the original German translation) to measure those electrical waves at the body's surface. EEGs (electroencephalograms) placed on a patient's skull measure the constant waves of electrical activity that wash over the brain many times per second, these cycles per second are measured as hertz. One hertz is one cycle per second; these were named after the German scientist Heinrich Hertz who was the first scientist to conclusively prove the existence of electromagnetic waves.

The human body, like all living things, has its own magnetic field and the only way an electric current can be generated by the body is by passing a flow of electrically charged material through a magnetic field. By the way, that is the same way electricity is generated.

We have only in recent times become aware of the importance of the electromagnetic spectrum of the body and its importance to health, so it is only natural that we will learn ways to manipulate those same magnetic fields to treat certain diseases. Scenar is the first step in that direction and is rapidly proving itself to be very useful for a variety of medical conditions.

SCENAR AND ALTERNATIVE MEDICINE

I think these electromagnetic devices are certainly just in their infancy and so at this point "we don't know what we don't know". From my perspective that is a great opportunity for those of us interested in alternative medical treatments for pain and orthopedic injuries etc.

There are various models available in many price ranges, and many are advertised on eBay and other internet sites. I would stick to the Scenar and not buy any cheaper inferior models that may or may not work. The Russians took a long time to develop the software that is the heart of this machine, I am not sure that the many Scenar knockoffs out there have taken the same time and therefore will probably not work as well, but that is just my humble opinion and might not have any basis in reality. The only device that I think is equally valuable is the Tennant Biomodulator, which I will describe in the following section.

The Scenar is something that probably should be included in any alternative medicine chest due to its amazing versatility and totally noninvasive nature.

PART TWO: THE TENNANT BIOMODULATOR

The Tennant Biomodulator (TBM) is a handheld device very similar to the Scenar, developed and manufactured in the United States by Dr. Jerry Tennant. Dr. Tennant also has written a superb book on the subject of electricity and its treatment of various diseases called *Healing is Voltage* that I highly recommend for anyone interested in this fascinating subject.

You can get a Tennant biomodulator for home use, but you need a prescription from a doctor; I try to only mention things that do not require a prescription, but occasionally some do, like EpiPen's and some others. I am not sure why this requires a prescription.

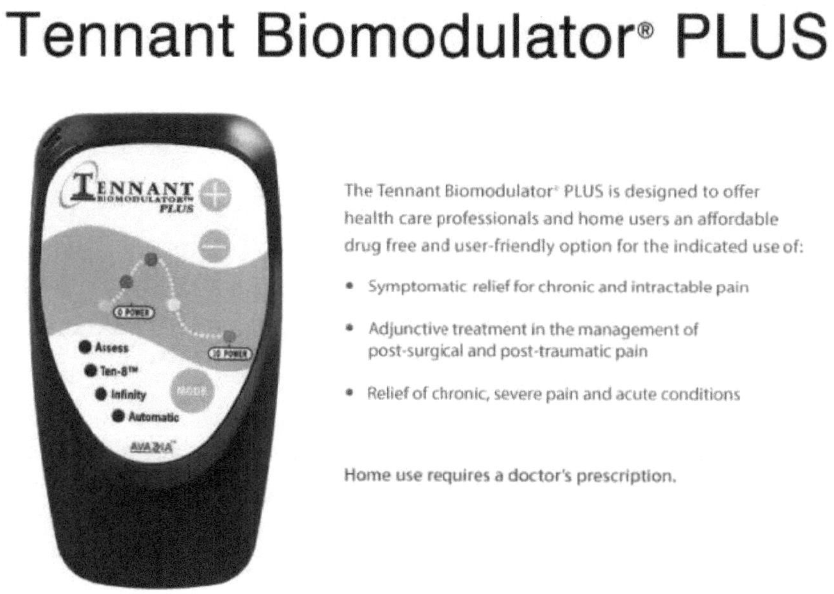

How Does The Tennant Biomodulator Work?

Similar to the Scenar, the TBM is a handheld electrical device that is a transcutaneous (crosses the skin) electrical nerve stimulator coupled with a biofeedback machine. TBM's primary role is in pain relief, but unlike a TENS unit, it transmits over various frequencies finding the exact frequency that matches the body part involved and donates electrons and helps raise voltage and pH of those cells, therefore promoting healing.

Electricity And Your Cells

What does raising the voltage actually do for your cells? The cells of your body are designed to run optimally at -20 mv (millivolts or a thousandth of a volt, microvolts are a millionth of a volt). In order to produce new cells or for healing cells the body needs to raise their voltage to -50 mv. When the voltage of a cell drops below -20 mv you begin to develop chronic diseases. At less than -20 mv the energy of the cells drops and they do not have the available energy to perform all their normal tasks and functions. There have been more than 70 published medical studies confirming that pain also begins when the cell's voltage or pH drops below -20 mv. Both a drop in voltage or pH will decrease the amount of oxygen in the cells.

This causes a switch from aerobic (with oxygen) metabolism to anaerobic (without oxygen) metabolism. So, why does that make you tired? The reason is that aerobic metabolism is much more efficient than anaerobic metabolism and aerobic metabolism produces sixteen times more ATP, which is the molecule your body utilizes for its energy. Also anaerobic metabolism is that which is favored by harmful microorganisms (germs) and allows them to flourish and therefore cause disease.

What Is The Voltage Of My Cells?

How do you know what your cells' voltages are? This can be easily done with the TBM using its access mode and applying the electrodes to the skin above the target organ. You can also measure the voltage with a voltmeter, however it is difficult due to the fact that the electricity of the body pulses and is not a steady stream.

What Causes Low Cell Voltage?

How did your cells get low in voltage? There are four primary reasons for low cellular pH and voltage, and they are:

Hypothyroidism

Thyroid disorders, especially low thyroid function or hypothyroidism is an epidemic in this country and is severely under diagnosed. The tests for thyroid function are not very good and other factors are contributing to this such as lack of iodine in the soils and consequently our diets, the wide use of bromines and fluorine that displace iodine and produce worthless inactive thyroid hormone. Hypothyroidism used to be diagnosed by clinical findings rather than lab tests. Since body temperature is controlled by the thyroid's effect on stimulating metabolism, a low-functioning thyroid will result in decreased body temperature. This method was utilized for the diagnosis of hypothyroidism before the advent of blood tests by checking body temperature in the morning before getting out of bed. Hypothyroidism also causes fatigue, constipation, hair loss, periorbital (around the eyes) swelling and cold intolerance (you always feel cold).

Supplying your body with a steady supply of supplemental iodine is a good idea with little downside if done properly and can be done with 5 drops of nascent iodine daily in a glass of fresh water or by using kelp or Iodoral daily (12.5 mg).

For you west coasters this also has the benefit of protecting your thyroids from the steady stream of radiation still coming from Fukushima or has everyone already forgotten that there are still hot reactors there that the Japanese cannot control. The prevailing winds and currents blow west towards Hawaii, Alaska and the west coast of the United States.

Trans Fats

Trans fats are vegetable oils that are treated through an industrial process that adds hydrogen to them which transforms them to a solid at room temperature, thus their other name "partially hydrogenated fats". Food manufacturers use trans fats because they are less likely to spoil and thus have a longer shelf life. Fast food restaurants also use trans fats in their fryers because the oils do not to be changed as frequently.

Trans fats such as margarine and other abnormal fats are horrible for your health. These trans fats get incorporated in the cell walls and cannot function like normal body fat, they are closer in structure and function to plastic than fat! Since they have an abnormal structure they cannot conduct electrical impulses properly and therefore cause a drop in the voltage of the cells and promote pain and disease. Avoid these trans fats as much as possible.

Canola oil is another example of an unhealthy trans fat and should not be part of your diet. Fat is essential for our health and the current war against fat is very misguided; without enough essential fats you cannot survive much less be healthy. They are called essential for a reason.

Heavy Metal Poisoning

Since the modern environment in which we live is heavily polluted with a wide variety of heavy metals, we have absorbed these harmful substances which poison our bodies and prevent adequate cell function and thereby decrease the voltage of our cells. Heavy metals are harmful because they damage the mitochondria, which is the powerhouse of the cell that produces ATP or the energy molecules our cells utilize. Heavy metals such as mercury, lead, and cadmium all destroy mitochondria and drop the voltage of the cells affected. Unfortunately 80 percent of the mercury in our bodies comes from dental fillings! I personally hate going to the dentist and having any dental procedures done, especially getting a filling; there is no way I am going to have all my fillings redone even though it is highly recommended! Bottom line, there are certain things I will do to help my health and others that are just too painful, this is one of the latter.

Be careful of products originating in China, many of which are contaminated with lead and other heavy metals, it has even been found in children's toys. Sometimes there are unlikely sources of heavy metals such as mercury found in fish like tuna; if you love tuna sandwiches like I do, then you have to keep in mind that you might develop toxic levels of mercury. Chelation therapy helps remove heavy metals and other toxins from our bodies.

Chronic Dental Infections

Bacteria and fungi do not have digestive systems; in order for them to digest food they must release powerful digestive enzymes that dissolve substances from the surrounding body parts they are infecting. As you can imagine in the case of dental infections these enzymes need to be much more powerful than if the bacteria were infecting your skin. For bacteria to infect teeth they must release two very powerful types of enzymes or toxins called gliotoxins and thioethers. These two powerful enzymes have far-reaching effects, well beyond the teeth, reaching many distant areas of the body and causing the mitochondria to shut down. Root canals are done by removing the artery and nerve of a tooth; this in effect leaves a dead tooth. Any dead tissue left inside the body is prime territory for colonization and infection by bacteria and fungi and is therefore a source of decreased voltage and disease. Studies have shown that up to 95 percent of all focal infections in the body are caused by infections originating in either the teeth or tonsils. In my medical practice of over twenty-five years I have never seen a patient with bad teeth in good health, the two just do not go together, bad teeth always equals bad health. Therefore once again I cannot stress to brush your teeth, gargle with a mixture of half peroxide and half water daily, and then floss your teeth.

How Are pH And Voltage Related?

Since pH is an indirect measurement of voltage, any solution is either an electron donor or an electron scavenger (stealer). If a solution is an electron donor, then it is giving up electrons, since electrons carry a negative charge, if you are giving up a negative then you in effect are becoming more positive, so electron donors carry a positive voltage or charge. When a solution is an electron stealer then it is taking on negative charges and therefore carries a negative voltage or charge.

Voltage is converted on a logarithmic scale to pH ranging from 1-14, with 7 being neutral. Anything less than seven is acidic anything greater than 7 is alkaline or basic.

Our bodies' cells are designed to run in a range from a pH of 7.35 (-20 mv) to a pH of 7.45 (-25 millivolts). In order to heal or produce new cells the voltage must be raised to about -50 mv. Diseases and cancer begin at levels below -20 mv. All disease is characterized by having low voltage, therefore it stands to reason that correcting low voltage will cure disease; using the various methods I have outlined below will help energize and alkalinize the body and thereby raise the pH and voltage of the cells and cure disease. Remember, in order for your body to heal itself it needs not only the proper pH or voltage, but it also needs all the right parts to build the cells needed for healing. When I say right parts, what I mean is all of the minerals and trace elements, vitamins and fresh water and healthy, unprocessed foods for all the essential amino acids (proteins) and essential fatty acids and carbohydrates. You can correct the voltage and pH all day long, but without the right building blocks your body cannot properly construct the new cells it needs.

How Can You Correct Electrical Problems In Your Body?

So, that begs the question of how do we correct this drop in energy in the body's cells? There are various means of doing so such as:

The Tennant Biomodulator

The Tennant biomodulator will donate a steady stream of electrons that will recharge the cells involved and raise their voltage and pH, changing the internal environment of the cells thus promoting health and healing chronic disease states, as well as decreasing pain.

Sun Exposure

Exposure to sunlight is healthy for you, it just has to be done with moderation and if you have fair skin it will need to be done in stages. Early morning and late day sun are the best ways to get your skin acclimated to receiving the benefits of sunshine. I would suggest a half hour daily for the first week or two and then increase to twice daily, morning and late day. During these sessions you will not be wearing sunblock of any type and will apply a moisturizer such as pure Aloe Vera gel after each session to help protect your delicate skin. The best way to get all the benefits of sunshine is by placing your feet on dirt or bare ground, this helps ground your body and helps the beneficial flow of electrons.

My fellow tree huggers will like to hear this, hugging other living things like a tree or another human or pet also helps a healing flow of electrons into your body. This is something we all intuitively felt when hugging someone or your pet; it just makes you feel good and now you know why.

Alkalinize Your Body

Alkalinize (raise the pH) of your body by drinking alkaline water. You can make your own alkaline water by adding a teaspoon of baking soda to water daily and drinking it. There are also alkaline water products on the market, one I personally like is Noah's Water…this is not only alkaline but contains increased magnesium and oxygen. I don't think you need one of these gadgets that attach to your sink and alkalinize your water, they are very expensive and I think you would get just as much benefit from drinking baking soda mixed with your water.

You can also use certain minerals to alkalinize your body. Minerals such as magnesium, potassium, calcium, and sodium are all alkalinizing and will help raise the pH of your body. These minerals also complement each other; for example, you need calcium to help muscles contract and conversely you need magnesium to help muscles relax, so these two have to be in balance to prevent dominance of contraction or relaxation to occur. The cells of our body have a pump that maintains high levels of sodium outside of the cells and potassium inside, this pump needs magnesium to function properly. The calcium concentration inside of cells requires sodium to be maintained properly. As you can see these four minerals have to be both abundant and in balance within your body to maintain good health and an alkaline environment or terrain for your cells to float in.

An important concept to keep in mind when supplementing with vitamins or minerals is that nutritious food trumps supplements every time. Food that is grown in organic, mineral and trace element-rich soils teeming with healthy soil microbes is by far the best way to get your vitamins and minerals. The microorganisms in soil will transform inorganic minerals and trace elements into organic forms by chelating them, plants are then able to better absorb them and in turn we eat the plants that are chock-full of the minerals we need, in a form we too can absorb. Feeding your soil with rock dust, sea solids, or Azomite as well as humus and manure and keeping it organic should provide the perfect environment for your soil microbes to produce the fulvic acid as well as minerals and trace elements in organic form.

One other concept to keep in mind is if you are taking mineral supplements to correct a deficiency or to alkalinize your body, the best way is with acidic foods such as cooked tomatoes, citrus fruits, and vinegar.

Vitamin C also helps because it is an acid. Taking minerals with acidic foods helps increase their absorption, especially in the elderly who have decreased stomach acid and anyone who is taking antacids or medications such as Zantac, Pepcid, Prevacid, Protonix, Prilosec, Aciphex, etc. Also keep in mind that sometimes minerals will compete with each other for absorption, such is the case with calcium and magnesium supplements. If you are taking more than 250 mg of either calcium or magnesium then it is best to take them separately so as not to compete with absorption sites.

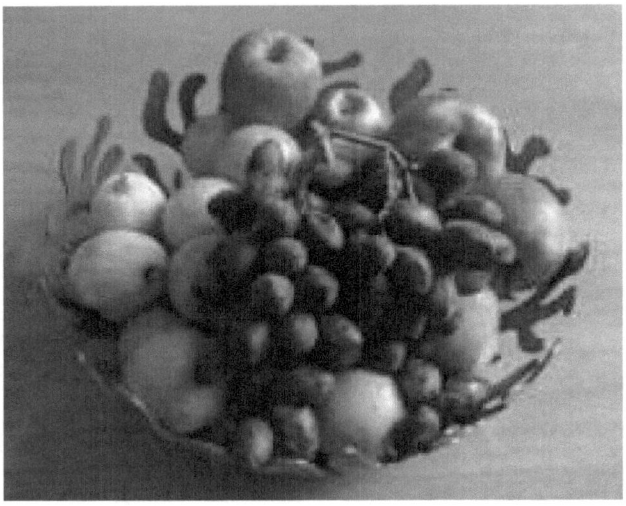

Raw Fruit and Vegetables

Raw fruits and vegetables should also be organic whenever possible. Organic fruits will have higher levels of minerals and trace elements and most importantly will contain fulvic acid which helps all nutrients enter the body's cells by its positive effect on the permeability of the cell wall. Fulvic acid opens up the cell walls allowing the entrance of all types of nutrients essential to the body. Raw fruits and vegetables also contain all of the enzymes that nature packed into them, so they are readily available to your body to help in the digestion of these foods, thereby helping your body absorb them. Many of my patients also express concerns about eating fruit because of the high carbohydrate content. It is true that high carbohydrates cause insulin to spike, but it is related to the glycemic index. What the glycemic index measures is how rapidly glucose enters the blood stream. A rapid spike in glucose or a high glycemic index food will spike insulin as a response to the sudden elevation of glucose.

Most fruits and vegetables are usually not too bad (with the exception of watermelon and a few others) because they are packaged along with lots of soluble and insoluble fiber and other plant nutrients that slow the release of glucose thus avoiding spiking insulin. See the chart below for some common foods and their glycemic indexes.

Glycemic Index / Glycemic Load Chart

Glycemic Index is a measure of how fast a food increases the blood sugar.
Glycemic Load is the measure of the blood sugar raising power per serving of food.

	Glycemic Index (glucose =100)	Carbs (grams per serving)	Glycemic Load Per serving
High	70 or more		20
Medium	56 to 69		11 to 19
Low	55 or less		10 or less
Fruits			
Apple, 1 average	38	21.0	8
Apple pie	44	29.5	13
Banana, 1 whole	51	26.5	14
Banana cake	47	37.5	18
Cantaloupe	63	13.5	9
Orange	42	16.0	7
Pineapple	65	19.0	12
Raisins, 1/2 cup	64	44.0	28
Watermelon	72	6.0	4
Vegetables			
Asparagus (6 spears)	8	4.0	1
Broccoli, 1/2 cup steamed	6	2.0	1
Cabbage, 1 cup raw	6	7.5	1
Carrots, 1 cup raw	47	6.0	3
Corn on the cob, 1 ear	53	29.0	15
French Fries, 1/2 cup	75	29.0	22
Green Beans, 1/2 cup boiled	28	5.0	1
Green Peas, 1/2 cup boiled	48	6.0	3
Baked Potato, white	85	30.5	26
Spinach, 1/2 cup steamed	6	3.5	1
Sweet Potato	61	28.0	17
Tomatoes, 1 cup raw	6	5.0	1
Grains			
Bagel, white, 2 oz.	72	32.0	23
Corn tortilla	52	23.0	12
Hamburger bun	61	15.0	9
Macaroni and Cheese	64	50.0	32
Pumpernickel bread, 1 slice	50	15.0	8
Rice, brown, 1 cup cooked	55	33.0	18
Rice, white, 1 cup cooked	64	40.0	26
Spaghetti, boiled, 1 cup	61	45.0	27
Waffles, one 7" round	76	27.0	21
White bread, 1 slice	73	14.0	10
Whole Grain bread, 1 slice	51	14.0	7

Essential Oils

Essential oils each vibrate at a certain range of frequencies. In order for them to produce their healing effect the target organ also has to be vibrating at a similar frequency; if not then there will be no communication between them and hence no effect. Think of the cells as radio stations, if the station frequency is FM 101 and you are trying to hear it by turning your dial to another number you will not pick up that station because your radio's receiver is not set at the right frequency. It is the same way with the human body; each organ vibrates at a particular range, for example the brain operates between 70 and 78 megahertz frequency. If you try to cure a headache with Rose oil, which has a frequency of about 320, you will get no effect at all. However, if you use Peppermint oil, which vibrates at about 78, it will work because it is at the same frequency as the brain. When you study the medicinal uses of various essential oils there are lists of their frequencies that will help you match them up to the frequencies of the organs involved. The mismatch of frequencies between the essential oils used and their target organs is probably one of the greatest reasons for patients not getting the benefit they should from the use of those oils.

Dr. Tennant has taken the use of essential oils to an entirely new level by developing blends of various oils which vibrate at different frequencies in order to target specific areas of the body. He has a pelvic blend for problems with the pelvic area organs; a problem in the chest uses a chest blend. The use of the TBM alleviates the pain and corrects the voltage of the cells involved and when combined with essential oils helps correct their frequencies and the information carried within each cell. The combination of the two modalities is very effective and he has had great success in treating many otherwise incurable conditions.

PART FIVE

ODDS AND ENDS

ALTERNATIVE/NATURAL MEDICINE CHEST

ALPHABETICAL LIST OF ITEMS TO INCLUDE IN YOUR ALTERNATIVE/ NATURAL MEDICINE CHEST

A:

Ace bandages: At least a dozen, these come in very handy for multiple uses.

Acetaminophen (Tylenol): Stockpile a large supply of these, they are inexpensive and the government, in their infinite wisdom, will eventually reduce the dosing of these for fear of liver toxicity.

Activated Charcoal: I recommend getting an ample supply of both the loose powder and the capsules. You can use it for medical treatments and also there is no better material to make a water filter.

A and D ointment: An excellent barrier cream, for diaper rash as well as any skin irritation. It is made of Vitamins A and D as well as Lanolin. I suggest the one pound jars, especially if you have sensitive skin or young children.

Afrin nasal spray: Never use for more than a week or it will worsen the nasal obstruction by causing rebound (comes back worse), however nothing works better short-term for a blocked nose.

Alcohol: Rubbing and swabs, very useful and inexpensive. Can also be mixed 50/50 with water and put in a plastic bag and then frozen into a slush to make inexpensive cold packs.

Aleve (Naproxen): Stockpile a large supply of these, great painkillers, fever reducers (don't use it for this unless it is 103 F and you are miserable, see fever section for explanation), inflammation and stiffness.

Allegra: A non-sedating antihistamine, great for allergies, allergic reactions, vertigo, and sinus problems.

Alka-Seltzer: This is an effervescent combination of aspirin, sodium bicarbonate (baking soda), and citric acid. It helps pain, indigestion, inflammation, and stomach aches. Do not take this if you have any bleeding problems; the aspirin in it will worsen them.

Almond Oil: Made from almonds, this works very well as a skin softener for rough, dry, chapped skin.

Aloe Vera (gel and liquid): Try to get the closest you can get to pure. CVS carries a 99 percent pure gel. Do not waste your money on low percentage gels, it is also very easy to grow and use directly from the plant. Use it for any skin irritation, excellent for sunburns, chapped, raw skin, and frostbite. Also works to soothe the digestive tract in modest amounts and will help constipation.

Alpha-Lipoic acid (Lipoic acid): See Lipoic acid below for full details.

Amaranth: A grain-like plant that is easy to grow in the United States and has wonderful nutritional value, it is also an excellent treatment to prevent radiation damage by using oil pressed from its tiny seeds. See the section of seed oils for full details.

Amino Acid supplements: Amino acids are the building blocks of proteins. There are two groups; essential amino acids are those that cannot be manufactured by the human body and nonessential which can be manufactured from other nutrients. There are over 40,000 different proteins your body has to manufacture from its pool of amino acids, hence their critical importance to your health.

Anbesol (Benzocaine): Topical anesthetic that works well for tooth, mouth pain as well as sore throats.

AndrographisPaniculata: Andrographis is an annual herb that is a very potent stimulator of immunity by boosting the power of the immune system. It is very effective as such against viral illnesses of all types.Andrographis is also a strong anti-inflammatory agent. It is sometimes marketed under the name Kan Jang. It should not be used by pregnant women.

Anise (seed and oil): An essential oil made from the anise plant, see section on essential oils for complete details. Anise contains many phytonutrients including a phytoestrogen that helps soothe women's cramps and calms the intestinal tract when the seeds are made into a tea.

Antivert (Meclizine): Great treatment for vertigo (dizziness) and to prevent vomiting.

Aspirin: Get both 81 mg baby aspirin (misnamed, never give to a child under12) and full dose 325 mg. Use the enteric coated form (Ecotrin) so as not to cause GI upset, it does not break down in the stomach but rather bypasses the stomach and is broken down and absorbed in the intestines.

Astaxanthin: Astaxanthin is a carotenoid (hence its orange/red color) and a powerful antioxidant. In fact it is 6,000 times as powerful as vitaminC. Astaxanthin stays active far longer than any other antioxidant and continues to neutralize free radicals, which helps to support the body's natural immunity. Astaxanthin is also a very potent anti-inflammatory agent and will help stiff joints and other inflammatory problems. It helps athletic strength and endurance and helps athletes recover quickly when exhausted. It also helps macular degeneration, helps slow the development and progression of dementia and Alzheimer's disease. It also helps lower blood pressure and protects the heart.

Astragalus (Astragalusmembranaceus): Astragalus is an herb that has anti-inflammatory properties as well as helps to regulate the body's immune system. It is useful in asthma.

Avocado Soybean Unsaponifiables(ASU): This is an extractof theunsaponifiable portion of both avocado and soybean oils. It helps reduce inflammation in the joints as well as protecting existing cartilage and promoting the growth of new cartilage, all of which helps osteoarthritis and other arthralgia's(joint problems causing pain).

Azo (phenazopyridine hydrochloride): An analgesic (painkiller) for burning urination and urinary tract discomfort. It is excreted by the kidneys and passes through the bladder, numbing it up and taking away your pain. Note: It will turn your urine reddish orange in color; no worries, this is a normal effect of it, since chemically it is a dye. Another name for it is Pyridium.

AZOMITE: I would buy several of the 45 lb. size packages of these. You will need them to take orally and for your medicinal garden. (I am not screaming the name, it is always written in capital letters).AZOMITE stands for 'A to Z of minerals and trace elements'. It is harvested from an ancient seabed and has all the minerals and trace elements that are in our blood and hence what we need for optimal health.

It is outstanding as a fertilizer for plants and they will have all the nutrients they need for your medicinal garden, and therefore will be incorporated in organic form in your foods.

B:

B complex Vitamins: Water soluble vitamins that are essential for your health. Take one a day. They are excellent for nerve damage, as well as helping all psychological illnesses like ADD, depression, and anxiety.

Baby Shampoo: Cheap and good to clean wounds, shampoo, clean body.

Bacopa: A water-dwelling plant used by many to increase memory, mental acuity (sharpness), help treat ADD.

Bacitracin: Good topical antibiotic cream for wounds, cuts, and scrapes. It is active against both staph and strep infections. It is also one of three components of triple antibiotic or Neosporin. I recommend Neosporin as a better topical antibiotic, but both will work to keep wounds clean and uninfected. Both Neosporin and Bacitracin are over the counter. By the way, the name comes from a patient named Tracy who had a compound fracture of her tibia and this bacillus was isolated from that wound, hence the name Bacillus of Tracy ....or Bacitracin.

Bag Balm: Great for chafed or dry skin, or skin that is raw from boots, etc., officially a Veterinarian medicine.

Baking Soda (sodium bicarbonate): Buy as much of this as you can afford.

Multiple uses.

Bandages: I would buy a large supply of sterile bandages of various sizes.

Band-Aids: I would buy the cloth kind, not plastic, and as many as you can. Also buy various sizes.

Basil: An herb that also is used in its oil form as an essential oil, see that section for full details.

Baster (as in turkey baster): Can be used for ear lavage or cleaning, as well as wound cleaning, washing out debris.

Bee Propolis: See Propolis.

Benadryl (Diphenhydramine): It is a sedating antihistamine, buy several bottles of this, it is cheap and has multiple uses like insomnia, allergic reactions, hives, itchiness, and sinus congestion. Like all antihistamines it will also work for nausea and vertigo or dizziness.

Bentonite Clay: An aluminum silicate absorbent clay whose primary constituent is Montmorillonite. There are different subtypes of Bentonite clay named after their dominant minerals...potassium, sodium, calcium, or aluminum. It is formed from weathered volcanic ash. It is very absorbent and is used to dry wet rashes, orally for constipation, and any toxin exposure due to its ability to absorb toxins on its surface. Helps protect skin from the urushiolthe toxic oil of poison ivy, sumac, and oak. It will work on any contact dermatitis or itchy rash.

Benzocaine anesthetic ointment or liquid (Anbesol): It is an effective topical anesthetic.Great for toothaches.

Berberine: Berberine is a plant alkaloid derived from many plants including barberry, goldenseal, and Oregon grape. It acts as a potent antibiotic as well as a very effective treatment for diabetes, with potency identical to metformin. The best dose for diabetes is 500 mg tid (three times daily). If you are diabetic this is essential to stockpile for your medicine chest. It is also reported to have positive anti -cancer effects.

Bergamot: This is an Italian citrus fruit similar to an orange, an oil is made from its rind. See essential oil section for full details.

Bergamot Oil: It is a cold pressed essential oil made from the rind of the bergamot orange. It is the essential oil used to flavor Earl Gray Tea.

Betadine (povidone-iodine): It is an effective anti-microbial agent that will also provide iodine for radioactive protection, thyroid support. Excellent for disinfecting animal and other bites and for wound protection.

Bitter Melon (Momordicacharantia): A tropical vine related to watermelon, pumpkin, squash, and zucchini. Bitter melon is used in the treatment of diabetes. See section on diabetes for full details. Never use this plant in pregnant women since it will induce bleedings, contractions, and abortion.

Bitter Orange: A type of essential oil, see section of the same name for full details.

Black Cohosh: Also known as black bugbane and black snakeroot and fairy candles. It is good for hot flashes, PMS problems, menopausal and menstrual problems.

Black Elderberry: Black Elderberry (Sambucusnigra) is a small tree whose flowers and berries are used to treat fever.

Black Pepper Oil: An essential oil, see that section for full details.

Black Seed (Nigella sativa): An annual plant with great nutritional value,oil can be made from its seeds that are useful to treat and prevent many medical conditions. See section on seed oils for full details.

Bleach: This is very useful but has a limited shelf life, it rapidly weakens after 6 months. Helps disinfect water, with multiple other uses.

Blood pressure cuff (sphygmomanometer): Get the manual kind, not the electronic.

Borage: A pretty annual plant that is important as a medicinal plant, used for PMS, hot flashes, and menopause problems as well as GI disturbances such as intestinal flu and GI upset.

Borax: Borax is a natural mineral found in ancient dried salt lake beds. It is primarily mined as is and packaged as such; most of the mines are either in Turkey or the western United States. It is a wonderful source of the mineral boron (see below). It is used in solution to treat fungal infections and also to treat arthritis.

Boric Acid: This is a weak acid made from boron. NEVER TAKE THIS ORALLY IT IS A POISON. However, it works well topically as a wound antiseptic, and for wound cleansing. Helps in the treatment of burns as a wound dressing or a salve. It is also useful in the treatment of eye wash; however you have to use it in a very dilute form. It can also be used for acne and to prevent athlete's foot by sprinkling it in your socks.

Boron: A chemical element, it is mined as borax. At a dose of 3 mg of boron a day it is excellent to build strong bones in growing children and adults, especially helpful in menopausal women for protection and treatment of osteopenia and osteoporosis. In this form it is nonpoisonous to humans and generally considered harmless. It is however harmful to insects and can be used as a potent insecticide. It is very effective in treating arthritis, raising testosterone and estrogen levels, and fungal infections of all types.

Bovine Colostrum: Bovine colostrum is the pre-milk substance made by cows, it is followed by production of normal cow's milk, and is chock full of antibodies to protect the newborn calf. Those same antibodies are very active against bacterial, viral, and protozoal organisms that cause diarrhea, which can rapidly kill a newborn calf. Strangely enough it contains very little lactose. See Stolle's Milk.

Brewer's Yeast: A yeast used to ferment sugars into ethanol (the alcohol we drink). Brewer's yeast originates from the fungus Saccharomyces cerevisiae. Brewer's yeast is a rich source of B complex vitamins and minerals and is sometimes used as a supplement.

Bromelain: Bromelain is an extract derived from the stems of pineapple plants, and has been found to be useful in the treatment of gout. It has also been used as an anti-inflammatory and is very useful in the treatment of all types of joint pain.

Bulb syringes: Excellent to clean ears with a 50/50 mix of water and hydrogen peroxide. Helps irrigate wounds.

Bungee cords: Get various sizes, they have multiple uses. Medically they can be used to bind splints, help support a limb, wrap wound dressings, etc.

Butterbur: Butterbur is a common European weed that has strong antihistamine effects, is non-sedating and as strong as prescription Zyrtec. Butterbur is also used in the treatment of migraine headaches when combined with white willow.

BZK wipes (Benzalkonium chloride): Used as hand sanitizers and wound disinfectants, can also be used for sore throats. It is a potent antiseptic compound.

C:

Calamine lotion: It is made from a combination of zinc oxide and ferric oxide or a zinc carbonate compound. It is effective for treating any of the skin irritations from any of the poison ivy, oak, or sumac. It will work to soothe the skin from sunburns, any rashes, chickenpox, insect bites and stings, and eczema. It can be used on oozing rashes, blisters, and abscesses. It also has mild antiseptic properties and can be used on chafed, scratched skin to prevent infections.

Calcium: Calcium is an important mineral and has multiple vital functions in the human body. It helps build strong bones in osteoporosis and in growing children (along with strong teeth), it helps the heart function properly especially in its contraction and electrical conduction, helps nerves function properly and along with magnesium will help lower blood pressure. Just like our bones and teeth contain a lot of calcium, so do eggshells, you can pulverize an eggshell into fine powder and put it in a glass of water and drink it to get your calcium, or sprinkle it on food. Oyster shells also contain a lot of calcium and one of the popular brands is Oscal which actually stands for Oyster Shell Calcium. Dairy products contain a lot of calcium as does seaweed, spinach, kale, almonds, sesame seeds, beans, black strap molasses, figs, and rhubarb.

Calendula herb (Marigold) Oil: This is known to have antiviral properties as well as being anti-inflammatory as well as aiding in the healing of wounds.

Celery Seed Extract: Celery Seed Extract has been shown to lower uric acid levels and thus is useful for the treatment of gout.

Calmoseptinecream: A wonderful combination of zinc oxide and menthol, hence it is very soothing for burning rectum/anal areas. Excellent barrier cream around an ostomy.

Capsaicin pepper powder (chili pepper powder): It works as a topical anesthetic for sprains, joint pain, back aches, and muscle injuries. It also works in psoriasis to help burning and painful areas, in peripheral neuropathy (nerve pain of diabetes and other nervous injuries). It works by leaving it on the skin or rubbing it into the skin until it starts to burn, then wipe it off.

It is also the active ingredient in pepper spray. **Note:** The only way to stop the burning from this pepper is to neutralize it with whole milk or cream.

Carrot Seed Oil: An essential oil made from the seeds of carrots. See section on essential oils for complete details.

Cascara Sagrada (Rhamnuspurshianus): Cascara Sagrada is a small woody shrub, native to the western United States. It is Spanish for sacred bark. It is a very potent reliever of constipation, and has to be used with caution.

Castor Oil: I would buy a large bottle of this, it has multiple uses. Keep some flannel with it and a heating pad or a hot water bottle to make your castor oil packs. Useful treatment for sprains and muscle and joint pain.

Cayenne Pepper Powder: A plant relative of capsaicin pepper with similar uses.

Celery and celery extract: Celery works well to control blood pressure. Celery contains a phytochemical (plant derived chemical) that causes the arterial walls to relax and thereby lowers blood pressure. It is also very healthy to eat. I would stockpile the seeds of several open pollinated (non-hybrid) varieties in your seed vault.

Cepacol: Contains both benzocaine and menthol to help soothe sore throat, will numb and soothe it.

Combat application tourniquet (CAT): Excellent tourniquet that you can even self-apply. Go online and check out the excellent films on how to use the CAT; that will give you a much clearer idea as to how to use them.

Chaga Mushrooms (Inonotusobliquus): Chaga mushrooms are medicinal mushrooms that grow on trees mostly in northern climates. They are wonderful immune system boosters and a powerful antioxidant, known to the Chinese as the King of Plants.

Chamomile Oil: Used for its antiseptic and anti-inflammatory properties.

Chamomile Tea: A double strength version of this tea can be made and cooled, using an eyecup can be instilled into the eye to treat conjunctivitis.

Chlorhexidine: See Hibiclens below.

Chromium: Chromium is a mineral that is very important for glucose control and is considered an essential trace element. It is often referred to as Glucose Tolerance Factor. It helps insulin drive glucose into the cells thus lowering blood glucose levels. Since it lowers insulin requirements, it also lowers insulin levels in your blood and the resulting insulin resistance is improved. The dose varies from 1,000 mcg (micrograms) or a millionth of a gram, as opposed to milligrams, which are one thousandth of a gram, to four thousand mcg daily.

Chelated minerals: These are inorganic minerals that are converted into organic form by their chelation or combination with amino acids. Inorganic minerals cannot be absorbed by the body until they are made organic and this can either be done in the soil by microorganisms, in the plants, or in our intestines by beneficial probiotics.

Cheese cloth: I would buy several packages of these, many uses especially to filter material.

Chondroitin: A natural substance made by the body, it is part of cartilage and retains water molecules, helping to moisten and keep cartilage flexible. See Glucosamine and Chondroitin.

Cinnamon: Especially useful if you are a diabetic or there are diabetics in your family. Cinnamon has been proven to be quite effective in the lowering of blood glucose levels in diabetic patients. The dose for diabetics is approximately 500 mg bid or twice daily. The best type of cinnamon is cassia cinnamon or Chinese cinnamon. Cinnamon can also be used in its oil form, and as such has been used as an insect repellent.

Citronella Oil: Citronella oil is a natural insect repellent made from the leaves and stems of the lemongrass family of plants. It can be combined with either a carrier oil or alcohol and made into an effective natural insect repellent. Citronella oil is also an antifungal agent and has even been used to calm barking dogs!

Cloves: Cloves are the aromatic buds of the clove tree, which is a member of the myrtle family. Cloves contain clove oil, when the fresh buds are mashed they release the oil and can be placed directly against a sore tooth. See clove oil.

Clove Oil: An essential oil that has wonderful analgesic effects and is an excellent oil to numb up tooth and gum pain. It is one of the essential ingredients in Tiger Balm and is used to treat hangovers. See section on essential oils for complete details. See cloves.

Coconut Oil: Get several large bottles, it has medicinal as well as nutritional uses. Helps provide essential fats to your diet and especially your brain. Helps in any psychological illness including dementia, ADD, anxiety and depression. It is a wonderful source of beneficial fats known as medium chain triglycerides, which cross the blood-brain barrier and have positive effects upon the brain.

Cod Liver Oil: Cod liver oil is a nutritional supplement made from the liver of cod fish. Like most fish oils it is rich in omega-3 fatty acids such as DHA and EPA, it is also rich in vitamins A and D and historically was used medicinally for these vitamins in children to prevent rickets. It can be made by filling a barrel with cod livers and sea water and allowing it to ferment for up to a year. Cod liver oil is different from other fish oils due to its higher content of vitamins A and D. If you have children this is a good thing to have, especially during the winter months when their vitamin D content will plummet, leaving them susceptible to the flu and other illnesses.

Coffee filters: Multiple uses, great for filtering water for drinking.

Colace (docusate sodium): Excellent stool softener, good for any constipation or irritable bowel problems. Also useful in patients with hemorrhoids, it softens your stool and makes passage across the anus less painful.

Colostrum: Colostrum is the first milk produced by a lactating humans and all other mammals. It is chock-full of beneficial nutrients and antibodies to help protect the infant from infections. It is useful at any age to prevent infections and boost the immune system. See the entire section under how to treat an infection.

Cold packs: Multiple uses, headaches, swollen body parts and painful areas etc.

Colloidal Minerals: Excellent easily assimilated form of minerals and trace elements. These come in liquid preparations.

Colloidal Silver: Colloidal silver is a preparation of silver that can be ingested to control internal infections. It is best used for a short period of time.

Colostrum: See Bovine Colostrum.

Comfrey: This is an excellent medicinal garden plant, much loved by bees. Its leaves are full of minerals and make an excellent compost or mulch. Can also work as a compost activator. The leaves can be soaked in water for about five weeks to make a "tea" to fertilize your organic garden. Medically it should never be ingested due to poisonous alkaloids that it contains, however topically it helps heal all skin conditions from acne to psoriasis and helps sprains and supposedly helps broken bones heal, hence its nickname knit bone.

Compost: This is made of decomposing organic matter, it helps build healthy soil and helps water retention and plant health and growth. All your vegetable and fruit kitchen scraps should be composted and"fed" to your garden torecycle all those valuable nutrients. **Note:** The easiest compost tomake is by taking all your leaves in the fall and shredding them and placing them in a pile or a container, even tomato cages will work fine. After several months or in the spring you will have nice compost on the bottom of the pile. Adding coffee grounds to it is a good way to supercharge your compost pile, they need to be used coffee grounds, not fresh.

Compost starter or activator: This is a mix of bacteria that will start the digestion of your raw compost. Traditionally comfrey has also been utilized for this. Nothing works better than used coffee grounds; save a bunch of them and add them to shredded leaves for great compost.

Compound W: A wart-removing compound useful for those suffering with warts, made from salicylic acid from the white willow tree, it is also what aspirin comes from.

Co Q10 (Coenzyme Q10): This is a fat-soluble, vitamin-like substance that is responsible for energy generation by the mitochondria (the powerhouse of every cell in the body) and hence is very helpful in treating fatigue and low energy problems. It also is part of the antioxidant cascade and helps regenerate vitamin E and therefore helps in immunity. Reported to be helpful in radiation injury and especially useful in congestive heart failure (along with selenium).

Useful in diabetes along with zinc and vitamin E for the production of insulin. CoQ10 also helps to lower blood pressure. Take between 100 and 200 mg daily, always with a fatty meal since it is fat soluble and won't otherwise be properly absorbed.

Copper tablets: You will need these if you are on any zinc tablets for a long period; zinc depletes copper.

Corn starch: Numerous uses besides cooking.

Cotton balls: I would buy several bags of these.

Cordyceps (Cordycepssinensis): Cordyceps is a Chinese medicinal mushroom that has been found to both reduce bronchial secretions and also to expand the airways, hence its usefulness in asthma.

Cranberry tablets: Great for persistent urinary tract infections or burning upon urination, frequent urination, and nocturia (getting up at night to urinate). Cranberry contains a chemical which preventspathogenic (disease causing) bacteria from sticking to the bladder or urethral walls and therefore preventing their infecting humans.

Crutches: Save any old ones or try to buy a used pair, most are adjustable. These invariably will come in handy. Look at garage sales and flea markets for a used pair or two.

Cucumber: The vegetable cucumber's juice can be squeezed into an eye, and used to treat conjunctivitis.

Cumin: An herb with many medicinal qualities, it is also used as an essential oil; see that section for full details.

Curcumin: Curcumin is an ingredient in Tumeric, a popular south Asian spice. Curcumin is both a strong anti-inflammatory agent as well as a potent antioxidant. It also stimulates contraction of the gallbladder, thus aiding in digestion.

Cypress Oil: An essential oil that has medicinal uses.

D:

Dakins Solution: Dakins solution is a wound care solution devised by an American chemist named Harold Dakin during WWI. It is made of a combination of bleach, baking soda, and sterile water, and is quite effective in cleansing wounds and promoting healing. It only has a shelf life of about two days. It is also known as diluted sodium hypochlorite solution 0.05%.

Dandelion Leaf (Taraxacumofficinale): Dandelion is everywhere and has potent uses as a diuretic or water pill to help increase your urination, and thus lowers your blood pressure. It can also be used to make a great wine, if you are so inclined.

DEET: DEET is a wonderful insect repellent that is critical to have in a large supply if you spend a lot of time outdoors. I would recommend getting the 30 percent; this will last about 24 hours when applied.

Apply it to clothes when possible and skin when no other choice is available. Do not use it on infants.

Dental floss: This is important. If you are like me and just don't have the coordination to floss well, then buy the pre-made spears; these are very useful. I personally love the small, battery powered dental flosser called the Hummingbird. It uses a AAA battery and it lasts a long time. It vibrates and slips the floss easily even between those tight molars in the back. Flossing is critical to good dental care.

Dents Toothache Drops: A benzocaine-containing liquid that numbs up toothache pain; it also comes in gum form. Useful to have especially if you have children or adults in your family with poor dentition (teeth).

Desenex (miconazole nitrate): This is a useful over-the-counter antifungal powder, cream, or spray. I prefer the powder; very useful for jock itch, fungal infections of the skin, and athlete's foot.

DGL (deglycyrrhizinated licorice): Made from licorice, this is useful for the treatment of stomach problems like gastric and duodenal ulcers; it also works as an antacid.

Diphenhydramine (Benadryl): See Benadryl for complete details.

Distilled water: Several uses especially when mixing medicinals.

DMSO (Dimethyl Suffixed): Very useful topically as a pain reliever. It also has endless uses as a solvent to dissolve various medicines that you want to apply topically, since DMSO crosses the skin without harming it. It has been used as a liniment for horses to treat their injuries. It works very well for fungal infections when the antifungal medicines are dissolved in it. Depending on your state, it may or may not be legal for human use.

Droppers: You will need an ample supply of these, especially if you are making essential oils.

Duct tape: I would buy at least two dozen rolls of this. It has endless uses in the home and even has been used for severe toe and fingernail infections. It can also be used to close wounds when cut into thin strips and used similar to steri strips or butterfly bandages.

Dulcolax tablets and suppositories (bisacodyl): It is a stimulant laxative useful for constipation. I prefer Epsom salt in a glass of water, but Dulcolax also works.

E:

Echinacea Oil: This oil is made from plants of the same name, also known as coneflowers. In all of its forms it is used to boost the immune system and shorten the length of colds and flu like illnesses. It is controversial whether it is truly effective for this use. It should not be used in children under twelve due to its effect upon their immature immune systems.

Elderberry (Sambucusnigra): Elderberry is a perennial shrub that grows all over the United States, and if possible should be part of your medicinal garden.Elderberry is antibacterial, antiviral, and anti-inflammatory in addition to which it boosts your immune system.

Emergen-C: It is an effervescent drink made from a powder and has mixed types of mineral ascorbates (vitamin C) and B vitamins as well as other vitamins and minerals. This is an excellent way to boost your immune system if you are sick or feel like you are getting sick. I personally like the raspberry, but hey, to each his own.

Enema bags: These can be either disposable or non -disposable, with the tubing and clamps to control the flow. These can also be used as hot water bottles and as douche bags.

Enzymes: I would buy both digestive enzymes and metabolic or systemic enzymes. These are especially useful if you find yourself relying on processed, packaged or canned foods. After a half an hour cooking at 125 F, the enzyme content of most food is destroyed, enzymes are essential for your health hence the benefits of raw foods and fermented foods which are loaded with enzymes.

Epinephrine: Epinephrine is also known as adrenaline, and is a hormone secreted by the adrenal gland. It is involved in the fight-or-flight response and causes vasoconstriction (tightens up blood vessels), brochodilitation (opens up bronchioles or airways), increased energy and alertness and to treat anaphylaxis (life threatening allergic reactions). For our purposes it is useful to control bleeding and for anaphylaxis, see EpiPen below.

EpiPen and EpiPen Jr.: EpiPens contain epinephrine or adrenaline. Depending on your allergy problems, I would keep a pair of these, EpiPenjr. if you have children. They could be lifesaving with bee stings and severe allergic reactions.

Epsom Salt (magnesium sulfate): I would keep a lot of this in your medicine chestdue to its multiple uses. For medical uses, there are very few therapeutic substances like this. It can be used for sprains, muscle pain, muscle spasm, constipation, cardiac conditions and even as a sedative.

Essential Oils: A good variety of these will be invaluable. If you plan on making them, get all the bottles, etc. now along with the droppers. There are several excellent books on the subject, well worth the money. These oils are very good at treating a variety of conditions.

Eucalyptus Oil: An essential oil made from the tree of the same name. Please see full details in the essential oil section.

Everlasting Oil (Helichrysum Oil): An essential oil with many uses, also is long lasting without spoiling, hence the name. It can be used for treating bruises, asthma, bronchitis, irritable bowel, anxiety, and depression, and pain relief. See text for complete details.

Excedrin: A combination of aspirin, Tyenol, and caffeine.This is a very effective painkiller especially for migraines. Note: Excedrin Migraine is no different than extra strength Excedrin. Excedrin is inexpensive and I would buy several large bottles. If you have migraines or if people in your family have migraines.

Eyebright (Euphrasiaofficinalis): Eyebright is an herb that grows at high altitudes primarily in alpine meadows. It gets its name from its use for eye infections, but it also is very useful to treat the congestion associated with colds and allergies.

Eye cup: Pretty self-explanatory, it is used to deliver medicines to an eye. I don't know how much more I can say about this without sounding like an idiot.

F:

Fennel: Fennel is a very useful plant. In the medicinal garden it attracts many pollinators and beneficial insects. It also grows into a delicious vegetable, much loved by my Italian family. It also is useful in nausea and vomiting.

Fenugreek: Fenugreek can be found as seeds, capsules, powder, and tea. Made from the herb that grows primarily in the Mediterranean area. It contains a compound called diosgenin that has properties similar to estrogen. Hence its use especially in women for hot flashes, PMS symptoms, menstrual problems as well as increasing the libido of women. At about 3 grams a day, women have used it for breast enlargement, it also aids in breastfeeding. It also is useful in the treatment of diabetes at 500 mg bid (twice daily) since it helps lower glucose levels. It is also useful in digestive problems, bronchitis, and inflammation like arthritis. It will cause a distinctive odor several days after its use.

Fermentation supplies: These will come in handy if you want to ferment any foods to preserve them. Old crocks and fermentation jugs are easy to find at flea markets or buy online. Learning to ferment foods is a wonderful way to enhance their nutritional value and also to preserve them. There are several good books, I would advise picking one up, see the bibliography at the end of this book for references.

Feverfew (Tenacetumparthenium): This is a perennial herb, a member of the daisy family. It is used for the treatment of migraine headaches.

Fish Oil (Omega-3 Fatty Acids): I would buy the best brand you can afford, the inexpensive brands sometime contain mercury so be careful. Fish Oil is excellent for overall health, great for squelching the flames of joint inflammation in conditions like arthritis. It is good for your brain, memory and immune system. Is very helpful in ADHD and ADD and anxiety and depression. See text for complete details.

Flaxseed Oil: Another high omega-3 fatty acid source, like fish oil, krill oil, and walnut oil. Same properties as fish oil above. Useful to use as a condiment on salads and vegetables, it will deliver some good fat (oils are just fats that are liquids at room temperatures) content to your diet and will make you feel full due to its fat content.

Frankincense: An aromatic resin made from trees of the same name from the Middle East. Its name comes from the old French for Frankish incense (or French incense). In its oil form it has many medicinal uses, see essential oil section for full details.

Fulvic Acid: See Supreme Fulvic.

G:

GABA (gamma aminobutyric acid): GABA is an inhibitory neurotransmitter in the brain and as such causes relaxation and helps relieve anxiety.

Garlic (Allium sativum): In its many forms, as the plant, garlic powder, capsules, oil, and an aged extract form of garlic known as Kyolic (see Kyolic below). Garlic has many uses as a plant/nutraceutical and a medicinal herb as well as an essential oil. Garlic oil has antiseptic qualities and was used as recently as WWII to treat wounds. It also lowers cholesterol. A day or two after using garlic oil the unmistaken stink of garlic will permeate your skin and your breath, due to the volatile acetones and other odiferous components of garlic.Garlic is also used to lower blood pressure. The dose of aged garlic extract is 600 mg bid (twice daily). You can always eat it straight from the garden as well; all plants in the same family, such as leeks, chives, and onions all have positive medicinal effects as well from their common compound, allicin. Garlic is good for the heart due to its effect on lowering triglycerides and cholesterol, preventing platelet clumping, as well as lowering homocysteine levels If you are eating garlic to get its beneficial effects, you need to eat 5 or 6 cloves of fresh garlic daily.

Gentian Root (Gentianalutea): Gentian root is a European herb that comes from the root of the yellow gentian plant. Gentian root stimulates appetite and aids digestion by helping promote bowel movements, thus aiding in constipation. It also helps alleviate reflux (heartburn) and vomiting.

Gentian Violet: Gentian violet is an organic pigment that has excellent bacteria- killing properties and is used for wounds and wound care. See Hydrofera.

Geranium Oil (Pelargonium graveolens): This essential oil is very useful for acne and skin infections like cellulitis. It will also treat lice and help menopausal problems. It is a very powerful antimicrobial and oftentimes is combined with lavender oil for the treatment of wounds.

German Chamomile Oil (Matricariachamomilla): It has many medicinal uses, especially for skin abscesses, boils, and infections, scalp problems, nausea and vomiting, PMS, earaches, and headaches.

Ginger: In its various forms as well as tablets for nausea and the oil. It is also very useful for motion sickness.

Ginko (Ginkobiloba): Ginko has both antioxidant and anti-inflammatory properties and also helps mental function and is widely used to support memory.

Gloves: We all will need medical gloves or surgical gloves for disease protection if we are involved in any type of medical care that involves body fluids.

Glucosamine and Chondroitin: Glucosamine is a natural substance made by the body and not found in any foods except the shells of crabs, lobsters, shrimp, and the bones of animals. It helps build and heal cartilage. Chondroitin is also made by the body and helps moisten cartilage and keep it flexible, also helps it heal.

Glutamine (L-glutamine): This amino acid is the most abundant free (non bound to a protein) amino acid in the human body. It is useful to accelerate the body's healing after trauma, burns, injuries, and wound healing. It also helps build muscle. As you can see, all of its uses are for building and repair of the body. It comes in a powder form or in capsules. Useful to have around, after all, you don't have to be Nostradamus to predict that there will be a lot of opportunities to use something to repair and rebuild an injured body.

Glutathione: Glutathione is the most important antioxidant made by the human body, and is manufactured by every cell in the body. It is an essential part of the water soluble arm of the immune cascade, and is regenerated by both vitamin C and alpha-lipoic acid.

Glycerin: Glycerin is also known as Glycerine and Glycerol, is a viscous (thick), colorless and odorless sugar alcohol compound. It is unusual in that it is water soluble and also hygroscopic (it draws water towards it). It is basically a triglyceride (fat) with three hydoxyl molecules attached to it, thus it is water soluble. It is used medicinally to moisturize and as a lubricant, it is also put into suppositories to treat constipation. It is also used to soften earwax.

Gold Bond (powder or cream): The primary active ingredients in Gold Bond are menthol to heal itch and zinc oxide for skin protection. This is very useful for chafed, raw skin, odor control, and to reduce moisture. I find it useful in warm weather when applied to the groin to prevent jock itch and to feet to prevent athlete's foot. It also works to prevent diaper rash.

Goldenseal (Hydrastis Canadensis): Goldenseal is a perennial herb native to the eastern United States and Canada. It is also known as orange root due to the color of its yellow/orange root. It is used topically (on the skin) as an antimicrobial (antibiotic) and internally as a digestive aid. It contains berberine which is useful in the treatment of diabetes. It also has other chemical components that are useful in the treatment of inflammation in arthritis.

Green Tea: Green tea is made from tea leaves that are unfermented and thus preserve most of their beneficial plant compounds such as polyphenols. They have many health benefits and should be included in your daily regimen to maintain good health. See the section on treatment of infections for complete details, but green tea has many health benefitsespecially its antibacterial, antiviral, and antifungal effects.

Gymnasia (Gymnemasylvestre): A tropical herb that originated on the Indian subcontinent and has been used traditionally in Ayurvedic medicine. It is currently used for diabetes by its action on raising insulin levels, thus lowering glucose or sugar levels and helping diabetes.

H:

Hawthorn (Crataegusoxycanthae): Hawthorn is a small tree or shrub, the dried fruits of which are used as either a digestive aide or to help lower blood pressure. It can easily be grown in most of the United States. For hypertension the dose is 250 mg of the extract tid (three times daily).

Hazelnut Oil: Hazelnuts (also known as filbert nuts and cobnuts) and their oils are wonderful nutritional products and medicinal oils. They are easy to grow in the United States and Canada. They grow abundantly with little care needed and have few pests. They are rich in protein and unsaturated fats as well as B vitamins. It is used for skin problems as well as to help nutritionally.

Helichrysum Oil: See Everlasting Oil.

Hemp Oil: This is an essential oil manufactured from the ever useful marijuana plant. Besides the obvious uses for marijuana as a recreational drug, the plant has been cultivated since the earliest times for hemp to make rope. Hemp oil is very nutritional and contains an abundant supply of essential fatty acids like omega-3 fatty acids (like in fish oil), it also contains all the essential amino acids that man needs to survive. It can be added to foods, but using it for frying destroys much of its nutritional properties. It helps restore wasted bodies and helps boost immunity. It is highly recommended for daily intake in order to correct any underlying nutritional deficiencies. It is useful in helping anyone recover from injuries.

Huereque: A type of Mexican cactus, where the root is used to produce this compound. It is very useful in the treatment of diabetes since it has the property of lowering blood glucose levels. It should be cycled, six months of taking it, then one month off of it and then repeat the cycle. This prevents the development of tolerance to the active ingredient, and allows it to keep working indefinitely.

Hibiclens (chlorhexidine): Hibiclens is a topical antiseptic that is active against most bacteria and also against fungi and some viruses. It is currently used as a preoperative (before surgery) cleansing scrub to prevent post- operative (after surgery) infections. It is also used in mouthwashes to help cleanse the mouth and prevent cavities as well as a treatment for gum disease or gingivitis. It is also useful to clean the mouth after trauma and also after the extraction of teeth to prevent infections. It may cause a brownish discoloration of teeth and gums if used for a prolonged period due to the destruction of the bacteria in the mouth and the proteins they release.

Honey: I would buy a large supply of this in its raw unfiltered form, and also the Manuka honey. This will never spoil and has multiple uses. It can be used both for food and medicinally especially important in treating wounds and skin tears and ulcers. It also has value as a sweetener and for nourishment, with a high mineral content, especially the raw honeys made from wild floral sources. The great news is that it never spoils because it inhibits the growth of bacteria, fungi, and viruses to its antimicrobial activity and its osmotic effect.

Horsetail (equisetum): Horsetail is a living fossil, meaning it is the only surviving member of a large class of plants from over a hundred million years ago, where it dominated the forest floor. It is the only plant today that reproduces from spores rather than seeds. It is shaped like a horse's tail and thus its name. Medicinally its primary use is as a diuretic and also in the treatment of bladder and kidney infections and disorders. It is found on all continents except Antarctica; be careful planting it, it can be invasive. It is a weed growing all over the place here on my Connecticut property.

Hot packs: These will come in handy for treatment of muscular injuries, back problems, etc.

Hot water bottles: Same as above.

Humus: Humus is the organic matter in soil that has reached the point of stability and cannot break down any further; it provides fertility to the soil and is very important. If you have poor soil, now is the time to buy humus and add it to your soil. It lasts for centuries and will help poor soils function better. Humus contains both humic and fulvic acids.

Hurricaine Topical Anesthetic Gel (benzocaine): This can be used for any topical anesthetic needs.

Hyaluronic acid (hyaluronan): This acid is found throughout the body, especiallyin the extracellular matrix (the fluid surrounding and between all the cells of the body, it is basically what cells are immersed in). Medicinally it is used topically for both wound healing and eczema and normally there are large amounts of this acid in the skin.

Hydrocortisone cream: This is very useful, keep a large supply of this, get the strongest percentage you can find. It is useful for the treatment of poison ivy, sumac, and oak as well as any contact dermatitis (itchy rash). It can also be used to shrink swollen hemorrhoids. It will help any allergic skin reaction.

Hydrofera: This is a wound dressing impregnated with both Methylene blue and gentian violet organic pigments, both of which have excellent bacterial killing properties.

Hydrogen Peroxide: Buy a very large supply of this. It is inexpensive and has multiple uses. Buy the higher percentages than the 3% pharmacy variety and dilute it down to three percent.

5-HTP (5 hydroxytryptophan): This is an intermediate metabolite of tryptophan in the eventual production of serotonin. It should be given along with B vitamins which are involved in the reaction as well. It is very useful for the treatment of ADD, ADHD, anxiety, and depression. A good replacement for the SSRIs (selective serotonin reuptake inhibitors) like Prozac, Zoloft, and Paxil.

Hyssop Oil: This oil comes from the hyssop plant (hyssop officinalis), it is often used in herbal preparations along with liquorice to treat lung diseases. Hyssop is very useful in the garden to attract bees and other pollinators. Odd fact: Hyssop has also been found to increase the yield from grapes when planted along side of them. It also helps cabbage by repelling an insect pest known as the cabbage white butterfly.

I:

Ibuprofen (Motrin): Very useful painkiller will also lower fevers but only do that if it is greater than 103 F and the patient is delirious. It works well for pain, headaches, menstrual cramps, sprains, and other joint and muscle injuries. Always take it with food to prevent upsetting your stomach. The usual dose is about 400 mg three times a day and that can be doubled for severe aches and pains.

Ice packs: A small collection of these are very useful to have and are inexpensive.

Imodium (Loperamide): Imodium is an opioid derivative and like all opiates it decreases theperistalsis (thewave-likemotionthatmovesfoodfromyour mouth to your anus). It is used therefore in the treatment of diarrhea. Avoid its use if the patient has a high fever or if there is bloody stool. It has no effect in cholera, Shigella, or Campylobacter infections. It should also not be used if the patient is in liver failure or cirrhosis of the liver, like in end-stage alcoholics since it may cause hepatic encephalopathy (the patient gets very confused and may even lead to coma). It also should not be used in cases of C. difficile infections, because they release toxins and a slowing of the gut will increase absorption of toxins and may lead to toxic mega colon.

Inositol: Inositol is a type of carbohydrate found in the cell membrane of all cells. It formerly was included in the B complex group of vitamins. It aids the liver in processing fats and is also important for the proper functioning of nerves and muscles. It is useful in the treatment of anxiety and depression.

Iodoral tablets: See iodine below.

Iodine: Buy it in nascent form, betadine, SSKI, and iodoralfor your medicine chest since it is so versatile. It is especially useful in the prevention of thyroid cancer with nuclear radiation exposure due to the release of radioactive iodine by nuclear bombs. The saturation of the thyroid with good iodine will prevent the uptake of the radioactive form and therefore prevent thyroid cancer, especially in growing children.

Ipecac syrup (Syrup of Ipecac): It is made from the root of the ipecac plant. It is a syrup that induces emesis (it causes vomiting). It does this by causing irritation to the gastric mucosa or stomach lining. It also has action as an expectorant (helps you cough up mucous or phlegm from your lungs.

Israeli Battle Dressing: It is unlikely you will ever need these, but if you want your medicine chest to be complete then I would stock a couple of these. They are very useful and can even be applied by yourself if no one is around to help you. I would recommend going to their website and watching a few of their excellent instructional videos.

J:

Jasmine Oil: An essential oil made from the jasmine plant's flower. It has many medicinal uses please see the section of the same name for full details.

K:

Kan Jang: See Andrographispaniculata.

Kaolin clay: A mineral clay that is used for upset stomachs and for diarrhea, it was the active ingredient in Kapopectate, but no longer. It is also used by organic farmers to spray on crops to prevent insect damage; it is especially helpful in apples to prevent sun scald.

Kaopectate: Is used in the treatment of diarrhea. It got its name from its original use of Kaolin clay to soothe the stomach and the digestive tract, it no longer contains kaolin but is useful for diarrhea.

Kava (Piper methysticum): Kava is also known as Kava Kava. It is a plant from the Pacific islands of Polynesia. It has both sedative and anesthetic properties and is used extensively throughout those islands by the natives. The roots are taken and ground up into a fine powder and used in its preparation. It is useful for sleep and anxiety. It is also a mild painkiller and has psychoactive properties (it gets you high) if used in strong enough doses.

Kefir: A liquid nutritional drink made using kefir grains and fermenting milk. Kefir grains contain more than twenty types of yeast and bacteria. Kefir, unlike most probiotics, helps permanently colonize your intestines with probiotic bacteria.

Kling wound dressing: Kling is very useful gauze wound dressings that cling to the body's contours which helps keep them in place.They are very useful and I would keep several rolls handy in your medicine chest. It is inexpensive and very useful. If you need to bandage several injured people quickly and efficiently, this is the way to go.

Kombucha: Kombucha is a sweetened tea that has been further fermented by the addition of SCOBY or symbiotic colonies of bacteria and yeast. It is a wonderful source of B vitamins, antioxidants and other nutrients.

Krill Oil: Krill oil is similar to fish oil, and is made from shrimp-like crustaceans called krill. Krill oil has the added benefit of high phospholipid content as well as containing astaxanthin, a very potent antioxidant. The astaxanthin comes from the algae the krill eat as their primary food source. It has numerous health benefits including increasing strength and endurance. Krill oil is very high in omega-3 fatty acids similar to fish oil, and is a strong anti-inflammatory. Krill oil also contains a lot of EPA which helps elevate moods. Since the omega-3 fatty acids in krill oil is contained in phospholipids it is more easily absorbed by the body than fish oil and hence has more bioavailability to the cells of the body.

Kristalose: Kristalose is also known as Lactulose, a manmade sugar in a powder form. It is used in the treatment of constipation, and does so by drawing water into the bowels and softening the stool. A softer stool is more compliant and will pass through your bowels more readily. It can also be used in the treatment of hepatic encephalopathy (a condition of end-stage alcoholics, where they become progressively confused and disoriented). Kristalose is indigestible by the human body due to a lack of the specific enzymes to perform the task and thus exits the bowels unchanged.

Kyolic: Kyolic is a brand name for a wonderful, potent but odor free aged garlic extract. It is very potentgarlicextractthatisveryusefulforthetreatment of infections such as the common cold to MRSA. It will be useful to have if your supply of fresh garlic runs out. It also comes in a powder form. Note:Kyolic contains no allicin, the most active ingredient in garlic, but it does contain over 200 other sulfur-rich compounds in garlic and hence still has many of the health benefits associated with raw garlic.

L:

Lactaid: Lactaid is an enzyme supplement which is made of lactase, which is the enzyme that humans use to digest the milk sugar lactose. Lactose is the milk sugar that gives milk its sweet taste.

Many nonwhites (and some whites as well) cannot produce this enzyme and thus are lactose intolerant and cannot digest milk. Ingesting Lactaid with a milk-containing meal will therefore provide the lactase enzyme necessary to digest the milk.

Lactase: Lactase is the enzyme necessary for the digestion of milk. See Lactaid, above.

Lactobacillus Acidophilus: Key probiotic to have; a decent supply of this is important. It is especially important after any antibiotic use, to recolonize the intestines and prevent pathogenics(disease causing) bacteria from overgrowing the intestines.

Lactoferrin: Lactoferrin is a protein excreted primarily in colostrum and mother's milk as well as in most bodily secretions such as tears, saliva, and nasal secretions. It binds up iron, making it unavailable to bacteria which need it to survive. Lactoferrin also has potent antibacterial, antiviral, antifungal, and antiparasitic properties and boosts the immune system. It is also useful in the treatment of ulcers and intestinal conditions like Crohn's disease and ulcerative colitis. In an emergency situation it can be used to help after significant blood loss and to treat any anemias or iron deficiencies.

Lactulose: This is a synthetic disaccharide or double sugar. It is made from lactose and works on the gut by drawing in fluid and thus relieving constipation. See Kristalose.

Lanacane (Benzocaine): Topical anesthetic ointment. It is also used as an anti- itch medication.

Lavender Oil: Lavender oil is one of the most important of the essential oils for your medicine chest. It is made from the distillation of lavender flowers. It has many medicinal uses such as an antiseptic and also a pain reliever for stings, bites, and minor burns. It also helps in joint and muscle pain and can be massaged into the skin overlying those sore muscles. It helps in sunburn and also helps repel lice. It is also used extensively for relaxation and stress relief and also to help tension headaches where it can be massaged into the scalp of the temporal area (temples) and neck.

Lectins: Lectins are proteins produced by the body that attach themselves to the glycoprotein coat of viruses and other microorganisms, thus incapacitating them. See Mannose Binding Lectins (MBL).

Legumes: Legumes is the botanical term for beans. Beans are an excellent source of lean protein as well as having many other benefits when included in a diet. Climbing beans are also one part of the"three sisters" that Native Americans used to provide all of the essential amino acids one needs in their diet. They are easy to grow, come in countless varieties, and I recommend you having several varieties for your medicinal garden. They also are very useful as a non-animal protein source.

Lemon Balm (Melissa officinales): Lemon balm is also known as balm or balm mint. It is a member of the mint family and can be used medicinally either as a tea and taken internally or as an oil and massaged into the skin. As a tea it is used for anxiety and sedation. As oil it is used for Graves' disease or hyperthyroidism (overactive thyroid) because of its effect on the thyroid. It is the main ingredient in Carmelite water, which is popular in Germany.

Lemongrass Oil: Lemongrass oil is made from the plant Cymbopogonflexuous. It is in the grass family and is so named due to its lemon fragrance. It has many medicinal uses for a variety of infections; it also helps with edema and digestive problems and improves circulation.

Lemon Myrtle Oil (Backhousiacitriodora): Lemon Myrtle oil is made from the tree of the same name. It is not only a strong antiseptic, but also has strong antiviral, antibacterial, and antifungal properties, and as such is excellent for wounds and infections.

Lemon juice: Useful for cooking, added to drinks it makes them healthful and refreshing. It is excellent when applied to insect bites and stings. Added to water daily it helps prevent kidney stones.

L-Glutamine: L-glutamine is an amino acid that helps heal burns, it also prevents infections and promotes healing.

Lidocaine ointment or gel (xylocaine): Lidocaine is a local anesthetic (numbs up and kills pain). It is useful when muscles are sore, it also can be found in a liquid form that can be injected locally for pain control.

Linden Oil: This is an essential oil made from the flowers of the linden tree. It is a useful essential oil, see the essential oil section for complete details.

Lipoic acid (Alpha-Lipoic acid): This is often abbreviated ALA. See text for full details but this is essential for the antioxidant cascade and supporting your immune system. It also gives much needed energy when a patient is fatigued. ALA is also very useful in the treatment of diabetes and diabetic peripheral neuropathy. The dose varies between 300 - 1200 mg daily. Like many substances it comes in two forms, essentially mirror images of each other, the R and S forms. Some ALA is labeled R/S when it contains both forms. The active form in the body is the R form, so try to purchase R-ALA.

L-Lysine (amino acid): Lysine uses a receptor on the surface of the cell that is very similar to that of arginine. The herpes family of viruses…chickenpox, herpes [genital and labial (lip)] infections and herpes zoster (shingles) all require arginine for the replication of the virus. If you take L-lysine when you have a herpes infection or to prevent one, it will flood the receptors and prevent the uptake of arginine and will help stop the virus dead in its tracks. I always give it along with vitamin C to boost your immune system.

Lobelia (Lobelia inflate): Lobelia is also known as Indian tobacco, due to the fact that Indians used to smoke this herb, ironically to treat respiratory problems. It works well to dilate the lungs and improve breathing and as such is useful in asthma attacks. It is potentiated by mixing it in tincture form with tincture of cayenne pepper.

Lomatiumdissectum: Lomatium is a plant in the carrot family. It has strong antibacterial and antiviral properties and is even active against tuberculosis. It is the strongest native antiviral plant that we have, and as such is very useful against colds, flu, and other viral illnesses.

Lycopene: Lycopene is a red plant pigment in the carotene family, found in tomatoes and many other red fruits (but not all red fruits). It is an antioxidant but it also has been found to be useful in exercised-induced asthma.

Lye: Lye is made from the burning of wood, which creates ashes; these ashes are then soaked in water and the water soluble alkaline substance produced is lye. Lye can be used to make soap by adding it to animal fat.

M:

Maalox: Maalox is an antacid used for relief of stomach upset and heartburn. It is made of calcium carbonate and can also be used for a source of calcium. It is also a laxative and will relieve constipation. It is useful for the treatment of ulcers.

Magnesium Oil: Magnesium oil is a misnomer, it is not an oil but a supersaturated magnesium chloride in water. Applied to the skin, it bypasses the intestines and helps relax the area where it is applied. It is excellent to use for orthopedic injuries.

Magnesium tablets: Slow-Mag, magnesium oxide, etc. These are very useful for nutrition and leg cramps, migraine headaches, muscle spasms, constipation, and especially to lower blood pressure in patients with hypertension. The usual dosage range is between 300 and 1,000 mg daily. If you are taking too much you will experience some diarrhea.

Magnesium Oxide: A form of magnesium, see above.

Magnesium sulfate (Epsom salt): I would buy a large supply of this, multiple uses. It has multiple uses for severe constipation, muscle aches, joint aches, and sore feet and is very effective when made into a poultice and applied to sore areas of the body.

Maitake Mushrooms (Grifolafrundosa): Another medicinal mushroom that is an important immune system booster and antioxidant. It is loaded with many phytonutrients including B vitamins, minerals, fiber, and amino acids, thus it is a wonderful food as well.

Majestic Earth plant-derived minerals: A large supply of these as well. These are an excellent source of all minerals and trace elements in colloidal form, so they are well assimilated (absorbed and used by your body).

Mannose Binding Lectins (MBL): Mannose Binding Lectins are one of the most important lectins, or proteins, that attach themselves to invading microorganisms like viruses and prevent their entry into cells; thus they are potent as antiviral proteins. Red algae contain large amounts of MBLs and is useful in the treatment of viral diseases.

Manuka honey: This is the most potent medicinal honey; it is from New Zealand. In fact, the healing power of honeys is compared using a scale called the Unique Manuka Factor. Manuka honey is useful to help heal all types of wounds, burns, ulcers, and other skin problems. See the section in the text on honey. Manuka honey amazingly comes from the same Manuka tree that Tea Tree Oil is made from.

Marshmallow Root: Marshmallow root is a mucilaginous herb, like psyllium and slippery elm. It contains a lot of soluble fiber, and when dissolved in water, it forms a gel that absorbs water and helps diarrhea.

Marijuana: Illegal; Excellent for anxiety, loss of appetite, stress relief, and general relaxation. Highly recommended as an aphrodisiac as well as a euphoric (something that induces euphoria or happiness), but I never told you that...LOL. Its medicinal uses have been recognized by many states which have legalized medicinal marijuana use.

Meadowsweet (Spiraeaulmaria): Meadowsweet is a perennial herb in the rose family, found in damp meadows, it contains salicin, which is the active ingredient in aspirin, and thus helps fevers.

Melatonin: Melatonin is a hormone secreted by the pineal gland deep inside the human brain. It controls your biological clock that in turn controls your body's natural rhythms of sleep and wakefulness. It helps sleep and is naturally released by the body with the onset of darkness, its release declines with age. It is also a very potent antioxidant, thus has been found to be protective from cancer. It also helps decrease blood pressure at night and also helped reduce the frequency and severity of migraine headaches.

Metamucil: Great laxative and fiber supplement, contains psyllium husk. Its use as a fiber supplement can decrease the absorption of vitamins, minerals, and proteins.

Methylene Blue: Methylene blue is a organic pigment that has antiseptic qualities and is used along with Gentian violet in an excellent wound care product called Hydrofera which is very effective in prevention of wound infections.

Methylsulfonylmethane (MSM): See MSM below.

Milk of Magnesia (Magnesium hydroxide): When you suspend magnesium hydroxide in water, it develops a milky appearance and hence the name Milk of Magnesia. It is used as an antacid as well as a laxative. It has a strong osmotic effect, meaning it draws fluid to itself and therefore pulls fluid into the intestines and helps the dryness of constipation. It does interfere with the absorption of both folic acid and iron and therefore you should be cautious with its long-term usage.

Mineral clays: See Bentonite and Kaolin.

Mineral Oil: Mineral oils are mostly made from petroleum. They have medicinal uses for vaginal dryness and skin dryness. They are also used to remove impacted earwax.

Mint: Mint is a perennial herb (comes back every year, as opposed to an annual which only lives one season). Mint is unusual in the plant world for having a square stem instead of round. It is used to treat stomach aches. Menthol is made from mint and works as a decongestant. It also has many uses as an essential oil, see that section in the text for complete details. Mint is very easy to grow and is also very invasive. You only need to buy one or two plants and you will have mint for life. If you have a small garden area, plant it in pots to prevent it from taking over your garden.

Mirrors: Small dental type will come in handy to view inside the mouth, especially in hard-to-reach corners in the back.

MMS (miracle mineral solution): Multiple anti-infective uses when antibiotics run out. See text for details. Highly controversial substance, banned for human use in the Unites States and Canada.

Mole pads: Buy a stock of these; useful for any foot problems such as blisters, corns , bunions etc.

Moringaoleifera: An African tree with a multitude of health benefits. It can be grown in the United States and treated as an annual, harvested for its multiple health benefits. It is also known as the Ben oil tree. It is full of protein, vitamins A and C, potassium and calcium to name but a few of its nutrients. See text for complete details.

Motrin (Ibuprofen): Stockpile as much of this as you can. It is a very useful painkiller, fever reducer, and to reduce soft tissue swelling.

Mountain Savory Oil (Satureja Montana): This is a essential oil that also has strong antimicrobial effects as well as positive effects on both the digestive and immune systems. It also works well against skin infections and genitourinary tract infections. Like almost all essential oils other than lavender oil, it needs to be diluted with a carrier oil and can be irritating to the mucous membranes of the mouth.

MSM (methylsulfonylmethane): MSM is a medicinal supplement that is an organic sulfur-containing compound that supposedly works by its contribution of organic sulfur to the body. It is especially useful in joint aches, as my wife will readily attest to its use for joint pain. It is frequently combined with glucosamine chondroitin for osteoarthritis and joint complaints. It is also used for its anti- inflammatory effects.

Mucilaginous Herbs: Mucilaginous herbs are herbs that become a slippery, gel- like mass when mixed with water and are excellent in the treatment of diarrhea. Three of the best are slippery elm, marshmallow root, and psyllium. They are full of soluble fiber and thus it absorbs water, and helps diarrhea.

Mullein Oil: This essential oil is made from the very common weed of the same name. Look up a photo of it online and you will immediately recognize it from your garden. See section on essential oils for full details.

Mycorrhizal fungi: Another very essential item for the medicinal garden. This soil fungus is utilized by the vast majority of the world's plants. It is a normal inhabitant of healthy soil. This fungus enters the roots of plants and feeds the plant minerals and other soil nutrients in exchange for sugar from the plant. This fungus greatly enlarges the surface area of plant roots, enabling them to be much more effective. I sprinkle some powdered form of this onto the roots of everything I plant.

Mylanta: Useful antacid and for intestinal gas relief.

Myrrh Oil (Commiphoramyrrha): This is made from the resin of Myrhh, which is from Egypt. It has both antiviral and antibacterial properties. It also is a strong astringent and will contract skin and help contract blood vessels and slow bleeding, it also slows hair loss. It is also antifungal and will help athlete's foot, ringworm, and jock itch. It should be used carefully in people with hypertension (high blood pressure), taken internally it may take away your appetite, cause stomach aches, and nausea and headaches.

N:

N-Acetylcysteine (NAC): NAC is a derivative of the amino acid cysteine. It is a strong antioxidant but its best use is to liquefy mucus in the sinuses and bronchioles, helping to mobilize those secretions. For that reason it is very effective in allergies and sinus problems, but will also help colds and congestion.

Nail clippers: I would recommend avoiding the small size, they are weak and annoying. Get the largest clippers you can find; buy a couple, they are always useful to have around.

Naproxen (Aleve): Essential painkiller, anti-inflammatory, reduce high fevers, stockpile a large supply of this. Be careful always to take it on a full stomach to prevent GI upset. It is also very useful in the treatment of migraine headaches and hangovers.

Neosporin ointment: This is a combination antibiotic cream used to treat minor cuts and scrapes as well as minor skin infections.

You don't usually need this to heal a wound, most will heal without infection, unless from a bite or other germ-filled source. When you use it, apply it tid or three times a day until the wound heals. It is also known as triple antibiotic ointment because it is a combination ofPolymyxin B, Neomycin, and Bacitracin.

Neroli Oil: This is an essential oil made from the fragrant blossoms of orange trees, please see essential oil section for full details. It is the one of the most expensive oils.

Neti Pot: If you suffer with allergies or sinus problems this is key. Using this pot to flush out your sinuses will keep them clear of allergens (allergy causing substances) as well as flushing out any mucous sinus drainage. The solution used to clean your sinuses is a combination of saline (salt water) and sterile water. There is some potential danger in not using sterile water because of possible contamination with parasites, etc. I find that I enjoy a good nasal irrigation every night before bed with a saline solution; it moisturizes my nasal passages and washes out any debris and allergens. If you suffer with severe allergies or dry, cracked nasal mucosa (the lining of your nose) then you too should consider this practice daily.

Nettle Root: An extract of this plant root has been shown to have uricosuric properties and helps gout by promoting the excretion of uric acid. It can be taken as a tea or in capsule form.

Niacinamide (vitamin B3): Niacinamide is one of the members of the family of B vitamins known as B complex. Niacinamide is a metabolite of niacin but without any of the side effects like flushing. It is as effective as benzodiazepines in the treatment of anxiety, but without any addiction problems.

Noxzema: An emulsion made of fats and beeswax, very useful as a moisturizer and to rub on to sore muscles, helps irritated skin as well.

Nutmeg Oil: This is an essential oil made from the seeds of the plant Myristicafragrans. See the essential oil section for full details.

O:

Occlusive dressing: Good to have for trauma and to keep a wound dry.

Oil of Cloves (clove oil): Originally from India, it is an important painkiller, especially for dental problems. It helps moisturize skin and reduces skin inflammation; it also helps cough medicine taste better. It helps a toothache by either using a leaf directly on the tooth or some oil; a little rubbed on the gums of an infant will help teething. It will work as a painkiller rubbed directly into your skin, helps foot pain the same way. It will heal raw, irritated skin from bed sores to poison ivy or oak. It also has the effect of dilating blood vessels, so it helps with tension headaches. For a headache apply some oil to a rag and apply that to the forehead and temples. Or just rub a few drops into your forehead and temples (temporal area). For stomach pain put a few drops in a glass of juice or water and drink it.

Olive Leaf: Olive leaf in the United States usually comes in a powdered form. It is beneficial in the lowering of blood pressure and the usual dose for that is 500 mg qid or four times daily. Note: Like many botanicals it may take three or four months to take full effect.

Olive Oil: Multiple uses, food, nutrition, and you can even put a shoelace wick in it and make a candle. As a medicinal I would recommend Extra Virgin Olive Oil, which is made from the first pressing of the olives or drupes. It is excellent for dry skin; the Romans used it for this for centuries. Olive oil is a potent anti-inflammatory, as potent as ibuprofen, thus has a role in the reduction of breast cancer rates. It also helps lower blood pressure and cholesterol and triglycerides (bad fats in your blood). It is rich in antioxidants, especially vitamin E. Among plant oils, olive oil is the highest in monounsaturated fats, which is beneficial because it does not oxidize like the polyunsaturated fats. Olive oil has been shown to help bone mineralization and calcification by helping in calciumabsorption; thus it is helpful in osteopenia (the stage betweennormal and osteoporosis) and osteoporosis

Omega-3 Fatty Acids (Fish oil): I would stockpile the best quality you can find, multiple uses.

Works for heart health, lowers blood pressure, helps your brain and your skin, and helps depression and ADD, ADHD, and anxiety disorders. It helps inflamed muscles and joints especially in arthritis. Helps lower cholesterol and triglycerides and raises good HDL cholesterol.

Omeprazole (Prilosec): Over-the-counter potent acid reducer. See Prilosec for full details.

Oragel (Benzocaine): Topical painkiller for dental problems.

Oregano Oil: Useful essential oil with multiple medical uses. It can be used in a vaporizer to open up a stuffed head; several drops can be added to juice or water for a sore throat treatment. It is reported to have both antifungal and antiviral effects. You can mix it with a carrier oil such as jojoba, grape seed, or almond oil, at a rate of twelve drops of oregano oil to one ounce of carrier oil. Do not use it on broken skin, it will burn. It will work like a natural insect repellent just like mint or thyme; mix it with a carrier oil and apply it before going outside. It is very strong and tastes horrible, so be prepared. You can also use it with a carrier oil like olive oil and rub it on your skin, helps with psoriasis. It is not advised to use oregano oil on pregnant women or nursing women, children, and people with hypertension or heart problems.

P:

Para cord (Parachute cord): Multiple emergency uses, including tying splints, etc.

Parsley Oil: An essential oil made from the plant Petroselinumsativum, please see essential oil section for complete details. Be very careful with this, it can be very toxic.

Passionflower (Passifloraincarnata): Passionflower works its magic in a similar fashion as Valerian, it calms and soothes nerves and is mildly sedating. It is useful in anxiety, insomnia, and also hypertension.

Patchouli Oil: An essential oil that was and is still very popular with "hippy chics". See essential oil section for full details.

Pepcid AC or Pepcid Complete: These are H2 blockers, as is Zantac, and are useful to cut down stomach acid. This class is not as strong as the PPIs like Prilosec, but they work fine and are inexpensive. Sodium bicarbonate (baking soda) works very well to neutralize stomach acid and is a lot cheaper; you just cannot take it for too long due to pH changes.

Peppermint (Tea or Oil): An essential oil that works very well for pain and sore muscles and headaches. You should dilute it in a carrier oil to prevent any skin irritation. Peppermint tea also soothes the stomach and intestines and is useful for nausea and vomiting. See text for complete details.

Peru Balsam: An essential oil made from a balsam tree of the same name; please see section on essential oils for full details.

Pine Oil: An essential oil made from pine tree resin; see section on essential oils for full details.

Plantain (PlantagoMajor or PlantagoLanceolata): A family of weeds that have naturalized all over the world. Plantain, when chewed and made into a poultice or a paste, is wonderful to treat bites, stings, and wounds and will prevent infections and promote healing as well as easing pain, itching, and stinging.

Plastic Food Wrap: Useful for occlusive dressings for wounds, besides food uses.

Pond's Cold Cream: An emulsion made of fats and beeswax; it is an excellent moisturizer and can be used in the nose to moisten the cracked, dry mucous membrane lining the nose when you have nose bleeds.

Potash: Potash is a water soluble, potassium-containing compound made from wood ash. After the burning of wood, the ashes are soaked in water and this creates lye, which is very alkaline. The liquid lye was placed in large pots and the water was boiled off; the remaining substance is potash, which is a wonderful fertilizer, but like lye, it is very alkaline.

Potassium: The mineral potassium is one of the most important electrolytes in the human body. It can be used to lower blood pressure, along with magnesium and calcium. It helps muscle cramps, Charlie horses, and actually helps sleep if given at bedtime. It also helps with restless leg syndrome (that feeling as if your legs cannot relax and you are moving them under your covers at night). It should be given with care in patients with renal disease. Bananas and all dried fruit like raisins, dates, cranberries, and prunes are high in potassium.

Potassium Iodide: Potassium iodide is a reduced form of iodine that is very useful to take as a supplement when there is a suspicion of impending radiation exposure, it will protect your thyroid gland from the uptake of radioactive iodine and prevent thyroid cancer.

Prilosec (Omeprazole): Prilosec is an over-the-counter PPI or proton pump inhibitor; another is Prevacid. They work to decrease the production of stomach acid in patients with reflux (heartburn), gastritis, and ulcers. If you suffer with these problems you should probably stockpile a supply of these. Sodium bicarbonate or baking soda in water helps as well, as does an apple twice a day.

Propolis: Propolis is the resinous mixture that bees gather from tree sap, tree buds, and other floral sources, and they use it to seal gaps and problem areas within their hives. Propolis is very useful in the treatment of herpes infections of all types. It is also known as bee propolis.

Psyllium seed: Psyllium is a plant originally from India called Plantagoovata. Psyllium seed is full of soluble fiber that forms a gel in the intestine and promotes good flow of stools, thus helping constipation, as well as lowering cholesterol. See Metamucil.

Q:

Q-tips: I would stockpile a large supply of these, very useful and inexpensive. Be very careful when placing Q-tips in the ear, to prevent perforation of the eardrum.

Quinton Marine Plasma: A wonderful, health enhancing drink made from plankton blooms in the world's oceans. Buy the isotonic, not the hypertonic form. It is wonderful for your overall health and provides all the minerals and trace elements found normally in ocean water. See text for full details.

Quercetin: Quercetin is a flavonoid which is a class of plant pigments. It is found in fruits, vegetables, and grains. It works as an antihistamine and an anti-inflammatory agent and is very useful in the treatment of allergy problems.

R:

Ranitidine (Zantac): See Zantac below for complete details.

Red Algae: Red algae is used to treat viral infections, due to its high content of Mannose Binding Lectins, preventing the viral particles from adhering to and crossing into cells. See Mannose Binding Lectins, Lectins.

Red Cross Toothache Medicine: A great over-the-counter toothache powder.

Reishi (Ganodermalucidum): Reishi is a type of medicinal mushroom that has many beneficial effects, such as activating the immune system to fight viral and bacterial infections, lowering blood pressure and cholesterol levels, and protecting the body from cancer. Most of its positive effects come from its high beta-glucan content.

Resveratrol: Resveratrol is a plant-derived polyphenol that is found in the skin of grapes and other plants. It has multiple health enhancing properties such as decreasing the stickiness of platelets, lowering insulin resistance, lowering cancer rates, and even helping in weight loss. It is also a strong antioxidant.

Rhodiolarosea: Rhodiola is a perennial plant also known as Golden Root and Russian Rhodiola. It works well against fatigue, anxiety, depression, and helps to increase attentiveness.

Rock dust: Approach a local quarry to see if you can buy a large supply of this. Fabulous for your medicinal garden. Rock dustprovides a great source of minerals for soil microorganisms and results in large, robust, and very healthy plants. The plants will convert the inorganic minerals into a colloidal organic form that can be readily utilized by your body. Add a generous quantity of this to your soil annually and watch your vegetables flourish and convert all those minerals into tasty health-giving vegetables.

Roman Chamomile Oil: An essential oil different in its uses from German chamomile. Please see essential oil section for full details.

Rose Oil: An essential oil made from roses. Very often the very fragrant Damascus rose is used in its production. See section on essential oils for full details.

Rosemary Oil (Rosmarinusofficinales): Naturally this is made from rosemary (did that really surprise you?), which is a perennial herb with evergreen- type, aromatic leaves. It is a wonderful garden plant and will give you the raw material to make this essential oil. It is used to help sooth sore muscles, help gout, and it also helps memory, hence the reason rosemary was thrown into graves as people were buried, to help remember them after their death. If you like to cook, especially Italian food (which, let's face it, is the best food on the planet), it is used as an ingredient for flavoring various dishes. It is easy to grow in well drained, good soil with a lot of sun exposure, and I would include it in any medicinal garden.

S:

Safety Pins: Useful for holding ace bandages, etc.

Saint John's-wort: Saint John's-wort is a perennial flowering herb that has naturalized all over the world. It is used as a treatment for both anxiety and depression and also has antimicrobial properties as well as anti- inflammatory properties. It is also made into oil and is useful in the treatment of otalgia or ear pain.

Saline Spray: This is another name for salt water. It is inexpensive and good for wound irrigation as well as sinus irrigation. See neti pot above.

SAM-e (S-adenosyl methionine): This compound is made from the enzymatic conversion of the body's energy molecule ATP with the amino acid methionine. It is produced and consumed primarily in the liver and is involved in many of the body's metabolic pathways. It originally was thought to be useful in the treatment of Alzheimer's disease, but it was later discovered that the problem was a B12 deficiency. However, it is very useful in the treatment of arthritis, fibromyalgia, and joint complaints. SAM-e is best absorbed on an empty stomach and it also requires the ingestion of vitamins B6, B12, and folate all of which are in B complex vitamins). Do not take SAM-e if you are taking levodopa for Parkinson's disease since it will reduce its effectiveness.

SAM (structural aluminum malleable): Great for splints, these are very useful and come in various sizes and are easily molded to whatever needs arise. Smaller sizes are great for fingers.

Salicylic Acid: Nature's aspirin, from a willow tree bark. It has many medicinal uses, same as aspirin. Aspirin is so inexpensive and so readily available without a prescription, so I would recommend stockpiling aspirin instead of this. Also, the doses of aspirin will be more precise.

Scalpels: I would recommend getting both #11 and #15, and a good supplyof them. Number 11 scalpels are for lancing (piercing) and the #15s are for cutting.

Scenar: This Russian handheld device is wonderful for helping pain and disease. It stands for Self Controlling Energy Neuro Adaptive Regulator. What it is in essence is an electrical nerve stimulator coupled to a biofeedback energy generator that sends specific frequencies back into the body to raise the voltage and heal the cells.

Scissors: Get various sizes, including those heavy duty ones that cut through everything. Small surgical ones are good as well as medium sizes for cutting hair.

Sea Salt (Celtic Sea Salt): This is salt derived from dehydrated sea water. It is much better for you than traditional table salt which is just sodium chloride, which does not contain these other minerals and trace elements and is unnatural and foreign to your body.

Selenium (Selenium methionine): Essential mineral for your thyroid and your overall health. It helps reduce cancer rates when high in soil, helps boost your immune system, and helps joint pain. The recommended daily dose is 200 mcg (micrograms) daily. It is available in the vitamin section of most health food stores and pharmacies. Selenium methionine is the chelated form of selenium, and thus better absorbed and utilized by the body. See Brewer's Yeast.

Serratiopeptidase: Serratiopeptidase is an enzyme produced in the intestines of silk moths. The moth uses this enzyme to dissolve its cocoon so it can escape. It is a protease enzyme, meaning it digests proteins and as such is used to dissolve circulating immune complexes in allergies.

Sesame Oil: Sesame oil is an oil derived from sesame seeds. It is used in cooking in India and parts of Asia and the Middle East. It also has medicinal uses as a stress reliever for massages, as well as lowering blood pressure. It is very rich in antioxidants and healthy polyunsaturated fats and especially in vitamin E. It also is rich in calcium, magnesium, zinc, copper, and vitamin B6.

Shiitake Mushrooms (Lentinulaedodes): A medicinal, edible mushroom from Asia. Like many other medicinal mushrooms it is an immune system booster and a strong antioxidant. It also has many wonderful phytonutrients.

Silvadene Burn Cream (silver sulfadiazine): A very useful cream to have for burns; prevents infection and promotes healing. Silver is a strong antimicrobial. Many people use colloidal silver to treat systemic infections.

Simethicone: Good for intestinal gas. It has many brand names, Gas-X, for example.

Sleepytime Tea: Made with Valerian root and is excellent for insomnia.

Sling: You can make these, but ask friends for old ones they no longer use, or save your own. Flea markets and garage sales are excellent sources of used medical equipment like slings, crutches, immobilizers, etc. You should stock up on all of these for your medicine chest.

Slippery Elm: Slipperyelmisamucilaginousherb, like psylliumandmarshmallow root. It contains a large amount of soluble fiber that forms a gel-like mass and absorbs water, thus helping diarrhea.

Soap: Liquid and hard soaps are useful for disinfection. You will need a good supply of these. Stock up on both types whenever you see a sale; they will come in handy and are inexpensive.

Soft Cervical Collar: If you or a friend has one of these from a neck injury, then save them. You can also improvise one from those neck pillows they sell for airplanes or roll up a towel and bind it with duct tape.

Sodium bicarbonate (baking soda): Buy a large supply of this for your medicine chest, multiple uses. See text for complete details.

Spenco Second Skin: I would buy both the blister kits and the burn pads, very useful stuff. You can go online and see the various product lines they offer.

Stethoscope: Get one of these; even if you don't know how to use it, you may find a doctor or nurse who does. It is relatively easy to master and allows you audible access to the chest, lungs, heart, and abdomen to access problems.

Stinging Nettle: Stinging nettle is an annual weed that is a strong antihistamine without the sedation or dry-mouth side effects of pharmaceutical antihistamines.

Stolle's Milk: Stolle's milk is a special preparation of milk enhanced by exposing the cow to different infections so it will produce antibodies that are naturally concentrated in its milk. See the entire section on it under the 'how to treat any infection' section.

Supreme Fulvic: The brand name of a wonderful natural powder made from deposits on an ancient seabed that had volcanic ash deposited into it, resulting in a mix of all minerals and trace elements as well as amino acids and fulvic acid. Fulvic acid causes cell membranes to become more permeable (open to) the absorption of these same minerals, trace elements, and amino acids and has many other health benefits.

Surgical Masks: You will need these to protect the patient and yourself, also if epidemics occur.

Surgical Tape: Get a good supply of this, it is inexpensive and very valuable. It comes as either paper or cloth tape; both have their uses.

Syntra5: This is an all-natural proprietary herbal mix that is very useful in treating diabetes. See the diabetes section for complete details. It is a little expensive, but if you are a brittle diabetic (poorly controlled), then this could prove life saving for you.

Syringes: The large 50 cc syringes are especially useful for wound irrigation as well as cleaning ears. I would buy at least three of these.

T:

Tallow: Tallow is made from raw beef or mutton fat known as suet. Suet usually comes from nearby the kidneys and loin of these cows and sheep. The fat is rendered,which just means the process by which this hard fat is processed into either lard or tallow. Rendering also means utilizing almost everything from a slaughtered animal. The difference between lard and tallow is that lard is made from pork (pig) fat and tallow is either from beef or sheep. Tallow is high in both Vitamins A and D (Vitamins E and K in lesser amounts), both of which are very healthy for your skin. You have to get organic, grass fed animals for your tallow, these are full of minerals and trace elements and vitamins along with omega-3 fatty acids. Industrially raised animals are full of hormones and toxic chemicals which get concentrated in their fatty tissue and therefore are further concentrated in their fat and the tallow. Tallow is wonderful for all skin ailments, especially psoriasis and eczema, and for burns of all types, including sunburn.

Taurine: Taurine is an amino acid or a building block to a protein. Like many amino acids it has a profound effect when used to target a problem, in this case to lower blood pressure, at a dose of six grams a day.

Tea Tree Oil: Tea tree oil comes from the leaves of the melaleuca tree from Australia. It is a very potent antimicrobial and is very useful for all kinds of infections. There is a word of caution about using it too diluted where it will be too weak to work and may lead to microbial resistance. This is not a problem when used at the proper strength.

Tecnu: Tecnu is the brand name for an alcohol-based solution which removes urushiol, the oil substance that is contained in the plant tissues of poison ivy, poison oak, and poison sumac. It is the substance which causes the allergic reaction responsible for those rashes. Fortunately it is soluble in alcohol, benzene, and ether, meaning that it is dissolved by those substances. Tecnu contains alcohol which removes this oily resin and helps prevent the allergic reaction. Note: You should always use cold water to remove urushiol, and do it ASAP after exposure. Hot water will open your skin pores and facilitate the entry of urushiol deeper into the skin where the body attacks it and the allergic reaction causes the rash and the insufferable itch.

Tennant Biomodulator: The Tennant biomodulator is a handheld electrical device similar to the Scenar. It is an electric nerve stimulator coupled with a biofeedback device that generates healing frequencies back to the body. It is outstanding for promotion of pain control and healing of tissues.

Theanine: Theanine is a non-protein amino acid found in green tea. Theanine works by its effects on several neurotransmitters in the brain, causing relaxation and relief of anxiety. It is potentiated by co-administration with GABA.

Thermometer: Do not get the digital electronic versions, eventually the batteries will die. Get a couple of the old fashioned mercury thermometers, they will last forever if you don't drop them.

Thyme Oil (Thymus labiatae): Originally a Mediterranean area plant, it is now grown all over the world. The oil of this plant has very strong antimicrobial properties and works against MRSA, VRE, anthrax, TB, and typhoid among many other infections. Keep a good supply of this oil in your medicine chest, few other oils compare to it in its disease fighting abilities.

Tick Twister: A wonderful small plastic device that easily removes ticks. These only cost a few dollars and are wonderful to have. If you ever have tried to remove a tick you realize how tenacious they are.

Tinactin (Tolnaftate): This is an antifungal agent, comes in cream, spray, and powder; also called Absorbine, Odor Eaters, etc. Useful for athlete's foot, jock itch, and ringworm (which is a fungus, not a worm).

Tincture of Iodine: Very useful for small cuts and scrapes to prevent infection. Like all tinctures it is made with alcohol, combined with elemental iodine. It is about 50 % alcohol and thus it is about 100 proof. It is a useful topical antiseptic for wound cleaning. It can also be used in a pinch to disinfect water at a rate of 5 drops of the 2 % tincture per liter of water. This contains about 1 mg of free iodine per drop. Other than this purpose, which I would recommend Lugol's solution for rather than tincture of iodine, it should never be taken orally.

Tolnaftate: See Zeasorb. It is an antifungal agent. It is also the active ingredient in Lamisil AF, Tinactin, Tinaderm, Absorbine, and Odor Eaters.

Tongue Depressors: These are valuable for a you to be able to visualize a person's throat. Another good trick is to ask the person to yawn, as this opens up their mouths and depresses their tongues. They can also be cut down and used for finger splints; keep the round end on the bottom so it will not cut the skin between fingers.

Transglucosidase enzyme: An enzyme that blocks the metabolism of dietary starches to glucose, hence its usefulness in both diabetes and weight loss. See diabetes section for complete details.

Turmeric (Curcuma longa): Turmeric is a perennial herb from India. It is a powerful antioxidant and also has antimicrobial properties and can be used as a wound paste to prevent infections. It also has powerful anti- inflammatory properties and thus helps in asthma.

U:

UvaUrsi (ArctostaphylosUva-ursi): UvaUrsi is the botanical name for bearberry. It has strong antimicrobial properties and is excellent for the treatment of urinary tract infections. It works best in alkaline urine, so make sure not to take anything that may acidify your urine, like vitamin C.

V:

Valerian Root (Valerianaofficinalis): The primary ingredient in Sleepytime Tea, very relaxing and sedating and non-habit forming. Valerian helps relax and soothe nerves; in many people this constant anxiety is the cause of their hypertension and thus Valerian lowers blood pressure nicely. It can also be used for anxiety and insomnia.

Vanadium: Vanadium is an essential trace element that has the effect of mimicking the action of insulin and thus is useful in the treatment of diabetes. The dose is between 5 and 20 mg daily.

Vanilla Oil: An essential oil made from the seed pods of the vanilla plant. It has many medicinal uses, please see essential oil section for complete details.

Vaseline Petroleum Jelly (Petrolatum): Very useful stuff, not only for lubrication, toenail fungus, nosebleeds, and chest colds. Since it is a petroleum product it can also be used to start a fire, as it is very flammable.

Vicks VapoRub: Vicks VapoRub is a mentholated topical cream, made with an oil base. This works great for chest congestion for children and adults. It should not be used in infants where it increases inflammation and chest congestion. It should not be used in the nose or mouth where it potentially could be inhaled into the lungs. It contains camphor, eucalyptus oil, and menthol as its primary active ingredients. These all act as cough suppressants as well as having topical analgesic effects.

Vinegar: Keep a ready supply of this on hand. It has multiple nutritional and medicinal uses. See text for complete details.

Vitamins: Stockpile these as well, including A, B complex, C, D3 (the best form of D), E, K2 (best form of K), CoQ 10, alpha lipoic acid, and a good multivitamin with minerals and trace elements. Remember that only B and C can be taken on an empty stomach because they are water soluble. All the others need to be taken with a fatty meal or they will not be absorbed; that includes the multivitamin.

VSL #3: Currently this is the strongest probiotic on the market and very useful to recolonize an intestinal tract that has been ravaged by the use of antibiotics as well as being very useful in inflammatory bowel diseases like Crohn's and ulcerative colitis.

W:

Walnut Oil: Walnut oil is extracted from English walnuts (also called Persian walnuts). It is used in cooking as well as nutritionally. It is a wonderful source of healthy polyunsaturated and monounsaturated fatty acids. It also contains large amounts of Linoleic acid and alpha Linoleic acid which are converted by the body to omega-3 fatty acids. Hence, along with Flaxseed oil it is a good source of omega-3 fatty acids from sources other than fish oil. I happen to think that it also tastes very good, so add it to your salads and vegetables. If you have any skin conditions, like psoriasis and eczema, essential fatty acids and vitamin D are very helpful in their treatment.

White Petrolatum: Petroleum jelly same as Vaseline. Note: Like all petroleum products this will work well to start a fire.

White Tea: White tea is made from young, unopened tea buds and young tea leaves. It is the most potent of all the teas in its anticancer, antifungal, antibacterial, and antiviral effects. It promotes good health overall and should be included in your daily regimen. Please see the section on treatment of infections without antibiotics for complete details.

White Vinegar: Also known as distilled vinegar, which is a misnomer; it is not made by distillation but rather by fermentation of distilled alcohol. The fermentate is then diluted to a 5 - 8% acetic acid solution, with a pH of 2.4. White vinegar is used medicinally as well as in cooking,baking, meat preservation, and pickling.

White Willow: See Willow Bark.

Willow Bark: All types of willows love wet soils, consequently they all have very watery bark sap which contains large amounts of salicylic acids. It is the source for aspirin, and thus is used in the treatment of pain and fever. Willow bark has been used for thousands of years for this purpose by people throughout the world. It has also been used topically for the treatment of acne, seborrhea of the scalp, and psoriasis. As a 6% solution it has been mixed in petroleum jelly and used topically on calluses, warts for one hour at a time and then washed off, twice daily at most due to its potential to irritate skin. It helps to soften and moisturize, which can be fatal. It should also not be used if you have bleeding or clotting problems, since just like aspirin it will increase bleeding.

Witch Hazel: A good astringent, use on hemorrhoids to shrink them. It is also a useful medicinal small shrub easyto grow in your medicinal garden. Witch hazel is produced from the leaves and bark.

Y:

Yarrow (Achilleamillefolium): Yarrow is also known as common yarrow. It is very useful in stopping bleeding and hence its other common name staunchweed. It is also useful in the treatment of fever.

Z:

Zantac (ranitidine): Zantac is an H2 blocker or a medication to cut down on heartburn (reflux) and gastritis, etc. by decreasing the production of stomach acid. Since the H in H2 means histamine, it is also useful along with antihistamines in the treatment of hives and other allergic reactions. Since it interferes with the production of intrinsic factor in the stomach, if used for a long period of time it will cause vitamin B12 deficiency.

Zeasorb Powder (tolnaftate): It is a topical antifungal agent. It is an excellent foot and groin powder for athlete's foot, ringworm, and jock itch. It also soothes sore feet. Tolnaftate is the active ingredient in Lamisil AF, Tinactin, and Absorbine, as well as Odor Eaters.

Zinc (in its various forms): Zinc oxide cream to help protect your skin from sun and helps burns. Zinc lozenges, great for cold sores, cankers, sore tongue and mouth. Zinc tablets to help raise zinc levels, good for wound healing. Also helps raise testosterone levels and is necessary for the production of insulin. There are several hundred enzyme systems in the body dependent upon zinc for their actions. Zinc also boosts the immune system, thus its beneficial effect upon infections. The usual dose is about 25 mg daily. This can be doubled in a patient who is severely injured, burned, or infected, who will require more. Remember, if you give zinc for any length of time you will also need to supplement with 3 mg of copper daily, since zinc will lower copper levels.

Zyrtec (Ceftirizine): It is an antihistamine, works well for itch, nausea, and vomiting, dizziness (vertigo), hay fever, and allergies of all types as well as hives. It is mildly sedating, so I often advise patients to take it at bedtime so the sedation wears off by morning.

BIBLIOGRAPHY AND SUGGESTED READING LIST TO FURTHER EXPLORE SOME OF THE CONCEPTS DISCUSSED IN THIS BOOK

1,801 Home Remedies: Trustworthy Treatments for Everyday Health Problems, published by Readers Digest Books, authored by various contributors, 2004.

Acupressure's Potent Points: A Guide to Self-Care for Common Ailments, by Michael Reed Gach, published by Bantam Books, 1990.

Acquiring Genomes: A Theory of the Origins of Species, by Lynn Margulis and Dorion Sagan, published by Basic Books 2002.

Advanced Aromatherapy: The Science of Essential Oil Therapy, by Kurt Schnabel, PhD, Healing Arts Press, 1995. This German author does a wonderful job on a difficult subject.

Alternative Medicine: The Definitive Guide, second edition, by Larry Trivieri, Jr. and John W. Anderson, editors, Celestial Arts Books, 2002. This is "The Handbook" to alternative medicine cures, exhaustively researched and written.

An Alternative Approach to Allergies: The New Field of Clinical Ecology Unravels the Environmental Causes of Mental and Physical Ills, by Theron G. Randolph, MD and Ralph W. Moss, PhD, published by Harper Row Publishers, revised edition 1989.

An Epidemic of Absence: A new way of understanding Allergies and Autoimmune Disease by Moises Velasquez-Manoff, published by Scribner, 2012. An excellent overview of the causes of disruption of the human immune system against a background of evolution and human history.

Aromatherapy for Health Professionals, 4th edition, by Shirley and Len Price, Churchill Livingstone Elsevier Publishers, 2013. An excellent work on aromatherapy and its uses medically.

Ascorbate: The Science of Vitamin C, by Dr. Steve Hickey and Dr. Hilary Roberts, 2004, no publisher listed.

The Backyard Homestead: produce all the food you need on just a ¼ acre edited by Carleen Madigan, Storey Publishing LLC, 2009.

Baking Soda, by Vicki Lasnky, published by Book Peddlers, 2004. This short book covers over 500 uses for baking soda.

Biochemical Individuality: The Key to Understanding What is Shaping Your Health, by Roger J. Williams, PhD, published by John Wiley and Sons, 1956. A book about our personal biochemical uniqueness and its ramifications for our health.

Biological Inorganic Chemistry: An introduction by Robert R. Crichton, published by Elsevier, 2008.

The Blue Book Guide to Preserving, printed by Ball, who is the manufacturer of ball bottles for canning and preserving. This is a concise but extensive review of canning techniques for a variety of foods, very useful book.

The Body Electric: Electromagnetism and the Foundation of Life, by Robert O. Becker, MD and Gary Selden, published by William Morrow and Company, 1985. This is a classic on the emerging field of energy medicine, using electric and electromagnetic forces as medical treatments.

Bottom Lines Prescription for Natural Cures by James F. Balch, MD and Mark Stengler, ND, published by Bottom Line Books, 2004.

Breakthrough: the Miracle Mineral Solutions of the 21st Century, parts 1 and 2, 4th edition, by Jim Humble.

Breed Your Own Vegetable Varieties: a gardener's and farmer's guide to plant breeding and seed saving by Carol Deppe, 2nd edition, published by Chelsea Green Publishing Company, 2000. In case you are want to store food long term, this book will teach you all you need to improve upon the varieties of vegetables that you have stashed in your medicinal seed vault.

Cancer and Vitamin C, by Linus Pauling and Ewan Cameron, revised edition, published by Camino Books, 1993. This is a classic, Linus Pauling at his best. This was one of the first alternative medical texts I ever read and it fascinated me, and still does.

Cancer Is a Fungus: A Revolution in Tumor Therapy, by Dr. T. Simoncini, Edizioni Lampis, 2005. This book is written by the courageous Dr. Simoncini and details some of his successes in treating cancer as the fungus that it might likely be.

Charcoal Remedies.com, by John Dinsley, by Gatekeeper Books, 2005. An excellent review of the multiple uses of activated charcoal.

The Chemistry of Essential Oils Made Simple, by David Stewart, Care Publications, 3rd printing, 2010. This is one of the best books you will ever find on this subject as well as chemistry in general.

The Chemistry of Man, 2nd edition, by Bernard Jensen, PhD.

Clinical Nutrition of the Essential Trace Elements and Minerals: The guide for health practitioners, edited by John D. Bogden, PhD, and Leslie M. Klevay, MD, Humana Press Publishers, 2000.

Colloidal Minerals and Trace Elements: How to Restore the Body's Natural Vitality, by Marie-France Muller, MD, ND, PhD, published by Healing Arts Press, 2002. This is hands down the best book written on this subject. I have a very worn, dog-eared copy. It is getting difficult to find.

Colloidal Silver: Medical Uses, Toxicology, and Manufacture, 3rd edition, by John Hill, published by Clear Springs Press, LLC.

Colloidal Silver Today: The All Natural Wide Spectrum Germ Killer, by Warren Jefferson, published by Healthy Living Publications, 2003.

Complete Book of Minerals for Health, by J.I. Rodale and staff, 6th printing, Rodale Books, Inc., 1967.

The Complete Guide to Edible Wild Plants, authored by The Department of the Army, Skyhorse Publishing, 2009.

The Complete Home Healer, by Angela Smyth, published by Harper Collins, 1994. A little dated but still informative.

Craft Cider Making, by Andrew Lea, published by The Good Life Press, Ltd, revised edition 2010. A very handy little guide to cider making, an great skill to have and a lot of fun.

Curing the Incurable: Vitamin C, Infectious Diseases, and Toxins, by Thomas E. Levy, MD, 3rd edition, published by LivOn Books, 2009. Dr. Levy is the world's expert on the various uses of vitamin C. This book is fascinating and compelling.

Dead Doctors Don't Lie, by Dr. Joel D. Wallach and Dr. Ma Lan, by Wellness Publications LLC, 1999. This is a classic that started as a series of lectures on cassette tapes. For someone new to the idea of mineral deficiencies, this will be very eye opening, although I am not particularly fond of the title!

Deep Nutrition: Why Your Genes Need Traditional Food, by Catherine Shanahan, MD and Luke Shanahan, published by Big Box Books, 2009. The author of this book has outstanding insight into real food and the need to eat wholesome, unadulterated foods and how they truly nourish our bodies.

Degeneration, Regeneration, by Melvin E. Page, DDS, Biochemical Research Foundation, 1949.

DHA: The Magnificent Marine Oil: Health Learning Handbook, by Beth M. Ley-Jacobs, PhD, published by BL Publications, 1999.

The Disease Delusion: Conquering the Causes of Chronic Illness for a Healthier, Longer, and Happier life, by Dr. Jeffrey S. Bland, Harper Collins Books, 2014.

Disease Prevention and Treatment, expanded 4th edition, by Life Extension Foundation, published by Life Extension Media, 2003. The Life Extension Foundation is a wonderful organization involved with cutting edge nutritional treatments and groundbreaking research. They also produce a very extensive line of vitamins, minerals, and nutraceuticals which are true to their labeling. They also publish a magazine that I highly recommend which is jam-packed with new and exciting information. This is a 1500 page tome full of scientific information easily read by your average nonmedical reader.

DMSO: Nature's Healer, by Dr. Morton Walker, published by Avery, 1993. A great overview of DMSO and its varied medical uses old but a classic nevertheless.

Dr. Mark Stengler's Natural Healing Library, by Dr. Mark Stengler, publisher, Bottom Line Books, 2011.

The Doctor's Book of Home Remedies: by the editors of Prevention magazine. Rodale Press, 2009.

Earth Clinic Presents: Nature's Best Remedies, edited by Daniel P. Kray, published by Body Axis, LLC, 2011. A handy little book for various illnesses and symptoms that can be treated naturally.

Earthing: the most important health discovery ever? by Clinton Ober, Stephen Sinatra, MD and Martin Zucker, published by Basic Health Publications, 2010.

Edible: An Illustrated Guide to the World's Food Plants, published by the National Geographic Society, 2008.

Empty Harvest: Understanding the Link between our Food, our Immunity, and our Planet, by Dr. Bernard Jensen and Mark Anderson, published by Avery Publishing Group, 1990.

The Encyclopedia of Medical Breakthroughs and Forbidden Treasures, by Medical Research Associates, which also published by them. Years 2004 - 2011. An excellent, well-written book, full of wonderful insights into a variety of medical conditions.

Energy Medicine: the Scientific Basis, by James L. Oschman, published by Churchill Livingstone Books, 2000. A great book for someone wanting to fully understand the relationship between energy and cellular health.

The Enlivened Rock Powders, by Harvey Lisle, published by Acres USA, 1994. This book examines the use of rock dust in agriculture as a method of remineralization of the soil.

Enzymes Enzyme Therapy: How to jump-start your way to lifelong good health, by Dr. Anthony J. Cichoke, 2nd edition published by Keats Publishing, 2000.

Enzymes: The Key to Health, Volume 1, the Fundamentals, by Howard F. Loomis, Jr., DC, published by the American Printing Company, Inc., 2012. I have looked high and low and it appears that he never wrote any subsequent volumes. This first volume is very well written.

The Enzyme Treatment of Cancer and Its Scientific Basis, by John Beard, DSc, reissued by New Spring Press, 2010.

Enzymes: What the Experts Know: The role of enzyme therapy in restoring, promoting, and maintaining optimal health, by Tom Bohager, published by One World Press, 2006.

Epigenetic: The Ultimate Mystery of Inheritance, by Richard C. Francis, published by W.W. Norton and Company, Inc., 2011. This is a very well-written book on a very exciting new field in genetics and inheritance.

The Everything Hard Cider Book: All you need to know about making hard cider at home, by Drew Beechum, published by Adams Media, 2013.

Everything You Need to Know About Enzymes: A simple guide to using enzymes to treat everything from digestive problems and allergies to migraines and arthritis, by Tom Bohager, published by Greenleaf Book Group Press, 2008.

The Fast Diet: Lose weight, stay healthy, and live longer with the simple secret of Intermittent Fasting by Dr. Michael Mosley and Mimi Spencer, published by Atria Books, 2013. This is by far one of the best and easiest diet plans to follow for sustained weight loss. It has a profound insulin-lowering effect, which turns your body from fat storage to fat metabolism and weight loss.

Fertility from the Ocean Deep, by Charles Walters, Acres USA, 2005. A good look at the use of sea solids in agriculture and its amazing results.

Fighting Radiation and Chemical Pollutants with Foods, Herbs, and Vitamins: Documented natural remedies that boost your immunity and detoxify, by StevenR. Schechter, ND, published by Vitality Ink, 1990.

Folk Medicine: A Vermont doctor's guide to good health, by D.C. Jarvis, MD, published by Henry Holt and Company, 1958. Some weird theories, but also some interesting insights into folk healing.

Food Forensics: The Hidden Toxins Lurking in Your Food and How You Can Avoid them for Lifelong Health : by Mike Adams. Published by BenBella Books 2016. An eye opening expose of our foods, and how they are destroying our health.

The Foragers Harvest: A guide to identify, harvest, and prepare edible wild plants, by Samuel Thayer, published by The Foragers Harvest Press, 2010. This is a very well-written guide to finding and eating wild plants.

The Fourth Phase of Water: Beyond Solid, Liquid, and Vapor, by Gerald H. Pollack, Ebner and Sons Publisher, 2013. This is a mind-blowing look at water like you have never seen it before.

The Free Man's Declaration for Health and Longevity, by William Campbell Douglass II, MD, published by New Market Health Publishing, 2013. Dr. Douglass is a fascinating physician who has spent his entire career seeking the "truth" in medicine and challenging conventional medical dogma.

From Soil To Supplement: A course in food, diet, and nutrition, by Dr. Royal Lee, reprinted by Serene River Press, 2005.

Gaia's Garden; A Guide to Home Scale Permaculture, 2nd edition, by Toby Hemenway, published by Chelsea Green Publishing Company, 2009. This is an excellent introduction to the vital skill of permaculture.

Gardening for The Future of the Earth, by Howard Yana Shapiro, PhD and John Harrisson, published by Bantam Books, 2000. This book is a compilation of chapters each written by a master of organic gardening, full of very useful information.

Gardening When It Counts: growing food in hard times, by Steve Solomon, published by New Society Publishers, 2005.

Geotherapy: Innovative methods of Soil Fertility Restoration, Carbon Sequestration, and Reversing Co2 Increase: Edited by T. Goreau, R. Larson and J. Campe. Published by CRC Press, 2015

The Germ That Causes Cancer, by Doug A. Kaufmann with Beverly Thornhill Hunt, PhD, published by Media Trition, 2002.

The Green Pharmacy Guide to Healing Foods: Proven Natural Remedies to Treat and Prevent More than 80 Common Health Concerns, by James A. Duke, PhD, published by Rodale, 2008.

Gut and Psychology Syndrome: Natural Treatments for Dysphasia, Autism, ADD, Dyslexia, ADHD, Depression, and Schizophrenia, by Dr. Natasha Campbell McBride, MD, published by Medinform Publishing, 2004.

Harnessing the Earthworm, by Thomas J. Barrett, Shields Publications, 1947. A classic on earthworms and their utilization and breeding. Earthworms are indispensable to a healthy garden, and a fun skill to develop.

The Healing Intelligence of Essential Oils: The Science of Advanced Aromatherapy, by Kurt Schnabel, PhD, Healing Arts Press, 2011. A very complete work on essential oils and their use.

The Healing Nutrients Within: Facts, Findings, and New Research on Amino Acids, by Eric R. Braverman, MD, with Carl C. Pfeiffer, MD, PhD, published by Keats, 1987.

The Healing Power of Fever: Your Body's Natural Defense Against Disease, by Christopher Vasey, ND, Healing Arts Press, 2008.

Healing is Voltage: The Handbook, by Jerry Tennant, MD, 3rd edition, no publisher or date of publication listed in the book, therefore it is presumably self-published. Nevertheless it is an interesting point of view and he does a very good job of explaining a difficult idea to grasp. A good introduction to energy medicine and how it works at the cellular level.

The Healing Powers of Vinegar: A complete guide to nature's most remarkable remedy, by Cal Orey, published by Kensington books, 2006.

The Healing Sun: sunlight and health in the 21st century, by Richard Hobday, PhD, Findhorn Press, 1999. This is an excellent overview of the healing power of sunlight on the human body.

Health Benefits of Vitamin K2: A revolutionary natural treatment for heart disease and bone loss, by Larry M. Howard and Anthony G. Payne, PhD, published by Basic Health Publications, Inc., 2006.

Health from the Sea and Soil: How to Keep Healthier, Feel Better, and Live Longer Using Nature's Vital Nutrients, by Charles B. Ahlson, published by Exposition Press, 1962.

Health From the Seas: Freedom from Disease, by John Croft, Vital Health Publishing, 2003.

Helping Yourself to Health From the Sea, by Howard H. Hirschhorn, Parker Publishing Company, 1979.

Herbal Antibiotics: Natural alternatives for treating drug resistant bacteria, 2nd edition. Stephen Harrod Buhner. Storey Publishing 2012.

The Herbal Medicine-Makers Handbook: A Home Manual, by James Green, by Crown Publishing Group, 2000.

Herbolution: New Discoveries in Detoxification Using Herbal Enzymes, by Kevin Sullivan, ND, published by Tate Publishing and Enterprises, 2011.

The Honey Revolution: Restoring the Health of Future Generations, by Ron Fessenden, MD, MPH, and Mike McInnes, MRPS, published by World Class Emprise, LLC, 2008. This is a very well-researched and -written book on the health benefits and uses of honey.

How to Effectively Use Honey as Medicine: what doctors don't tell you, 2nd edition, by Ruth Tan. No publisher listed in book.

How Soils Work: A study into the God-Plane Mutualism of Soils and Crops, by Paul Syltie, PhD, published by Xulon Press, 2002.

How to Grow Food, by Richard Gianfrancesco, A step by Step Guide to growing all kinds of fruits, vegetables, herbs, salads, and more, published by Firefly Books 2011.

How to Stay Alive in the Woods: A complete guide to food, shelter, and self- preservation that makes starvation in the wilderness next to impossible, by Bradford Angier, originally published in 1956, revised edition by Fireside, 1998.

Humus and the Farmer, by Friend Skyes, published by Rodale Press, 1949. An early classic text on organic farming methods and their superiority.

Hydrosols: The Next Aromatherapy, by Suzanne Catty, Healing Arts Press, 2001. Hydrosols, or hydrolates, are the pure, water-based solutions created when essential oils are steam distilled. The resulting hydrosols can be ingested or applied topically, without significant side effects, considered to be the homeopathic version of aromatherapy.

Hypothyroidism: The Unsuspected Illness, by Broda O. Barnes, MD and Lawrence Galton, Harper and Row Publishers, 1976. A classic on hypothyroidism.

Identifying and Harvesting Edible and Medicinal Plants in Wild and not so Wild Places, by "Wildman" Steve Brill with Evelyn Dean, Harper Collins Publishing, 1994. This is the essential guide to finding and using delicious wild, edible plants for nutrition and better health. This book will teach you how to identify and utilize many plants growing right under your nose. Full of very practical information.

The Illustrated Encyclopedia of Healing Remedies, by C. Norman Shealy, MD, Harper Collins Publishers, 1998, 2002. A very complete handbook, which includes aromatherapy, Ayurveda cures, homeopathy, and others.

Into the Light, by William Campbell Douglass II, MD, 4th edition published by Rhino Publishing, S.A, 2003. A very interesting book making a compelling argument for the use of light as a medical treatment through a process known as Photoluminescence, which looks like it may hold the answer to the current antibiotic overuse and resistance.

Introduction to Permaculture by Bill Mollison with Reny Mia Slay, 2nd edition, published by Tagari Publications, 1994. Bill Mollison is the originator of permaculture and this is an excellent handbook on a subject.

Iodine: Why You Need It 3rd edition, by David Brownstein, MD, published by Medical Alternatives Press, 2008. I am a big fan of Dr. Brownstein, who has courageously championed the correct use of iodine as well as the pervasive epidemic of undiagnosed hypothyroidism. He has written several books and they are all a very good read and very informative.

Iodine: Bringing Back the Universal Medicine, by Dr. Marc Sircus, e-book. Available at his website: www.Dr.Sircus.com.

The Iodine Crisis: What you Don't Know About Iodine Can Wreck Your Life, by Lynne Farrow, published by Devon Press, 2013. A fun read about iodine and how the current crisis situation has developed.

Know Your Fats: The Complete Primer for Understanding the Nutrition of Fats, Oils, and Cholesterol, by Mary G. enig , PhD. A great book on lipids (fats) and their impact on human health.

Living Clay: Nature's Own Miracle Cure Calcium Bentonite Clay, by Perry A., Print and Bind Books, 2006. A simple review of various medicinal uses of bentonite clay.

The Machinery of Life, 2nd edition, by David S. Goodsell, published by Springer Science and Business Media, LLC, 2009. This book is an outstanding introduction to biochemistry.

The Macrobiotic Way: 3rd edition, by Michio Kushi, Stephen Blauer, and Wendy Esko, by Avery Trade Publishers, 2004. This is the definitive guide to a macrobiotic diet and life style.

Mayo Clinic: Book of Home Remedies, published by Time Home Entertainment, 2010.

Medicine for the Outdoors: The essential guide to first aid and medical emergencies, 5th edition, by Paul S. Auerbach, MD, published by Mosby, Inc., 2009.

The Merck Manual of Medical Information, 2nd Home Edition, published by Pocket Books, 2003.

Micro-Cosmos: Four Billion Years of Microbial Evolution, by Lynn Margulis and Dorion Sagan, published by Summit Books, 1986.

Micro Miracles: Discover the healing power of enzymes, by Ellen W. Cutler, DC, with Jeremy E. Kaslow, MD, published by Rodale, 2005.

Minerals: Key to Vibrant Health and Life Force, by Jacob Swilling, PhD, published by Know Your Options, Inc., 2003.

Mini Farming: Self-Sufficiency on a ¼ Acre, by Brett L. Markham, published by Skyhawk Publishing, 2010. This is a wonderful book which covers everything from healthy soil to seed saving and lots more along the way.

Miracles from the Vault: An Anthology of Underground Cures, by Jenny Thompson and Health Sciences Institute, published by Health Sciences Institute, 2013. A good review of recent discoveries and cures.

The Miraculous Properties of Ionized Water: The definitive guide to the world's healthiest substance, by Bob McCauley, published by Spartan Enterprises, Inc., 2006.

The Missing Diagnosis II, by C. Orian Truss, MD, 2009, appears to be self- published. This is a fascinating look at the role of candida infections and our health. This is the sequel to the 1983 edition.

Morphic Resonance: The Nature of Formative Causation, by Rupert Sheldrake, published by Park Street Press, 1981. A very deep book on the organization of biological systems, with a very unique perspective.

The Most Effective Natural Cures on Earth, by Jonny Bowden, PhD, Fair Winds Press, 2008. A really well-written and -researched book with outstanding explanations and lots of clinical information.

The New Self-Sufficient Gardener: The complete illustrated guide to planning, growing, storing, and preserving your own garden's produce, by John Seymour, published by Dorling Kindersley, Ltd., 2008.

Nutrient Power: Heal Your Biochemistry and Heal Your Brain, by William J. Walsh, PhD, published by Skyhorse Publishing, 2012. Fascinating book full of incredible insight into the effects of nutrition on behavior.

Nutrition, Health, and Disease, by Gary Price Todd, MD, published by Whitford Press, 1985.

Natural Health Remedies, by Janet Maccaro, PhD, published by Siloam, Strang Publishing Group, 2006.

Natural Medicine, Optimal Wellness: The Patients Guide to Health and Healing, by Jonathan V. Wright, MD, and Alan R. Gaby, MD, published by Square One Publishers, no date of publication listed in the book. A well-researched book with excellent commentaries by the authors.

Nature's Garden: A guide to identifying, harvesting and preparing edible wild plants, by Samuel Thayer, published by The Foragers Harvest Press, 2010. A follow-up to his earlier "The Foragers Harvest", but replete with new information.

Nature's Robots: A History of Proteins, by Charles Tanford, and Jacqueline Reynolds, Oxford University Press, 2001.

The New Mineral Cure, by Dr. Michael Kessler, by Doctors Health Press, 2007.

The Nutraceutical Revolution, by Richard Firschein, ND, Riverhead Books, 1998.

Nutrition and Mental Illness: An Orthomolecular Approach to Balancing Body Chemistry, by Carl C. Pfeiffer, PhD, MD, published by Healing Arts Press, 1987.

The Oil That Heals: A Physician's Successes with Castor Oil Treatments, by William A. McGarey, MD, 16th printing published by A.R.E. Press, 2010.

The Omega Rx Zone: The Miracle of the New High Dose Fish Oil, by Dr. Barry Sears, published by Harper Collins Publishers, 2002.

The Omega Solution, by Jonathan Goodman, ND, by Prima Publishing, 2001. An excellent and well-written review of the benefits of omega-3 and omega-6 fatty acids.

The One Minute Cure: The secret to healing virtually all diseases, by Madison Cavanaugh, published by Think OutsideThe Book Publishing, 2008. This book delves into the therapeutic uses of hydrogen peroxide.

Oral Enzymes - New Approach to Cancer Treatment, by F. Klaschka, published by Forum Medizin, 1996.

Orthomolecular Medicine For Everyone: Megavitamin Therapeutics for Families and Physicians, by Abram Hoffer, MD, PhD, and Andrew W. Saul, PhD, published by Basic Health Publications, 2008. This is an excellent explanation and handbook of the use of the use of vitamins and other nutrients as medicines, very well written. A great introduction to the subject of orthomolecular medicine.

The Orthomolecular Treatment of Chronic Disease: 65 Experts on Therapeutic and Preventive Nutrition, edited by Andrew W. Saul, PhD, published by Basic Health Publications, 2014.

The Oxygen Prescription: The Miracle of Oxidative Therapies, by Nathaniel Altman, Healing Arts Press, 1995.

The Paleo Diet: Lose weight and get healthy by eating the food you were designed to eat, by Loren Cordain, PhD, published by Wiley, 2002.

Participating in Nature: Wilderness Survival and Primitive Living Skills, by Thomas J. Elpel, 6th edition published by HOPS Press, LLC, 2009.

PEMF: The 5th Element of Health, by Bryant A. Meyers, published by Balboa Press Books, 2014. A very well-written text on Pulsed Electromagnetic Field treatments, well documented, I highly recommend it to better understand magnetic fields and how they benefit our health.

The PH Miracle: Balance Your Diet and Reclaim Your Health, by Robert O. Young, PhD, and Shelley Redford Young, published by Warner Books, 2002.

A Planet of Viruses, by Carl Zimmer, published by the University of Chicago Press, 2011.

Pottenger's Prophecy: How Food Resets Genes for Wellness or Illness, by Gray Graham, NTP, and Deborah Kesten, MPH, and Larry Scherwitz, PhD, published by White River Press, 2011.

Primal Panacea, by Thomas E. Levy, MD, by MedFox Publishing, 2011. Another wonderful book by Dr. Levy on the many life-saving uses of high dose ascorbic acid or vitamin C.

Probiotics: Protection Against Infection, by Case Adams, PhD, Logical Books, 2012. This is a great review of probiotics and their amazing potential to benefit human health as well as their interactions with our bodies.

The Probiotics Revolution, by Gary B. Huffnagle, PhD, Bantam Books, 2007. Dr. Huffnagle is both a microbiologist and an immunologist and has wonderful insights into the fascinating world of our endogenous flora.

Radiation Survival: How to Prepare Now and Survive Radiation Exposure, by Larry and Cheryl Poole, 2011, no publisher listed. A good guide to radiation exposure and its effects. It is worth the price just for chapter seven on radiation neutralizers.

Rare Earths: Forbidden Cures, by Joel D. Wallach, DVM, and Ma Lan, MD, published by Double Happiness Publishing Company, 1994. This is a very informative text on the subject of various mineral and trace element deficiencies and their source...mineral depletion of the soils and its consequences to our bodies and our health.

Real Food: What to Eat and Why, by Nina Planck, published by Bloomsbury Publishing, 2006.

The Resilient Farm and Homestead: An Innovative Permaculture and Whole Systems Design Approach, by Ben Falk, published by Chelsea Green Publishers, 2007.

Rethinking Pasteur's Germ Theory: How to Maintain Your Optimal Health, by Nancy Appleton, published by Frog, Ltd., 2002. Written by a nutritionist, looks at disease from the viewpoint of the health of your immune system, not the germs that are attacking us.

Riddled with Life: Friendly worms, ladybug sex and the parasites that make us who we are, by Marlene Zuk, published by Harcourt, 2007.

Rife's World of Electromedicine: The story, the corruption, and the promise, by Barry Lynes, published by BioMed Publishing Group, 2009.

Rodale's Illustrated Encyclopedia of Herbs, by Rodale Press, 1987. A very comprehensive and well-written review of many different herbs.

Root Cellaring: The simple no processing way to store fruits and vegetables, by Mike and Nancy Bubel, published by Rodale Press, 1979.

Scatter, Adapt, and Remember: How Humans Will Survive a Mass Extinction, by Annalee Newitz, published by Anchor Books, 2013. This book is fun and full of interesting insights.

Sea Energy Agriculture: Nature's Ideal Trace Element Blend for Farm, Livestock, and Humans, by Maynard Murray, MD, revised second edition, by Acres Publishing, 2003.

Sea Salt's Hidden Powers: The Biological Action of all Ocean Minerals on Body and Mind, by Jacques de Langre, PhD, Happiness Press, 1994.

Secrets of the Soil: New Solutions for Restoring our Planet, by Peter Tompkins and Christopher Bird, published by Earth Pulse Press, Inc., 1998.

Secrets of an Alkaline Body: The New Science of Colloidal Biology, by Annie Padden Jubb and David Jubb, published by North Atlantic Books, 2004.

Seed Savers Exchange: Annual catalogue free at seedsavers.org. This is an outstanding source for open-pollinated heirloom seeds. A huge variety of vegetables, beans, garlic, potatoes, herbs, and flowers. Also an excellent source of organic seeds for your medicinal seed vault with wholesale pricing available.

Sepp Holzer's Permaculture: A practical guide to small scale integrative farming and gardening, by Sepp Holzer, published by Chelsea Green Publishers, 2004. A small book chock-full of valuable information for anyone interested in small scale farming and permaculture techniques. This man has mastered this in the Austrian Alps much to the amazement of his neighbors and visitors, and is flourishing.

Sick and Tired: Reclaim Your Inner Terrain, by Robert O. Young, PhD, and Shelly Redford Young, LMT, Woodland Publishing, 2001.

Sleep to Save Your Life: The complete guide to living longer and healthier through restorative sleep, by Gerard T. Lombardo, MD, Harper Collins Publisher, 2005.

Sodium Bicarbonate: Rich Man's, Poor Man's Cancer Treatment: second edition, e-book by Dr. Marc Sircus. Can be found at his website, www.DrSircus.com. Excellent textbook on the multiple medical uses of sodium bicarbonate.

Solved: The Riddle of Illness, by Stephen E. Langer, MD, and James F. Scheer, published by Keats Publishing, Inc., 1984.

Special Operations Forces Medical Handbook, 2nd edition, published by Skyhorse Publishing, 2011.

The Sprouting Book: How to Grow and Use Sprouts to Maximize Your Health and Vitality, by Ann Wigmore, published by The Avery Publishing Group, 1986.

Staying Healthy with Nutrition: The complete guide to diet and nutritional medicine by Elson M. Haas, MD, with Buck Levin, PhD, published by Celestial Arts, 2006. This is a wonderful book, very insightful and well researched and written. A good primer for healthy living habits.

Studies in Deficiency Disease, by Robert McCarrison, reprinted by Cornell University Library, 1921. A classic work reprinted on the relationship between vitamin and mineral and trace element deficiencies and various disease states.

The Sun, the Sea, and Tomorrow, by F.G. Walton Smith and Henry Chapin, published by Charles Scribner's Sons, 1954. The story of using the sea for food, energy, and minerals.

The Survival Medicine Handbook: A guide for when medical help is not on the way, by Joseph Alton, MD, and Amy Alton, 2nd edition, published by Doom and Bloom, LLC, 2013. A good introduction to the subject but overall rather incomplete.

Survival of the Sickest: The surprising connections between disease and longevity, by Dr. Sharon Moalem, published by Harper Collins Books, 2007. A fascinating review of diseases and how they ultimately impact mankind, very well written.

Today's Greatest Alternative Medicines, compiled by the Health Sciences Research Team, published by Health Sciences Institute, 2009.

Tomorrow's Cancer Cures Today: 25 secret therapies from around the world, by Allan Spreen, MD, published by Health Sciences Institute, 2009.

The Trace Elements and Man: Some Positive and Negative Aspects, by HenryA. Schroeder, MD, by the Devin Adair Company, 1973.

Treasury of Natural Cures, by Dr. Jonathan V. Wright, published by New Market Health Publishing, 2013. This is a very nice review of the latest and greatest natural cures, very well written.

Treating Ebola and Other Infectious Diseases, by Dr. Marc Sircus, International Medical Veritas Association, 2014. A very interesting, refreshing point of view, with some very good insights. Lots of good credible information on Ebola. Available as an e-book at his website, www.Dr.Sircus.com.

The Trophoblast and the Origins of Cancer: One solution to the medical enigma of our time, by Nicholas J. Gonzalez, MD, and Linda L. Isaacs, MD, published by New Spring Press, 2009. This is a fascinating insight into a very likely mechanism for the origins of many types of cancer, resurrected from the groundbreaking work of an English scientist, Dr. John Beard, from over one hundred years ago.

The Underground Health Reporter: Little Known Discoveries that Make a Dramatic Impact on Your Health. This book is a compilation of essays from a website that has been around since December of 2009, giving weekly insight into unusual health cures; very interesting. Date of publication 2009 to 2012 published by Think Outside of the Book Publishers.

Vibrational Medicine, by Richard Gerber, MD, published by Bear and Company, 2001. This is a great book to immerse yourself into and familiarize yourself with the exciting world of Energy Medicine. Dr. Gerber did a great job of making this complicated subject both easily understood and enjoyable.

Virgin Coconut Oil, by Brian and Marianita Jader Shilhavy, published by Tropical Traditions, 2004.

Viruses and the Evolution of Life, by Luis P. Villarreal, AMS (The American Society of Microbiology) Press, 2005. If you are interested in viral evolution, this is your book, very technical; not for a layman without extensive knowledge. That being said, it is a very interesting read.

The Vitamin D Revolution: How the power of this amazing vitamin can change your life, by Soram Khalsa, MD, published by Hay House, Inc., 2009.

The Vitamin D Cure, by James E. Dowd, MD, and Diane Stafford, by John Wiley and Sons, Inc., 2008.

Vitamin K2 and the Calcium Paradox: How a Little Known Vitamin Can Save Your Life, by Kate Rheaume-Bleue, ND, published by Harper Collins Publishers, 2012. A fun read on a vitamin that is virtually unknown in the medical world.

The Vitamins: Fundamental Aspects in Nutrition and Health, fourth edition, by Gerald F. Combs Jr., Academic Press Publishers, 2012. A very in-depth review of vitamins for medical professionals only.

Water and Life: The Unique Properties of H20, edited by Ruth M. Lynden-Bell, Simon Conway Morris, John D. Barrow, John L. Finney, and Charles L. Harper, Jr., published by CRC Press, 2010. This is a very technical book, basically a collection of papers written about the various properties of water, definitely not for a layman, but never the less very interesting.

When There Is No Doctor: Preventive and emergency home healthcare in challenging times, by Gerard S. Doyle, MD, published by Process Media, 2010.

Wilderness Medicine: Beyond First Aid, by William W. Forgey, MD, 6th edition published by Falcon Guides, 2012. A good first aid guide to keep handy.

The Wonderful World Within You: Understanding Your Individual Differences can be the Key to a Healthier more Vigorous Life, by Dr. Roger J. Williams, revised edition published by Bio-Communication Press, 1998.

The World's Healthiest Foods, by George Mateljan, GMF Publishing, 2007. This is a very exhaustively written book of almost 900 pages, jam-packed with wonderful facts and tidbits about the foods covered.

Your Natural Medicine Cabinet: A practical guide to drug free remedies for common ailments, by Burke Lennihan, published by Green Healing Press, 2012.

2 000045 356382
www.epubli.de